AANA Advanced Arthroscopy

The Knee

Series Editor

Richard K. N. Ryu, MD

President (2009-2010)
Arthroscopy Association of North America
Private Practice
Santa Barbara, California

AANA Advanced Arthroscopy

The Knee

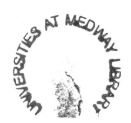

Robert E. Hunter, MD
Director, Orthopedic Sports Medicine Center
Heart of the Rockies Regional Medical Center
The Orthopedic Sports Medicine Center
Salida, Colorado

Nicholas A. Sgaglione, MD
Chief, Division of Sports Medicine
Associate Chairman, Department of Orthopaedics
North Shore University Hospital
Manhasset, New York
Associate Clincial Professor of Orthopaedics
Albert Einstein College of Medicine
New York, New York

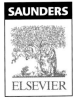

SAUNDERS

ELSEVIER

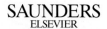

SAUNDERS
ELSEVIER

1600 John F. Kennedy Blvd.
Ste 1800
Philadelphia, PA 19103-2899

AANA Advanced Arthroscopy: The Knee

ISBN: 978-1-4377-0664-2

Library of Congress Cataloging-in-Publication Data
AANA advanced arthroscopy. The knee / [edited by] Robert E. Hunter, Nicholas A. Sgaglione. -- 1st ed.
    p. ; cm.
  ISBN 978-1-4377-0664-2
 1. Knee--Endoscopic surgery. I. Hunter, Robert, 1949- II. Sgaglione, Nicholas A. III. Arthroscopy Association of North America. IV. Title: Advanced arthroscopy. V. Title: Knee.
  [DNLM: 1. Arthroscopy--methods. 2. Knee Joint--surgery. WE 870 A112 2010]
  RD561.A 24 2010
  617.5'820597--dc22

2009043126

Publishing Director: Kim Murphy
Developmental Editor: Ann Ruzycka Anderson
Publishing Services Manager: Frank Polizzano
Senior Project Manager: Peter Faber
Design Direction: Ellen Zanolle

Working together to grow
libraries in developing countries

www.elsevier.com | www.bookaid.org | www.sabre.org

ELSEVIER BOOK AID International Sabre Foundation

DEDICATION

*To my wife, Patti, for her unconditional love and support,
and in memory of my father, Samuel W. Hunter, M.D.*

Robert E. Hunter, MD

---

*To Leslie, Nicholas, Caroline, Jonathan, and Matthew.
Thanks for all your patience and support.*

Nicholas A. Sgaglione, MD

Contributors

Annunziato Amendola, MD
Professor, Department of Orthopaedics and Rehabilitation, University of Iowa Hospitals and Clinics; Director, University of Iowa Sports Medicine Center, Iowa City, Iowa
Proximal Tibial Osteotomy

Robert Arciero, MD
Professor, Department of Orthopaedic Surgery, University of Connecticut School of Medicine; Director, Sports Medicine Fellowship, University of Connecticut Health Center, Farmington, Connecticut
Anatomic Reconstruction of the Posterolateral Corner

John D. Beck, MD
Orthopaedic Surgeon, Geisinger Medical Center, Danville, Pennsylvania
Multiple-Ligament Knee Injuries and Management of Knee Dislocations

Jack M. Bert, MD
Adjunct Clinical Professor, University of Minnesota School of Medicine, Minneapolis; Medical Director, Summit Orthopedics, St. Paul, Minnesota
Complications of Knee Arthroscopy; Degenerative Arthritis

Timothy M. Bert, MD
Department of Orthopedic Surgery, Campbell Clinic, Memphis, Tennessee
Complications of Knee Arthroscopy

James Bicos, MD
Department of Orthopedics, St. Vincent Orthopedics/St. Vincent Sports Performance Center, Indianapolis, Indiana
Anatomic Reconstruction of the Posterolateral Corner

Kevin F. Bonner, MD
Orthopaedic Sports Medicine, Jordan-Young Institute, Virginia Beach, Virginia
Transtibial Single-Bundle Posterior Cruciate Ligament Reconstruction

Thomas R. Carter, MD
Head, Orthopedic Surgery, Arizona State University; Orthopedic Surgeon, Orthopedic Clinic, Tempe, Arizona
Allograft Osteochondral Transplantation

Luke Choi, MD
Resident, Department of Orthopaedic Surgery, University of Virginia School of Medicine, Charlottesville, Virginia
Inlay Posterior Cruciate Ligament Reconstruction

James C. Y. Chow, MD
Clinical Assistant Professor, Southern Illinois University School of Medicine, Springfield; Founder, Orthopaedic Research Foundation of Southern Illinois, Mt. Vernon, Illinois
Arthroscopic Osteochondral Transplantation

James Campbell Chow, MD
Orthopaedic Surgeon, Arizona Center for Bone and Joint Disorders; Orthopaedic Surgeon, St. Luke's Medical Center, Phoenix, Arizona
Arthroscopic Osteochondral Transplantation

Brian J. Cole, MD, MBA
Professor, Department of Orthopedics and Department of Anatomy and Cell Biology, Rush University Medical Center, Chicago, Illinois
Meniscal Transplantation

Corey Edgar, MD, PhD
Orthopaedic Surgeon, Department of Orthopaedic Surgery, Boston Medical Center, Boston, Massachusetts
Reconstruction of the Medial Patellofemoral Ligament

Gregory C. Fanelli, MD
Orthopaedic Surgeon, Danville, Pennsylvania
Multiple-Ligament Knee Injuries and Management
of Knee Dislocations

Nicole A. Friel, MS
Research Fellow, Department of Orthopaedic Surgery,
Rush University Medical Center, Chicago, Illinois
Meniscal Transplantation

Nick Frost, MD
Modbury Public Hospital, Adelaide, Australia
Arthroscopic Osteochondral Transplantation

Freddie H. Fu, MD
David Silver Professor of Orthopaedic Surgery and Chairman,
Department of Orthopaedic Surgery, University of Pittsburgh
School of Medicine and University of Pittsburgh Medical
Center; Head Team Physician, Department of Athletics,
University of Pittsburgh; Adjunct Professor, School of Health
and Rehabilitation Science, University of Pittsburgh,
Pittsburgh, Pennsylvania
Double-Bundle Anterior Cruciate Ligament Reconstruction

John P. Fulkerson, MD
Clinical Professor of Orthopedic Surgery, University
of Connecticut School of Medicine; Orthopedic Surgeon,
Orthopedic Associates of Hartford, Farmington, Connecticut
Tibial Tubercle Transfer

Armando Gabrielli, MD
Department of Orthopaedic Surgery, University of Rome,
Tor Vergata, Rome, Italy
Proximal Tibial Osteotomy

Raffaele Garofalo, MD
Orthopaedic Surgeon, Department of Clinical Methodology
and Surgical Technologies, Orthopaedic and Trauma Clinic,
Università degli Studi di Bari, Bari, Italy
Multiple-Ligament Knee Injuries and Management
of Knee Dislocations

Vipool Goradia, MD
Go Orthopedics, Chester, Virginia
Knee Arthroscopy: Setup, Diagnosis, Portals, and Approaches

Jeffrey Halbrecht, MD
Medical Director, Institute for Arthroscopy & Sports Medicine,
San Francisco, California
Arthroscopic Medial Plication for Patellar Instability

Stephen Hendricks, MD
Alaska Orthopaedic Specialists, Anchorage, Alaska
Double-Bundle Posterior Cruciate Ligament Reconstruction

Robert E. Hunter, MD
Orthopedic Surgeon, Orthopedic Sports Medicine Center,
Salida, Colorado
Arthroscopic Treatment of Tibial Eminence Fractures

Darren L. Johnson, MD
Professor of Orthopaedic Surgery, University of Kentucky
College of Medicine; Professor and Chair, Department
of Orthopaedic Surgery, and Director of Sports Medicine,
University of Kentucky Medical Center, Lexington, Kentucky
Revision Anterior Cruciate Ligament Reconstruction

Donald H. Johnson, MD, FRCS(C)
Assistant Professor of Orthopaedic Surgery, University
of Ottawa Faculty of Medicine; Attending Physician,
Ottawa Hospital; Director, Sports Medicine Clinic,
Carleton University, Ottawa, Ontario, Canada
Meniscal Resection

Peter Jokl, MD
Professor, Vice-Chairman, and Section Chief, Department
of Sports Medicine, Yale University School of Medicine;
Attending Physician, Yale–New Haven Hospital,
New Haven, Connecticut
Microfracture

Jason Koh, MD
Clinical Associate Professor, University of Chicago Pritzker
School of Medicine; Vice Chairman, Department of
Orthopaedic Surgery, North Shore University Health System,
Evanston, Illinois
Approach to Chondral Damage in the Patellofemoral Joint

Eric J. Kropf, MD
Assistant Professor, Department of Orthopaedic Surgery
and Sports Medicine, Temple University School of Medicine;
Attending Physician, Temple University Hospital,
Philadelphia, Pennsylvania
Double-Bundle Anterior Cruciate Ligament Reconstruction

Peter R. Kurzweil, MD, MBA
Orthopaedic Surgeon, Memorial Orthopaedic Surgical Group,
Long Beach; Orthopaedic Surgeon, Memorial Prompt Care,
Westminster, California
Meniscal Repair

David W. Lemos, MD
Fellow in Sports Medicine, Detroit Medical Center,
Warren, Michigan
Arthroscopic Evaluation and Diagnosis of the Patellofemoral Joint

Mark J. Lemos, MD
Associate Professor, Boston University School of Medicine;
Lecturer, Tufts University School of Medicine, Boston;
Director of Sports Medicine, Lahey Clinic, Burlington,
Massachusetts
Arthroscopic Evaluation and Diagnosis of the Patellofemoral Joint

Stephen E. Lemos, MD, PhD
Team Physician, Detroit Lions and Detroit Pistons; Attending
Physician, Detroit Medical Center, Warren, Michigan
Arthroscopic Evaluation and Diagnosis of the Patellofemoral Joint

Emilio Lopez-Vidriero, MD, PhD
Fellow in Arthroscopy and Sports Medicine, University
of Ottawa Faculty of Medicine and Ottawa Hospital, Ottawa,
Ontario, Canada
Meniscal Resection

James H. Lubowitz, MD
Director, Taos Orthopaedic Institute, Taos Orthopaedic Institute
Research Foundation, and Taos Orthopaedic Institute Sports
Medicine Fellowship Training Program, Taos, New Mexico
Arthroscopic Management of Tibial Plateau Fractures

Bert R. Mandelbaum, MD, DHL
Director, Santa Monica Orthopaedic and Sports Medicine
Research Foundation, Santa Monica, California
Chondrocyte Transplantation Techniques

David McGuire, MD
Orthopaedic Surgeon, Alaska Orthopaedic Specialists,
Anchorage, Alaska
Double-Bundle Posterior Cruciate Ligament Reconstruction

Bart McKinney, MD
Orthopaedic Surgeon, Appalachian Orthopaedic Associates,
Johnson City, Tennessee
The Stiff Knee

Michael J. Medvecky, MD
Associate Professor, Department of Orthopaedics
and Rehabilitation, Yale University School of Medicine;
Attending Physician, Yale–New Haven Hospital, New Haven,
Connecticut
Microfracture

Chealon D. Miller, MD
Resident, Department of Orthopaedic Surgery, University
of Virginia School of Medicine, Charlottesville, Virginia
Inlay Posterior Cruciate Ligament Reconstruction

Mark D. Miller, MD
Orthopedic Surgeon, Sports Medicine and Arthroscopic Surgery,
Orthopedic Center of St. Louis, St. Louis, Missouri
Inlay Posterior Cruciate Ligament Reconstruction

Kai Mithoefer, MD
Orthopaedic Surgeon, Harvard Vanguard Medical Associates,
Chestnut Hill, Massachusetts
Chondrocyte Transplantation Techniques

S. L. Mortimer, MD
Clinical Instructor, Sanford School of Medicine, University
of South Dakota; Attending Physician, Black Hills Surgical
Hospital, Rapid City, South Dakota
Arthroscopic Treatment of Tibial Eminence Fractures

Roger Ostrander, MD
Orthopaedic Surgeon, Andrews Orthopaedic & Sports
Medicine Center, Gulf Breeze, Florida
The Stiff Knee

Lonnie Paulos, MD
Adjunct Professor, University of South Alabama College
of Medicine, Mobile, Alabama; Research Associate, University
of West Florida, Pensacola; Vice President/Medical Director,
Andrews-Paulos Research and Education Institute; Co-Medical
Director, Andrews Institute Surgical Center; and Orthopaedic
Surgeon, Andrews Orthopaedic & Sports Medicine, Center,
Gulf Breeze, Florida
The Stiff Knee

Daniel Purcell, MD
Resident, Orthopaedic Surgery, University of Connecticut
Medical Center, Farmington, Connecticut
Anatomic Reconstruction of the Posterolateral Corner

John C. Richmond, MD
Professor of Orthopaedic Surgery, Tufts University School
of Medicine; Chairman, Orthopedic Surgery, New England
Baptist Hospital, Boston, Massachusetts
Anatomic Single-Bundle Anterior Cruciate Ligament Reconstruction

Samuel P. Robinson, MD
Orthopaedic Sports Medicine, Jordan-Young Institute,
Virginia Beach, Virginia
*Transtibial Single-Bundle Posterior Cruciate Ligament
Reconstruction*

Eugenio Savarese, MD
Orthopaedic Surgeon, Genovese Rehabilitation Center
and San Carlo Hospital, Potenza, Italy
Proximal Tibial Osteotomy

Anthony A. Schepsis, MD
Professor and Director of Sports Medicine and Director
of the Sports Medicine Fellowship Program, Department
of Orthopaedic Surgery, Boston University School of Medicine;
Head Team Physician, Boston University Intercollegiate Athletic
Program; Head Team Physician, University of Massachusetts,
Boston Intercollegiate Athletic Program, Boston, Massachusetts
Reconstruction of the Medial Patellofemoral Ligament

Brian D. Shannon, MD
Orthopaedic Surgeon, Sharon Regional Health System,
Sharon; Orthopaedic Surgeon, Orthopaedic Center of Western
Pennsylvania, Hermitage, Pennsylvania
Meniscal Repair

J. Christopher Shaver, MD
Orthopaedic Surgeon, Fort Loudon Medical Center,
Lenoir City, Tennessee
Revision Anterior Cruciate Ligament Reconstruction

Walter Shelton, MD
Visiting Professor, University of Mississippi School of Medicine;
Fellowship Co-Director, Mississippi Sports Medicine and
Orthopaedic Center, Jackson, Mississippi
Anterior Cruciate Ligament Repair

Mark A. Slabaugh, MD
Department of Orthopaedics, Wilford Hall Medical Center,
San Antonio, Texas
Meniscal Transplantation

Matthew Stiebel, MD
Orthopaedic Surgeon, West Palm Beach, Florida
Reconstruction of the Medial Patellofemoral Ligament

Joon Ho Wang, MD
Department of Orthopaedic Surgery, Korea University Ansan
Hospital, Gyeonggi-Do, South Korea
Double-Bundle Anterior Cruciate Ligament Reconstruction

Peter Yeh, MD
Chief Resident and Clinical Instructor, Yale University School
of Medicine, New Haven, Connecticut
Microfracture

Preface

The Arthroscopy Association of North America (AANA) is a robust and growing organization whose mission, simply stated, is to provide leadership and expertise in arthroscopic and minimally invasive surgery worldwide.

Towards that end, this five-volume series represents the very best that AANA has to offer the clinician in need of a timely, authoritative, and comprehensive arthroscopic textbook. These textbooks covering the shoulder, elbow and wrist, hip, knee, and foot and ankle were conceived and rapidly consummated over a 15-month timeline. The need for an up-to-date and cogent text as well as a step-by-step video supplement was the driving force behind the rapid developmental chronology. The topics and surgical techniques represent the cutting edge in arthroscopic philosophy and technique, and the individual chapters follow a reliable and helpful format in which the pathoanatomy is detailed and the key elements of the physical examination are emphasized in conjunction with preferred diagnostic imaging. Indications and contraindications are followed by a thorough discussion of the treatment algorithm, both nonoperative and surgical, with an emphasis on arthroscopic techniques. Additionally, a Pearls and Pitfalls section provides for a distilled summary of the most important features in each chapter. A brief annotated bibliography is provided in addition to a comprehensive reference list so that those who want to study the most compelling literature can do so with ease. The supporting DVD meticulously demonstrates the surgical techniques, and will undoubtedly serve as a critical resource in preparing for any arthroscopic intervention.

I am most grateful for the outstanding effort provided by the volume editors: Rick Angelo and Jim Esch (shoulder), Buddy Savoie and Larry Field (elbow and wrist), Thomas Byrd and Carlos Guanche (hip), Rob Hunter and Nick Sgaglione (knee), and Ned Amendola and Jim Stone (foot and ankle). Their collective intellect, skill, and dedicaton to AANA made this series possible. Furthermore, I sincerely thank all the chapter contributors whose expertise and wisdom can be found in every page. Elsevier, and in particular Kim Murphy, Ann Ruzycka Anderson, and Kitty Lasinski, was a delight to work with, and deserves our gratitude for a job well done. I would be remiss if I did not acknowledge that the proceeds of this five-volume series will go directly to the AANA Education Foundation, from which ambitious and state-of-the-art arthroscopic educational initiatives will be funded.

RICHARD K.N. RYU, MD
Series Editor

Contents

Basics

Knee Arthroscopy: Setup, Diagnosis, Portals, and Approaches

Vipool Goradia

Performing successful arthroscopic surgery with a low complication rate begins during the preoperative planning phase. When evaluating a patient for arthroscopy, the surgeon must consider the preoperative diagnosis, anatomic variants, and risk factors for complications. Each of these can be ascertained by obtaining a careful history and performing a thorough physical examination, as well as appropriate diagnostic testing. Depending on surgeon preference, the planning phase will likely affect operating room setup, request for special instruments, patient positioning, and portal placement.

Although some surgeons prefer to use the same setup and portals for every arthroscopic procedure, it can be more efficient to customize these based on the planned procedure and the pathology identified during diagnostic arthroscopy. Failure to do so may result in greater length of operation and risk for perioperative morbidity.

ANATOMY

The knee joint, as other joints, is composed of a synovial lining within the capsule. Superior to the patella the synovium extends to form the suprapatellar pouch (Fig. 1-1).[1] Superior medial or lateral portals are commonly placed within this pouch. A layer of fat separates the pouch from the distal anterior femoral shaft. The pouch extends medially and laterally along the femoral condyles into the medial and lateral gutters. The suprapatellar pouch and gutters are frequent locations for loose bodies.

Articular cartilage covers the tibial plateau and anterior, distal, and posterior condyles of the femur, along with the patella. Iatro-

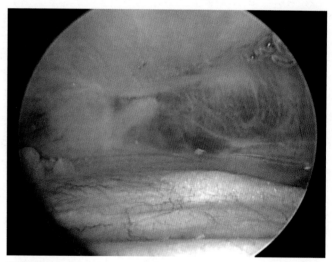

FIGURE 1-1 Arthroscopic view of suprapatellar pouch from high anterolateral portal.

genic injury to articular cartilage should be avoided at all times. Most injury is caused by forceful insertion and movement of the arthroscopic camera and/or instruments during arthroscopy. A knowledge of anatomy, portal placement, and constant visualization of instruments is also required to avoid iatrogenic injury to articular cartilage and other structures.

The bony anatomy of the knee relevant to arthroscopic knee surgery includes the distal femur, the proximal tibia, and the patella. With the knee at 60 degrees of flexion, the inferior pole of the patella is located above the lateral joint line and is an important guide for anterolateral portal place-

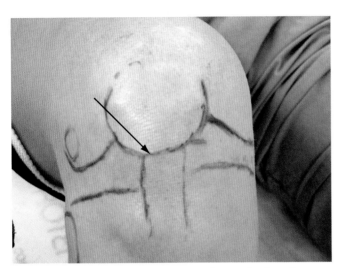

FIGURE 1-2 Photograph of knee showing inferior pole of patella relative to high anterolateral portal placement.

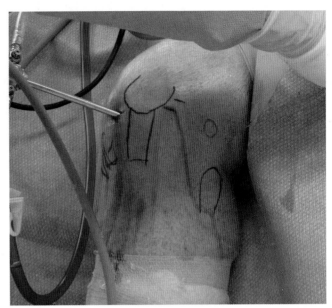

FIGURE 1-3 Direction of camera insertion toward intercondylar notch.

ment (Fig. 1-2). Exceptions to using this landmark, however, occur in cases of patellar alta, baja, dysplasia, or congenital absence. These conditions should be identified preoperatively with physical examination and standard radiography.

The femoral trochlea consists of medial and lateral trochlear ridges that arise from the corresponding femoral condyle.[1] The medial femoral condyle is larger than the lateral from proximal to distal and anterior to posterior. The lateral femoral condyle, however, is wider at the level of the femoral notch. Distally, the femur opens into a notch that contains the femoral origins of the anterior and posterior cruciate ligaments. The notch serves as a target for careful, controlled introduction of cannulas and instruments from anterior portals to avoid injury to articular cartilage (Fig. 1-3). When using the scalpel for anterior portal placement, the blade should be pointed toward the notch but blind insertion beyond the skin and capsule should be avoided, because this would risk injury to the cruciate ligaments.

The medial tibial plateau is larger than the lateral plateau; the two are separated by an intercondylar sulcus or fossa.[1] Adjacent to the fossa is a medial and lateral tibial spine that separates the fossa from the corresponding tibial plateau. The femoral condyles and tibial plateaus are incongruous without the medial and lateral menisci. The fibula, although extra-articular, has direct relevance to arthroscopic knee surgery, because it serves as a landmark for portals and surgical approaches. The proximal fibula forms a joint with the proximal posterior surface of the tibia (tibiofibular joint). It also serves as an insertion for the lateral collateral ligament and biceps femoris tendon.

A knowledge of neurovascular anatomy around the knee joint is important for preventing iatrogenic injury during portal placement and surgical approaches.[2] Posteriorly, in the midthigh, the sciatic nerve branches into the tibial (or popliteal) and common peroneal nerves. At the posterior joint line of the knee just posterior to the joint capsule, the tibial nerve passes between the two heads of the gastrocnemius muscles, along with the popliteal artery and vein. From medial to lateral, the structures include the nerve, artery, and vein (Fig. 1-4).[1] Although Matava and colleagues[3] have shown that knee flexion increases the distance between the tibial insertion of the posterior cruciate ligament (PCL) and the popliteal neurovascular structures, other studies have not confirmed this. At 100 degrees of knee flexion, they reported a maximum distance of slightly less than 1 cm between the popliteal artery and PCL insertion.

The common peroneal nerve passes posterior to the biceps femoris tendon and courses between it and the lateral head of the gastrocnemius toward the fibular head (Fig. 1-5).[1,2] It then courses laterally around the fibular neck and into the peroneus longus tendon. In most individuals, the biceps femoris tendon insertion onto the fibular head can be palpated in 90 degrees of knee flexion. Placing incisions, portals, and retractors anterior to this landmark will help avoid injury the common peroneal nerve.

On the medial aspect of the knee, the saphenous nerve and its infrapatellar branch are at risk for injury during placement of medial and posteromedial portals, as well as during all medial approaches to the knee. The nerve and its branch have a variable course and number of terminal branches.[1,2] In general, the saphenous nerve passes between the gracilis and sartorius muscles approximately 3 cm posterior to the medial femoral epicondyle. The infrapatellar branch courses beneath the sartorius (i.e., posterior to it) and runs along the anteromedial aspect of the knee, where it can terminate medially or laterally to the medial border of the patellar tendon (Fig. 1-6).

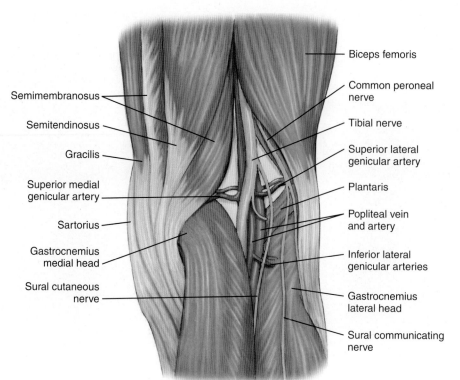

Semimembranosus

Semitendinosus

Gracilis

Superior medial
genicular artery

Sartorius

Gastrocnemius
medial head

Sural cutaneous
nerve

Biceps femoris

Common peroneal
nerve

Tibial nerve

Superior lateral
genicular artery

Plantaris

Popliteal vein
and artery

Inferior lateral
genicular arteries

Gastrocnemius
lateral head

Sural communicating
nerve

FIGURE 1-4 Posterior aspect of knee showing tibial nerve, popliteal artery, and vein within popliteal fossa.

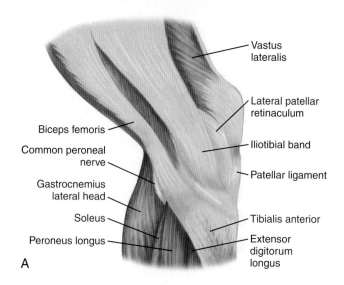

Biceps femoris

Common peroneal
nerve

Gastrocnemius
lateral head

Soleus

Peroneus longus

Vastus
lateralis

Lateral patellar
retinaculum

Iliotibial band

Patellar ligament

Tibialis anterior

Extensor
digitorum
longus

A

FIGURE 1-5 Lateral aspect of knee. **A,** Common peroneal nerve passing posterior to biceps femoris tendon. **B,** Common peroneal nerve passing laterally around the fibular neck.

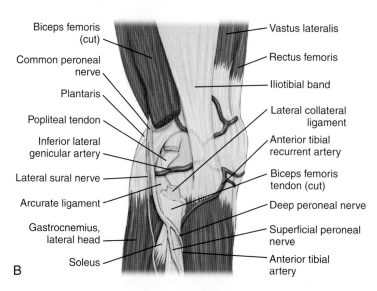

Biceps femoris
(cut)

Common peroneal
nerve

Plantaris

Popliteal tendon

Inferior lateral
genicular artery

Lateral sural nerve

Arcurate ligament

Gastrocnemius,
lateral head

Soleus

Vastus lateralis

Rectus femoris

Iliotibial band

Lateral collateral
ligament

Anterior tibial
recurrent artery

Biceps femoris
tendon (cut)

Deep peroneal nerve

Superficial peroneal
nerve

Anterior tibial
artery

B

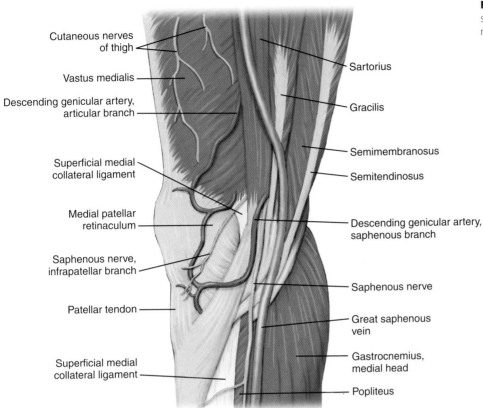

Cutaneous nerves of thigh

Vastus medialis

Descending genicular artery, articular branch

Superficial medial collateral ligament

Medial patellar retinaculum

Saphenous nerve, infrapatellar branch

Patellar tendon

Superficial medial collateral ligament

Sartorius

Gracilis

Semimembranosus

Semitendinosus

Descending genicular artery, saphenous branch

Saphenous nerve

Great saphenous vein

Gastrocnemius, medial head

Popliteus

FIGURE 1-6 Anteromedial superficial structures of knee showing saphenous nerve and its infrapatellar branch.

PATIENT EVALUATION

History And Physical Examination

Each patient undergoing knee arthroscopy should have a complete history, physical examination, and informed consent that are well documented. Anesthetic, medical, and deep venous thrombosis risks should be identified and addressed preoperatively. Details of the history and examination for specific diagnoses will be covered in the appropriate chapters elsewhere in this text.

Diagnostic Imaging

At a minimum, all patients should have preoperative radiography, including a standing posteroanterior (PA) view with the knees flexed 45 degrees, a lateral view, and a Merchant or sunrise view. These x-rays can be useful for identifying degenerative joint disease, osteochondral or other fractures, tumors, loose bodies, and patellar pathology, such as patella alta or baja, bipartite, or dysplasia.

The need for magnetic resonance imaging, computed tomography, and other imaging is based on the initial history, examination, radiographs, and response to prior treatment and will be discussed in the appropriate chapters.

TREATMENT

Anesthesia Options

Knee arthroscopy can be performed under general, spinal, or local anesthesia. The choice primarily depends on surgeon and patient preference, but in some cases may be influenced by the patient's medical history. In a prospective randomized study of

400 patients, Jacobson and associates[4] compared three anesthesia options and concluded that local anesthesia was technically feasible in 92% of patients undergoing elective knee arthroscopy. However, when comparing patient satisfaction, the local anesthetic group had 90% satisfaction versus 97% for the general anesthesia group. Horlocker and Hebl[5] performed an evidence-based review of published studies comparing various anesthetic methods for knee arthroscopy. They reported that the results of most studies were biased by surgeon and patient expectations as well as by differences in postoperative management. They concluded that a single method of anesthesia could not be recommended for all surgeons performing or patients undergoing knee arthroscopy.

Arthroscopic Technique

Operating Room Setup

One or more video monitors are required. Traditionally, cathode ray tube (CRT) monitors have been the standard. New flat screen liquid crystal display (LCD) monitors are increasingly being used (Fig. 1-7) and currently most manufacturers of arthroscopic video equipment also offer high definition (HD) monitors. Although only one monitor is needed, many operating rooms use two or more monitors (see Fig. 1-8). Although there is less benefit of multiple monitors for knee arthroscopy, they can be very useful for shoulder and hip arthroscopy.

The control boxes for the arthroscopic camera, shavers, pump, and other devices can be placed on a mobile tower (Fig. 1-8A) that is easily moved from room to room or can be con-

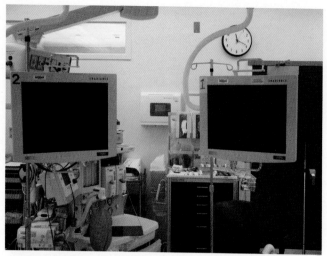

FIGURE 1-7 The use of two LCD video monitors permits the surgeon and assistant to work and comfortably view the arthroscopic video.

tained on a boom (see Fig. 1-8B). The advantage of the boom is that there are less electrical cords across the floor and that the monitor(s) can be positioned independently of the tower.

Most basic arthroscopic knee procedures, such as meniscectomies, chondroplasties, lateral releases and loose body removals, can be performed by the surgeon with the assistance of a single surgical scrub technician. More advanced procedures such as ligament reconstructions, meniscal repairs, cartilage restoration, and osteotomies, can be easier to perform with a second surgical assistant.

Similarly, all members of the operating room team should be informed well in advance of possible variations in the planned procedure(s) and the instruments required. It is important to discuss required instruments in advance with the surgical team and/or coordinator. Staff in the room must also know where instruments are located in case they are requested during the surgery.

Proper patient positioning is extremely important in terms of patient safety and surgical efficiency. A standard operating room bed is needed, with a leg portion that lowers. If fluoroscopy is planned, a radiolucent table may be needed. It is important to make certain that you can obtain the needed fluoroscopic images prior to prepping and draping the patient. It is the surgeon's responsibility to oversee the positioning of the patient. In situations in which you frequently perform surgery at a given center or hospital, you may want to train the staff to position patients for you. Even if you delegate this task, it is still your responsibility to make sure that they are positioned correctly. When training staff, it is important to explain your rationale for patient positioning instructions because they may not readily understand the importance of specific instructions relative to surgical efficiency and patient safety.

The use of leg holders or posts is determined by the preoperative diagnosis, surgical plan, and surgeon preference. A variety of different commercial leg holders are available for the operative and nonoperative leg. When operating on both knees, bilateral leg holders are also available (Fig. 1-9A). In most cases, a unilateral leg holder (see Fig. 1-9B and C) or lateral post (see Fig. 1-9D) is used for the operative leg. Leg holders may include padding, and some others require you to apply padding to the leg prior to securing it within the holder. Some holders are designed to hold the leg with a tourniquet (see Fig. 1-9B) and others require the tourniquet to be outside the holder (see Fig. 1-9C). If you prefer a unilateral holder or lateral post, it will be important to determine how to protect the contralateral leg. The use of a leg holder for the nonoperative leg has been shown to increase the risk of compression to the peroneal nerve as courses around the fibular neck.[2] Nonoperative leg holders can also cause a stretch injury to the femoral

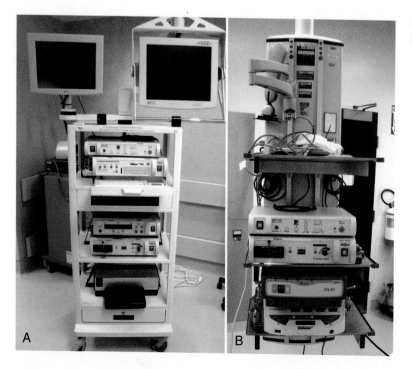

FIGURE 1-8 A, Arthroscopic boom. **B,** Mobile arthroscopic tower.

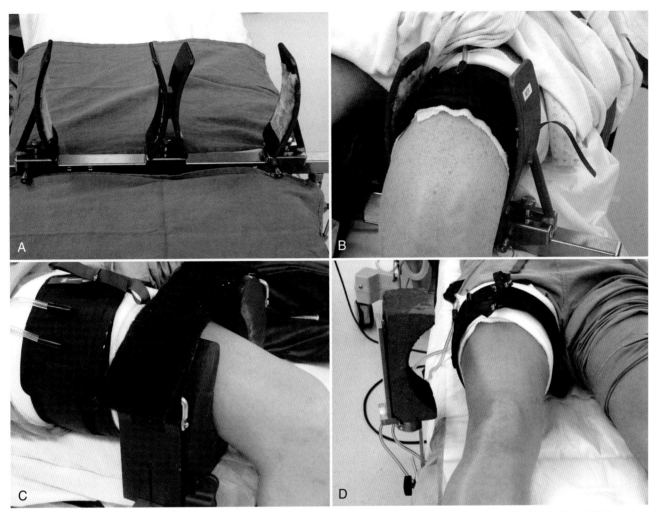

FIGURE 1-9 Leg holders and lateral post. **A,** Bilateral leg holder. **B,** Unilateral leg holder with tourniquet positioned within holder. **C,** Unilateral leg holder with tourniquet outside of holder. **D,** Lateral post.

nerve if the hip is held extended. If the foot of the bed is left up for a lateral post, then positioning the nonoperative leg does not require anything special. If the foot is dropped, it is often easiest to place a large pad under the nonoperative thigh to keep the hip flexed (Fig. 1-10). If there is concern about pressure on the peroneal nerve, additional foam padding can be applied in this region, particularly in thin patients.

Other issues related to the leg holder include the position of the foot of the bed and the use of hip bumps. For lateral post use, the foot of the bed can remain up (see Fig. 1-9D) or it can be lowered. The advantage of the lateral post is faster setup and positioning, ability to move the leg freely during surgery, ability to hyperflex the knee, and ease of placing the knee in a figure-of-four position. The primary disadvantage is that the leg tends to slide over the post when placing valgus stress on the knee for access to posterior horn of medial meniscus. This can be prevented, however, by having an assistant place downward pressure on the thigh (Fig. 1-11). The major disadvantages associated with a fixed leg holder is the risk of rupturing the medial collateral ligament with excess valgus stress[2]; knee flexion is limited by the lowered portion table and inability to move the leg freely. The

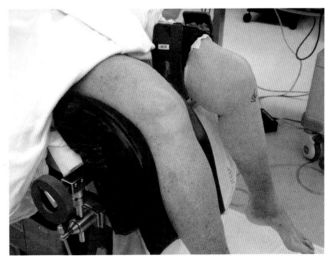

FIGURE 1-10 Pad for nonoperative leg used during knee arthroscopy.

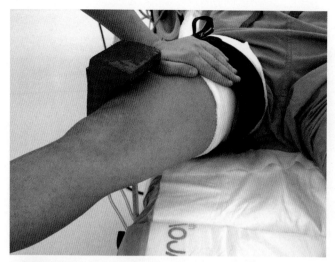

FIGURE 1-11 Valgus stress to knee joint with lateral post and assistant applying downward pressure on thigh. This prevents the thigh from sliding over the post.

inability to abduct the leg can sometimes pose difficulties in posteromedial portal placement. If this occurs, you can have an assistant carefully abduct the nonoperative leg or the leg holder can be loosened or even removed beneath the sterile drapes. Femur fractures have also been reported with the use of a leg holder, but these are rare.[6] Regardless of choice of leg holder, a small sandbag or other hip bump may be helpful for larger patients who tend to rotate their legs excessively externally when lying supine.

The next consideration is the decision on tourniquet usage. There are conflicting reports in the literature as to the usefulness of tourniquets in improving visualization and potential decreased recovery of muscle strength. Johnson and coworkers,[7] in a randomized prospective evaluation of 109 patients undergoing knee arthroscopy, reported that routine knee arthroscopy could be performed adequately without a tourniquet. Kirkley and colleagues.[8] in a similar evaluation of 120 patients, reported no complications associated with tourniquet use, with a slight trend toward less early postoperative pain and better isokinetic strength at 2 weeks postoperatively in the group in whom a tourniquet was not used. Tourniquets with a wide and/or curved cuff have been shown to decrease the risk of muscle and nerve injury. Rodeo and associates[9] have recommended that tourniquet time under 2 hours and pressures less than 350 mm Hg lower the risk of neuropraxia. Several authors have also shown that a tourniquet should not be reinflated during an operative procedure after it is deflated for a period of reperfusion.[10,11]

Potential Problems with Setup.   If the tourniquet is placed too low on the thigh, or if the leg holder is too low, the sterile operative field may be limited during the surgery. If a two-portal knee arthroscopy is planned but suprapatellar pathology is found and cannot be accessed via anterior portals, then a superior portal may be needed. The limited sterile field superiorly may prevent portal placement and could require repeat prepping and draping. Similarly, it may not be possible to create a posteromedial portal if posterior pathology is identified (see earlier).

Any potential need to convert a routine arthroscopic procedure to an open surgery or to a more involved procedure, such as anterior cruciate ligament (ACL) reconstruction, meniscal repair, or osteochondral transplantation, must be anticipated in advance to avoid repeat prepping and draping. The use of a lateral post may make conversion to more involved procedures simpler.

Arthroscopy Equipment

Gravity inflow, in which multiple bags of fluid are raised to 8 to 10 feet, is a common method for infusing the joint with fluid. Although more popular in the early days of arthroscopy, it continues to be used today by many surgeons. As technology has improved, the fluid pump has gained popularity. It provides the advantage of improved hemostasis and higher pressures.[2] There are a variety of different pumps available, so it is important for the surgeon to have a thorough understanding of the pump that he or she is using. Each pump has different controls for pressure and flow maintenance and the surgeon cannot assume that a set pressure on one pump is equal to the same pressure on another pump. It is also important to recognize that intra-articular pressures can be increased by simply manipulating the knee in flexion or extension.[12] Muellner and coworkers[13] have compared four pump systems and concluded that there is a significant difference among pumps in the pressure that was set and the actual measured intra-articular pressure. They also noted that all pumps were accurate at pressures below 60 mm Hg but not above this setting.

Selection of outflow methods also plays an important role in distention of the joint and providing a clear view. The options include suction or gravity outflow through the arthroscope sheath or through a separate outflow cannula. Continuous outflow, whether gravity or suction, will result in greater fluid use; therefore, intermittent outflow controlled by the surgeon or an assistant may be preferable. My preferred technique is presented later in this chapter.

Suction is also be connected to the shaver or burr and, similar to another type of outflow, can be used continuously or intermittently. Again, it is generally preferable to use suction on an intermittent basis to clear debris; continuous use can make it difficult to maintain joint distention. Although different manufacturers have small variations in shavers and burrs, they are usually available in different sizes and levels of aggressiveness. In general, the smallest, least aggressive instrument should be used. However, some smaller shavers and burrs tend to become clogged more easily from debris, which can require frequent cleaning. Regardless of which instrument is selected, it is important for the surgeon to be familiar with its characteristics. In particular, the surgeon should always know which side of the burr or shaver is the cutting side and which is the noncutting side. The surgeon should always maintain a clear view of the cutting side so as not to cause iatrogenic injury (Fig. 1-12). The instrument must be carefully placed (without force) into the joint, moved with the joint, and removed. Minimal if any torque should ever be applied to the shaft, and you should never shave or burr blindly. The surgeon also should not select the most aggressive burr just because is will perform faster. Slow, steady controlled movements are necessary when using a shaver, but especially a burr.

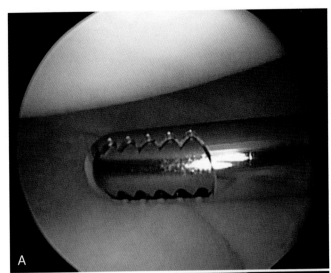

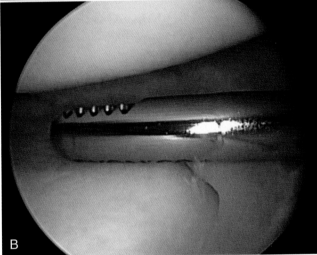

FIGURE 1-12 A, Arthroscopic view of the working end of a shaver. **B,** Arthroscopic view of shaver without view of shaver end.

The selection and proper use of an arthroscopic camera allow the surgeon to examine all areas of the knee joint efficiently. The arthroscope is available in 0, 30, and 70 degrees, although the 0-degree arthroscope is rarely used today because it provides the smallest field of view. As the light cord is rotated, the end of the arthroscope also rotates, resulting in a wide field of view. Most surgeons prefer the 30-degree arthroscope for most procedures. The 70-degree arthroscope should be available if a larger view is needed (e.g., looking around a corner), such as in the posterior aspect of the knee. Although it is important to use rotation of the arthroscope to increase the field of view, it is also important to maintain the orientation of the arthroscope with the anatomic position of the joint. For example, with the leg hanging off the end of the bed, the arthroscope power cord and camera should be maintained in a vertical orientation. This orientation should be maintained, even as the arthroscope is moved throughout the joint.

Most systems allow the surgeon to document the arthroscopic findings and treatment with photographs and/or video. Documentation can serve as an important reference for the surgeon, educational tool for the patient, and support for the charges to the insurance carrier. However, you should discuss giving videos to your patients with your malpractice carrier because some recommend against it.

Cannulas are not used as frequently in the knee as in other joints, but they can be useful for posterior portals. Disposable cannulas come in a variety of sizes. You should have several sizes available and should know in advance the minimum cannula diameter required by various instruments that you plan to use. Metal cannulas are useful for posterior portals because shavers can screw into the cannula directly and, with the use of an adapter, the camera can also be exchanged between cannulas.

With repeat use and normal wear, it is common to have to repair or replace cameras and light cords. It is therefore important to have extra cameras and light cords available during surgery. Other basic working instruments needed for knee arthroscopy include a probe, spinal needle, basket punches (narrow, wide, straight, upbiting, up curved, left , right, and back), graspers, cutters, and varying types of shavers, burrs, and cautery. Basket punches are available in various shapes and their selection largely depends on surgeon preference. More important than the shape, a variety of different angled and curved basket punches should be available so that all areas of the joint can be accessed.

Portals

Vertical versus horizontal portal incisions are primarily based on surgeon preference. A vertical portal provides greater options for extension in situations in which the pathology cannot be accessed because the initial portal is too high or low.

High Anterolateral Portal. The high anterolateral portal is the most common initial diagnostic portal. It is located above the lateral joint line, adjacent to the patellar tendon's lateral margin.[14] The inferior pole of the patella with the knee in 60 degrees of flexion is a good landmark for the inferior margin of this portal (Fig. 1-13A). It is important, however, to review the preoperative x-rays to make certain that the patient does not have patella alta

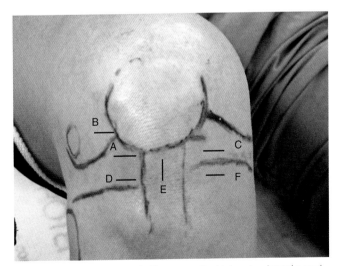

FIGURE 1-13 Anterior portals. Shown are the high anterolateral portal (A), patellofemoral axillary portal (B), standard anteromedial portal (C), accessory low anterolateral portal (D), transpatellar tendon portal (E), and accessory low anteromedial portal (F).

or baja. The anterolateral portal is useful for examining the medial, lateral, and patellofemoral compartments, visualizing the notch during ACL reconstruction, and treating medial meniscus pathology.[15] In addition to a viewing portal, it can be also used for fluid inflow.

In general, basic knee arthroscopy can be performed with a two- or three-portal technique. The two-portal technique requires inflow through the arthroscopic camera sheath while the three portal technique requires a separate superior portal for inflow. Most commonly, this superior portal is placed superolaterally. Stetson and Templin[16] have shown faster return to activities and return of quadriceps strength with the two-portal technique.

When pathology is expected in the lateral compartment based on the preoperative diagnosis, Kim and Kim[15] have recommended that the initial portal be placed more laterally and higher (patellofemoral axillary portal) than a standard high anterolateral portal. The patellofemoral axillary portal is at the junction or axilla of the lateral edge of the patella and the anterior edge of the lateral femoral condyle (see Fig. 1-13B). The authors stated that this portal allows excellent visualization of the popliteal hiatus, lateral gutter, and lateral compartment.

Anteromedial Portal.   A second working portal is created after performing an initial diagnostic examination through the first portal. Most often, the second portal is the anteromedial portal. The exact position of the portal is determined by the pathology (see Fig. 1-13C). As with all working portals, a spinal needle is used to determine its precise location. If access to the posterior horn of the medial meniscus is needed, the portal should be just above the anterior horn of the medial meniscus. If lateral compartment access is needed, the portal should be high enough to pass over the tibial spines. Alternatively, if pathology in the posterior horn of the lateral meniscus cannot be accessed through the anteromedial portal, a low anterolateral portal (see Fig. 1-13D) can be placed just above the anterior horn of the lateral meniscus.[15]

Accessory and Other Portals.   A transpatellar tendon or central portal can be created as an accessory working or viewing portal. The portal must be made vertically in line with the tendon fibers to avoid transecting the tendon. The portal is placed at the inferior pole of the patella (see Fig. 1-13E). It can be particularly useful in situations in which the anterolateral portal is too lateral and/or the anteromedial portal is too medial. In these cases, the transpatellar tendon portal can provide excellent visualization and access to the notch. Even when the other portals are placed appropriately, the transpatellar portal can be used as an accessory portal during ACL reconstruction.[14]

Additional anterior accessory portals can be placed at any location necessary for working or viewing. Most commonly, they are used to access a torn meniscus, articular cartilage defect, loose body, or the femoral tunnel placement for ACL or PCL surgery. The landmarks to avoid for accessory anterior portals are the menisci, articular cartilage, and inferior branch of the saphenous nerve. An accessory low anteromedial portal (see Fig. 1-13F) is often used for placement of a femoral tunnel via a medial portal.

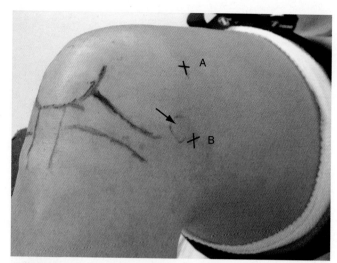

FIGURE 1-14 Anteromedial view of knee. Shown are the superomedial portal (A) and posteromedial portal (B). *Arrow,* medial femoral epicondyle.

The superomedial portal is placed 3 to 4 cm superior to the superior pole of the patella (Fig. 1-14A). It should be in line with the medial border of the patella or just posterior to it. The cannula and obturator should aim toward the suprapatellar pouch, just posterior to the patellar articular cartilage. This is an excellent portal for viewing patellofemoral tracking or the lateral retinaculum during release. Because the portal does violate the vastus medialis obliquus, it can affect return of postoperative knee function and quadriceps strength.[16] The superolateral portal is placed 3 to 4 cm superior to the superior pole of the patella and in line with the lateral border of the patella (Fig. 1-15A). It also provides excellent visualization of patellofemoral tracking. Either superior portal can also be used for fluid inflow.

All arthroscopic knee surgeons should be comfortable with access to the posterior compartments of the knee via posteromedial and posterolateral portals (see Figs. 1-14B and 1-15B, respectively). If unfamiliar with these portals, they should be

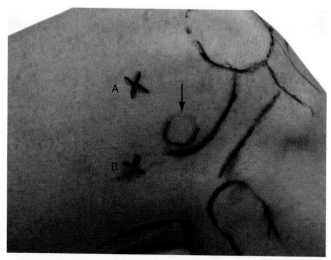

FIGURE 1-15 Anterolateral view of knee. Shown are the superolateral portal (A) and posterolateral portal (B). *Arrow,* lateral femoral epicondyle.

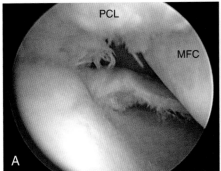
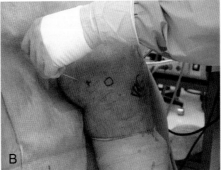
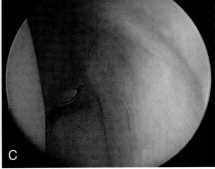

FIGURE 1-16 A, Arthroscopic view of interval between medial femoral condyle (MFC) and posterior cruciate ligament (PCL) used for passage of arthroscope into the posteromedial compartment of knee. **B,** External view of needle insertion for posteromedial portal. **C,** Arthroscopic view of needle entering posteromedial compartment.

practiced in the laboratory setting prior to attempting them in the operating room. With the arthroscope in the high anterolateral portal, the camera is advanced into the notch at the interval between the medial femoral condyle and PCL (Fig. 1-16A). Next, the arthroscopic sheath is held in place while the camera is replaced with a blunt trocar. The sheath and trocar are then gently advanced into the posteromedial compartment with the knee in 45 to 60 degrees of flexion. It is helpful to have the index finger of the hand holding the sheath positioned along its shaft. As the sheath is advanced, the index fingertip can be positioned so that it abuts the outside of the knee prior to penetrating the posterior capsule with the sheath and trocar. If difficulty is encountered during attempted passage, a limited inferior medial notchplasty can be performed, taking care to avoid injury to the PCL. This notchplasty may be required in cases of osteoarthritic spurs or otherwise stenotic notches.[17] Once in the compartment, the trocar is replaced with the camera and the posteromedial knee is palpated with a gloved finger. This will help in identifying the general area for placement of a spinal needle. The posteromedial portal is approximately 2 cm superior to the medial femoral epicondyle and 1 cm posterior (see Fig. 1-14B). With the knee in 90 degrees of flexion, the needle is directed toward the posterior aspect of the intercondylar notch (i.e., where the camera is located; see Fig. 16B and C). The exact position is dependent on the pathology present. Care should be taken to avoid injury to the popliteal neurovascular structures with transverse insertion

of the needle posterior to the posterior capsule.[3] Once the correct needle position is attained, a small skin incision is created. A hemostat is then used for blunt separation of soft tissues. This is helpful to prevent injury to the saphenous nerve or its branches. Next, a blunt obturator and cannula are inserted along the same direction as the spinal needle. The entry through the capsule can be directly visualized with the camera. In some cases, the blunt obturator will slide off the capsule in a posterior direction. If the capsule cannot be penetrated after a few careful attempts, the sharp obturator may be needed. This can be safe if you are confident in the direction required to penetrate the capsule. Once the obturator is against the capsule, it can be more easily pushed through it. The sharp obturator, however, increases the risk of injury to neurovascular structures if directed incorrectly.

In a similar fashion, a posterolateral portal can be established with the camera in the anteromedial portal. It is advanced through the notch between the ACL and lateral femoral condyle (Fig. 1-17A). This can often be done without replacing the camera with a trocar, but do not use excessive force. If the camera does not pass easily, it is safest to use a blunt trocar. A spinal needle is again used posterolaterally 2 cm superior to the lateral femoral epicondyle and anterior to the biceps femoris to avoid injury to the common peroneal nerve (see Figs. 1-15B and 1-7B). The needle is directed toward the tip of the camera (see Fig. 1-17C), a skin incision is created, and the cannula is inserted.

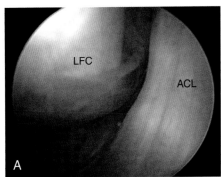
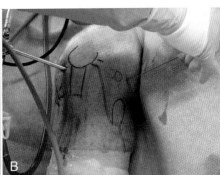
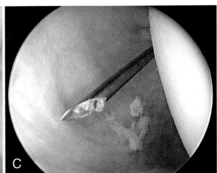

FIGURE 1-17 A, Arthroscopic view of interval between lateral femoral condyle (LFC) and anterior cruciate ligament (ACL) used for passage of the arthroscope into the posterolateral compartment of knee. **B,** External view of needle insertion for posterolateral portal. **C,** Arthroscopic view of needle entering posterolateral compartment.

Diagnostic Arthroscopy Technique

A standard leg holder is used for most arthroscopic procedures, and a lateral post is used for cruciate ligament reconstruction, patellofemoral realignment, and osteochondral autograft transfer (OAT) procedures requiring extreme knee flexion. If the leg holder is limiting the procedure in any way, it is removed by the circulating nurse during surgery, beneath the sterile drapes.

A routine knee examination for range of motion and ligament stability is performed. The tourniquet is placed over soft cotton roll approximately one handbreadth above the patella. The extremity is exsanguinated with an Esmarch bandage and the tourniquet pressure is increased to 300 mm Hg for most patients. For children or those with very small legs, the tourniquet pressure may be increased to 250 mm Hg. For obese patients, or those with elevated blood pressure, the tourniquet pressure may be increased to 350 mm Hg.

A large foam pillow is placed beneath the contralateral leg. After sterile prepping and draping, a horizontal high anterolateral portal is created. The arthroscopic camera sheath and blunt obturator are then carefully inserted through the capsule. The knee is extended and the sheath is further inserted into the suprapatellar pouch, just lateral to the patella. Care is taken to avoid injury to the femoral or patellar articular cartilage. A fluid pump is used for inflow through the arthroscopic sheath. Suction is also connected to the arthroscopic sheath and controlled by the surgeon. Suction is only used to clear cloudy fluid on an intermittent basis. Routine continuous suction of gravity outflow is not used.

Next, a quick initial diagnostic examination is performed. This should be a routine that works for the surgeon. My preference is first to examine the suprapatellar pouch, lateral gutter, patellofemoral joint, and medial gutter. The knee should be flexed and extended during examination of the patellofemoral joint. The knee is then flexed with gentle valgus stress applied as the camera is moved from the medial gutter into the medial compartment. The camera is then rotated to view the posterior horn, body, and anterior horn of the medial meniscus. The knee is flexed and extended to view the entire articular cartilage of the medial femoral condyle.

The camera is then pulled back slightly as the notch is entered. In some cases, it may be difficult to visualize the ACL fully because of a thick ligamentum mucosum. In this case, gently pass the camera over the top of the ligamentum and then push it slightly so that there is a close view of the medial portion of the lateral femoral condyle. The knee is then gently placed into a figure-of-four position and rested on the surgeon's thigh. This provides excellent visualization of the posterior horn of the lateral meniscus. As the knee is slowly extended, the lateral femoral condyle, body of the lateral meniscus, and anterior horn can be examined.

At this stage, an anteromedial working portal is created for most pathology. The superior-inferior position depends on the location of the pathology in the medial versus lateral compartments (see earlier). A spinal needle is inserted prior to creating a horizontal portal incision under direct visualization with the camera.

Next, a probe is inserted through the anteromedial working portal into the medial compartment. Although some have suggested that routine examination of the posterior compartment may be unnecessary,[18] result in increased morbidity, and decrease efficiency of the procedure, I prefer to examine posteromedially

and posterolaterally through the notch in all knee arthroscopies to avoid missing pathology.[19] Usually, this pathology includes a loose body or section of torn meniscus that is flipped posteriorly and not seen from an anterior view of the meniscus. The posteromedial compartment is examined while the arthroscope is still in the high anterolateral portal. If complete visualization is difficult, a 70-degree arthroscope is used, but this is extremely rare.

While the arthroscope is in the anteromedial viewing portal, it is passed into the posterolateral compartment for examination. If any additional pathology is identified from the anteromedial viewing portal, it is addressed at this time with existing portals or new portals as needed.

PEARLS & PITFALLS

PEARLS

- Risk of injury to branches of the saphenous nerve may be diminished with horizontal portals, careful dissection during meniscal repair, and hamstring tendon harvest and transillumination of the skin with the arthroscope. Light from the arthroscope may improve visibility of the nerve branches in their subcutaneous location.
- Prior to surgery, it is important for the surgeon to notify the operating room about assistants that will be required for the planned procedure(s) and their expected roles.
- The best system is to have a list of instruments absolutely needed for the planned surgery, along with a second list of instruments that should be available.
- Rather than having a set protocol for "always" or "never" using a tourniquet, it may be more important to use a tourniquet judiciously based on the planned procedure, patient-specific risk factors, and bleeding conditions during surgery.
- The arthroscopic field of view is not improved by changing the orientation of the camera but by rotating the light source.
- It is important to use the correct instrument for the required task and to examine the joint prior to placement of a working portal, because the location of this portal may be affected by the pathology identified.
- The no. 11 blade is inserted *completely through* the capsule for greater ease in passing instruments in and out of the working portal (Fig. 1-18).
- A second diagnostic examination is performed with the probe. Menisci, articular cartilage surfaces, and cruciate ligaments are carefully probed to identify pathology.
- While viewing from the anterolateral portal, perform any required work through the anteromedial or other working portals. Once the work is completed, the arthroscope is moved to the anteromedial portal or other viewing portals. This limits movement of the arthroscope back and forth and improves efficiency.

PITFALLS

- Injury to sensory nerves can result in loss of sensation and painful neuromas.
- Failure to have the needed instruments during surgery may result in inefficiency, complications, and poor outcomes.
- If the orientation of the camera is continuously changed, the surgeon will have difficulty triangulating instruments.
- Trying to use an instrument to perform a task that it is not designed for can result in iatrogenic injury to the joint and/or damage to the instrument.

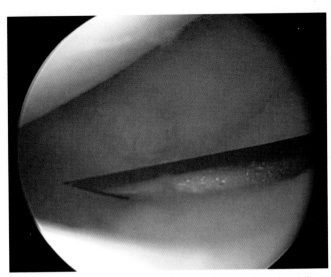

FIGURE 1-18 Arthroscopic view with camera in anterolateral portal viewing the scalpel-creating anteromedial portal.

- The tourniquet portion of the thigh is placed and secured within the leg holder with the leg in slight internal rotation. This helps prevent external rotation of the knee during placement of valgus stress.
- Proceeding immediately to the expected pathology based on the preoperative diagnosis, treating it, forgetting to examine the rest of the joint, and missing unexpected pathology should be avoided.
- If the scalpel is not inserted at the same orientation as the spinal needle, and if the tip of the scalpel is not viewed arthroscopically as it is inserted, iatrogenic injury to the meniscus and/or articular cartilage can result.
- The initial quick diagnostic examination may have been limited because of synovitis, thickened ligamentum, or hypertrophic fat pad. Failure to go back, remove obstructions as needed, and perform a thorough examination can result in missed pathology.
- Do not eliminate moving the camera into another portal just to complete the procedure faster. Complete examination and treatment often require viewing from different portals.

POSTOPERATIVE MANAGEMENT

At the end of the arthroscopic procedure, the joint is thoroughly irrigated and fluid is suctioned. The portals are each closed with a nylon suture. The joint is injected for postoperative pain control with 30 mL of 0.5% bupivacaine (Marcaine). Dressings are applied, the tourniquet is deflated, and a warm pink foot is confirmed. The postoperative protocol is based on the specific pathology treated and is discussed in the relevant chapters elsewhere in this text.

REFERENCES

1. Clarke HD, Scott WN, Insall JN, et al. Anatomy. In: Scott WN, ed. *Insall & Scott Surgery of the Knee*. Vol 1. 4th ed. Philadelphia: Churchill Livingstone; 2006:3-66.
2. Kim TK, Savino RM, McFarland EG, Cosgarea AJ. Neurovascular complications of knee arthroscopy. *Am J Sports Med*. 2002;30:619-629.
3. Matava MJ, Sethi NS, Totty WG. Proximity of the posterior cruciate ligament insertion to the popliteal artery as a function of the knee flexion angle: implications for posterior cruciate ligament reconstruction. *Arthroscopy*. 2000;16:796-804.
4. Jacobson E, Forssblad M, Rosenberg J, et al. Can local anesthesia be recommended for routine use in elective knee arthroscopy? A comparison between local, spinal, and general anesthesia. *Arthroscopy* 2000;16:183-190.
5. Horlocker TT, Hebl JR. Anesthesia for outpatient knee arthroscopy: Is there an optimal technique? *Region Anesth Pain Med*. 2003;28:58-63.
6. Cautilli R. Introduction to basics of arthroscopy of the knee. *Clin Sports Med* 1997;16:1-16.
7. Johnson DS, Stewart H, Hirst P, et al. Is tourniquet use necessary for knee arthroscopy? *Arthroscopy* 2000;16:648-651.
8. Kirkley A, Rampersaud R, Griffin S, et al. Tourniquet versus no tourniquet use in routine knee arthroscopy: a prospective, double-blind, randomized clinical trial. *Arthroscopy* 2000;16:121-126.
9. Rodeo SA, Forster RA, Weiland AJ. Neurological complications due to arthroscopy. *J Bone Joint Surg Am*. 1993;75:917-926.
10. Mohler LR, Pedowitz RA, Myers RR et al. Intermittent reperfusion fails to prevent post tourniquet neuropraxia. *J Hand Surg [Am]*. 1999;24:687-693.
11. Rorabeck CH, Kennedy JC. Tourniquet-induced nerve ischemia complicating knee ligament surgery. *Am J Sports Med*. 1980;8:98-102.
12. Funk DA, Noyes FR, Grood ES, et al. Effect of flexion angle on the pressure-volume of the human knee. *Arthroscopy*. 1991;7:86-90.
13. Muellner T, Menth-Chiari WA, Reihsner R, et al. Accuracy of pressure and flow capacities of four arthroscopic fluid management systems. *Arthroscopy* 2001;17:760-764.
14. Cohen SB, Fu FH. Three-portal technique for anterior cruciate ligament reconstruction: use of a central medial portal. *Arthroscopy* 2007;23:325e1-325e4.
15. Kim SJ, Kim HJ. High portal: practical philosophy for positioning portals in knee arthroscopy. *Arthroscopy*. 2001;17(3):333-337.
16. Stetson WB, Templin K. Two- versus three-portal technique for routine knee arthroscopy. *Am J Sports Med*. 2002;30:108-111.
17. Ojeda León H, Rodríguez-Blanco CE, Guthrie TB, et al. Intercondylar notch stenosis in degenerative arthritis of the knee. *Arthroscopy* 2005; 21:294-302.
18. Lubowitz JH, Rossi MJ, Baker BS, et al. Arthroscopic visualization of the posterior compartments of the knee. *Arthroscopy* 2004;20:675-680.
19. Amin KB, Cosgarea AJ, Kaeding CC. The value of intercondylar notch visualization of the posteromedial and posterolateral compartments during knee arthroscopy. *Arthroscopy*. 1999;15:813-817.

SUGGESTED READINGS

Cole B J, Sekiya JK, eds. *Surgical Techniques of the Shoulder, Elbow, and Knee in Sports Medicine*. Philadelphia: WB Saunders; 2008.
McKeon BP, Bono JV, Richmond JC, eds. *Knee Arthroscopy*. New York, Springer, 2009.
Miller MD, Cole BJ, eds. *Textbook of Arthroscopy*. Philadelphia: WB Saunders; 2004.
Stoller DW, ed. *MRI, Arthroscopy, and Surgical Anatomy of the Joints*. Philadelphia: Lippincott-Raven; 1999.

Arthroscopic Treatment of Tibial Eminence Fractures

S. L. Mortimer ● Robert E. Hunter

Tibial eminence fractures are intra-articular fractures that can be a challenging injury for orthopedic surgeons to manage. These represent an avulsion injury of the insertion of the anterior cruciate ligament (ACL) at the tibia and are considered the equivalent of an ACL tear.[1,2] Poncet first described the tibial eminence fracture in 1875 and, since then, the treatment algorithm has changed significantly, from nonoperative management to what is now considered contemporary arthroscopic management.[3] This chapter will discuss in detail a current review of the anatomy, mechanism of injury, diagnosis, treatment, rehabilitation, and potential complications that can occur with tibial eminence fractures.

ANATOMY

The tibia is the primary weight-bearing bone of the knee joint. The most proximal aspect of the tibia is comprised of the medial and lateral tibial condyles. The articular surfaces of the condyles are the medial and lateral tibial plateaus, which articulate with the corresponding medial and lateral femoral condyles. The plateaus are separated by the intercondylar eminence, which serves as the site of attachment for the anterior and posterior cruciate ligaments and the fibrocartilaginous menisci.[4] Specifically, the midpoint of the intercondylar eminence serves as the distal attachment of the ACL.

The mechanism of injury for tibial eminence fractures is similar to an ACL tear; however, it involves an avulsion fracture at the ACL insertion. The injury may be associated with valgus and external rotation. It is often seen in skiers and is related to a boot-induced injury after the skier lands on the tail of the ski or to the phenomenon referred to as a "phantom foot" injury, which involves forced internal rotation with knee flexion. Although seen frequently in skiers, it is also seen in other sports, bicycle accidents, motor vehicle accidents, and pedestrian versus motor vehicle injuries.

Tibial eminence fractures are seen in children usually between the ages of 8 and 15 years.[3,5,6] Although this fracture pattern is commonly associated with a childhood injury, it is also seen in adults.[2,7,8] It is theorized that this occurs more commonly in children because of the relative weakness of the incompletely ossified tibial eminence as compared with the fibers of the ACL. It has also been proposed that the injury occurs secondary to greater elasticity of the ligaments in younger people.[9]

PATIENT EVALUATION

History And Physical Examination

Similar to patients with other fractures involving the knee joint, patients presenting with fractures of the tibial eminence present with a painful swollen knee and have difficulty bearing weight. Initial examination is often difficult secondary to pain and may limit evaluation of the ligaments. A complete neurologic and vascular examination must be performed. Careful assessment of the soft tissues is crucial when first examining the patient. The compartments must be evaluated for compartment syndrome and any neurovascular deficit must be identified immediately. Recognizing the presence of an open or closed fracture also is important when trying to determine a treatment plan.

Diagnostic Imaging

Plain radiographs are usually diagnostic and involve anteroposterior, lateral, and oblique views. Computed tomography (CT) scanning may be used to define bony architecture better and magnetic resonance imaging (MRI) is useful for determining additional injuries to chondral surfaces, menisci, and ligaments. Arteriography and vascular surgery consultation must be considered in the presence of diminished pulses or abnormal vascular examination. We prefer to obtain an MRI in all pattients in whom tibial avulsion is suspected to confirm the diagnosis and determine the amount of displacement and presence of associated pathology.

Classification

Meyers and McKeever first described the classification scheme for tibial eminence fractures in 1959.[2] Their classification divides these fractures into three types based on displacement of the avulsed fracture fragment (Fig. 2-1). Type I represents a nondisplaced or minimally displaced fracture at the anterior margin. Type II fractures involve the anterior third or half of the avulsed bone displaced proximally, with an intact posterior hinge resembling a bird's beak. Type III fractures have a completely displaced fracture. These have been further subdivided into IIIA and IIIB fracture classifications.[10] Type IIIA fractures involve the ACL insertion only, whereas the IIIB type includes the entire intercondylar eminence. Some have labeled comminuted fractures as type IV.[10]

Associated injuries with fractures of the tibial eminence are common. Meniscus injuries are the most common injuries seen; however, these fractures may be associated with chondral and ligamentous injuries as well.[11,12] In an unpublished study, we found an interposed intermeniscal ligament in 80% of types II and III injuries. This has profound implications for treatment strategies. In addition, tibial eminence fractures are also seen with tibial plateau fractures, specifically Schatzker types V and VI fractures.[13]

TREATMENT

The goal for management of tibial eminence fractures should be no different than for any other intra-articular fracture. Anatomic reduction and rigid fixation that allow for early range of motion should be the treatment for these fractures. Debate has ensued over anatomic reduction versus overreduction. It has been proposed that overreduction may result in excessive tension of the ACL, which results in limited knee range of motion.[14] Others have countered this by stating that plastic deformation of the ACL occurs prior to the avulsion fracture and thus overreduction would result in a better outcome.[9] Numerous studies have documented residual laxity in well-reduced tibial eminence fractures, and most have concluded that the laxity is not symptomatic.[15-17] More studies are needed to answer the question of anatomic versus overreduction, but there is consensus that any displacement requires at least an anatomic reduction.

Management has been based on the Meyers and McKeever classification, with recommendations for immobilization in extension for type I fractures. Some controversy exists in regard to what degree the knee is to be extended for nonoperative management. Meyers and McKeever have recommended immobilization in 20 degrees of flexion.[2,8] Similarly, Beaty and Kumar have recommended immobilization in 10 to 15 degrees of flexion.[18] Fyfe and Jackson based their recommendations of flexing the knee to 30 to 40 degrees because the ACL is taut in extension and, with some flexion, the tension on the avulsion fragment would be less.[19] These authors favor immobilization in full extension to avoid a flexion contracture, which can occur if the knee is kept in a flexed position. We encourage straight leg raises and quadriceps isometrics and allow full weight bearing, as tolerated, in a brace locked in full extension. The knee should not be immobilized in hyperextension because extensive stretch on the popliteal artery may result in a compartment syndrome.[13] Regardless of the position of immobilization, close follow-up with radiographs weekly for 4 weeks should help confirm maintenance of reduction.

Treatment of type II fractures has been controversial. Closed reduction may be attempted by aspiration of the hemarthrosis and knee extension performed to allow the femoral condyles to help reduce the fracture.[20] Anteroposterior and lateral radiographs should be taken to verify reduction and, with difficult visualization, CT or MRI should be performed. Often, anatomic reduction is not achieved secondary to interposition of the medial meniscus, lateral meniscus, or intermeniscal ligament. Persistent displacement, despite attempted reduction maneuvers, warrants arthroscopic evaluation and treatment. Many reports have identifed associated soft tissue injuries, including chondral, meniscal, and ligamentous structures. The need for anatomic reduction of

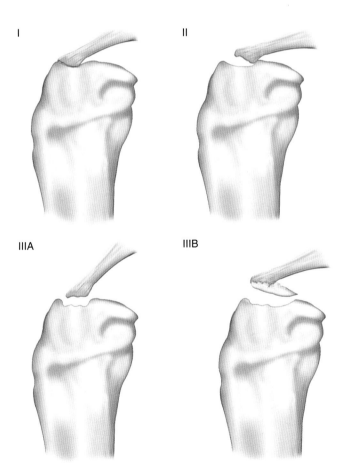

FIGURE 2-1 Meyers and McKeever classification of tibial intercondylar eminence fractures. *(Adapted from Lubowitz JH, Elson WS, Guttman D. Part II: Arthroscopic treatment of tibial plateau fractures: intercondylar eminence avulsion fractures. Arthroscopy. 2005;21:86-92.)*

these fractures to allow for postoperative stability and motion, combined with the need to identify and treat these associated injuries, make arthroscopic evaluation necessary for successful treatment of most type II and all type III fractures.[16,21-24] These authors also think that most, if not all, type II fractures were likely a type III level of displacement at the time of disruption. Based on that, we take an aggressive operative approach to most type II injuries.

Closed reduction may be attempted for type III injuries, but anatomic reduction and maintenance of reduction are difficult. Most experts agree that type III fractures require reduction and fixation.[13,25,26] Arthroscopic reduction and fixation of these injuries have become the standard of care and has made open reduction and internal fixation a treatment that is infrequently necessary or used.

Techniques involving the use of cannulated screws or suture have been described and the results with either method have been excellent. Risks of cannulated screw placement involve comminuting the fracture fragment, crossing the physis with a screw, hardware impingement necessitating removal, and posterior neurovascular injury. Repair using nonabsorbable suture fixation provides the benefit of eliminating these risks and still maintaining an excellent reduction and result.

Arthroscopic Technique

General or epidural anesthesia may be used. The leg is secured in an arthroscopic leg holder and the foot of the bed is flexed. The contralateral leg is supported with a foam pad and abducted to the side to allow fluoroscopy of the involved extremity in both anteroposterior and lateral projections. A tourniquet is placed around the thigh, but is not routinely used. After prepping and draping, an superomedial portal is established. A fluid pump is used to promote hemostasis and adequate visualization. Care is taken to keep pressure relatively low to avoid fluid extravasation. This has not been found to be a problem

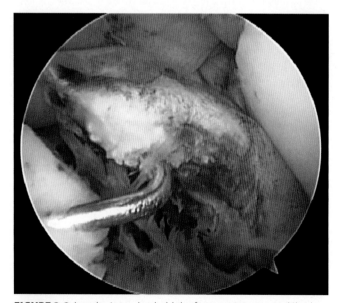

FIGURE 2-2 A probe is used to hold the fracture site open to débride the clot, intermeniscal ligament, or other debris.

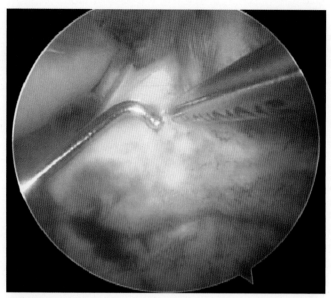

FIGURE 2-3 A probe and Steinmann pin are used to reduce the fracture anatomically.

nor have elevated compartment pressures. An anterolateral portal is established for the arthroscope. The hematoma is evacuated until reasonable visualization is possible. Once pathology can be visualized, an anteromedial portal is established after localization with a spinal needle. An arthroscopic probe is then used to dislodge any clotted blood or debris at the site of fracture (Fig. 2-2).

A synovial resector (4.5 mm) is used to débride the region further and to remove any debris from the fracture bed. Once the fracture site has been débrided, the probe is used to attempt a reduction. Interposition of the intermeniscal ligament or the menisci requires use of the probe to hold the soft tissue structures out of the way while attempting to reduce the fragment with an ACL guide or probe. An accessory medial portal is created 1.5 to 2.0 cm medial to the anteromedial portal for the probe. In patients in whom the intermeniscal ligament prevents reduction and also cannot be mobilized, resection is performed. Once the fracture has been reduced, a 0.062-inch Steinmann pin is placed percutaneously from a medial parapatellar position to hold the fracture reduced (Fig. 2-3).

If there is a large fragment and the piece is large enough to consider placing a cannulated screw, fixation is achieved by using one or two 4.0-mm cannulated screws (Synthes USA, Paoli, Pa). If the Steinmann pin that is holding the reduction is in good position, it may be used as the guide pin for the cannulated screw. If not, a second wire may be placed under fluoroscopic control. The goal is to have the pin(s) just penetrate the posterior cortex of the tibia. Frequent use of fluoroscopy is recommended to ensure accurate placement of the wire and screw and also to make sure that the wire is not being advanced as the screw is placed.

Suture fixation should be used when the fracture is small or comminuted, or in the presence of open growth plates. Some have advocated using the suture methods for all patients because these result in less risk (neurovascular bundle) and less

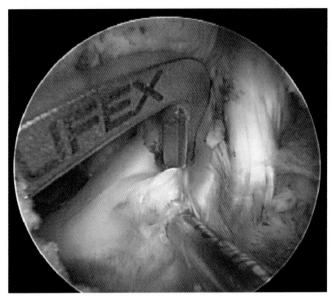

FIGURE 2-4 The ACL tibial tunnel guide is used to pass a 2.4-mm wire on the medial side of the fragment.

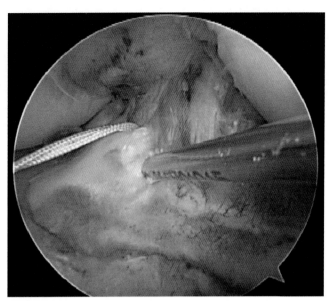

FIGURE 2-6 The medial 2.4-mm wire is withdrawn, a suture passer is placed in the hole, and two Ultrabraid sutures (Smith & Nephew Endoscopy, Andover, Mass) are passed.

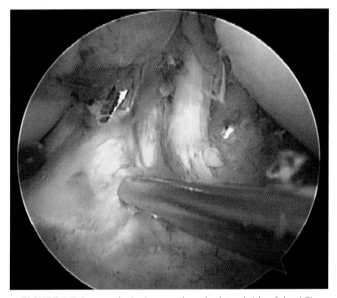

FIGURE 2-5 A second wire is passed on the lateral side of the ACL.

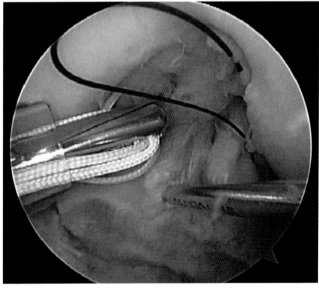

FIGURE 2-7 The lateral 2.4-mm wire is removed, the Hewson suture passer (Smith & Nephew Endoscopy) is passed, and the other ends of the sutures are brought out of the tibial cortex.

secondary procedures (hardware removal) [25,26] These authors favor the suture technique in all cases. After the fracture is reduced and held in position with the Steinmann pin, the ACL tibial tunnel guide is used to pass a 2.4-mm guide pin through the anteromedial tibial metaphysis, entering the joint on the medial side of the fragment (Fig. 2-4). A second wire is passed starting 1 to 2 cm lateral to the first hole on the tibial cortex, entering the knee at the lateral side of the fragments (Fig. 2-5). The first wire is removed and, immediately after removal, a Hewson suture passer (Smith & Nephew Endoscopy, Andover, Mass) is passed up the hole and two Ultrabraid sutures (Smith & Nephew Endoscopy) are delivered into its loop through the anteromedial portal and pulled out the anteromedial tibia (Fig. 2-6). The second wire is taken out and the Hewson suture passer is immediately placed into the joint (Fig. 2-7). The opposite end of the ULTRABRAID suture(s) are delivered into its loop and pulled out the tibia (Fig. 2-8). A crochet hook or blunt probe is passed into the subcutaneous tissue through one of the suture holes, hooking the opposite sutures, and pulling them out the same hole. A knot is tied and passed through the skin puncture hole and subcutaneous tissue and is secured tightly to the tibial cortex. Each suture is tied and secured individually (Fig. 2-9). This provides firm fixation of the fracture fragment and can be visualized directly.

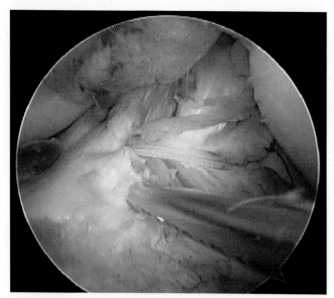

FIGURE 2-8 The suture has been passed through both tibial holes. It now holds the ACL and its fracture fragment reduced.

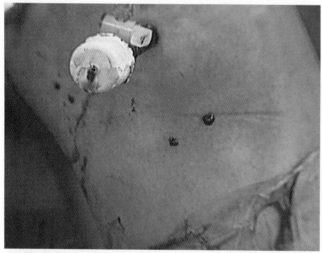

FIGURE 2-9 The sutures are tied through one of the wire holes, leaving no incision along the tibia.

PEARLS & PITFALLS

PEARLS

- Intra-articular fractures result in more bleeding and larger, more painful effusions than ligament or cartilage injuries. Therefore, when an acute knee trauma presents with a tense effusion, look carefully for an intra-articular fracture.
- Intermeniscal ligament interposition occurs in a high percentage of types II and III injuries. Left unattended, this will preclude reduction and healing.
- Meyers and McKeever type II injuries underwent more displacement at the time of injury and were likely type III in most cases.
- Indications for arthroscopic intervention are the presence of radiographic or MRI displacement or pathologic laxity of an examination.

- Hold reduction with a Steinmann pin placed percutaneously from a medial parapatellar position; use fluoroscopy.
- Suture fixation is the preferred method in the skeletally immature and with comminuted or small fragments.
- When passing the sutures through the anteromedial portal to secure the avulsion, using a small (5.5-mm) cannula for suture passage will eliminate the chance of entrapping subcutaneous and capsule tissues.
- If having difficulty pulling sutures out through the puncture created by the 2.4-mm guide pin, make a small longitudinal incision between the two guide pin puncture wounds, retrieve all sutures through this incision, and tie each suture individually.

PITFALLS

- Failure to remove debris from the fracture site will result in nonanatomic reduction and more laxity.
- Poor placement of Steinmann pins or screws may result in injury to the neurovascular structures; use fluoroscopy for all fixation pins and screws.
- Screw fixation may cause physeal arrest; be aware of open physes.

POSTOPERATIVE MANAGEMENT

Patients are placed in a hinged knee brace locked in 0 degrees of flexion for the first 4 weeks and allowed to perform passive or active-assisted range of motion exercises in the prone position through an arc of 0 to 90 degrees. Patients may bear weight as tolerated, with the brace locked at 0 degrees. Crutches are generally discontinued by postoperative day 10. At 4 weeks, the brace is removed, and closed-chain quadriceps exercises are begun. At 8 weeks, easy straight-ahead running is initiated and pivot-twist maneuvers are avoided until at least 12 weeks after surgery.

COMPLICATIONS

Although a good outcome is usually expected for fractures of the tibial eminence, complications do occur. Residual laxity after fixation is commonly found after arthroscopic reduction and fixation. Although multiple studies have reported results verifying positive Lachman tests and a difference in laxity from the contralateral uninjured extremity, most patients have functional stability and are not adversely affected.[7,15-17,27] Evidence of clinical instability warrants revision with ACL reconstruction.

Arthrofibrosis is a potential complication, but is rare if the patient undergoes arthroscopic reduction with fixation, because the goal of the operation is to promote early range of motion. Development of arthrofibrosis warrants aggressive therapy and possible manipulation under anesthesia, with arthroscopic lavage and débridement of adhesions. Loss of full extension can be avoided by immobilization in full extension and attention to quadriceps and hamstring strengthening.

Painful or symptomatic hardware is common with the use of cannulated screws. Loss of full knee extension can occur secondary to scar tissue or a prominent screw in the intercondylar notch. It has been demonstrated that at the time of hardware removal, soft tissue interposition is the rule, and that excision combined with implantation removal results in excellent outcomes.[28]

CONCLUSIONS

Arthroscopy is a safe and preferable alternative to closed management of types II and III tibial eminence fractures. The arthroscopic examination, reduction, and fixation can be accomplished in almost all patients. In addition, this technique provides superior reduction and fixation when compared with closed or open methods. Almost all patients return to sports at their previous level when treated with arthroscopic reduction and internal fixation, which further supports this as the approach that best predicts a good result.

REFERENCES

1. Kendall NS, Hsu SYC, Chan K. Fracture of the tibial spine in adults and children. *J Bone Joint Surg Br.* 1992;74:848-852.
2. Meyers, MH, McKeever FM. Fracture of the intercondylar eminence of the tibia. *J Bone Joint Surg Am.* 1959;41:209-222.
3. Gronkvist H, Hirsch G, Johansson L, et al. Fracture of the anterior tibial spine in children. *J Pediatr Orthop.* 1984;4:465-8.
4. Wiss DA, Watson JT. Fractures of the tibial plateau. In: Rockwood CA, Green DP, Bucholz RW, Heckman JD, eds. *Rockwood and Green's Fractures in Adults.* Philadelphia: Lippincott-Raven; 1996:1920-1953.
5. Chandler JT, Miller TM. Tibial eminence fracture with meniscal entrapment. *Arthroscopy.* 1995;11:499-502.
6. Owens BD, Crane GK, Plante T, et al. Treatment of type III tibial intercondylar eminence fractures in skeletally immature atrhletes. *Am J Orthop.* 2003;33:103-105.
7. Wiley JJ, Baxter MP. Tibial spine fractures in children. *Clin Orthop Relat Res.* 1990;(255):54-60.
8. Meyers MH, McKeevor FM. Fracture of the intercondylar eminence of the tibia. *J Bone Joint Surg Am.* 1970;52:1677-1683.
9. Noyes FR, DeLucas JL, Torvik PJ. Biomechanics of anterior cruciate ligament failure: an analysis of strain-rate sensitivity and mechanism of failure in primates. *J Bone Joint Surg Am.* 1974;56:236-253.
10. Zaricznyj B. Avulsion fracture of the tibial eminence treated by open reduction and pinning. *J Bone Joint Surg Am.* 1997;59:1111-1114.
11. McLennan JG. The role of arthroscopic surgery in the treatment of fractures of the intercondylar eminence of the tibia. *J Bone Joint Surg Br.* 1982;64:477-480.
12. Falstie-Jensen S, Sondergard Peterson PE. Incarceration of the meniscus in fractures of the intercondylar eminence of the tibia in children. *Injury.* 1984;15:236-238.
13. Schatzker J. Tibial plateau fractures. In: Browner BD, Jupiter JB, Levine AM, Trafton PG, eds. *Skeletal Trauma.* Philadelphia: WB Saunders; 1992;1745-1770.
14. Lubowitz JH, Elson WS, Guttmann D. Part I: arthroscopic management of tibial plateau fractures. *Arthroscopy.* 2004;20:1063-1070.
15. Baxter MP, Wiley JJ. Fractures of the tibial spine in children. *J Bone Joint Surg Br.* 1988;70:228-230.
16. Willis RB, Blokker C, Stoll TM, et al. Long-term follow-up of anterior tibial eminence fractures. *J Pediatr Orthop.* 1993;13:361-364.
17. Lee Y, Chin L, Wang N, et al. Anterior tibial spine fracture in children: follow-up evaluation by biomechanical studies. *Chin Med J.* 1996;58:183-189.
18. Beaty JH, Kumar A. Fractures about the knee in children. *J Bone Joint Surg Am.* 1994;76:1870-1880.
19. Fyfe IS, Jackson JP. Tibial intercondylar fractures in children: a review of the classification and the treatment of malunion. *Injury.* 1981;13:165-169.
20. Lubowitz JH, Elson WS, Guttman D. Part II: arthroscopic treatment of tibial plateau fractures: intercondylar eminence avulsion fractures. *Arthroscopy.* 2005;21:86-92.
21. Mah JY, Otsuka NY, Mclean J. An arthroscopic technique for the reduction and fixation of tibial-eminence fractures. *J Pediatr Orthop.* 1996;16:119-121.
22. Janarv P, Westblad P, Johansson C, et al. Long-term follow-up of anterior tibial spine fractures in children. *J Pediatr Orthop.* 1995;15:63-68.
23. Osti L, Merlo F, Bocchi L. Our experience in the arthroscopic treatment of fracture-avulsion of the tibial spine. *Chir Organi Mov.* 1997;82:295-299.
24. Matthews DE, Geissler WB. Arthroscopic suture fixation of displaced tibial eminence fractures. *Arthroscopy.* 1994;10:418-423.
25. Hunter RE, Willis JA. Arthroscopic fixation of avulsion fractures of the tibial eminence: technique and outcome. *Arthroscopy.* 2004;20:113-121.
26. Lubowitz JH, Grauer JD. Arthroscopic treatment of anterior cruciate ligament avulsion. *Clin Orthop Relat Res.* 1993;294:242-246.
27. Smith JB. Knee instability after fractures of the intercondylar eminence of the tibia. *J Pediatr Orthop.* 1984;4:462-464.
28. Senekovic V, Veselko M. Anterograde arthroscopic fixation of avulsion fractures of the tibial eminence with a cannulated screw: five-year results. *Arthroscopy.* 2003;19:54-61.

Arthroscopic Management of Tibial Plateau Fractures

James H. Lubowitz

The first preoperative consideration is nonoperative management. However, articular irregularities cannot be accepted and associated meniscal or ligamentous pathology must be evaluated and treated. Cast treatment also has the disadvantage of stiffness.

Open reduction and internal fixation (ORIF) is a historical option, and arthroscopic reduction and internal fixation (ARIF), with possible skin incision but no capsulotomy or arthrotomy, is the emerging gold standard.

ANATOMY

As reviewed by Lubowitz and colleagues,[1,2] the knee is anatomically designed well to achieve its function—providing stability, bending and rotational range of motion, and transmission of load. The tibia is the major weight-bearing bone of the knee joint. At its proximal articular surface, the tibia widens to form medial and lateral condyles. Between the condyles, the intercondylar eminence serves as the attachment for the menisci and the anterior and posterior cruciate ligaments. The relatively flattened condylar portions of the proximal tibia compromise the weight-bearing aspects of the plateau. The medial and lateral condyles articulate with corresponding medial and lateral femoral condyles.

With regard to pathoanatomy, the medial plateau is larger and stronger, explaining why lateral condylar tibial plateau fractures occur more frequently than medial condylar fractures. Additionally, with regard to intercondylar eminence avulsion fracture pathoanatomy, the anterior cruciate ligament (ACL) distal attachment is the midpoint of the tibial intercondylar eminence. Obviously, tibial intercondylar eminence fractures result in effective disruption of the ACL.

PATIENT EVALUATION

History and Physical Examination

Classic patient history is trauma as a result of a fall or motor vehicle versus a pedestrian accident.[1,2] Tibial plateau fractures are common in sports, particularly in skiers. Avulsion fractures commonly occur in children and adolescents, with 50% caused by a fall from a bicycle. However, it is sometimes misunderstood that this condition occurs only in the young. Although less common, ACL avulsion also occurs in adults.

On physical examination, patients present with painful swollen knees and generally are unable to bear weight. Careful history differentiates high- or low-energy injuries and a careful examination notes any evidence of a fracture blister, compartment syndrome, meniscal or ligamentous disruption, or neurovascular injury. To re-emphasize this key point, attention must be paid to peripheral pulses, neurologic function, and the status of the compartments of the injured extremity. Any open wounds must also be evaluated to ascertain a relationship to the fracture site or joint space.

Diagnostic Imaging

Standard radiologic knee trauma views usually reveal plateau fractures, but displaced fractures and compression fractures can be missed. X-rays are not accurate for determining the amount of depression when a compression fracture component is visible. Computed tomography (CT) with three-dimensional reconstruction provides precise information regarding the extent and pattern of articular and extra-articular components of the fracture. In addition to CT scanning to assess bony pathology, magnetic resonance imaging (MRI) is also recommended. MRI is the examination of choice for soft tissue injuries associated with tibial plateau fractures.

Arteriography should be considered when any suspicion for knee dislocation or arterial injury exists. High-energy injuries are associated with higher risks of compartment syndrome and arterial injury.

TREATMENT

Indications and Contraindications

The goal of tibial plateau fracture treatment is joint stability, with articular congruity and normal alignment. Preservation of full range of motion is also vital. Surgery is indicated for unstable or malaligned knees or articular incongruity. Surgery should also be considered to allow early range of motion for active patients, particularly athletes. The key point is articular compression or fracture displacement is the indication for surgery. Historically, 4 to 10 mm of fracture displacement or compression was considered acceptable, but today a 3- or 4-mm displacement should be considered as a relative indication for ARIF, particularly in active patients.

Contraindications to surgical intervention, when indicated, are rare. In older adult, debilitated, sedentary, and/or osteoporotic patients, the risks of surgery may outweigh the benefits. Surgical timing depends on associated soft tissue injury mechanism, including level of energy, neurovascular status, and open fracture. External fixation is usually temporizing.

The key point is that surgery is generally indicated based on fracture classification. The Schatzker classification of tibial plateau fractures is illustrated in Figure 3-1. I recommend ARIF for all type III fractures, and ARIF should be considered for types I, II, and IV fractures. Arthroscopy-assisted surgery for Schatzker type V and VI fractures (skin incision and plating, with arthroscopy but no arthrotomy), can also be considered. Chen and associates[3] have reported 85.1% and 90% satisfactory results for types V and VI fractures, respectively (Table 3-1).

The Meyers and McKeever classification of tibial intercondylar eminence fractures is illustrated in Figure 3-2. Surgery is indicated for type I fractures if they are associated with meniscus tears or other concomitant pathology that requires arthroscopy. Otherwise, these may be immobilized at or near full extension. Aspiration of hemarthrosis may result in substantial pain relief. There is sufficient evidence that surgery should be strongly considered for type II bird's beak pattern fractures because of the high association of anterior horn of the medial (or occasionally the lateral) meniscus lodged within the fracture site.[2,4-7] Closed reduction may be attempted for large type IIIB fractures because associated condylar contact may allow bony reduction after aspiration and hyperextension. For displaced type III fractures, ARIF is the state of the art procedure.[2]

An impressively large series by Chan and coworkers[3] is summarized in Table 3-1. The key point is that fracture types I, II, III, and IV had 100% satisfactory results. Fracture type V had 87.5% satisfactory results and Schatzker type VI had 90% satisfactory results.

Hunter and Willis[8] have described the outcome of suture or screw fixation of Myers and McKeever types II and III tibial intercondylar eminence fractures. At 32.6-month follow-up, the mean Tegner score was 6.35 and mean Lysholm score was 94.2. The best outcomes were seen in younger patients. No significant differences were seen in outcome with regard to type of fixation.

Conservative Management

As noted,[1] not all fractures of the tibial plateau require surgery. Fractures that are stable and minimally displaced may be amenable to cast immobilization, or bracing may allow early motion (but with delayed weight bearing). Other indications for nonoperative treatment may include injuries to the peripheral (submeniscal) rim of the plateau, a unique fracture pattern, and fractures in older adult, low-demand, or osteoporotic patients.

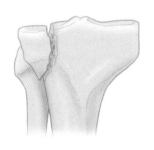

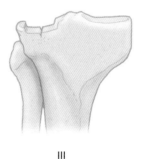

I

II

III

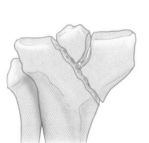

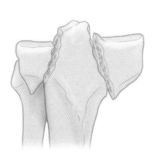

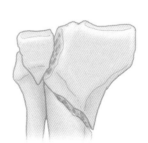

IV

V

VI

FIGURE 3-1 Schatzker classification of tibial plateau fractures. *(Adapted from Lubowitz J, Elson W, Guttmann D. Part I: arthroscopic management of tibial plateau fractures. Arthroscopy. 2004;20:1063-1070.)*

TABLE 3-1   Results of Arthroscopic Reduction and Internal Fixation of Schatzker Types V and VI Tibial Plateau Fractures*

Fracture Type	No. of Patients	Mean Clinical Score (Range)	Excellent	Good	Fair	Poor	Satisfactory Results (%)
I	1	29	1 (100%)	0	0	0	100
II	21	28.7 (26-30)	21 (100%)	0	0	0	100
III	4	28 (26-30)	4 (100%)	0	0	0	100
IV	10	25.3 (19-30)	9 (90%)	1 (10%)	0	0	100
V	8	27-6 (23-30)	6 (75%)	1 (12.5%)	1 (12.5%)	0	87.5
VI	10	26.8 (26-30)	3 (30%)	6 (60%)	0	1 (10%)	90
Total injuries	54	28.4	44 (81%)	8 (15%)	1 (2%)	1 (2%)	96% (52/54)

*Clinical assessment in 54 patients with 2- to 10-year follow-up results.
From Chan Y, Chiu, C, Lo Y, et al. Arthroscopy-assisted surgery for tibial plateau fractures: 2- to 10-year follow-up results. Arthroscopy. 2008;24:760-768.

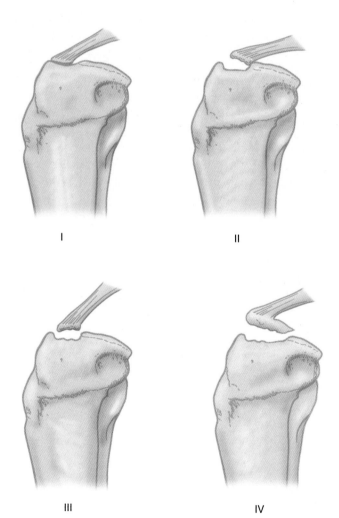

FIGURE 3-2 Meyers and McKeever classification of tibial plateau fractures. *(Adapted from Lubowitz, J, Elson, W, Guttmann, D. Part II: arthroscopic treatment of tibial plateau fractures: intercondylar eminence avulsion fracture. Arthroscopy. 2005;21:86-92).*

Meyers and McKeever type I tibial intercondylar eminence fractures may be immobilized near full extension. Aspiration may relieve pain in patient with intense hemarthrosis.

Arthroscopic Technique

My recommended ARIF technique was inspired by Caspari and colleagues,[9] Jennings,[10] and Buchko and Johnson.[11] Operative treatment must be specifically determined for each fracture type.

A circumferential leg holder and tourniquet are used, with the leg off the end of the table. The fluoroscope (C-arm) is turned upside down, so the flat (image acquiring) plate may be used as an operating table under the proximal tibia. Blunt double-hooked retractors may be used in a self-retaining mode with a spring-loaded suction cup designed to prevent fluid extravasation from accessory portals.

Arthroscopic lavage removes hemarthrosis. Dry arthroscopy decreases fluid extravasation and the risk of increased compartment pressure. A key point is to monitor compartment pressure, particularly in split fractures, in which extravasation occurs directly through the fracture line, to avoid fluid extravasation into the compartments. If an incision and plating is planned (ARIF without capsulotomy), these incisions should be made before arthroscopy in a location where the plate is planned; thus, fluid leak will occur via the incision rather than into the muscle compartments. To summarize, compartment pressure is monitored, measured if indicated, and thoughtful consideration given to fasciotomy if pressure is elevated.

Note that split fractures should be reduced first. For type I fractures, percutaneous, cannulated lag screws may be placed over a guide wire. In types II, III, and IV patterns, compression is first elevated using an angled tamp placed over a guide wire (Fig. 3-3). An ACL guide with a modified spoon-shaped tip to mimic the curve of the femoral condyle is used to place the guide pin in the center of the compressed fragments through a small incision in the proximal anteromedial tibial metaphysis. A coring reamer circumferentially penetrates the tibia cortex while removing as little bone as possible. A cannulated tamp is used to elevate the fracture site under arthroscopic visualization

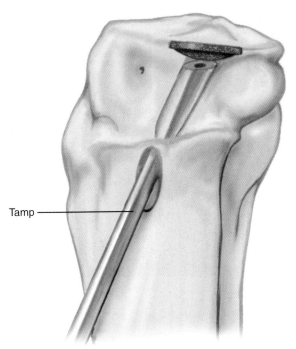

Tamp

FIGURE 3-3 Cannulated angled tamps reduce compression fracture elements via transtibial guide wires placed with an ACL guide and a modified, spoon-shaped marking hook. *(Adapted from Lubowitz J, Elson W, Guttmann D. Part I: arthroscopic management of tibial plateau fractures. Arthroscopy. 2004;20:1063-1070.)*

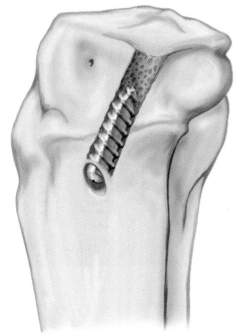

FIGURE 3-5 A cannulated, bioabsorbable interference screw reduces and then buttresses the tibial plateau compression fracture via the metaphyseal window. *(From Lubowitz J, Vance K, Ayala M, et al. Interference screw technique for arthroscopic reduction and internal fixation of compression fractures of the tibial plateau. Arthroscopy. 2006;22:1359e1-1359e3.)*

(Fig. 3-4). The underlying metaphyseal bone and cortical disk serve as autograft. A calcium- or hydroxyapatite-impregnated bioabsorbable cannulated interference screw of large diameter is then advanced through the cortical window to elevate the fracture further under direct arthroscopic visualization (Fig. 3-5). The screw first provides elevation. Next, the screw provides rigid internal fixation of the compressed fracture.[12] More-over, for type III patterns, the screw obviates the need for percutaneous placement of subchondral, metal, cannulated buttress screws, which radically reduces morbidity. For type III fractures, using this new technique, fluoroscopy is not required. Locked buttress plating (ARIF with arthroscopy without arthrotomy) has been reported for types V and VI fractures (Figs. 3-6 to 3-8).

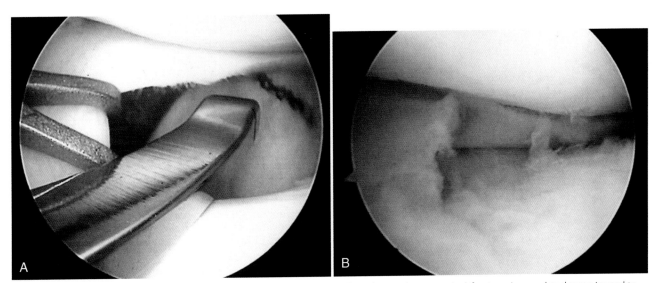

FIGURE 3-4 Prereduction (**A**) and postreduction (**B**) views of Shatzker type III (lateral central compression) fracture. A cannulated tamp is used to elevate the fracture site under arthroscopic visualization (arthroscopic anterolateral portal view, right knee, lateral compartment). *(From Lubowitz J, Vance K, Ayala M, et al. Interference screw technique for arthroscopic reduction and internal fixation of compression fractures of the tibial plateau. Arthroscopy. 2006;22:1359e1-1359e3.)*

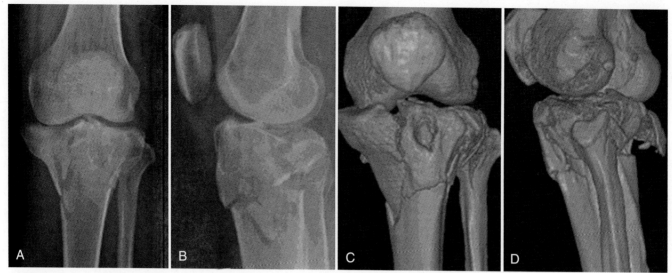

FIGURE 3-6 Schatzker type VI tibial plateau fracture in a 35-year-old man involved in a motorcycle accident. **A, B,** Plain radiographs showing bicondylar fractures with diaphyseal extension(anteroposterior and lateral views). **C,** Anterior view of three-dimensional CT reformation showing comminuted articular surface. **D,** Lateral view of three-dimensional CT scan showing severe depression of bicondylar articular surface. *(From Chan Y, Chiu, C, Lo Y, et al. Arthroscopy-assisted surgery for tibial plateau fractures: 2- to 10-year follow-up results. Arthroscopy. 2008;24:760-768.*

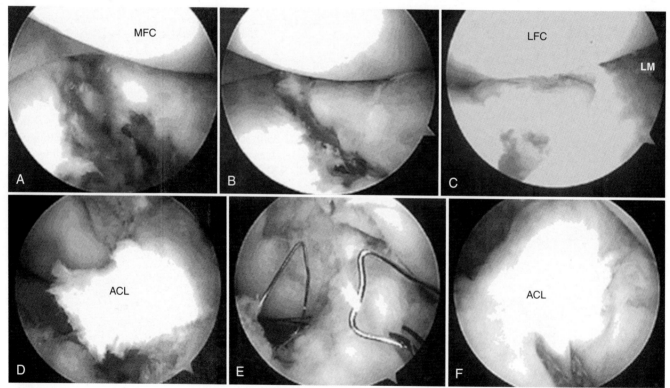

FIGURE 3-7 A, Preoperative arthroscopic view. A depressed medial tibial plateau is evident with a large bony gap. **B,** The depressed portion of the tibial articular cartilage is elevated by the technique of arthroscopy-assisted reduction with bilateral buttress plate fixation. **C,** The depressed portion of subchondral bone and the lateral tibial articular surface is elevated and reduced. **D,** Final management of ACL avulsion fracture with displacement. **E,** Arthroscopically assisted fixation by pullout suture. **F,** Four no. 5 Ethibond sutures (Ethicon, Somerville, NJ) were tied firmly at the proximal tibial site, and well reduction of ACL avulsion fracture could be visualized by arthroscopy. LFC, lateral femoral condyle; LM, lateral meniscus; MFC, medial femoral condyle. *(From Chan Y, Chiu, C, Lo Y, et al. Arthroscopy-assisted surgery for tibial plateau fractures: 2- to 10-year follow-up results. Arthroscopy. 2008;24:760-768.*

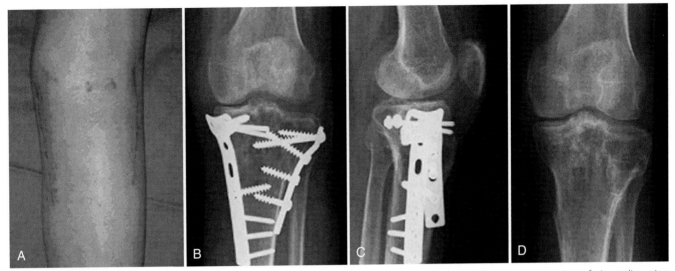

FIGURE 3-8 A, Only two longitudinal wounds appear on either side of the leg postoperatively. No knee arthrotomy or extensive soft tissue dissection was performed in the patient. **B, C,** Plain radiographs showed solid bone union with normal alignment (anteroposterior and lateral views). The knee joint was very stable. **D,** After more than 7 years' follow-up, no joint surface depression or post-traumatic osteoarthritis. Satisfaction with treatment (arthroscopy-assisted reduction with bilateral buttress plate fixation) was high. *(From Chan Y, Chiu, C, Lo Y, et al. Arthroscopy-assisted surgery for tibial plateau fractures: 2- to 10-year follow-up results.* Arthroscopy. *2008;24:760-768.*

Surgical Management: Tibial Intercondylar Eminence Avulsion Fractures

ARIF of ACL avulsions with screws was first described in 1993 by Lubowitz and Grauer,[13,14] but I now acknowledge disadvantages, including risks of comminution of the fracture fragment, posterior neurovascular injury, and the need for hardware removal. Because of these risks, ARIF using non-absorbable sutures passed through drill holes and tied over the tibial tubercle is now my preferred technique.

The patient is placed in a circumferential leg holder, with the knee off the end of the table. A tourniquet facilitates visualization, and the most recently published technique concludes that no fluoroscopy is needed for this procedure.[12] Calf compartments must be continually palpated to ensure that fluid extravasation does not result in compartment syndrome. Although intercondylar eminence avulsion fractures are contained injuries, they may be associated with capsular disruption.[2]

Standard anterolateral and anteromedial portals are used. A central transpatellar tendon vertical portal can be used as an accessory portal when indicated. Cannulas are recommended during suture passage to prevent soft tissue interposition.

Thorough lavage removes hemarthrosis. The fracture is reduced. Fibrous tissue or clot must be removed from the fracture bed. Entrapped meniscal tissue is retracted and dislodged.

A 90-degree suture lasso may be placed percutaneously (or via an accessory portal) through the fibers of the ACL in its midcoronal plane and as close to the bony fragment (distally) as possible. The wire loop within the lasso is secured with an arthroscopic grasper (Fig. 3-9) and pulled via a cannula through either of the portals and loaded with a no. 2 high-strength suture. The high-strength suture is pulled back through the ligament fibers and out through the skin and accessory portal.

An ACL guide is used to placed medial and lateral drill holes to pull the ends of the suture and fragment down into

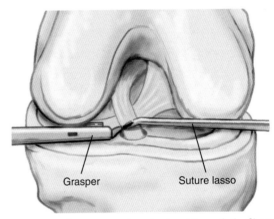

Grasper   Suture lasso

FIGURE 3-9 A 90-degree suture lasso is placed through the fibers of the ACL. The wire loop within the lasso is secured with an arthroscopic grasper. *(Adapted from Lubowitz, J, Elson, W, Guttmann, D. Part II: Arthroscopic treatment of tibial plateau fractures: intercondylar eminence avulsion fracture.* Arthroscopy. *2005;21:86-92).*

the fracture bed. A longitudinal incision is centered over the tibial tubercle. The medial pin enters the tibia just medial to the tubercle, and the lateral pin just lateral. The guide places two 3-mm cannulated retropins at the medial and lateral edges of the fracture bed in the midcoronal plane under direct arthroscopic visualization.

A Nitinol wire loop is passed up through the cannulated retro pins, medially and laterally, respectively. Routine suture passage brings the suture ends out through the medial and lateral drill holes. Distal traction reduces the fracture. The sutures are tied under tension while an assistant performs a reverse Lachman maneuver. With the use of supersutures, only one suture is usually required (Fig. 3-10).

Postoperative radiographs may suggest a few millimeters of superior displacement of the fracture fragment. This is usually

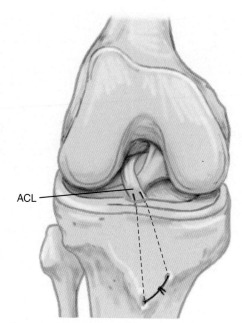

FIGURE 3-10 The fracture is reduced by pulling down on the suture ends, which are tied over the tibial tubercle. *(Adapted from Lubowitz, J, Elson, W, Guttmann, D. Part II: arthroscopic treatment of tibial plateau fractures: intercondylar eminence avulsion fracture. Arthroscopy. 2005;21:86-92).*

not seen on the arthroscopic view, and as long as the surgeon is certain that the meniscus is not entrapped, this should not be considered a failure of surgical treatment. Despite this radiographic finding, which is often subtle, excellent functional outcome and knee stability are the rule.[2]

PEARLS & PITFALLS

- High-energy injuries are associated with higher risks of compartment syndrome and arterial injury.
- On physical examination, pay careful attention to peripheral pulses, neurologic function status of the compartments of the injured extremity, and open wounds.
- Articular compression or fracture displacement is the indication for surgery; 3- or 4-mm displacement should be considered a relative indication for ARIF, particularly in active patients.
- I recommend ARIF for all Schatzker type III fractures, and ARIF should be considered for types I, II, and IV fractures. Reported 2- to 10-year results are satisfactory in 100% of cases.
- Arthroscopy-assisted surgery for Schatzker types V and VI fractures (skin incision and plating), but no arthrotomy, generally results in satisfactory 2- to 10-year results.
- Split fracture elements are reduced first, and then compressed fracture elements.
- During surgery, plan to prevent and monitor for iatrogenic leg compartment syndrome.
- ARIF of tibial intercondylar eminence avulsion fractures using nonabsorbable sutures passed through drill holes and tied over the tibial tubercle is my currently preferred technique.
- Radiographs of well-performed ARIF of tibial intercondylar eminence avulsion fractures may show a few millimeters of fracture displacement. Functional outcomes are excellent.
- Arthroscopic reduction with rigid internal fixation allows early motion for rehabilitation. Weight bearing is delayed.

POSTOPERATIVE MANAGEMENT

The key points of the rehabilitation protocol are that arthroscopic reduction with rigid internal fixation allows early motion and weight bearing is delayed.

For ARIF of tibial plateau fractures, continuous passive motion is recommended. Early range of motion is encouraged, with the goal of 0 to 90 degrees at 2 weeks and full range of motion at 6 weeks. Weight bearing is not permitted for 3 months. Partial weight bearing is recommended during the fourth month, especially in the case of compressed fractures. Hinged bracing for 6 weeks is recommended for patients with associated collateral ligament injuries.[1]

For intercondylar eminence avulsion fractures, the patient can be discharged on the day of surgery. Crutches are optional and recommended at first, and patients are permitted to bear full weight with the knee locked in a brace in full extension. The brace is unlocked or removed for CPM. Formal physical therapy is recommended to achieve and monitor the goal of 90 degrees of knee flexion at 2 weeks and full range of motion by 6 weeks. Isometric quadriceps and hamstring and abductor and adductor strengthening with the knee locked in the brace are permitted during the first 6 weeks. After 6 weeks, the brace is discontinued. Resisted flexion is permitted through full range of motion, and resisted extension is permitted through a range of 30 to 90 degrees. Terminal resisted extension is not performed until 3 months.[2]

CONCLUSIONS

As noted,[1,2] arthroscopy is a valuable tool for the assessment of tibial plateau fractures and is the treatment of choice for associated intra-articular pathology. ARIF of selected tibial plateau fractures allows anatomic reduction and rigid internal fixation with less morbidity than with ORIF, and has the advantage of superior visualization of the entire joint. I recommend ARIF for type III fractures and consideration of ARIF for types I, II and IV. Some authors have applied ARIF to more complex (type V or VI) fracture patterns, with satisfactory outcomes.[3]

With regard to tibial intercondylar eminence avulsion, ARIF is recommended for all displaced type III fractures and should be considered for all cases of displaced type II fractures. Fractures without displacement after closed reduction require careful evaluation to rule out meniscal entrapment. Repair using nonabsorbable super suture fixation allows early range of motion and has the advantages of eliminating the risks of comminution of the fracture fragment, posterior neurovascular injury, and the need for hardware removal, as compared with ARIF using screws.

REFERENCES

1. Lubowitz, J, Elson, W, Guttmann, D. Part I: arthroscopic management of tibial plateau fractures. *Arthroscopy.* 2004;20:1063-1070.
2. Lubowitz, J, Elson, W, Guttmann, D. Part II: Arthroscopic treatment of tibial plateau fractures: intercondylar eminence avulsion fracture. *Arthroscopy.* 2005;21:86-92.
3. Chan Y, Chiu, C, Lo Y, et al. Arthroscopy-assisted surgery for tibial plateau fractures: 2- to 10-year follow-up results. *Arthroscopy.* 2008;24: 760-768.

4. Burnstein DB, Viola A, Fulkerson JP. Entrapment of the medial meniscus in a fracture of the tibial eminence. *Arthroscopy*. 1998;4:47-50.

5. McLennan JG. The role of arthroscopic surgery in the treatment of fractures of the intercondylar eminence of the tibia. *J Bone Joint Surg Br*. 1982;64:477-480.

6. Falstie-Jensen S, Sondergard-Petersen PE. Incarceration of the meniscus in fractures of the intercondylar eminence of the tibia in children. *Injury*. 1984;15:236-238.

7. Zaricznyj B. Avulsion fracture of the tibial eminence treated by open reduction and pinning. *J Bone Joint Surg Am*. 1997;59:1111-1114.

8. Hunter RE, Willis JA. Arthroscopic fixation of avulsion fractures of the tibial eminence: technique and outcome. *Arthroscopy*. 2004;20:113-121.

9. Caspari RB, Hutton PM, Whipple TL, Meyers JF. The role of arthroscopy in the management of tibial plateau fractures. *Arthroscopy*. 1985;1:76-82.

10. Jennings JE. Arthroscopic management of tibial plateau fractures. *Arthroscopy*. 1985;1:160-168.

11. Buchko GM, Johnson DH. Arthroscopically assisted operative management of tibial plateau fractures. *Clin Orthop Relat Res*. 1996;(332):29-36.

12. Lubowitz J, Vance K, Ayala M, et al. Interference screw technique for arthroscopic reduction and internal fixation of compression fractures of the tibial plateau. *Arthroscopy*. 2006;22:1359e1-1359e3.

13. Lubowitz J, Grauer, J. Arthroscopic treatment of anterior cruciate ligament avulsion. *Clin Orthop*. 1993;294:242-246.

14. Lubowitz J, Grauer J. *Arthroscopic Treatment of Anterior Cruciate Ligament Avulsion*. Chicago: Mosby-Year Book; 1994.

The Stiff Knee

Bart McKinney ● Roger Ostrander ● Lonnie Paulos

Arthrofibrosis of the knee is a serious problem that can be difficult to treat. The process begins when the traumatic stimulus of an injury and/or surgery causes the formation of extensive, internal scar tissue. This is followed by shrinkage and tightening of the knee's joint capsule. This fibrotic tissue leads to loss of joint motion and, in some cases, articular cartilage degeneration. The patient with a stiff knee will have altered gait mechanics, which can then affect the hip or contralateral knee. If a stiff knee is not appropriately treated, the loss of motion may become permanent, leading to significant disability.

The purpose of this chapter is to review the normal functional range of motion of the knee with relevant anatomy and discuss possible causes of arthrofibrosis and treatment options in an effort to help manage the complicated stiff knee patient effectively.

ANATOMY AND PATHOANATOMY

Anatomy

Normal Knee Range of Motion

The knee has been described as having 6 degrees of freedom—internal-external rotation, compression-distraction, medial-lateral translation, abduction-adduction, anterior-posterior translation, and flexion-extension. Normal extension is 0 degrees, but some individuals may have slight hyperextension of up to 5 degrees. Normal knee flexion is 140 degrees in men and 143 degrees in women. Knee flexion up to 165 degrees is seen in certain groups.[1] The functional range of motion for most activities of daily living is 10 to 120 degrees. Loss of knee flexion or extension can lead to significant disability and inability to perform simple every day activities. Studies looking at gait patterns have shown that 67 degrees of knee flexion is required in the swing phase of walking, 83 degrees to ascend stairs, 90 degrees to descend stairs, 93 degrees to rise from a standard chair, and 110 degrees to cycle upright.[2]

The knee joint is a complex articulation among the femur, tibia, and the patella. The knee consists of two menisci, two collateral ligaments, and two cruciate ligaments. There are multiple specific areas within the knee that have the potential to develop fibrosis leading to stiffness. The treatment of a stiff knee is based on these specific areas that are most often affected. It is important to understand the anatomy and pathoanatomy associated with each of these areas.

Potential Locations of Entrapment

Suprapatellar Pouch. The suprapatellar pouch, also referred to as the suprapatellar bursa, is the superior continuation of the knee joint. This area is posterior to the quadriceps tendon and anterior to the femur. It continues on either side of the patella as the medial and lateral gutters. This area is covered by a synovial membrane. The suprapatellar pouch should extend 3 to 4 cm above the patella. It is the most common area of arthrofibrosis. With extensive scarring of the suprapatellar pouch, knee flexion is typically lost (Fig. 4-1). Terminal extension is usually not affected as much.

Medial and Lateral Gutters. The suprapatellar pouch is continuous, with two spaces on either side of the patella. These are the medial and lateral gutters. Structures found contiguous to the medial and lateral gutters include the medial and lateral patellofemoral ligaments and thickened synovial folds, or plicas. Distally, the gutters are continuous with the medial and lateral compartments. Much like the suprapatellar pouch, scarring in the medial or lateral gutter will lead to flexion loss only. However, if a large medial plica is present, the knee could develop peripatellar contraction and fat pad impingement, leading to both flexion and extension loss.

Medial and Lateral Compartments. The medial and lateral compartments contain deep capsular ligaments and menisci. Loose

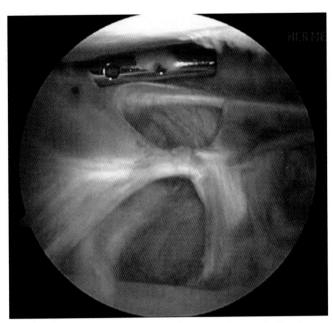

FIGURE 4-1 Arthroscopic view of suprapatellar pouch fibrosis.

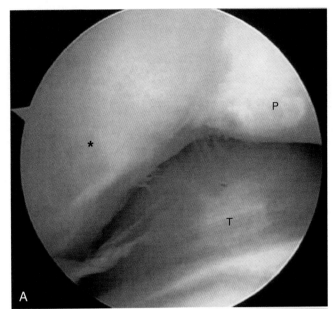

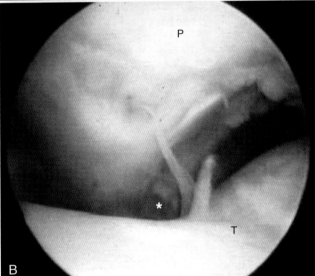

FIGURE 4-2A,B Arthroscopic views of infrapatellar entrapment. P, patella; *, scar tissue forming a pseudotendon between patella and tibia; T, trochlea.

bodies or bucket handle meniscal tears in these compartments may lead to restricted range of motion. It is important to evaluate these at the time of surgery and address any pathology found.

Anterior Interval.   This potential site of entrapment includes the fat pad, patellar tendon, and retropatellar recess. The anterior interval is bordered anteriorly by the fat pad and patellar tendon, posteriorly by the intracondylar notch and anterior border of the tibial plateau, superiorly by the patella, and inferiorly by the tibial tubercle. The retropatellar recess is a space between the insertion of the patellar tendon and anterior border of the tibia. Extracapsular structures in this area include the medial and lateral patellotibial ligaments. These structures can become contracted, leading to progressive arthrofibrosis of the knee. When fibrosis and scarring occur in the anterior interval, the patella may be drawn inferiorly, creating patella baja. However, patella baja, or patella infera, may not always occur with arthrofibrosis unless a dense band of scar forms between the inferior pole of the patella and anterior aspect of the tibial plateau (Fig. 4-2). This pseudopatellar tendon can severely hinder knee motion and lead to patella tendon resorption. Loss of flexion and extension may be present in those patients with anterior interval involvement (Fig. 4-3).

Intracondylar Notch.   The intracondylar notch is bordered anteriorly by the fat pad and patella, posteriorly by the posterior capsule, medially by the medial femoral condyle, laterally by the lateral femoral condyle, and inferiorly by the medial and lateral tibial eminence. The superior aspect of the intracondylar notch is also referred to as the roof of the notch. This area is devoid of articular cartilage. Contained within the intracondylar notch is the anterior cruciate ligament and posterior cruciate ligament. Two accessory ligaments may be seen, the ligament of Humphry and ligament of Wrisberg. Malpositioned ligament reconstruc-

tions, fibroproliferative tissue, or loose bodies in this area may contribute to decreased knee range of motion.

Posterior Compartments.   The posterior compartment is bordered anteriorly by the posterior horns of the medial and lateral menisci, the posterior cruciate ligament insertion, and the posterior aspect of the medial and lateral femoral condyles. The posterior border is the posterior capsule. Contracture of these posterior knee structures or posterior capsule from prior trauma, surgery, or prolonged immobilization may lead to arthrofibrosis. Loose bodies within this area may also lead to limited knee motion.

Pathoanatomy

To treat arthrofibrosis successfully, the surgeon must identify the cause. Failure to indentify the cause and correct it will most likely lead to recurrence of the stiffness.

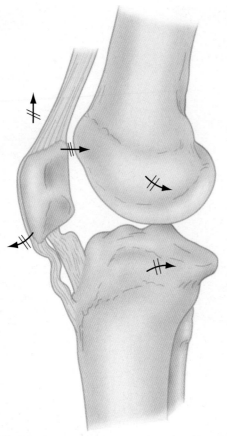

FIGURE 4-3 Limited patellar motion when pseudotendon is present *(arrows).*

Potential Causes of Knee Stiffness

Immobility. The effects of immobility, regardless of the cause, are always the same. Prolonged immobilization of the knee causes progressive contracture of the capsule and pericapsular structures. It also causes encroachment on the joint by fibrofatty connective tissue. The border between the cartilage and fibrous tissue may become indistinguishable. This can eventually lead to joint cavity obliteration. Pressure necrosis, erosion, and cysts occur where cartilage surfaces contact one another for prolonged periods. The subchondral plate is invaded by mesenchymal cells, destroying the deep cartilage layers.[3]

Ligament Reconstruction Technical Errors. Every knee that has had surgery or injury demonstrates decreased knee motion and patella tightness as it progresses through the normal healing process. However, certain factors can increase the chances of arthrofibrosis. Malposition of tunnels for ligament reconstruction can lead to a stiff postoperative knee. With anterior cruciate ligament (ACL) reconstruction, if the tibial tunnel is too anterior, the graft will impinge on the roof of the notch, thus limiting extension.[4] If the femoral tunnel is too anterior, the graft will become taught too early in flexion, limiting terminal flexion.[5] Overtensioning of the graft during ligament reconstruction can overconstrain the knee as well.

Rehabilitation. Arthrofibrosis can be caused by overly aggressive, painful postoperative rehabilitation. Forced painful motion

can lead to inflammation and scar tissue formation, creating a negative effect on the knee instead of the positive one that was intended.

Timing of Surgery. Acute ligament reconstruction of the knee has been shown to have a higher incidence of arthrofibrosis than delayed reconstruction. Shelbourne and colleagues found a statistical difference in postoperative range of motion in patients who had ACL reconstruction performed within 1 week of the injury compared with those who had reconstruction 3 weeks after the injury.[6] Harner and associates found the rate of arthrofibrosis to be 37% in the acutely reconstructed knee as compared with 5% of those who had delayed reconstruction.[7] Others have found no difference in arthrofibrosis rates and surgical timing. Bach and coworkers found no difference in the range of motion between acute and chronic reconstruction.[8] It is our opinion that the condition of the soft tissue dictates the timing of the surgery. If the patient has good active quadriceps control, near-normal preoperative range of motion, and no longer has a warm swollen knee, then surgical reconstruction may be undertaken safely, regardless of the time from injury.

Patient Factors. Some patients are more prone to scar formation. Patients with genetic disorders such as scleroderma are predisposed to arthrofibrosis. Other patients may not have a specific genetic disorder but have a higher likelihood of forming fibrotic tissue. These fibrotic healers are at an increased risk for arthrofibrosis, regardless of other potential causes. They tend to produce keloid scars. Careful attention at the time of the history and physical examination may lead the surgeon to recognize patients who may be at a higher risk for the development of a stiff knee. Some research has focused on finding specific genetic alleles responsible for arthrofibrosis. Skutek and colleagues looked at 17 patients who developed arthrofibrosis after ACL reconstruction. They found that patients with arthrofibrosis were less likely to have allelic group HLACw*07 and more likely to have allelic group HLACw*08 on human leukocyte antigen (HLA) loci.[9]

Infection. Infection is one of the leading causes of arthrofibrosis. It is important that the surgeon always remain suspicious of infection as a cause for slowed postoperative progression. The human body's natural defense against an infection is to enclose the infection with a wall of fibrotic tissue, which can limit the knee's range of motion.

Hemarthrosis. Significant bleeding into the knee joint can cause capsular distention. With a large enough effusion, the quadriceps can become inhibited. In the acute setting, a hemarthrosis may result in no unwanted sequelae. However, if a large hemarthrosis persists, the knee will remain in a slightly flexed posture for a prolonged period. This, combined with the quadriceps inhibition, may lead to arthrofibrosis. Aspiration of the hemarthrosis with a large-bore needle can increase patient comfort and hasten the return of full active extension.

Fat Pad Trauma. Albert Hoffa, a German surgeon, first described a condition characterized by traumatic and inflammatory changes occurring in the infrapatellar fat pad in young athletes. These changes may lead to pain, swelling, and restricted motion of the knee. Hypertrophy of the fad pad may cause it to become entrapped between the tibia and femur. Catching of this hypertrophied fat pad may occur when the flexed knee is extended suddenly. If this condition persists for a significant period, fibrosis may develop.

PATIENT EVALUATION

History and Physical Examination

A detailed history should be obtained from the patient. The examiner must inquire about any previous trauma, infections, fractures, or surgery to the knee. It is important to get details about past treatments, including the duration of immobilization and postoperative rehabilitation. The surgeon should try to determine the cause of the stiffness. In many cases, potential causes of the stiff knee can be identified based on the patient's history. The examiner also must determine whether there is any associated pain. If there is significant pain associated with the stiffness, then the location may provide a clue about the site of greatest entrapment. For example, a patient with an infrapatellar entrapment and stiffness will most often complain of anterior knee pain.

The physical examination should begin with a generalized inspection of the patient. Contralateral knee motion should be assessed. The examiner should evaluate the ipsilateral hip and ankle for any concurrent pathology. The patient may have an antalgic gait because of a painful knee that won't fully extend. The affected knee should be inspected thoroughly. It is important to note any previous incisions or scar. As noted earlier, some patients are fibrotic healers and may produce abundant scar or keloids. Muscle atrophy is common and should be noted if present.

Palpation of the knee should follow. The temperature of the knee should be determined and compared with the contralateral knee. The surgeon will need to evaluate the knee for any intraarticular effusion present. Warmth and swelling are important findings that will guide treatment options. If a significant effusion is present, consideration should be given to knee aspiration to rule out infection as a possible cause. Range of motion should be measured with a goniometer in a consistent fashion that can be replicated during subsequent physical examinations. The contralateral knee range of motion should also be measured. A standard knee ligamentous examination should be carried out. The location of any pain elicited should be documented. Joint line tenderness may be present if the patient has significant arthritis or a concurrent meniscus tear.

One of the most important structures to examine in the stiff knee patient is the patella. The patella is the centerpiece of knee motion and is almost always involved in the stiff knee. Medial and lateral patella glide should be assessed. Medial and lateral patellar tilt should be measured and compared withthe contralateral side. Decreased medial or lateral tilt compared with the contralateral side is suggestive of medial or lateral gutter involvement. Anterior patellar tilt should also be assessed (Fig. 4-4). If the patient has infrapatellar entrapment, he or she will usually lose the anterior patellar tilt. With moderate to severe infrapatellar entrapment, the patient will usually develop a shelf sign,

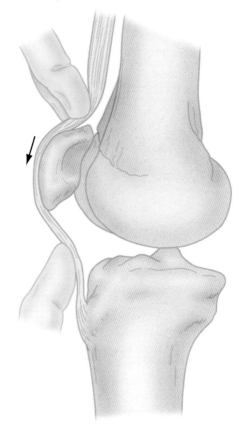

FIGURE 4-4 Anterior patellar tilt *(arrow)*.

which denotes loss of the retropatellar tendon bursa and adherence of the patellar tendon to the tibia (Fig. 4-5).

Diagnostic Imaging

A standard series of radiographs should be taken on initial evaluation of the stiff knee. Weight- bearing anteroposterior and 45-degree anteroposterior flexion views should be obtained to assess for any degenerative changes. Bilateral 30-degree lateral views should be obtained to evaluate for any degenerative changes as well as any patella baja. A Merchant or sunrise view

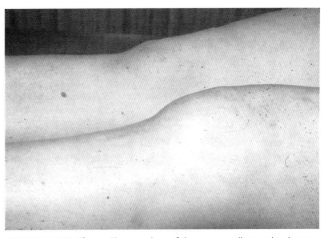

FIGURE 4-5 Shelf sign. Shown is loss of the retropatellar tendon bursa with adherence of the patellar tendon to the tibia.

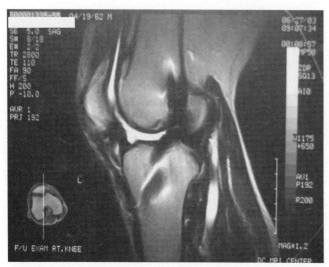

FIGURE 4-6 MRI scan of infrapatellar entrapment and pseudotendon formation.

Box 4-1 Indications, Contraindications, and Relative Contraindications for Treatment

INDICATIONS

1. Extension loss ≥5 degrees
2. Flexion <125 degrees
3. Failure to progress in a physical therapy program with a minimum duration of 3 mo
4. Suspected intra-articular cause of the arthrofibrosis

CONTRAINDICATIONS

1. Persistent knee inflammation with warmth or swelling
2. Any active quadriceps muscle lag
3. Noncomplaint patient or patient seeking secondary gain
4. Severe multiple compartment degenerative joint disease
5. Active infection
6. Complex regional pain syndrome

RELATIVE CONTRAINDICATIONS

1. Moderate to severe infrapatellar entrapment
2. Patella infera

---

of the knee should be obtained to evaluate patella tracking as well as any patellofemoral degenerative changes. Long leg alignment or scanograms should be obtained if any significant varus or valgus malalignment is suspected. Computed tomography and ultrasound have little use in the evaluation of the stiff knee, but magnetic resonance imaging (MRI) may be of some benefit. A MRI scan can evaluate the structures within the knee, including the location and integrity of any previously reconstructed ligament. It can also help quantify the degree of any cartilage loss or injury. Loose bodies within the intracondylar notch will be evident by MRI. An MRI scan will give a detailed evaluation of the fat pad, which may have contracted, calcified, or formed a pseudotendon (Fig. 4-6).

TREATMENT

The key to treating arthrofibrosis of the knee successfully is identifying the cause. Once the cause has been identified, a treatment plan can be created and carried out to correct it. If the cause is not corrected and only the stiffness is treated, the arthrofibrosis will undoubtedly recur.

Indications and Contraindications

It is important for the surgeon to understand the indications and contraindications for arthroscopic or open lysis of adhesions (Box 4-1). The most common mistake is to operate too soon on a stiff knee. Although short-term range of motion may improve, this second hit only worsens the arthrofibrosis in the long run. The knee must not be warm and swollen when proceeding with any treatment. It may take from 2 to 12 months before the knee has returned to a noninflamed state. Regardless of the cause, the quadriceps muscle must be contracting normally prior to proceeding with surgery. If the patient does not have adequate quadriceps strength to maintain extension after the surgery, the procedure will have a poor outcome.

Infrapatellar entrapment is an extremely difficult condition to treat arthroscopically. Although a mild degree of infrapatellar entrapment may respond to arthroscopic release, moderate to severe cases usually require an open release, with or without a retropatellar interposition patch. To correct patella infera, elevate the patellar tendon away from the anterior tibia, and restore the alpha angle, it is sometimes necessary to move the tubercle both superiorly and anteriorly. The DeLee-Paulos osteotomy is designed to accomplish this. A large shingle of anterior tibia (including the tubercle) is created. A 5-mm deep cut is made above the tubercle. A second 15-mm deep cut approximately 3 cm distal to the tubercle is also made. These two cuts are connected medially to laterally and the bone fragment is then moved superiorly, enough to correct the patella baja. As the bone fragment moves superiorly, it automatically proceeds anteriorly. It is fixated with one to two screws. The defect created by the osteotomy is then bone-grafted (Fig. 4-7).

Conservative Management

Prevention is the best treatment for arthrofibrosis. Range-of-motion (ROM) exercises should be initiated as soon as possible after surgery. Other postoperative measures that can be taken to prevent stiffness include immediate quadriceps exercises, patellar mobility exercises, and obtaining early extension. Once arthrofibrosis has occurred, conservative treatment is based on the degree of involvement. Mild to moderate motion loss is treated initially with more active and passive ROM exercises, patellar glides, anti-inflammatories, analgesics for pain control, and extension bracing at night. If moderate to severe motion loss is present, it is critical to stop any painful treatments. Painful aggressive therapy at this point will only worsen the problem. A tapered dose of oral steroids may also be used for those who do not have contraindications. Muscle stimulation may be used and can be helpful. The most important part of this waiting period, during which the knee is still swollen and warm, is to avoid aggressive physical therapy and forceful manipulation. Swimming and cycling are activities that may be started during this time, with low risk of worsening the vicious cycle of pain, inflammation, and stiffness.

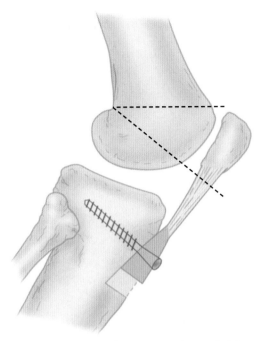

FIGURE 4-7 DeLee-Paulos osteotomy for patella infera.

Arthroscopic Technique

Before considering surgery, the patient must have minimal swelling, no warmth, improving pain, and good quadriceps function. Common findings at the time of surgery usually include degeneration of the articular cartilage, abundant fibrous tissue, soft tissue transformation, and patella infera.[10] The surgeon must be prepared to address these at the time of surgery if found.

Anesthesia

In the ideal situation, the patient is placed under general anesthesia with a regional nerve block and indwelling catheter. This allows for good pain control postoperatively, resulting in better patient compliance with immediate postoperative rehabilitation. An alternative strategy is to use epidural anesthesia with an epidural catheter for intraoperative and postoperative pain control.[11]

Equipment

Standard knee arthroscopy equipment is used. We have 30- and 70-degree arthroscopes available for adequate visualization, and 4.5- and 5.5-mm full-radius arthroscopic shavers are frequently used. An electrocautery hook is used for scar releases. Arthroscopic biters and graspers should be present in case any concurrent pathology is found at the time of arthroscopy.

Positioning

We position the patient supine on the operating room table in a slight Trendelenberg. A small bump is placed under the ipsilateral hip. A nonsterile tourniquet is placed on the operative leg as high as possible. A foot rest is applied to the end of the operating room table to allow for maintained flexion during the procedure. A lateral post is used. Ideally, the surgeon will have an assistant available to help with leg positioning during the procedure.

Capsular Distention

We use a similar technique as described by Millett and Steadman.[12] We distend the capsule initially with 60 mL of normal saline through a superolateral injection. Fluid should follow easily into the suprapatellar pouch. If resistance is felt, the needle is redirected until the knee is easily distended. An additional 60 mL of normal saline is then injected slowly to allow for some additional distention of the contracted capsule.

Portal Placement

The surgeon should be familiar and comfortable making multiple portals for the treatment of knee arthrofibrosis. We make a standard anterior lateral portal at the level of the inferior pole of the patella using a no. 11 blade scalpel. Once the camera is inserted and driven down into the medial compartment, we approximate the anteromedial portal using an 18-gauge spinal needle. The anteromedial portal should be medial to the patellar tendon and just superior to the anterior horn of the medial meniscus. Under direct visualization, we create the anteromedial portal using a no. 11 blade scalpel. A superolateral portal is created just superior and lateral to the superior pole of the patella. This portal should be at the inferior edge of the vastus lateralis. A superomedial portal may also be needed and is created just medial and superior to the superior pole of the patella. If posterior capsular release is required, a posteromedial portal is also created.

While looking in the posterior medial compartment, an 18-gauge spinal needle is inserted under direct visualization. The needle is inserted anterior to the medial head of the gastrocnemius to avoid the neurovascular structures. Once the portal site is approximated, a no. 11 blade scalpel is used to incise the skin. A hemostat may be needed to spread the subcutaneous tissue down to the level of the capsule. A blunt trocar is then inserted under direct visualization, creating the posteromedial portal. Occasionally, a posterolateral portal may be needed for complete release. We first insert a spinal needle under direct visualization anterior to the biceps femoris, anterior to the lateral head of the gastrocnemius, and posterior to the fibular collateral ligament. If the portal is too far posterior, the peroneal nerve is in danger. In a manner similar to that for the posteromedial portal, the skin is incised with a scalpel. A hemostat is used to dissect bluntly through the soft tissue down to the capsule. The capsule is then entered with a blunt-tipped trocar.

Locations of Entrapment

Suprapatellar Pouch.   It is important to examine the suprapatellar pouch for adhesions (see Fig. 4-1). Use electrocautery to lyse any adhesions or plica seen. If the suprapatellar pouch appears to be small, then scar tissue has likely encroached on the superior part of the pouch. It may be necessary to débride the superior part of the pouch with an arthroscopic shaver. The pouch should extend at least 3 cm proximal to the patella. If significant débridement using the arthroscopic shaver is required, we recommend cauterizing the tissue afterward to achieve hemostasis.

Medial and Lateral Gutters.   As with the suprapatellar pouch, the medial and lateral gutters should be inspected. Lyse any adhesions visualized in this area with electrocautery. Typically, the adhesions will form between the capsule and femoral condyle. If the medial or lateral patellofemoral ligament is contracted, release of these ligaments is usually required. If limited medial glide and lateral patellar tilt are present on physical examination, we usually proceed with a lateral retinacular release. Starting at the inferior aspect of the vastus lateralis, the lateral release is performed using an electrocautery hook. The release is carried down to the level of the anterior lateral portal site. Once the release is complete, the patella should be able to be tilted 45 to 70 degrees. Additionally, the patellotibial ligament may require release distal to the lateral portal. If limited lateral glide and limited medial tilt are present, a medial release may be performed as well.

Medial Compartment.   As with any knee arthroscopy, the surgeon should inspect the medial compartment and address any pathology found. In the severely contracted knee, significant chondromalacia may be present.

Infrapatellar Area.   Inspection of the fat pad should be performed. In severe arthrofibrosis, a dense wall of scar may be present, making it difficult to visualize the fat (see Fig. 4-2). The fat pad should never be fully resected. The fat pad should be released using electrocautery on the medial and lateral sides. It is also important to release scar and the fat pad from the anterior tibia. In a normal knee, a retropatellar recess or bursa is usually present. An anterior recess release should be performed by use of electrocautery. The wall of scar should be released just proximal and anterior to the anterior horns of the medial and lateral meniscus. The release should be carried out distally 1 cm below the articular surface of the tibial plateau. Occasionally, a distinct pseudopatellar tendon will form between the inferior pole of the patella and anterior tibia. Resection of this dense band of tissue may be necessary. Care should be taken to avoid overzealous resection in this area. If the tendon is exposed to bone, then recurrence is likely. If retropatellar tendon fibrosis is present, but not patella infera, the use of a barrier to prevent adhesions of the patellar tendon to the anterior tibia may be needed. A nonreactive barrier such as the Bard hernia patch is an excellent choice. It can be cut to the approximate size and sutured to the anterior tibia directly posterior to the patellar tendon. The polyethylene surface faces the tendon. The patch may be left in place and does not require removal (Fig. 4-8). Care should also be taken to avoid abrading or severely cauterizing the bone, because this will increase the chances of recurrence.

Intercondylar Notch.   The notch should be inspected for any signs of impingement. If a cyclops lesion is present, it should be resected. Any loose bodies should be removed. If prior ligament reconstruction has been performed, evaluation of the graft in full flexion and extension should be carried out. If the graft appears to impinge on the roof of the notch, a notchplasty should be performed. If the graft is malpositioned, resection or staged revision ligament reconstruction may be required to achieve improved range of motion. It is important that the surgeon discuss this possible situation with the patient preoperatively in case it is encountered during the surgery.

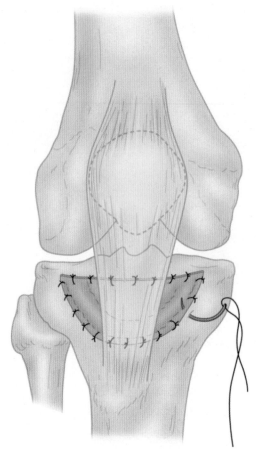

FIGURE 4-8 Polyethylene patch placement for severe patella infera and entrapment.

Lateral Compartment.   The lateral compartment should be inspected and any pathology found addressed at the time of arthroscopy.

Posteromedial and Posterolateral Compartments.   It is important to visualize the posterior compartments to look for loose bodies that may be impinging and limiting flexion. Posterior capsular release is rarely indicated unless the inciting injury or surgery involved the posterior capsular structures. If a posterior release is to be performed arthroscopically, we recommend releasing the posterior medial capsule only using an electrocautery hook through an accessory posteromedial portal. It is important to release the capsular tissue only. The surgeon must be extremely cautious during this part of the procedure. Directly posterior to the posterolateral capsular is the popliteal vein. We do not recommend the routine release of the posterolateral capsule arthroscopically because of the high risk associated with this procedure.

Manipulation

Manipulation of the knee may be carried out at the time of arthroscopy or as a stand-alone procedure. After the selected anesthetic is administered, the knee is examined and gently manipulated. We recommend hand placement closed to the knee joint to obtain short lever arms and decrease the risk of fracture. We apply a slow steady pressure as the knee is manipulated. In most cases, you will feel and hear some tearing as the scar gives way. Manipulation for flexion only is generally successful. Closed manipulation for extension loss is rarely indicated and should be preceded by an arthroscopic release.

Open Release

There are many cases in which arthroscopic release may not be enough to regain full motion. An open release may be required in revision surgery, severe contractures, moderate to severe infrapatellar entrapment, and patella infera.

We place the incision in the midline or slightly medially, depending on the previous surgical incision sites. A medial parapatellar arthrotomy is then used. Similar to arthroscopic débridement, a systematic approach should be used. The medial gutter and suprapatellar pouch are released from any adhesions. A lateral retinacular release is then performed. The intracondylar notch is evaluated and any pathology addressed. Osteophytes or cyclops lesions may be present. If the ACL has been reconstructed, position and isometry are evaluated. Débridement of the ACL is sometimes necessary in severe cases. Any heterotopic ossification or soft tissue calcifications encountered during this procedure are excised. The fat pad is then released from any adhesion. The fat pad must never be excised completely or recurrence is almost guaranteed. The retropatellar recess is then reestablished. If moderate to severe infrapatellar entrapment or bone to tendon contact in this area is present, we place an interposition polyethylene barrier in the retropatellar recess (see Fig. 4-7). This barrier will prevent recurrence of the adhesion between the anterior tibia and inferior patellar tendon. If significant patella infera is present (>1 cm), we perform a DeLee osteotomy, in which the tibial tubercle is moved anteriorly and superiorly. One or two screws are then placed to secure the tubercle back to the anterior tibia.

If persistent motion loss is still present, we proceed with an open posterior capsular release. A posterior medial incision is made. The superficial dissection is between the medial patellar retinaculum and sartorius. The infrapatellar branch of the saphenous may cross over this incision and needs to be protected. Dissection is then carried out posterior to the superficial MCL and anterior to the medial head of the gastrocnemius to reach the posterior medial capsule. The capsule is superior and deep to the semimembranosus. The posterior medial capsule is carefully released. If persistent extension deficit is still present, a posterior lateral capsular release can also be performed. However, the surgeon must be extremely cautious when releasing the capsule around neurovascular structures.

PEARLS & PITFALLS

PEARLS

1. Surgical treatment for knee stiffness should not be initiated until the acute inflammatory process has resolved, with absence of warmth and swelling.
2. The quadriceps muscle must be contracting normally prior to proceeding with surgery. If the patient does not have adequate quadriceps strength to maintain extension after the surgery, the procedure will have a poor outcome.
3. You must identify and correct the underlying cause of the stiffness to prevent recurrence.
4. The treatment of a stiff knee is based on which areas of the knee are most affected.
5. Following surgery to correct a stiff knee, postoperative rehabilitation must focus on restoring extension and quadriceps strength. Flexion exercises are initiated once these goals are achieved.
6. Prevention of motion loss is the best way to restore knee function after surgery

PITFALLS

1. The fat pad is often released during surgery but should never be completely excised.
2. Aggressive, painful postoperative rehabilitation should be avoided. Rehabilitation must be criteria-based, with low force, and be painless and patient-controlled.

POSTOPERATIVE REHABILITATION PROTOCOL

The patient is sent home with an indwelling pain catheter to control pain for 2 to 3 days. It is important to use adequate oral analgesic medication to help comply with postoperative protocols. The patient is started on an anti-inflammatory medication and a continuous passive motion machine (CPM) is used immediately after surgery. CPM settings vary based on the severity of the stiffness. The goal of the CPM is to maintain the motion that has been obtained surgically. The angle of the CPM is decreased if significant pain is produced during high flexion. If both the flexion and extension contractures have been addressed, we divide the postoperative regimen into two phases. In terms of motion, therapists are instructed to work on extension only. Straight leg raises, short quadriceps arcs (30 degrees), and patella mobility exercises are also initiated. Only after restoration of passive and active extension are flexion exercises started. It is not uncommon to require a second procedure to regain full flexion if both extension and flexion deficits are present initially. This should be discussed with the patient preoperatively.

The postoperative rehabilitation protocol is goal-based. Once the patient has reached a certain goal, she or he progresses to the next stage. At no point is any exercise or maneuver forced on the patient. In severe cases, we also start the patient on a postoperative course of steroids (e.g., methylprednisolone [Medrol Dosepak]) after all incisions are healed and chances of infection reduced. Hyperextension braces or casts are important adjuncts to the treatment of knee arthrofibrosis but must be used judiciously. Forced hyperextension while fat pad or scar tissue impingement is present may preclude an osteochondral lesion of the femur and increases patellofemoral arthrosis. These devices are best used early in the process, before any formation of anterior scar tissue and patella entrapment, or after surgical removal of all impinging tissue and structures.

CONCLUSIONS

Arthrofibrosis is a common but difficult condition to treat. The key to treating this problem successfully is to identify the cause. Knee ROM can be successfully restored with a directed approach.

Surgical treatment for knee stiffness should not be initiated until the acute inflammatory process has resolved, with absence of warmth and swelling. Arthroscopic release with or without manipulation is successful in treating many areas of fibrosis within the knee. However, open release may be required for more severe cases with infrapatellar entrapment. Aggressive, painful postoperative therapy must be avoided. Using the principles described in this chapter, the reader should have a better understanding of how to manage the complicated stiff knee patient.

REFERENCES

1. Freeman MA, Pinskerova V. The movement of the normal tibio-femoral joint. *J Biomech*. 2005;38:197-208.
2. Laubenthal KN, Smidt GL, Kettelkamp DB. A quantitative analysis of knee motion during activites of daily living. *Phys Ther*. 1972;52:34-43.
3. Enneking WF, Horowitz M. The intra-articular effects of immobilization on the human knee. *J Bone Joint Surg Am*. 1973;54A:973-985.
4. Yaru NC, Daniel DM, Penner D. The effect of tibial attachment site on graft impingement in an anterior cruciate ligament reconstruction. *Am J Sports Med*. 1992;20:217-220.
5. Markolf KL, Hame S, Hunter DM, et al. Effects of femoral tunnel placement on knee laxity and forces in an anterior cruciate ligament graft. *J Orthop Res*. 2002;20:1016-1024.
6. Shelbourne KD, Wilckens JH, Mollabashy A, DeCarlo M. Arthrofibrosis in acute anterior cruciate ligament reconstruction: the effect of timing of reconstruction and rehabilitation. *Am J Sports Med*. 1991;19:332-336.
7. Harner CD, Irrgang JJ, Paul J, et al. Loss of motion after anterior cruciate ligament reconstruction. *Am J Sports Med*. 1992;20:499-506.
8. Bach BR Jr, Jones GT, Sweet FA, Hager CA. Arthroscopy-assisted anterior cruciate ligament reconstruction using patellar tendon substitution: two-to four-year follow-up results. *Am J Sports Med*. 1994;22:758-767.
9. Skutek M, Elsner HA, Slateva K, et al. Screening for arthrofibrosis after anterior cruciate ligament reconstruction: analysis of association with human leukocyte antigen. *Arthroscopy*. 2004;20:469-473.
10. Cosgarea AJ, DeHaven KE, Lovelock JE. The surgical treatment of arthrofibrosis of the knee. *Am J Sports Med*. 1994;22:184-191.
11. Kim DH, Gill TJ, Millett PJ. Arthroscopic treatment of the arthrofibrotic knee *Arthroscopy*. 2004;20:187-194.
12. Millett PJ, Steadman JR. The role of capsular distention in the arthroscopic management of arthrofibrosis of the knee: A technical consideration. *Arthroscopy*. 2001;17:E31.

SUGGESTED READING

Magit D, Wolff A, Sutton K, Medvecky MJ. Arthrofibrosis of the knee. *J Am Acad Orthop Surg*. 2007;15:682-694.

Complications of Knee Arthroscopy

Jack M. Bert ● Timothy M. Bert

Complications of knee arthroscopy can be divided into three broad categories—clinical or medical patient complications, technical or iatrogenic complications, and material- or device-associated complications. Clinical or medical complications can occur in patients undergoing knee arthroscopy, which include deep venous thrombosis (DVT), pulmonary embolus (PE), wrong-site surgery, and infections. Technical or iatrogenic complications include nerve and vascular injury, chondral injury and idiopathic necrosis of the femoral condyle, overresection or incomplete removal of a torn meniscus, fluid extravasation as a result of pump failure, chronic postoperative synovitis, cold therapy skin injury, and anterior and posterior cruciate ligament reconstruction complications. Material- or device-associated complications include problems with the placement of screws or fixation devices and the use of bioabsorbable materials used to repair the meniscus, including failure to heal, breakage or migration of the implanted material, and persistence of pain subsequent to the placement of the device.

CLINICAL OR MEDICAL COMPLICATIONS

Deep Venous Thrombosis and Pulmonary Embolus

Deep venous thrombosis (DVT) has been reported to be as high as 17.9% after arthroscopy of the knee. Some authors have stated that without proper screening, fatal pulmonary embolus (PE) may be as high as 1.3% of cases.[1] At an advanced arthroscopic knee course in August 2006, the audience was surveyed; 4 out of 40 knee arthroscopic surgeons had experienced a fatal PE in their practice, with an incidence in this small group of 10%.[2] Although arthroscopy of the knee is considered to be a "benign" procedure, one study noted at least one risk factor for DVT in 37% of patients undergoing routine knee arthroscopy.[3] In 2004, Geerts and colleagues[4] reported on multiple risk factors contributing to DVT and PE, including obesity, history of prior DVT, cancer, use of oral contraceptives, and increased age. Anderson and Spencer[5] catego-

rized the top 10 factors causing DVT and ranked them in terms of risk. Age older than 40 years was the most significant causative factor followed by obesity, prior history of DVT, cancer, bed rest longer than 5 days, major surgery, congestive heart failure, varicose veins, hip or lower extremity fracture, and estrogen treatment. They further noted that one or more risk factors increased the incidence of development of subclinical DVT or PE to 96.3%.

Eynon and associates[6] were one of the first to suggest that all patients having routine knee arthroscopies should receive anticoagulant prophylaxis. One study has reported the incidence of DVT and/or PE when comparing a control group and a second group treated with low-molecular-weight heparin (LMWH) without any known risk factors to be as high as five times greater when diagnosed by ultrasound on days 7 and 10 postoperatively.[7] Another study noted a 10 times greater incidence of DVT and/or PE after preoperative and postoperative treatment with LMWH when diagnosed with ultrasound at 12 and 31 days postoperatively.[8] It is estimated that between 20% to 30% of calf thrombi propagate proximally to the popliteal and femoral veins, which have an increased chance of resulting in PE. Some have argued that pharmacologic DVT prophylaxis should be routinely prescribed to patients undergoing knee arthroscopy for that reason.[1,6] However, there are no agreed on recommendations in the literature about prophylaxis for arthroscopy of the knee, with or without prior history of DVT or PE.[1] We recommend that all those undergoing knee arthroscopy should be given acetylsalicylic acid (ASA) preoperatively and postoperatively for 4 weeks and that those with acquired, genetic, or hemostatic risk factors be placed on preoperative and postoperative warfarin (Coumadin) or LMWH for 3 to 4 weeks to reduce the possibility of PE or DVT.

Wrong-Site Surgery

Wrong-site surgery (WSS) accounts for approximately 2% of all orthopedic claims. However, 84% result in a mean court award to the plaintiff of $48,087. Most of these were knee arthroscopies.

The Physician Insurer's of North America recorded 331 WSS claims from 1985 to 1995, and 225 were against orthopedic surgeons.[9] The incidence of WSS reported to the American Academy of Orthopaedic Surgeons (AAOS) between January 1995 and December 2003 were 17% wrong knee, 12% wrong person, and 10% wrong procedure. Interestingly, hospital-based ambulatory surgery centers had the highest incidence of errors, 53%. The three most important factors to prevent wrong-site surgery errors were preoperative patient identification, surgical site indelible marking, and the physician's signature on the surgical site. When all three of these were done, there was a 0% failure rate. However, when only two of these three were done, there was a 12% incidence of failure.[10] Additional analysis of the complications that occurred estimated that an orthopedic surgeon has a 25% chance of performing wrong-site surgery during his or her career and that WSS tends to increase with increasing age and increased caseloads.[9,11]

In a survey presented at the AAOS in 2005, 1575 Arthroscopy Association of North America members reported an incidence of one WSS for every 26,581 arthroscopic procedures that were performed. The average age of the respondents was 48.2 years, with a practice mean of 15.8 years; 8.5% of respondents had performed wrong-site arthroscopy at least once during their careers. In this survey report, the risk of WSS increases with surgeon age, increasing years of practice, and increased surgical volume.[12] In Minnesota, in 2004, there were 22 adverse events reported—13 patients had the wrong body part operated on, in four cases the wrong patient was operated on, and in five cases the wrong procedure was performed. In 2005, in Minnesota, there were 26 adverse events—16 patients had the wrong body part operated on, in two cases the wrong patient was operated on, and in eight cases the wrong procedure was performed.[13]

Several requirements to reduce the risk of WSS significantly must be implemented in the hospital or ambulatory surgery center setting. Initially, the admitting nurse must identify the patient's correct name preoperatively by verbally asking the patient and correlating this with the wristband. The surgeon should also check the patient's name, either by directly asking the patient for his or her name and looking at the wristband. Second, the surgeon and patient should sign the site with an indelible marker within the operative site not covered by a drape. The patient should put "yes" on the operative knee and the surgeon should sign her or his initials directly over the operative site. Third, and finally, the circulating nurse must read the permit out loud and everyone in the operating room should acknowledge that this has been read, with the patient, procedure, and surgical site stated clearly. If these recommendations are followed 100% of the time, the incidence of wrong site surgery should be 0%.

Infection

The incidence of infection after knee arthroscopy has been reported to be from 0.04% to 0.42%.[14-16] Risk factors that have been reported to contribute to knee arthroscopy infections include intra-articular steroids given intraoperatively, increased surgical time, prior surgical procedures, chondroplasty, and soft tissue débridement.[17] The diagnosis of infection can be difficult to make immediately postoperatively. Persistent pain and swell-

ing after arthroscopy should have joint aspiration and culture despite the absence of fever, erythema, leukocytosis, or benign-appearing joint fluid. This diagnosis needs to be made immediately, if possible, and then treated with knee arthroscopy, lavage, and 2 to 6 weeks of intravenous antibiotics. Antibiotic prophylaxis in knee arthroscopy has been discussed and debated by several authors. Based on objective published literature, there is no statistical improvement in infection rates with preoperative IV antibiotics in routine arthroscopic surgery of the shoulder and knee.[18] However, in today's legal climate, others have argued that prophylactic antibiotics may be considered the standard of care in the local community and should be given regardless.[19] Suggestions to avoid infections include operating efficiently and using antibiotic prophylaxis on immunocompromised patients. Furthermore, avoid the use of intra-articular steroids immediately prior, during, or after surgery. Finally, treat a swollen extremely painful knee postoperatively with immediate aspiration, cultures, and then aggressive arthroscopic débridement if the culture is positive, followed by IV antibiotics.

TECHNICAL OR IATROGENIC COMPLICATIONS

Nerve and Vascular Injury

Early reported complications of meniscal repair were common; these included saphenous neuropathy medially and peroneal neuropathy laterally secondary to injury and for nerve entrapment. Other complications associated with open meniscal repair, including both outside-in and inside-out techniques, were arthrofibrosis, severe postoperative effusion, and superficial and deep infection. Combined complication rates were reported as high as 18%.[20] Nerve and vascular injury have also been reported secondary to lateral meniscectomy and posterior cruciate and anterior cruciate ligament reconstruction. Despite the use of guide pins for the placement of the tibial guide pin (Fig. 5-1) during both anterior

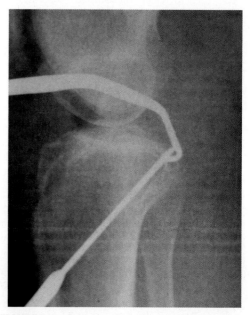

FIGURE 5-1 ACL guide with guide wire stop posteriorly.

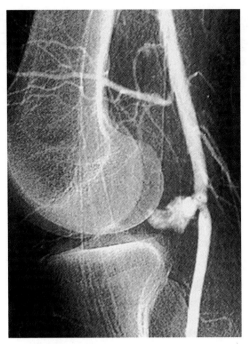

FIGURE 5-2 Perforation of popliteal artery.

and posterior cruciate ligament reconstruction, popliteal artery injury (Fig. 5-2) continues to be of concern.[21]

Chondral Injury

Iatrogenic chondral injury is common during routine meniscectomy, especially in a tight medial compartment . In our experience, the presence of articular scuffing will result in significant degenerative changes within a few years and sometimes even in a few months. Note the significant chondral injury at 1 year postoperatively in a 45-year-old patient after a routine meniscectomy (Fig. 5-3). After 4 years, significant changes can occur from a routine meniscectomy (Fig. 5-4). Articular cartilage is about 2000 μm

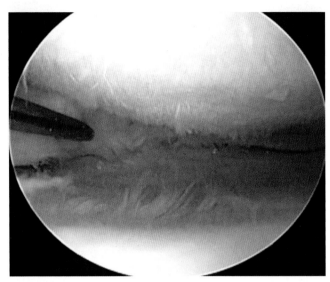

FIGURE 5-4 Result of chondral injury 4 years postmeniscectomy.

thick. A motorized shaver will shave up to 253 ± 78 μm and a radiofrequency (RF) thermal device will destroy up to 200 μm of articular cartilage. Some authors have argued that use of a RF device is more conservative than using a shaver.[22] In a series of 256 patients who had partial medial meniscectomies at a mean age of 47 years, with an average follow-up of 18.5 years, 63% had undergone grade I or II surface changes,[23] yet 83% had good to excellent clinical results. In this series, age, gender, and meniscal tear type did not influence functional results.[24] Factors such as the larger size of meniscal resection and female gender resulted in the most consistent associations with more x-ray evidence of osteoarthritis (OA) across multiple studies.[25]

Chondral injury is also dependent on the type of tear that occurs. Complex and horizontal cleavage tears are highly associated with an increased incidence and severity of cartilage degeneration compared with other types of meniscal tears.[26] In one study, 45 lateral meniscal tears were associated with another articular surface procedure within 13 years postmeniscectomy secondary to the development of OA.[27,28] Suggestions to avoid chondral injury during meniscectomy include removing as little meniscal tissue as possible, but still leaving a stable meniscal remnant. Also, avoid damage to the articular surface with the meniscal resector tools.[29] Furthermore, consider doing a partial intra-articular release of a portion of the medial collateral ligament (MCL) when the knee is too tight in the medial compartment before proceeding with meniscal resection, either using a pie crust technique with a spinal needle (Fig. 5-5) or cutting through the anterior portion of the MCL several millimeters from the meniscal rim with a cutting cautery (Fig. 5-6). Inadequate meniscal resection during meniscectomy with a retained superior or inferior horizontal cleavage flap has been implicated in causing long-term chondral damage (Fig. 5-7). Finally, not recognizing malalignment of the extremity will result in increasing failure rates subsequent to meniscectomy, with progressive OA of the meniscectomized compartment.[30]

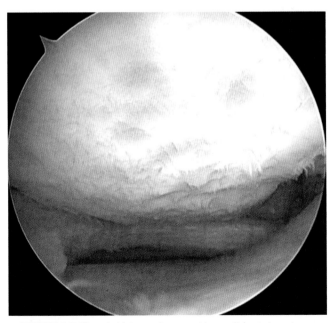

FIGURE 5-3 Chondral injury subsequent to medial meniscectomy.

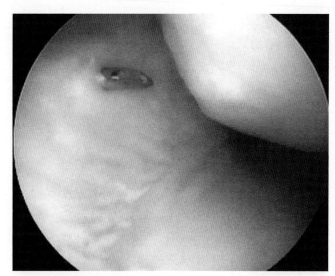

FIGURE 5-5 Pie crust technique for release of MCL.

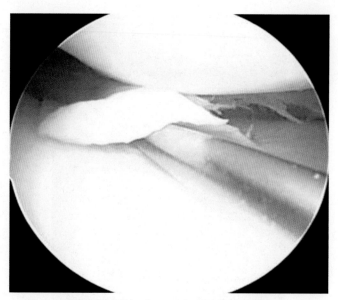

FIGURE 5-7 Inadequate meniscal resection.

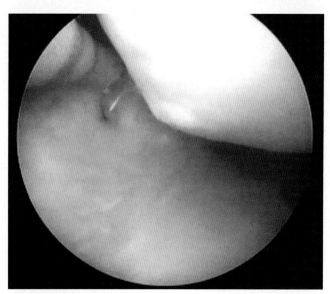

FIGURE 5-6 Electrocautery technique for partial release of anterior portion of MCL.

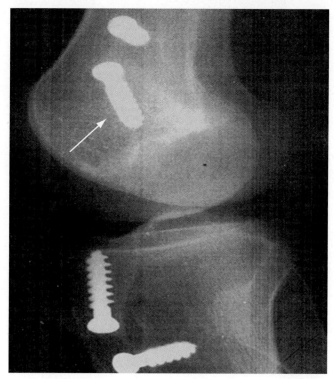

FIGURE 5-8 Anterior placement of femoral screw (*arrow*).

Anterior Cruciate Ligament Surgery Complications

Anterior cruciate ligament (ACL) reconstruction complications are not uncommon with single- or double-bundled techniques. Anterior placement of the fixation device in the intercondylar notch (Fig. 5-8) or posterior placement of the fixation device in the tibia (Fig. 5-9) are not uncommon. Cyclops lesions (Fig. 5-10) are also common as well. There appears to be no advantage of supplemental aperture fixation with screws or bone cores to reduce tunnel widening. It has been argued that supplemental aperture fixation is associated with increased tunnel widening.[31] Also, it has been suggested that leaving the stump of the ACL intact at the time of ACL surgery will reduce the incidence of cyclops lesions, because leaving the soft tissue in this area decreases the amount of debris that will surround the ACL in the tibia and reduce the amount of osteolysis that occurs next to the ACL.[32] Delayed laxity, recurrent tearing, and graft failure are not uncommon. Furthermore, poor preparation of the hamstring graft so that it loosens during stress can occur. The allograft must be thawed prior to preparation to avoid stretching prior to implantation. Other complications include premature tearing of the hamstring graft during harvesting (Fig. 5-11) and posterior wall blowout (Fig. 5-12). Patellar fracture after patellar tendon bone (PTB) harvesting is becoming less common because of increased usage of allograft material but chronic anterior knee pain secondary to

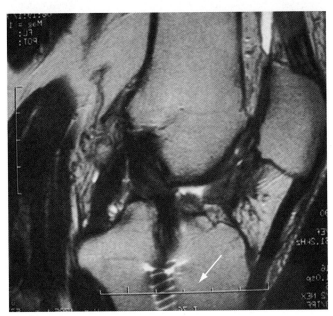

FIGURE 5-9 Posterior placement of tibial fixation device as noted on MRI scan (lateral view).

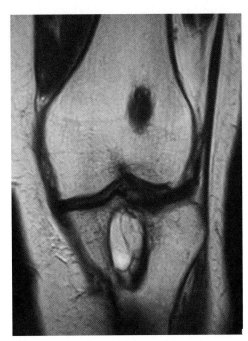

FIGURE 5-10 Cyclops lesion on AP MRI scan of tibia (AP view).

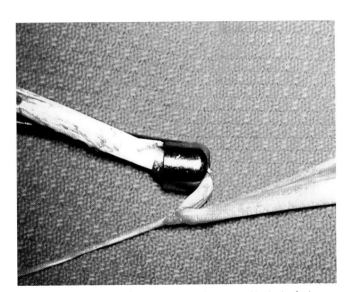

FIGURE 5-11 Premature hamstring resection caused by lack of release of adherent band. *(Courtesy of Dr. Don Johnson.)*

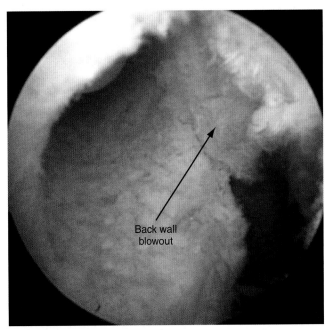

FIGURE 5-12 Posterior wall blowout. *(Courtesy of Dr. Don Johnson.)*

inadvertent infrapatellar nerve injury can occur subsequent to patellar tendon autograft harvesting. Double-bundle ACL reconstruction complications are primarily those of difficulty of placement of the double femoral tunnels. Also, fracture of the tunnel wall is not uncommon because it needs to be thin to place the tunnels in the anatomic position.[33]

MATERIAL- OR DEVICE-ASSOCIATED COMPLICATIONS

Biodegradable Implant Complications

Failed resorption of biodegradable implants has been reported with multiple designs. Meniscal arrows (Biofix; Bionx Implants, ConMed Linvatec, Pa) and Biostingers (ConMed Linvatec, Largo, Fla) have resulted in failure of repair with loosening and/or incomplete resorption at 5, 7, 9, and 13 months, resulting in persistent knee pain (Fig. 5-13). In all cases, the remnants of the biodegradable material were removed, synovectomies were performed, and all patients responded favorably. Several authors have described synovitis and chondral lesions up to 13 months postoperatively. On removal of implants and following synovectomy, patients ultimately did well. Chondral injury was present in all cases.[34-37] A case of the RapidLoc PLLA implant (DePuy Mitek, Raynham, Mass) loosening, resulting in chondral injury, was reported at 4 months postarthroscopy (Figs. 5-14 and 5-15). These patients most commonly present with mechanical symptoms at the time of device loosening.[38] The FAST-Fix meniscal repair system (Smith & Nephew, Andover, Mass) can cause a meniscal cyst at subsequent implantation prior to resorption of the device.[39] This was seen in one of the senior author's (JB) cases at 16 weeks postoperatively, with MRI confirming a meniscal cyst adjacent to a Fast-Fix meniscal repair device (Fig. 5-16).

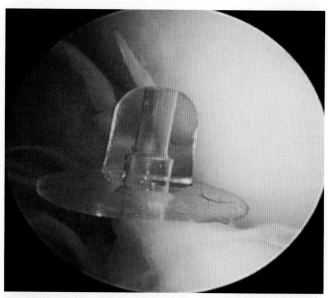

FIGURE 5-14 Dislodged RapidLoc fixation device (DePuy Mitek, Raynham, Mass). *(Courtesy of Dr. Alan Barber.)*

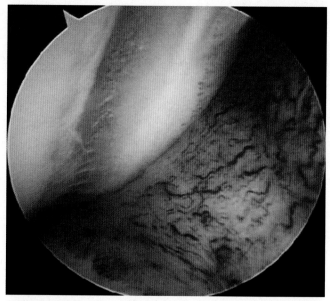

FIGURE 5-15 Femoral condylar injury secondary to RapidLoc device loosening. *(Courtesy of Dr. Alan Barber.)*

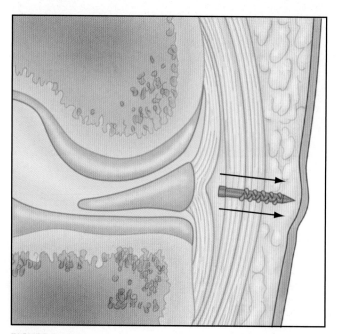

FIGURE 5-13 Posterior penetration of meniscal arrow, resulting in soft tissue irritation *(arrows)*. *(Courtesy of Dr. Alan Barber.)*

Miscellaneous Complications

Miscellaneous complications include fluid extravasation as a result of arthroscopy pump or tubing failure. If the pump continues to run without an egress cannula in the joint, and the joint becomes taut with fluid, the pump should be immediately shut down or extravasation of fluid into the thigh (Fig. 5-17) can occur.[40] Chronic synovitis after routine arthroscopy of the knee (Fig. 5-18) has been reported to be from 2% to 3%. Care must be taken not to overlook a postoperative infection. Treatment is prolonged oral anti-inflammatories or intra-articular steroid injections.[41]

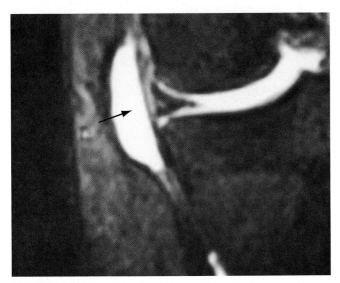

FIGURE 5-16 Meniscal cyst development 16 weeks after meniscal repair with Fast-Fix device (Smith & Nephew, Andover, Mass).

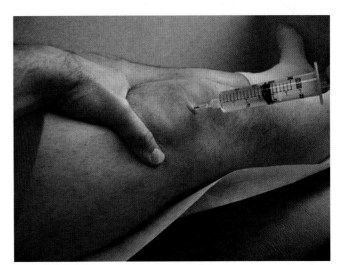

FIGURE 5-18 Severe synovitis postarthroscopic meniscectomy.

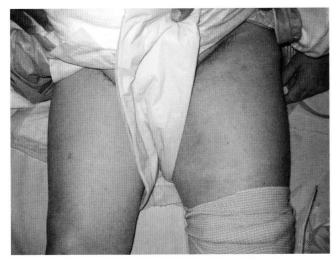

FIGURE 5-17 Fluid extravasation in left thigh caused by pump tubing failure.

- Always remember where the neurovascular anatomy is located laterally, posteriorly, and medially. Being meticulousness is crucial when performing ACL, PCL, posterolateral corner, and meniscal repairs to avoid neurovascular injury. If you even *think* that you have injured the popliteal artery, obtain a Doppler in the postoperative recovery area and a vascular surgeon's opinion immediately.
- It is better to avoid chondral injury by releasing a portion of the MCL in a tight knee than causing damage to the chondral surface. Patients who have a partial MCL release do well with conservative care when performing ACL or PCL surgery.
- Proper placement of the tunnels in the femur and tibia is critical to long-term results.

PITFALLS

- Ignoring predisposing risk factors for the development of DVT may lead to fatal PE survivorship of ACL surgery.
- Wrong-site, wrong- person, and/or wrong-procedure surgery is a very serious issue.
- Damage to the articular surface while performing a well-intentioned meniscectomy will cause more permanent articular surface damage than a poorly performed meniscectomy.

PEARLS*&*PITFALLS

PEARLS

- There are multiple common risk factors for DVT, including obesity and use of birth control pills. Seriously consider anticoagulation prophylaxis in patients with any risk factors, as well as the routine use of aspirin.
- Wrong-site, wrong-person, and/or wrong-procedure surgery occurred in every state in 2008. Make certain that you and the operating room personnel are compulsive about checking for the correct patient preoperatively, the correct procedure and the correct side. Do not make an incision without personally reading the consent out loud in the operating room.

CONCLUSIONS

Clinical, technical, and material-related complications are still present during or subsequent to routine arthroscopic knee surgery. Phlebitis and pulmonary emboli continue to be reported and are difficult to predict without a previous medical history. Prophylactic anticoagulation for routine arthroscopic procedures remains controversial. Technical complications are still common, including nerve and vascular injuries, despite improvements in instrumentation. Material complications have increased as a result of increased use of biodegradable implants. Suture technique complications are decreasing because of increased use of biodegradable devices, but still occur. It is important for the knee arthroscopist to be continuously aware of possible complications, even during the most routine arthroscopic knee procedures. Special vigilance is needed for the patient with a medical history that indicates a propensity to venous thromboembolism. There should be a continued awareness of knee anatomy when using percutaneous guide wires and performing suture repair techniques to avoid vascular and nerve complication.

REFERENCES

1. Bushnell B, Anz A, Bert J. Venous thromboembolism in lower extremity arthroscopy. *Arthroscopy.* 2008;24:604-611.
2. Hunter R, Sgaglione N, Carter T, Bert J. Treatment of articular cartilage injuries of the knee. Paper presented at: Orthopaedic Learning Center, Arthroscopy Association of North America Instructional Course; September 9-10, 2006; Rosemount, Ill.
3. Williams J, Hulstyn M, Fadale P, et al. Incidence of deep vein thrombosis after arthroscopic knee surgery: a prospective study. *Arthroscopy.* 1995;11:701-705.
4. Geerts WH, Pineo GF, Heit JA et al. Prevention of venous thromboembolism: the Seventh ACCP Conference on antithrombotic and thrombolytic therapy. *Chest.* 2004;126:338-400.
5. Anderson FA Jr, Spencer FA. Risk factors for venous thromboembolism. *Circulation.* 2003;107:9-16.
6. Eynon AM, James S, Leach P. Thromboembolic events after arthroscopic knee surgery. *Arthroscopy.* 2004;20:23-24.
7. Wirth T, Schneider B, Misselwitz F, et al. Prevention of venous thromboembolism after knee arthroscopy with low-molecular weight heparin (reviparin): results of a randomized controlled trial. *Arthroscopy.* 2001; 17:393-399.
8. Michot M, Conen D, Holtz D et al. Prevention of deep-vein thrombosis in ambulatory arthroscopic knee surgery: a randomized trial of prophylaxis with low-molecular weight heparin. *Arthroscopy.* 2002;18:257-63.
9. Canale T. Wrong-site surgery: a preventable complication. *Clin Orthop Relat Res.* 2005;433:26-29.
10. Wong D. AAOS patient safety: tools for implementation. Paper presented at: AAHKS 14th Annual Meeting; November 5-7, 2004; Denver.
11. Meinberg EG, Stern PJ. Incidence of wrong-site surgery among hand surgeons. *J Bone Joint Surg Am.* 2003;85:193-197.
12. Albright D, McDaniel S. The incidence of wrong-site surgery in knee arthroscopy. Paper presented at: Combined Meeting of Orthopaedic Associations; October 24-29, 2004; Sidney, Australia.
13. Minnesota Department of Health. Second Annual Public Report. Adverse Health Events in Minnesota; February 2006. Available at: http://www.health.state.mn.us/patientsafety/ae/aereport0206.pdf. Accessed December 14, 2009.
14. DeLee J. Complications of arthroscopy and arthroscopic surgery: results of a national survey. *Arthroscopy.* 1985;1:214-20.
15. Johnson L. Two per cent glutaraldehyde: a disinfectant in arthroscopy and arthroscopic surgery. *J Bone Joint Surg Am.* 1982;64:237-239.
16. D'Angelo G, Ogilvie-Harris D. Septic arthritis following arthroscopy, with cost/benefit analysis of antibiotic prophylaxis. *Arthroscopy.* 1988; 4:10-14.
17. Armstrong RW. Septic arthritis following arthroscopy: clinical syndromes and analysis of risk factors. *Arthroscopy.* 1992;8:213-23
18. Bert J, Giannini D, Nace L. Antibiotic prophylaxis for arthroscopy of the knee: is it necessary? *Arthroscopy.* 2007;23:4-6.
19. Lubowitz J, Kurzweil P. Editorial response to antibiotic prophylaxis for arthroscopy of the knee. *Arthroscopy.* 2007;23:1-3.
20. Small, NC. Complications in arthroscopic meniscal surgery. *Clin Sports Med.* 1990;9:609-617.
21. Austin K, Sherman O. Complications of arthroscopic meniscal repair. *Am J Sports Med.* 1993;21:864-869.
22. Voloshin I, DeHaven KE, Steadman JR. Second-look arthroscopic observations after radiofrequency treatment of partial thickness articular cartilage defects in human knees: report of four cases. *J Knee Surg.* 2005;18:116-122.
23. Outerbridge R. The etiology of chondromalacia patellae. *J Bone Joint Surg Br.* 1961;43:752-757.
24. Patel D, Bibbo C, Gupta M, Gehrmann R. Long-term results of arthroscopic partial medial meniscectomy in an otherwise normal knee. Paper presented at: American Academy of Orthopaedic Surgeons Annual Meeting; March 22-26, 2006; Chicago.
25. Meredith DS, Losina E, Mahomed NN, et al. Factors predicting functional and radiographic outcomes after arthroscopic partial meniscectomy: a review of the literature. *Arthroscopy.* 2005;21:116-122.
26. Christoforakis J, Pradhan R, Sanchez-Ballester J, et al. Is there an association between articular cartilage changes and degenerative meniscus tears? *Arthroscopy.* 2005;21:1366-1369.
27. Kuraishi J, Akizuki S, Takizawa T, et al. Arthroscopic lateral meniscectomy in knees with lateral compartment osteoarthritis: a case series study. *Arthroscopy.* 2006;22:878-883.
28. Alford JW, Cole BJ. Rapid progression of chondral disease in the lateral compartment of the knee following meniscectomy: a review of the literature and case reports. *Arthroscopy.* 2005;21:11-13.
29. Bert JM. Use of an electrocautery loop probe for arthroscopic meniscectomy: a five-year experience with results, indications, and complications. *Arthroscopy.* 1992;8:148-156.
30. Covall DJ, Wasilewski SA. Roentgenographic changes after arthroscopic meniscectomy: five-year follow-up in patients more than 45 years old. *Arthroscopy.* 1992;8:242-246.
31. Novak PJ, Wexler GM, Williams JS Jr. Comparison of screw post fixation and free bone block interference fixation for anterior cruciate ligament soft tissue grafts: biomechanical considerations. *Arthroscopy.* 1996;12:470-3.
32. Junkin L, Johnson D. ACL tibial remnant, to save or not. *Orthopedics.* 2008;31:154-159.
33. Howell S,Gittens M, Gottlieb J, et al. The relationship between the angle of the tibial tunnel in the coronal plane and loss of flexion and anterior laxity after anterior cruciate ligament reconstruction. *Am J Sports Med.* 2001;29:567-574.
34. Asik M, Sener N. Failure strength of repair devices versus meniscus suturing techniques. *Knee Surg Sports Traumatol Arthrosc.* 2002;10:25-29.
35. Ross G, Grabill J, McDevitt E. Chondral injury after meniscal repair with bioabsorbable arrows. *Arthroscopy.* 2000;16:754-756.
36. Seil R, Rupp S, Dienst M, et al. Chondral lesions after arthroscopic meniscus repair using meniscus arrows. *Arthroscopy.* 2000;16:E17.
37. Song EK, Lee KB, Yoon TR. Aseptic synovitis after meniscal repair using the biodegradable meniscus arrow. *Arthroscopy.* 2001;17:77-80.
38. Cohen SB, Anderson MW, Miller MD. Chondral injury after arthroscopic meniscal repair using bioabsorbable Mitek RapidLoc meniscal fixation. *Arthroscopy.* 2003;19:24-26.
39. Lombardi JA. Second-look arthroscopy with removal of bio- absorbable tacks. *Am J Orthop.* 2000;29:125-127.
40. McGuire D, Hendricks S. Incidence of frostbite in arthroscopic knee surgery postoperative cryotherapy rehabilitation. *Arthroscopy.* 2006;22: 1141e1-1141e6 *Arthroscopy.* 2002;10:25.
41. Rasmussen S, Lorentzen JS, Larsen AS, et al. Combined intra-articular glucocorticoid, bupivacaine and morphine reduces pain and convalescence after diagnostic knee arthroscopy. *Acta Orthop Scand.* 2002;73: 175-178.

Meniscal Procedures

Meniscal Resection

Emilio Lopez-Vidriero ● Donald H. Johnson

Joint line tenderness, locking, popping, or catching are the hallmark symptoms of the meniscal pathology. As the population becomes older and more active, the prevalence of degenerative meniscal tears increases. Meniscal injuries, mainly traumatic tears, represent one third of all athletic injuries. They usually involve a hyperflexion mechanism and prevent the patient from continuing his or her sports activity, and normal life. For these reasons, interest in the treatment of meniscal pathology has increased in the last century.

Knee joint stability is enhanced by the menisci in a similar manner to the glenoid or acetabular labrum. Basic and clinical research studies have shown that the main functions of the menisci are shock absorption and load transmission during knee joint movement and loading. In addition, the intact meniscus serves as a secondary restraint to anteroposterior knee motion. Finally, the menisci also have a role in proprioception and joint lubrication.

The menisci were once considered a vestigial tissue, without any function in the knee, and thus no treatment was required. Since then, in the last few decades, with the increasing information about the importance of the menisci, many treatment protocols have been described. The treatment options range from benign neglect to repair.

Meniscectomy is still the most frequent surgical procedure, almost 80% of operative cases. Arthroscopic meniscectomy achieves instant relief of pain caused by the mechanical symptoms resulting from the unstable fragments. The result is improvement of function of the knee joint.

The known advantages of arthroscopy over open surgery have now been widely recognized—day surgery without the need of hospital admission, less recovery time, less pain caused by the minimally invasive surgery, less global morbidity, more accurate resections because of better visualization, fewer complications, and less cost for the patient and/or the system. Thus, arthroscopic meniscectomy or repair has become the standard of care.

Arthroscopic surgery of the knee is a very common procedure. The American Academy of Orthopaedic Surgeons estimates that 636,000 are performed each year in the United States, and more than half are related to meniscal pathology.

This chapter reviews the main aspects of the basic science and clinical knowledge of the menisci. The classification of meniscal pathology related to the indications for its surgical treatment, emphasizing meniscectomy, are presented. We describe our surgical approach to the different configurations of meniscal tears, including special emphasis on the anterior cruciate ligament (ACL)–deficient knee with a meniscal tear. Rehabilitation programs and complications are also discussed. The literature on arthroscopic meniscectomy is reviewed to provide a scientific background to support the reader's clinical decisions.

ANATOMY

Menisci are discs of fibrocartilage interposed between the femoral condyles and tibial plateau. The articular surface of the medial condyle of the tibia is oval, with the longer axis being in the anteroposterior plane (Fig. 6-1). The central portion of the articular surface is not covered by meniscus and represents the articular area. The lateral meniscus plateau is almost circular and less concave. The menisci cover the peripheral two thirds of the tibia, and serve to deepen its articular surface and stabilize the joint. The upper borders of the menisci are concave and the undersurfaces are flat. Peripherally, the menisci thicken and are attached to the synovium and capsule. Centrally, the border is thin and exists as a free edge.

The medial meniscus is oval, 3.5cm in length, and wider posteriorly from its peripheral to its central aspects in the knee. Its anterior horn attaches to the tibial plateau just anterior to the attachment of the ACL. Some posterior fibers originating from the anterior horn cross the knee joint anteriorly, attaching to the lateral meniscus and forming the transverse ligament (see Fig. 6-1). Posteriorly, the meniscus is anchored to the intercondylar fossa of the tibia between the posterior cruciate ligament (PCL) and lateral meniscal attachment. Along its periphery, the medial meniscus is attached to the joint capsule and the deep medial collateral liga-

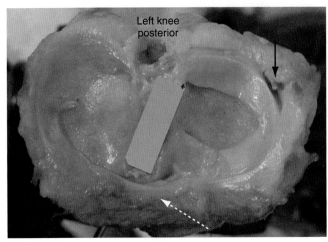

FIGURE 6-1 Axial view of the tibial plateau showing both menisci. Note that the cruciate ligament's insertion has been removed to allow better visualization *(grey rectangle).* Transverse ligament, *dashed arrow;* hiatus popliteus, *arrow.*

ment (MCL). The medial meniscus has less mobility than the lateral meniscus, and moves almost 10 mm from extension to flexion.

The lateral meniscus is circular, covering a larger portion of the articular surface than its medial counterpart. It is the same width anteriorly and posteriorly. The anterior horn attaches near the intercondylar spine posterior to the attachment of the ACL, with which it partially blends (Fig. 6-2). The posterior horn attaches just posteriorly to the intercondylar spines, anterior to the attachment of the medial meniscus. The lateral meniscus does not attach to the lateral collateral ligament but is attached loosely to synovium along much of its length. The anterior (ligament of Humphrey) and posterior (ligament of Wrisberg) meniscofemoral ligaments run from the posterior horn of the lateral meniscus to anterior and posterior, respectively, to the PCL attachment on the medial femoral condyle. Moreover, the tendon of the popliteus muscle, on its way to insert into the lateral condyle, crosses the joint through a hole on the lateral meniscus called the hiatus

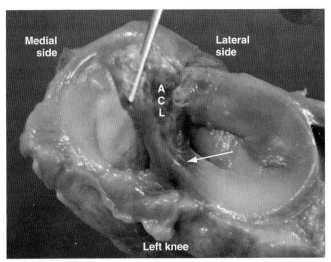

FIGURE 6-2 Oblique view of the tibia showing the insertion of the ACL. Note how the anterior horn of the lateral meniscus fibers blend with the ACL *(arrow).*

popliteus (see Fig. 6-1). This area along the popliteal hiatus is described as the avascular region.

Vascular Anatomy of the Meniscus

Menisci are relatively avascular, having a limited peripheral blood supply originating from the superior and inferior genicular arteries. Some of its branches form a premeniscal capillary plexus within the synovial tissue of the knee. This plexus forms a circumferential vascular pattern, with radial branches extending to the central portions of the menisci. The vessels penetrate readily into the peripheral 10% to 30% of the medial meniscus and into the peripheral 10% to 25% of the lateral meniscus. It is important to note that the vascular outer third of the meniscus is maintained throughout life, and does not significantly decrease with age.

Biomechanics and Meniscal Function

The menisci distribute stress over a large area of the articular cartilage. When the knee is loaded, the tensile strength of the meniscal matrix (hoop tension) counteracts extrusion of the meniscus. Therefore, the healthy meniscus responds to load mainly with compression.

The menisci have been shown to accept approximately 50% of the weight-bearing load with the knee in extension and 85% of the load with the knee at 90 degrees of flexion. The menisci increase the tibiofemoral contact area significantly, and thus reduce the stress on the articular cartilage.

A complete meniscectomy has been shown to decrease the contact area by approximately 50%.[1] A partial or total meniscectomy has been clinically demonstrated to result in degenerative changes in the knee.[2] This has been postulated to result from the increase in contact pressures in the knee. Even a minor meniscectomy, removing 15% to 34% of the meniscus, increases contact pressures in the knee by up to 350% and can result in degenerative changes. In meniscectomized knees, a significant reduction in contact area of about 55% is observed, and peak contact pressures increase an average of 260.4% compared with those of nonmeniscectomized knees.[3]

In addition, menisci also perform a role in absorbing forces or shocks during locomotion, where they dampen these forces by approximately 20%. The loss of this function may further contribute to the development of degenerative arthrosis of the knee.

Knee joint stability is enhanced by the menisci in a similar manner to the glenoid or acetabular labrum. The intact meniscus serves as a secondary restraint to anteroposterior knee motion.[4] The ACL-deficient knee can place abnormal stress on an intact medial meniscus, resulting in a meniscal tear. The increased anteroposterior motion created by meniscectomy in the ACL-deficient knee can lead to increased instability.

Thus, the function of the meniscus is to share in weight bearing, aid in lubrication, and help stabilize the compartment. The medial meniscus shares in 60% of the weight bearing of the medial compartment, compared with 70% of the lateral.

Regenerative Capacity of the Meniscus

King's 1936 experiment on a canine model represents the historical origin of the interest in meniscal healing.[5] Later experimentation demonstrated the necessity of a peripheral blood supply to support the inflammatory cascade required for meniscal healing.[6]

The reparative process of the meniscus involves a coalescence of blood from the peripheral vascular zone adjacent to the meniscal tear and formation of a fibrin clot. Undifferentiated mesenchymal cells accumulate in the clot, forming a cellular fibrovascular scar, which maintains the tear edges in a reduced position. The inflammatory reaction proceeds with ongoing invasion of cells from the synovial fringe and the fibrovascular scar tissue. This inflammatory cascade ultimately results in angiogenesis in the premeniscal capillary plexus, allowing vessels to proliferate throughout the repair tissue.

Studies have shown that when a radial tear extends into the synovium, it can heal spontaneously by 10 weeks.[7] The strength of this tissue is 33% normal at 8 weeks, 52% at 4 months, and 62% at 6 months. It is this inherent healing ability of the meniscus that clinical initiatives exploit in efforts to preserve as much meniscal tissue as possible.

CLASSIFICATION

A meniscal tear may be classified by its location relative to its blood supply and vascular appearance. The peripheral and central surfaces can be clinically graded as white (relatively avascular) or red (vascular) at the time of arthroscopy. This classification is based on anatomic studies that have depicted a peripheral vascular zone.

A red-red tear is defined as a peripheral capsular detachment, and has the best prognosis for healing. Unfortunately, a significant portion of tears occur in the white-white zone, which lies in the central avascular portion of the meniscus. This area of the meniscus has minimal blood supply, and theoretically is unable to heal. The remainder exist as red-white tears. These are meniscal rim tears through the peripheral vascular zone of the meniscus. The central portion of this tear exists in the avascular zone, so theoretically, these lesions should have sufficient vascularity to heal by fibrovascular proliferation.

Conventional wisdom dictates that meniscal repairs be limited to the peripheral vascular area of the meniscus (i.e., red-red and red-white tears). Both experimental and clinical studies have

Box 6-1 Criteria For Arthroscopically Defined Stability Using the Probe
• Cannot be displaced into the intercondylar notch
• Inner edge of meniscus cannot touch central part of the femoral condyle
• Length of the tear <10 mm

suggested that white-white tears are incapable of healing, even in the presence of a surgical suturing. This has thus provided the rationale for partial meniscectomy. In an effort to extend the zone of repair more peripherally, techniques such as the creation of vascular access channels by trephination, synovial abrasion, and use of a fibrin clot have been developed.

In addition, meniscal tears can be classified depending on their stability (Box 6-1). A tear is considered unstable when it is more than half the length of the meniscus and subluxes under the femoral condyle when probed with a hook (Fig. 6-3A). This concept is especially important to help decide the treatment options—left alone, trephinated, resected, or repaired.

Stable tears, which occur particularly in the posterior aspect of the meniscus and do not subluxate into the joint may be left alone (see Fig. 6-3B and C). Fitzgibbons and Shelbourne[8] have found that of 189 patients whose stable meniscal tears of the posterior horn of the medial meniscus were left alone, no patient was symptomatic at 2.6 years following surgery. Also, a stable longitudinal tear of the lateral meniscus, posterior to the popliteus, may be left alone, even in association with a torn ACL.

Tears can be described depending on their morphology and based on their configuration. Under these criteria, tears could be vertical or horizontal, according to whether the line of the lesion goes from superior to inferior (vertical) or from inside to outside (horizontal), commonly called open book or fishmouth tear (Fig. 6-4). Moreover, tears can be described as longitudinal if the pattern is from anterior to posterior (Fig. 6-5; also see Fig. 6-3), or transverse, also called a radial or parrot beak tear (Fig. 6-6). Combinations of these four basic patterns make up the others types of tears; the oblique tear is vertical and radial, and the so-called bucket

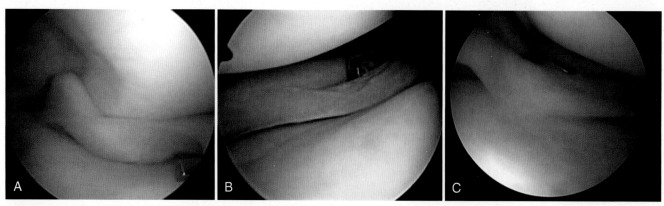

FIGURE 6-3 A, Unstable longitudinal vertical tear. Note how it subluxes under the femoral condyle when probed. **B,** Stable incomplete longitudinal vertical tear. Stability should be assessed continuously with the probe. **C,** Stable complete longitudinal vertical tear. Some tears although complete may also be stable.

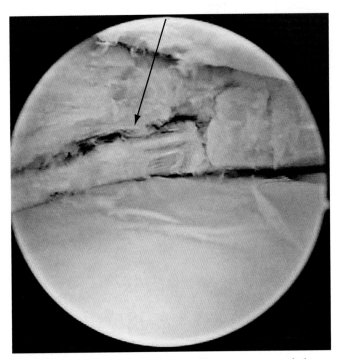

FIGURE 6-4 Horizontal degenerative tear. These tears may reach the vascular zone (*arrow*).

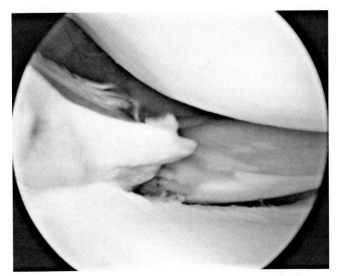

FIGURE 6-6 Radial tear. This is also called a parrot beak or flap tear.

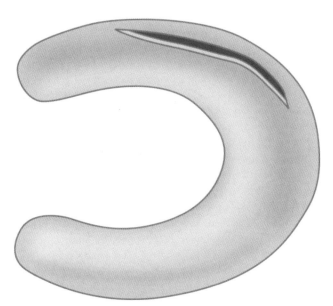

FIGURE 6-5 Diagram showing the longitudinal tear.

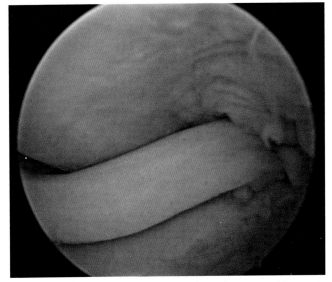

FIGURE 6-7 Bucket handle tear dislocated into the intercondylar notch.

handle tear is a vertical longitudinal tear that is unstable and subluxes completely under the condyle (Fig. 6-7; also see Fig. 6-3A). Finally, the complex tear is a combination of all of these, usually in a degenerative setting, located in the posterior horn of the medial meniscus (Fig. 6-8).

Longitudinal vertical tears usually occur in the young patient in association with an anterior ACL tear, and more frequently in the medial meniscus because of its lower mobility. Oblique tears tend to appear in between the medial and posterior thirds of the meniscus. They may cause mechanical symptoms of entrapment and pain caused by the tension on the meniscus–capsular junction.

Horizontal-shaped tears usually begin as intrasubstance degeneration in the middle of the meniscus, and migrate toward the free surface. Often, they also extend to the capsular junction and can cause the formation of a cyst. Because of the increasing size of the cyst over time, the patient may experience pain and tenderness. They usually appear more frequently in the lateral meniscus and are filled with a gel-like substance chemically similar to synovial fluid. These cysts have been reported to be 1% to 10% of meniscal pathology.[9]

Complex tears appear mainly in older patients and are usually associated with cartilage degeneration. They are considered to be part of the process of arthrosis and degenerative arthropathy.

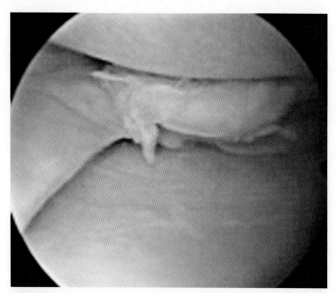

FIGURE 6-8 Complex tear. These tears are usually located in the posterior horn of the medial meniscus and are associated with degeneration.

Because of their complex pattern, the fragments can be unstable and cause mechanical symptoms. The pain associated with these tears is an added element to the generalized inflammation involved in the osteoarthritic knee. The associated histologic pathology is myxoid degeneration, hyaline acellular degeneration, and dystrophic calcification.[10]

Timing is also important in decision making. Tears can be acute, with more likelihood of healing, or chronic, which are usually associated with complex patterns and degeneration. These usually require resection. The time frame to consider a tear to be chronic is generally 8 to 12 weeks after the lesion has occurred.

The cause or mechanism of the tear should be determined. If the tear is traumatic, which usually happens in a young active patient, and is diagnosed acutely, there is an improved chance of success. On the other hand, degenerative complex tears usually occur in older patients and are associated with arthrosis. Whether they are a cause or consequence of the osteoarthritic process is still unknown.

Finally, tears can be classified depending on the side—that is, the medial or lateral meniscus. Metcalf and colleagues[11] have observed that 69% of tears affected the medial meniscus, whereas the lateral was affected 24% of the time. In their review, both menisci were torn at the same time in 7% of patients. Moreover, 80% of the tears were vertical or oblique and affected the posterior medial part of the meniscus.

In summary, the most common meniscal tears are as follows:

- Chronic, degenerative, horizontal, or complex in the medial meniscus (see Fig. 6-8)
- Acute, traumatic, longitudinal, and vertical in the medial meniscus (see Fig. 6-3)

The degenerative horizontal type tear usually occurs insidiously in older patients, and generally requires resection. On the other hand, the traumatic vertical or longitudinal tear is seen more often in the younger patient, and potentially can be repaired.

PATIENT EVALUATION

History

The meniscus is commonly injured in sports, but can occur as a sequel of age-related degeneration. In these cases, there may be no trauma but, more typically, patients give a history of a twisting hyperflexion injury followed by pain. This acute episode may involve locking of the knee and moderate swelling that usually develops over the first 24 hours. Recurrent episodes of pain and swelling are occasionally accompanied by complaints of mechanical symptoms such as catching, popping, or locking in the knee. The pain tends to localize along the joint line, especially with deep flexion and twisting motions.

Is also important to inquire about symptoms of instability, because the menisci are a secondary restraint to anteroposterior translation and certain tears can worsen in the setting of an ACL-deficient knee.

Physical Examination

The patient is examined for signs of an effusion, loss of quadriceps bulk, and decreased range of motion. Tenderness to palpation along the medial or lateral joint line is among the most sensitive signs of a meniscal tear (Fig. 6-9A). Studies have shown it to be as sensitive as 74%, with a positive predictive value of 50%.[12] The collateral and cruciate ligaments need to be assessed to determine whether additional injury is present. In the setting of an ACL-deficient knee the sensitivity of joint line tenderness has been shown to decrease to approximately 50%.

Special tests for assessing the meniscus, such as the McMurray, Steinmann, and Apley tests, are not conclusive but can aid in the diagnosis. The aim of all these maneuvers is to trap a fragment of meniscus between the tibia and femur, producing pain, a clunk, or both. Because the meniscus itself is fairly aneural, pain is caused by traction at the synovium-meniscal junction.

The McMurray test is preferred because it is easy, fast, and reliable. In addition, complementary knee tests may be done in the same position. This provocative test is performed with the patient supine, the hip flexed to 90 degrees, and the knee in forced maximal flexion. The foot is grasped by the heel, the knee is steadied, and the joint line is palpated with the other hand. As the knee is slowly brought into extension, an external rotation stress will test the medial meniscus and an internal rotation stress will test the lateral meniscus (see Fig. 6-9B). As a mnemonic rule, the heel of the foot points toward the injured meniscus. The test is considered positive when the patient feels pain in the appropriate joint line, accompanied by a thud or click. When the clunk is present, the test has a sensitivity of 98% but, because it is not always possible to evoke the clunk, its specificity is only 15%.[13]

In conclusion, the hallmarks of a meniscal tear are presence of an effusion, joint line tenderness, and a positive McMurray test. When the history and physical examination are considered together, the overall sensitivity to diagnose a meniscal tear, confirmed with arthroscopy, is approximately 95% and specificity is 88%.[14]

Diagnostic Imaging

Evaluation of the patient with a meniscal tear should include routine anteroposterior (AP) and lateral x-rays of the knee. If

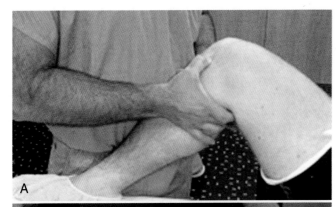

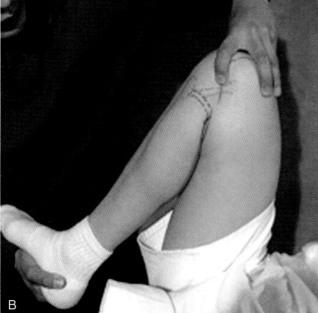

FIGURE 6-9 A, Palpating for joint line tenderness. This is the most sensitive sign for meniscal tear. **B,** The McMurray test. As a mnemonic rule, the heel of the foot points toward the injured meniscus. The test is considered positive when the patient feels pain in the appropriate joint line, accompanied by a thud or click.

degenerative changes are expected, standing views, including a 45-degree flexion AP view, should be obtained to assess the degree of joint space narrowing. Assessing osteoarthritis is important to counsel the patient about expectations of success. It has been proven that the degree of arthrosis before surgery correlates with worse postoperative results in the short- and long-term periods.[15,16]

Although not clinically indicated for all patients, magnetic resonance imaging (MRI) plays a valuable role in the evaluation of the full range of meniscal pathology, including the primary diagnosis of a meniscal tear, detection of a recurrent tear after resection or repair, and demonstration of associated injuries. MRI shows the relative locations of the tears, and is able to determine the presence of a meniscal tear with an accuracy of over 90%.[17] These results indicate that MRI is an accurate noninvasive technique for evaluating meniscal tears.

Image results should be combined with pertinent history and physical examination. It has been proven that meniscal tears in

young adults can be completely asymptomatic.[18] In these cases, MRI may modify the therapeutic plan. For example, if an athlete suffers an ACL during the season and the MRI demonstrates no tear, one may be inclined to let the athlete finish the season with a brace. If there is a meniscal tear associated with the ACL tear, the preference would be for early reconstruction.

TREATMENT

Indications and Contraindications

Meniscectomy is indicated when the type of tear has no chance to heal spontaneously or repair is not possible. Although technology is improving and the indications for repair are increasing, arthroscopic partial meniscectomy is currently still indicated in 80% of tears (Table 6-1).

Several factors should be taken into account when deciding whether to resect or repair a meniscal tear. These the location of the tear, morphology, size, chronicity, and inherent patient factors.

In terms of location, according to Arnoczky and Warren,[6] tears in the white-white zone have a low degree of vascularity and their chances of healing are very low. These are usually resected. If the tear is in the white-red zone, other factors should be considered to make a decision.

When morphology is taken into account, horizontal cleavage tears, radial lateral tears, and degenerative bucket handle tears of the meniscus are not usually considered reparable. Moreover, tears larger than 20 mm are normally resected.

Generally, tears are considered chronic after 8 to 12 weeks. Usually, the meniscus becomes shredded or degenerative with time, and is no longer suitable for repair.

Several patient factors can modify the decision. In terms of age, there may be less vascularity and cellularity in the older meniscus, and thus less healing potential. The older patient often has this type of degenerative tear that is nonreparable. There is no age limit to a meniscus repair, but most surgeons would favor meniscectomy over repair in patients older than 40 years.

TABLE 6-1 Indications for Meniscectomy: Situations in Which Meniscectomy Is Preferred Over Repair

Factor	Features
Meniscal Tear Factors	
Location	White-white
Morphology	Horizontal cleavage Radial lateral Degenerative bucket handle
Size	>20 mm
Chronicity	>8-12 wk
Patient Factors	
Age	>40 years old
ACL acute deficient knee	Small posterior flap tear in lateral meniscus
ACL chronic deficient knee	All types of tears
Rehabilitation	Noncompliant patient

Patients with an acute ACL injury often have a small posterior flap tear of the lateral meniscus. Although there is some controversy, most believe that this should simply be excised. In the chronic unstable ACL-deficient knee, a meniscus tear should be resected unless the ACL is reconstructed. Because of the abnormal kinematics of the ACL-deficient knee, the failure rate of meniscal repair in the unstable knee is much higher than in the stable or reconstructed knee.

If the patient is someone who will not be compliant with the rehabilitation program, then meniscectomy should be the first option over repair.

Conservative Management

The patient should be informed that some meniscal tears become asymptomatic after several months of protection of the joint. During this period, conservative treatment, including ice, non-steroidal anti-inflammatory drugs (NSAIDs), modification of activities, and protected weight bearing is prescribed. The best activity is use of an exercise bike. Full squats should be avoided. If the patient is willing to modify activity and has no pain or swelling, conservative management of the tear may be all that is required.

Arthroscopic Technique

If the patient continues to have pain, swelling, and locking or catching symptoms, and is willing to undergo surgical treatment, operative intervention is indicated. There are several surgical principles that should be followed to achieve a good outcome (Box 6-2). First, and following the Hippocratic principle of *primum non nocere* ("First, do no harm"), do not make the situation worse. If there is a stable, partial or total, vertical tear in a young patient, it should be left alone, and no resection is needed. Second, portal placement should be accurate enough to allow good visualization of the entire meniscus and tear configuration. In addition, portals should allow instruments of desired shapes to be introduced without scuffing the articular surface. Third, when resection is performed, the main objective is to achieve a stable peripheral rim and remove any unstable fragments that could cause mechanical symptoms or pain. During meniscectomy, it is important to contour the edges to have a smooth border and avoid progression to a second tear. The probe should be used continuously to assess stability of the rim. With bucket handle tears, 25% have a secondary tear of the rim that could be overlooked. If a complete meniscectomy is performed, care should be taken to prevent excessive bleeding from the meniscocapsular junction. After meniscectomy, or when the tear is left alone, stimulation of healing would help improve the results. This could be done by rasping the synovium, trephinating the meniscus to allow vascularization, and perforating the notch to cause bleeding. The penetration of the subchondral bone in the notch allows bone marrow mesenchymal cells in the field. Finally, adding autologous plasma rich in growth factors and cytokines may optimize the healing environment.

Preparation and Portal Placement

Patient positioning must allow circumferential access to the affected knee. The leg should be prepped and draped to allow posteromedial and posterolateral incisions if they are required in the case of a repair (Fig. 6-10). This can be done with the patient supine so that the break in the table is at the level of the tourniquet and the knee can be flexed to 90 degrees. Alternatively, a leg holder can be used that allows the surgeon to abduct the leg away from the operating table, allowing the knee to flex as needed for access.

The anterolateral portal is used to place the arthroscope for visualization. This portal is vertical, at the edge of the patellar tendon and at the inferior border of the patella. This high lateral portal allows the arthroscope to be above the fat pad, which avoids putting its tip into the fat pad—"fat padoscopy." It is also central enough to allow visualization of the posterior notch. A superolateral portal is made in the pouch to allow drainage and lavage to improve visualization.

Diagnostic arthroscopy is performed using a 30-degree arthroscope. This includes an evaluation of the suprapatellar pouch, both menisci, articular cartilage, and cruciate ligaments. After diagnosis, and based on the type of tear, the medial portal is established. With the help of the finger, the medial soft spot is

---

Box 6-2 Surgical Principles for Meniscectomy

- *Primum non nocere* ("First, do no harm.")
- Have good access for viewing and instruments.
- Achieve a stable rim and remove any unstable fragments of meniscus.
- Have a smooth border to contour the edges.
- Use the probe constantly.
- Protect the meniscocapsular junction.
- Stimulate healing by using a rasp, trephination, marrow, and plasma rich in growth factors.

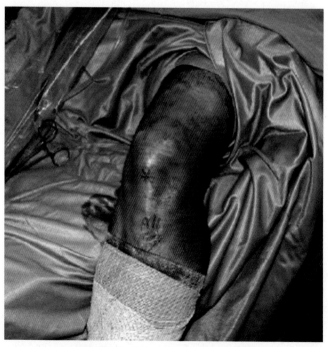

FIGURE 6-10 Setup for meniscectomy.

located. A spinal needle is placed to confirm the position of the new portal. The tip of the needle should be able to reach the area of the meniscal tear. The arthroscope is rotated to view the needle. It is essential to avoid cutting the meniscus or damaging the articular surface of the medial condyle. The medial portal is made with a no. 11 blade in an oblique direction to allow increasing the size of the portal, if needed. Making the incision oblique also reduces the potential to cut the articular surface with the blade. After the portals are established, the menisci are probed on the inferior and superior surfaces to identify any tears. In assessing meniscal stability, it is important to realize that the lateral meniscus is normally more mobile, up to 10 mm, than the medial meniscus,. The definition of an unstable meniscal tear is one that is half the length of the meniscus and subluxes under the condyle when probed with a hook (see Table 6-1). Although a tourniquet may be used to improve visualization during the procedure, some surgeons prefer to leave it deflated for the diagnostic arthroscopy to assess the vascularity of the meniscal tear after rasping. Meniscectomy in the medial meniscus is usually done close to extension and with valgus stress. In ACL-deficient patients, is important to take into account that the lateral compartment is usually subluxed anteriorly in internal rotation. The medial spine will obscure the visualization of the posterior horn of the medial meniscus. To get to the posterior horn of the medial meniscus, the assistant should perform external rotation of the tibia by holding the patient's ankle or the foot. On occasion, in a very tight knee, an 18-gauge needle may be used to "pie crust" the medial ligament over the tibia. When valgus stress is placed on the MCL, a large enough opening will allow access to the posterior horn.

On the lateral side, the best visualization is obtained with the knee flexed and the leg placed in the figure-of-four position. This position is also key in protecting the peroneal nerve, which lies posterior to the biceps femoris tendon and furthest from the joint capsule with the knee in flexion.

Resection Techniques

The technique is determined by the type of tear. The success of the resection is significantly affected by instrument access to the surgery site. The most common limiting factors are poor portal placement, a tight compartment, and/or instrument geometry. In general, the principles of partial meniscectomy are to remove the least amount of tissue possible to obtain stability of the remaining meniscal rim.

Approach to the Medial Meniscus.   We usually begin at the extreme posterior attachment. To view the resection directly, the arthroscope is passed into the medial compartment. Its tip is kept positioned against the tibia and the telescope is rotated to look up under the condyle. This throws light into the posterior area and prevents scuffing of the condyle with the arthroscope tip. Then, a meniscal up-curved punch, designed to fit under the curve of condyle, is used on tears of the posterior horn of the medial meniscus. When inserting the punch, it should be left closed until it is in place anterior to the meniscal tear and posterior to the curve of the condyle. It is then advanced posteriorly. This way the insertion is easier and iatrogenic lesions to the car-

tilage are avoided. The next step is to advance the upper jaw of the instrument just above the superior surface of the area intended for resection. Once the selected segment is positioned between the jaws, these are closed, resecting the tear vertically. This step should be repeated circumferentially until the leaflet is resected completely. The side-angled basket is also used as the resection proceeds anteriorly. To prevent the pushing away effect of the basket, certain maneuvers can be performed by the assistant. Our preferred maneuver is to apply digital pressure on the posterior capsule, stabilizing the superior leaflet so it can be seen, and resected if indicated.

Moving to the anterior aspect, a straight large basket is used to resect the length of a segment of approximately 1 cm. Then, the remaining fragments adjacent to the medial collateral ligament are resected with an angled basket. When the midportion of the medial meniscus is approached, it may be resected by changing the arthroscope to the medial portal and inserting the basket through the lateral portal. Between resections with hand instruments, a small-diameter intra-articular shaver can be used to smooth any rough scalloping and to develop a well-contoured rim between resected areas. The shaver with suction also removes semiattached fragments from the rim border to improve visualization and determine whether further resection is needed. Angled small and large baskets can also be used to resect the posterior third. It is advisable to monitor the resection carefully to ensure adequate resection.

Ideally, resection of the posterior medial meniscus leaves an approximate 2- to 3-mm rim. This is gradually beveled through the middle to the anterior third.

If resection of the anterior horn is required, back-biting cutters are available. Alternatively, place the arthroscope in the medial portal and the instruments in the lateral portal. Rotary basket cutters also can be used for resection of the anterior horn. Isolated anterior horn tears are relatively rare, occurring most often in combination with bucket handle tears.

Approach to the Lateral Meniscus.   The arthroscope is inserted through the anterolateral distal portal. The basket cutters are used through the medial portal to resect the midportion of the lateral meniscus. The posterior horn can not be approached this way. Thus, the lateral portal is used for instruments and the medial portal is used for the arthroscope. Resection of the anterior third of the right knee is performed by using the left rotary basket, inserted through the medial portal. The intra-articular shaver is used frequently, interspersed with the left or right rotary basket.

Resecting a Displaced Bucket Handle Tear.   In these cases, the anteriorly displaced fragment (see Fig. 6-7) obscures visualization of the medial compartment and the posterior region of the tear. The rim may be assessed before the tear is reduced to ascertain whether a repair is possible.

The first step is to reduce the fragment with the probe or the blunt trocar from the arthroscope to improve visualization. Valgus stress must be applied to perform the reduction.

Next, use the arthroscopic scissors to cut the posterior horn attachment. Cutting this first avoids the problem of the fragment displacing into the posterior compartment after cutting the anterior horn. The arthroscope may have to be placed into the intercondylar notch and the depth of the cut assessed from there. The anterior attachment is cut as close to the axilla of the tear as possible, leaving a minuscule attachment to prevent the fragment from moving away.

Finally, grasp the end of the fragment and remove it from the joint. The rim should be contoured with the 4-mm shaver. Be sure to hook the remaining rim, because there is a secondary tear in 25% of cases. If there is a tear in the rim, be sure to resect any unstable portion. If it is impossible to reduce the chronic displaced bucket handle on the medial side, the anterior attachment may be cut first. A grasper is used to place tension on the end of the bucket handle fragment, and cutting scissors are inserted through the same portal to cut under the posterior horn attachment. This cut is blind, and careful monitoring of the depth of the cut is important to prevent posterior neurovascular injury. The technique is similar to that for lateral displaced bucket handle tears.

Resection of a Radial Lateral Meniscus Tear. The radial tear of the lateral meniscus is approached with instruments from the medial portal. The straight basket is used to resect the posterior edge and the 90-degree basket is used to resect the anterior edge. The small shaver is used to contour the meniscus further. This has to be resected back to a normal-appearing rim. The body of the meniscus will often have a degenerative mucoid appearance that must be resected.

Resection of Lateral Meniscal Tears Associated with a Cyst. This tear is approached in much the same fashion as described for the radial tear (see earlier). The entrance to the cyst is usually below the meniscus and can be entered with a small shaver. Digital palpation of the cyst externally will cause some ganglion-like fluid to enter the joint through the entrance made by the shaver. The suction on the shaver is used to evacuate the cyst. No external excision of the cyst is necessary if the meniscectomy is adequate.

Resection of the Discoid Lateral Meniscus. Often, the central tear of the discoid meniscus will be difficult to visualize. The center of the meniscus is probed with a hook and the delamination or tear is then palpated. The basket forceps is brought through the medial portal and the central portion is resected back to a normal-appearing rim of lateral meniscus. It is important to probe the rim to be certain that it is attached, and not unstable. Rarely, a Wrisberg type of lateral meniscus will be encountered that does not have any peripheral attachments, and a suture repair of the rim must be performed.

Baker's Cyst and Degenerative Medial Meniscal Tears. In most cases, once the degenerative medial meniscus is resected, the recurrent effusions are controlled and the symptoms of pain and swelling caused by the Baker's cyst will improve. Occasionally, with a very large symptomatic cyst and a degenerative medial meniscal tear associated with degeneration of the medial compartment, the Baker's cyst must be addressed. A posteromedial portal is made with the arthroscope in the lateral portal and then advanced into the posteromedial compartment. The overlapping flaps of the Baker's cyst are identified and, with a shaver through the posteromedial portal, the inferior flap is resected to leave an opening into the cyst. The cyst will then drain into the joint and remain decompressed. Once the joint effusion is controlled, the Baker's cyst will gradually reduce in size.

Occasionally, with a chronic Baker's cyst, the shaver may have to be introduced into the cyst through a separate percutaneous puncture and the cyst walls resected. The arthroscope is introduced into the cyst through the opening made in the posterior capsule to monitor the progress of the cyst wall excision.

Special Considerations: Anterior Cruciate Ligament Reconstruction and Meniscectomy

Facing a meniscal tear during ACL surgery is not an uncommon situation. In some series, the incidence can be as high as 57%,[19] whereas some others have reported an incidence of approximately 30%.[20] A predominance of lateral meniscal tears has been demonstrated with acute ACL rupture, whereas the incidence of medial meniscal tears increases significantly with chronic ACL insufficiency. This suggests that lateral meniscal tears occur at the time of injury to the ACL or very soon after injury, whereas medial meniscal tears are acquired after the knee has been ACL-deficient.

A treatment decision is especially important in this scenario. Deciding to leave certain types of tears alone can result in saving time in these long procedures, with good outcomes. Definition of stability during arthroscopy, a tear that does not sublux under the condyles, or one less than 10 mm long, would be helpful in clarifying which tears could be saved. The bleeding environment along with the stable knee facilitates healing after surgery. Taking that into account, some surgeons consider that the radial tear of the lateral meniscus can also be saved in the setting of ACL reconstruction. Shelbourne[19] has advocated leaving alone the vertical tear located posterior to the popliteus tendon and the posterior horn avulsion, and has shown in a long-term follow-up that they are asymptomatic. In their series of stable peripheral vertical tears of the medial meniscus treated with trephination and abrasion, Shelbourne and Rask[21] have reported a 94% success rate.

Recently, Pujol and Beaufils[22] have proposed to leave alone those stable tears placed on the lateral side, based on a systematic review of the literature. On the other hand, they advised that tears in the medial meniscus, including the stable ones, should be repaired or resected because of the undesirable outcomes in the published series. This advice is based on literature results on medial meniscus tears left alone, which have been shown to fail in about 50% of cases. Failure is considered to be pain, locking, or any other clinical meniscal symptoms, along with proof of nonhealing in any image test, such as arthroscopic MRI, normal MRI, or arthroscopy.

In the setting of ACL reconstruction with a tear in the lateral meniscus that could not be left alone, more emphasis should be put on repairing it over resection because of its important role in stability. A repaired lateral meniscus has a potential role in reducing anterior translation and thus protecting the graft from undesirable stresses that could lead to failure.

In terms of timing of ACL surgery with a concomitant meniscal tear, it is advisable to perform the procedure before the third month postinjury, considering the findings of Papastergiou and associates.[20] They showed that the prevalence of a meniscal tear needing treatment increases significantly after this period. In their study, the prevalence of meniscal tear in the first 3 months after the traumatic injury was approximately 45%, increasing up to 69% after the sixth month. Considering that the prevalence of medial meniscal tears increases with time, they concluded that ACL reconstruction in the early period would reduce the risk of secondary meniscal tears.

PEARLS

PEARLS
- Use drainage from the superolateral portal to improve visualization.
- Use vertical oblique incisions in case portal augmentation will be needed.
- Use external rotation to get to the post horn of the medial meniscus.
- Use the figure-of-four position for the best approach to the lateral compartment, and use the probe constantly.
- Use the "pie crust" technique on the MCL to open the medial compartment.

Postoperative Rehabilitation

The goals of rehabilitation after meniscectomy are to diminish the swelling, regain full range of motion (ROM), and obtain similar thigh strength compared with that of the other knee. Some studies have supported physical therapy after partial meniscectomy over no treatment. These studies, which measured isokinetic knee extensor strength, have shown that the speed of strength recovery is significantly faster with physiotherapy (3 weeks) compared with no treatment (7 to 12 weeks).[23] Moreover, strength differences between groups were as large as 26% and the residual deficits of the untreated patients were two to three times greater than those of the treated patients.

In another study, a statistically significant improvement in return to sports activity ($P = .04$) and vertical and horizontal hop tests ($P = .04$ and $P = .02$, respectively) was reported for those who received physical therapy 4 weeks after surgery compared who the group who did not receive treatment.[24]

Controlled physiotherapy is advisable after surgery, especially in noncompliant patients. However, it has been shown in a systematic literature review that a supervised physiotherapy program, plus written and verbal advice after arthroscopic partial meniscectomy surgery, is no more effective than written and verbal advice alone.[25] In this same study, the authors concluded that for those patients who have undergone an uncomplicated arthroscopic partial meniscectomy, physical therapy is not necessary, because it will have little or no effect on their return to activities of daily living.

Rehabilitation after meniscectomy can be as aggressive as tolerated by the patient. Pain management during surgery and in the early postoperative period is crucial. The use of intra-articular and portal injections with long-lasting anesthetics (bupivacaine or ropivacaine), in combination with oral analgesics and anti-inflammatories, facilitates the beginning of ROM exercises as early as possible without pain. The use of local anesthetics is also beneficial to diminish the use of opioids, decreasing their side effects.

If no other procedures have been performed, the patient can progress to partial weight bearing immediately after the surgery. In case of concomitant chondral treatment or ACL surgery, individualized protocols should be followed.

The first days are focused on decreasing swelling. This can be performed with the assistance of the physiotherapist using draining massage, ROM exercises, electrotherapy, and cryotherapy. The use of self-controlled continuous passive motion (CPM) devices can also be helpful to aid in elevation of the knee. Some surgeons prefer not to use the physiotherapist for uncomplicated meniscectomies. In this case, the patient is instructed to use cryotherapy intermittently in the early postoperative period, along with elevation of the leg, and ambulation as tolerated. Oral anti-inflammatories are used for 5 days after surgery and other analgesics, such as acetaminophen, are authorized as needed.

In addition to swelling control, ROM exercises are encouraged. Once full ROM is achieved, strengthening exercises are introduced with the goal of obtaining normal muscular mass in the thigh. Usually, the other thigh is used as a control.

It has been shown that in the early postoperative period after partial meniscectomy, under a physiotherapist's supervision, the use of a bicycle ergometer equipped with an adjustable pedal arm improved gait performance at weeks 1, 2, and 4 after surgery compared with nonsupervised rehabilitation.[26] However, the most common protocol is to instruct the patient on how to perform the ROM and strengthening exercises by herself or himself.

Our protocol for meniscectomy is to visit the patient 1 week after surgery to examine the portals for infection, assess the ROM, and evaluate for deep venous phlebitis or septic arthritis. If there are no complications, and the ROM is good, the patient is advised to ride a stationary bike and begin a normal life. In addition, the patient is encouraged to resume unsupervised strengthening of quadriceps and hamstrings in the gym. Usually, the use of the bicycle is better tolerated in the first phase and muscle-specific exercises are recommended after several weeks. Once full strength compared with the other knee is obtained, sports-specific activities are authorized.

In the case of any problems such as stiffness or weakness, the patient is sent to supervised physiotherapy and individualized rehabilitation protocols are begun.

OUTCOMES

The menisci were once considered a vestigial tissue, without any role in the knee.[27] At that time, total open meniscectomy was considered the definitive treatment for its pathology. The short-term results of total meniscectomy are good because it eliminates the mechanical symptoms of locking immediately and achieves fast pain relief. On the other hand, the clinical results worsen with time, and osteoarthritis of the involved compartment appears sooner than age-matched controls without total meniscectomy.[28] In addition, total meniscectomy is associated with more radiographic osteoarthritis over time than partial meniscectomy.[16]

Because of the increasing information about meniscal function, surgical procedures have evolved with the objective of preserving as much tissue as possible. Thus, partial meniscectomy has become the elected treatment when repair is not possible. The American Academy of Orthopaedic Surgeons estimates that 636,000 arthroscopic procedures of the knee are performed each year in the United States.[29]

With the help of optical magnification and minimally invasive instruments, arthroscopic partial meniscectomy has become the gold standard over open surgery.[30] Numerous reports have commented on the beneficial effect of the use of arthroscopy over open surgery.

The advantages related to arthroscopic surgery are day surgery without the need of hospital admission, less recovery time, less pain caused by the minimally invasive surgery, less global morbidity, improved visualization with more accurate resections, resulting in better long-term outcomes, fewer complications, and lower cost for the patient and/or the system.

When analyzing partial meniscectomy results, various methods of determining surgical outcome have been used, ranging from clinical examination to patient satisfaction and radiographic measurements. In general, in the literature, uniformly good to excellent results have been documented in 80% to 95% of patients within the first 5 years after partial meniscectomy. Rockborn and coworkers[31] have reported a mean Lysholm score of more than 84 in the first year after meniscectomy. It has been shown that allowing the patient to watch the arthroscopic procedure increases his or her overall understanding and satisfaction in the early postoperative period. In addition, it decreases the anxiety and worries about the surgery and the postoperative period significantly.[32]

Clinical outcomes in the long term are also satisfactory. Burks and colleagues[33] have published overall Lysholm scores of 94 and average satisfaction index of 8.8. Moreover, the Tegner change of desired versus actual activity level was 0.3. This means that the subjective results were satisfactory 15 years after meniscectomy.

Higuchi and associates,[34] based on the criteria of Tapper and Hoover and the International Knee Documented Committee's evaluation form (IKDC), rated their results after 12.2 years postmeniscectomy as being excellent and good in 71% of their series.

Because of the variety of measuring tools used in the different studies, it is difficult to compare their results. Addressing that issue, the University of Western Ontario has developed, and validated the WOMET.[35] This is a simple, disease-specific tool designed to evaluate health-related quality of life in patients with meniscal pathology to be used in research or in clinical practice uniformly.

Meniscectomy is a well-known risk factor for secondary osteoarthritis (OA) of the knee. Traditionally considered as a result of joint injury and increased cartilage contact stress caused by the loss of meniscal tissue, wear and tear is a straightforward explanation for secondary knee OA. In addition, there is proof of an interaction between primary heritable OA and exogenous secondary OA caused by meniscectomy.[36] Moreover, there is a sixfold increased relative risk for the development of radiographic osteoarthritis after total meniscectomy compared with nonoperated controls.[2] However, as expected, partial meniscectomy induces less radiographic OA over time than does total meniscectomy.[16]

Is important to note that radiographic changes do not clearly correlate with clinical symptoms.[37] Thus, radiographic outcome appears to be a poor determinant of overall outcome from surgery.

Degenerative tears of the menisci have been associated with osteoarthritis. Whether degenerative tear is a cause or consequence of osteoarthritis is still unknown. Some studies have suggested that a degenerative tear could be the first sign of arthritis in the knee. Patients suffering a degenerative tear experience worse clinical outcomes than those with a traumatic lesion.[38] Partial meniscectomy of degenerative tears is associated with a high risk of radiographic and symptomatic tibiofemoral arthritis at 16-year follow-up.[2] Evaluating for pain after exercise at 8.5 years follow-up, patients with flap or horizontal tears had worse clinical outcomes after meniscectomy than those with bucket handle tears.[39]

Data regarding medial versus lateral partial meniscectomy are controversial. Although in vivo studies have not clearly shown significant differences between sides, laboratory studies have proven that lateral partial meniscectomy is more dangerous than the same procedure performed in the medial compartment. Englund and Lohmander[16] published worse radiographic outcomes in association with lateral meniscectomy 22 years after surgery than medial meniscectomy. The lateral meniscus carries a higher load in the knee compared with the medial meniscus. Consequently, its loss may result in increased cartilage contact stress.

To be able to inform the patient about expectations after surgery, it is important to be familiar with the predicting factors affecting the results. Intuitively, one might think that they would include the following: the compartment involved (lateral meniscectomy resection is worse than medial); the amount of resection (more removed equals more risk); the type of resection (radial resection of even a small portion may destroy the hoop stress function and probably is the equivalent of a near-total meniscectomy); associated conditions (ACL insufficiency and chondral pathology are probably overall even more significant indicators of probable degenerative progression); tibiofemoral alignment (varus alignment risk for medial meniscus, lateral for valgus); and body habitus, patient age, and activity level.

However, only some factors have proven to affect the outcome significantly. In the short term, only female gender and previous OA are associated with a slower rate of recovery from arthroscopic partial meniscectomy, whereas age, body mass index, depth of meniscal excision, involvement of one or both menisci, and extent of meniscal tear show no association.[15] In the long term, contributing risk factors for arthritis development after meniscal resection are similar to risk factors for common knee osteoarthritis. Systemic and local biomechanical factors interact. Younger patient age predicts a better long-term prognosis after meniscectomy, whereas, obesity, female gender, and preexisting early-stage OA are features associated with poor self-reported and radiographic outcomes.[16]

COMPLICATIONS

The overall complication rate of knee arthroscopy is relatively low.[40] It has been estimated in retrospective large series of 118,590 and 395,566 arthroscopies to be 0.8%[41] and 0.5%,[42] respectively. In those series, complications were more likely to occur with more complex procedures, such as meniscal repair, synovectomy, and intra-articular reconstruction of both the ACL and PCL. In a prospective study reviewing 10,262 procedures, Small[43] has found an overall complication rate of 1.68%. The most common complications in this study were hemarthrosis (60.1%), infection (12.1%), thromboembolic disease (6.9%), anesthetic complications (6.4%), instrument failure (2.9%), complex regional pain syndrome 1 (CRPS 1; 2.3%), ligament injury (1.2%), and fracture or neurologic injury (0.6% each).

In general, arthroscopic meniscectomy is an innocuous procedure. However, complications can arise during surgery or in the postoperative period. Operative complications are usually iatrogenic and may be avoided with careful surgical technique. During surgery, several structures may be damaged, such as the medial collateral ligament, neurovascular structures, and meniscal and cartilage tissues.

Medial collateral injury during arthroscopic maneuvers may occur. Leg holders or posts are commonly used to aid exposure, particularly of the posterior horn of the medial meniscus. To achieve better exposure, valgus force is applied. If force is not used judiciously, a medial collateral ligament injury may result. This is especially possible in a tight medial compartment in a middle-aged or older patient in whom the soft tissues are likely to be less flexible. Small[42] has reported a 0.003% incidence of medial collateral injury; ninety % of them were attributed to the use of the leg holder. Treatment is normally conservative by functional bracing, with initial restriction of extension.

Neurologic damage can occur during arthroscopic meniscectomy. Rodeo and coworkers have reported four possible mechanisms: (1) direct trauma; (2) pressure secondary to a compartment syndrome caused by extravasation of fluid; (3) damage related to the use of a tourniquet) and (4) dysfunction caused by the ill-understood condition of CRPS 1. Nerve injury to the sensitive branches innervating the knee can cause numbness and/or neuropathic pain. This can happen in the anterior part of the knee when preparing the portals. Occasionally, formation of a neuroma can be troublesome and it is possible that a relatively minor nerve injury can lead to CRPS 1.

On the medial side, the infragenicular branches of the saphenous nerve (IGBSN) can be affected more commonly. Sherman and colleagues[44] have reported an incidence of 22.2% of sensory changes in the distribution of the IGBSN after standard portals had been used. Although safe zones have been advocated, the wide variability in the course of the nerve precludes the absolute avoidance of damage. Mochida and associates[45] have recommended that arthroscopic portals should be positioned close to both the patella and patellar tendon if injury to the IGBSN is to be avoided. On the lateral side, there has been a report of injury to the common peroneal nerve during lateral meniscectomy,[46] but this complication usually occurs during meniscal suture.

A temporary paresis may occur after prolonged inflation of the tourniquet. In the series of Sherman and coworkers,[44] the incidence of complications was directly related to age and tourniquet time. However, the higher risk for major complications was in the group in which the tourniquet time was longer than 60 minutes regardless of age, with a predicted complication rate of 14.3%. To avoid this type of complication, it is important that regular checks be made on the accuracy of tourniquet pressure, which should be deflated after a maximum of 2 hours.

Another complication that can occur during portal preparation is iatrogenic section of the anterior horns of the menisci, which are especially vulnerable. This can be avoided by palpating the soft point for the anterolateral portal and creating the anteromedial portal under direct arthroscopic visualization. It is advisable to cut upward with the knife, away from the meniscus, rather than downward.

Iatrogenic lesions to the cartilage can also occur when inserting the different instruments. It is important not to use a sharp trocar to introduce the arthroscope into the knee. A portal of adequate size should be made so that a blunt obturator can be used. One way to avoid cartilage damage during the arthroscopic procedure is always to direct any instrument to the intercondylar notch gently. After that, use the arthroscope to control its position and then direct the instrument where needed under arthroscopic control.

Apart from intraoperative complications, postoperative complications may also occur, such as joint effusion, residual pain, infection, and thromboembolism. Joint effusion after surgery can be caused by hydrarthrosis or hemarthrosis. Hydrarthrosis is usually a consequence of synovitis. This could be caused by the presence of previous knee osteoarthritis or by aggressive use of the joint during rehabilitation or daily activities. On the other hand, hemarthrosis is usually a consequence of extended meniscal excisions reaching the vascular zone or even the capsule. This can cause intense pain and loss of ROM in the knee. If the joint is under high tension, evacuation might be needed. Infiltrating with local anesthetic and adrenalin may be helpful. Rarely, a second-look arthroscopy is needed to cauterize the bleeding vessel. To avoid this complication, some surgeons do not use a tourniquet or deflate it before finishing the arthroscopy. In this way, bleeding points can be controlled and cauterized with the aid of electrical devices. In addition, preserving as much of the meniscal tissue as possible, mainly the rim, and avoiding sectioning the capsule are also efficacious methods to prevent bleeding. Joint effusion, in general, is managed with evacuation, rest, elevation, and ice. If it is persistent, the judicious use of an injection of cortisone is indicated.

If postoperative pain is well managed, residual pain after surgery is usually related to the preexisting condition of the knee. The previous state of the femoral, tibial, and patellar cartilage plays a key role. The more wear the cartilage has had before the surgery, the less likely is it possible to achieve complete pain relief in the short term or long term. Moreover, the presence of mechanical symptoms such as locking after surgery can be also be attributed to the incongruence of the worn joint instead of an incomplete resection. The clinical situation of persistent pain can be evaluated with a contrast MRI. The dye may demonstrate a persistent cleft into the remaining rim, indicating incomplete resection.

Infection rates of arthroscopic meniscectomy are similar to those of other basic arthroscopic procedures. Kirchhoff[46a] has reported an incidence of infection in elected arthroscopy of 0.42%. In knee arthroscopy, Sherman and colleagues[44] have reported an incidence of 0.1%, DeLee[41] of 0.08%, D'Angelo and Ogilvie-Harris[47] of 0.23%, and Armstrong and associates[48] of 0.42%. This severe complication may be avoided with the use of antibiotic prophylaxis. Bert[47a] has shown that routine antibiotic administration does not reduce the rate of postoperative septic arthritis. Although some institutions do not routinely use antibiotic prophylaxis in arthroscopic meniscectomy procedures, D'Angelo and Ogilvie-Harris[47] have recommended its use based on their cost-effective analysis. On the other hand, the appearance of septic arthritis of the knee postmeniscectomy is a devastating complication that should be treated aggressively. The most common infecting organism is *Staphylococcus aureus*. In the treatment protocol, arthroscopic débridement, along with intravenous antibiotics, should be included. Continuous passive motion is recommended as soon as the patient tolerates it.

The overall incidence of thromboembolic disease in knee arthroscopy is approximately 0.1%. Thromboembolism is even more infrequent after meniscectomy because of the short duration of the procedure and the possibility of immediate mobility after surgery. There is no indication for routine thromboprophylaxis in arthroscopic surgery, but the operating and tourniquet times should be kept to a minimum and postoperative mobilization should be as rapid as possible. Chemoprophylaxis should be considered only for high-risk patients, particularly those with previous thromboembolism.

Some exceptional complications have been reported. Berndt and coworkers[49] have reported the appearance of heterotopic ossification of the medial portal after partial meniscectomy. Furthermore, MacDessi and colleagues[50] have reported a series of eight cases of osteonecrosis after meniscectomy. They attributed the cause to subchondral fractures and suggested that this complication should be treated successfully with arthroplasty.

CONCLUSIONS

The arthroscopic technique offers advantages and better outcomes over the open procedure, as does partial over total meniscectomy. In general, the literature has documented uniformly good to excellent results in 80% to 95% of patients who have undergone arthroscopic partial meniscectomy in the short term. In the long term, results are more controversial.

Although meniscectomy is still the most frequent current procedure, there is an increasing interest in preserving techniques because of more information about the role of the menisci. Moreover, new biologic enhancing techniques, along with tissue engineering, may be the future of the treatment of meniscal pathology.

REFERENCES

1. Ahmed AM, Burke DL. In-vitro measurement of static pressure distribution in synovial joints. Part I: tibial surface of the knee. *J Biomech Eng.* 1983;105:216-225.
2. Englund M, Roos EM, Lohmander LS. Impact of type of meniscal tear on radiographic and symptomatic knee osteoarthritis: a sixteen-year followup of meniscectomy with matched controls. *Arthritis Rheum.* 2003;48:2178-2187.
3. von Lewinski G, Stukenborg-Colsman C, Ostermeier S, Hurschler C. Experimental measurement of tibiofemoral contact area in a meniscectomized ovine model using a resistive pressure-measuring sensor. *Ann Biomed Eng.* 2006;34:1607-1614.
4. Levy IM, Torzilli PA, Warren RF. The effect of medial meniscectomy on anterior-posterior motion of the knee. *J Bone Joint Surg Am.* 1982; 64:883-888.
5. King D. The healing of semilunar cartilages. 1936. *Clin Orthop Relat Res.* 1990;(252):4-7.
6. Arnoczky SP, Warren RF. Microvasculature of the human meniscus. *Am J Sports Med.* 1982;10:90-95.
7. Arnoczky SP, Warren RF. The microvasculature of the meniscus and its response to injury. An experimental study in the dog. *Am J Sports Med.* 1983;11:131-141.
8. Fitzgibbons RE, Shelbourne KD. "Aggressive" nontreatment of lateral meniscal tears seen during anterior cruciate ligament reconstruction. *Am J Sports Med.* 1995;23:156-159.
9. Lantz B, Singer KM. Meniscal cysts. *Clin Sports Med.* 1990;9:707-725.
10. Ferrer-Roca O, Vilalta C. Lesions of the meniscus. Part I: macroscopic and histologic findings. *Clin Orthop Relat Res.* 1980;(146):289-300.
11. Metcalf R, Burks R, Metcalf M. Arrhroscopic meniscectomy. In McGinty J, Caspari R, Jackson R, eds. *Operative Arthroscopy.* Philadelphia: Lippincott-Raven; 1996:263-297.
12. Shelbourne KD, Martini DJ, McCarroll JR, VanMeter CD. Correlation of joint line tenderness and meniscal lesions in patients with acute anterior cruciate ligament tears. *Am J Sports Med.* 1995;23:166-169.
13. Evans PJ, Bell GD, Frank C. Prospective evaluation of the McMurray test. *Am J Sports Med.* 1993;21:604-608.
14. Terry GC, Tagert BE, Young MJ. Reliability of the clinical assessment in predicting the cause of internal derangements of the knee. *Arthroscopy.* 1995;11:568-576.
15. Fabricant PD, Rosenberger PH, Jokl P, Ickovics JR. Predictors of short-term recovery differ from those of long-term outcome after arthroscopic partial meniscectomy. *Arthroscopy.* 2008;24:769-778.
16. Englund M, Lohmander LS. Risk factors for symptomatic knee osteoarthritis fifteen to twenty-two years after meniscectomy. *Arthritis Rheum.* 2004;50:2811-2819.
17. Konan S, Rayan F, Haddad FS. Do physical diagnostic tests accurately detect meniscal tears? *Knee Surg Sports Traumatol Arthrosc.* 2009;17: 806-811.
18. Boden SD, Davis DO, Dina TS, et al. A prospective and blinded investigation of magnetic resonance imaging of the knee. Abnormal findings in asymptomatic subjects. *Clin Orthop Relat Res.* 1992;(282):177-185.
19. Shelbourne K. "Aggressive" nontreatment of lateral menical tears seen during anterior cruciate ligament reconstruction. *Knee.* 1996;3:201-237.
20. Papastergiou SG, Koukoulias NE, Mikalef P, et al. Meniscal tears in the ACL-deficient knee: correlation between meniscal tears and the timing of ACL reconstruction. *Knee Surg Sports Traumatol Arthrosc.* 2007;15: 1438-1444.
21. Shelbourne KD, Rask BP. The sequelae of salvaged nondegenerative peripheral vertical medial meniscus tears with anterior cruciate ligament reconstruction. *Arthroscopy.* 2001;17:270-274.
22. Pujol N, Beaufils P. Healing results of meniscal tears left in situ during anterior cruciate ligament reconstruction: a review of clinical studies. *Knee Surg Sports Traumatol Arthrosc.* 2009;17:396-401.
23. Moffet H, Richards CL, Malouin F, et al. Early and intensive physiotherapy accelerates recovery postarthroscopic meniscectomy: results of a randomised controlled study. *Arch Phys Med Rehabil.* 1994;75:415-426.
24. Vervest AM, Maurer CA, Schambergen TG, et al., Effectiveness of physiotherapy after meniscectomy. *Knee Surg Sports Traumatol Arthrosc.* 1999; 7:360-364.
25. Goodwin P, Morrisey M. Physical therapy after arthroscopic partial meniscectomy: is it effective? *Exerc Sports Sci Rev.* 2003;2:85-90.
26. Kelln BM, Ingersoll CD, Saliba S, et al. Effect of early active range of motion rehabilitation on outcome measures after partial meniscectomy. *Knee Surg Sports Traumatol Arthrosc.* 2009;17:607-616.
27. Bland-Sutton J. *Ligaments: Their Nature and Morphology,* 2nd ed. London: J Lewis; 1897.
28. Roos H, Laurén M, Adalberth T, et al. Knee osteoarthritis after meniscectomy: prevalence of radiographic changes after twenty-one years, compared with matched controls. *Arthritis Rheum.* 1998;41:687-693.
29. Praemer A, Furner S, Rice D. *Musculoskeletal Conditions in the United States,* 2nd ed. Rosemont, Ill: American Academy of Orthopaedic Surgeons; 1999.
30. Simpson DA, Thomas NP, Aichroth PM. Open and closed meniscectomy. A comparative analysis. *J Bone Joint Surg Br.* 1986;68:301-304.
31. Rockborn P, Hamberg P, Gillquist J. Arthroscopic meniscectomy: treatment costs and postoperative function in a historical perspective. *Acta Orthop Scand.* 2000;71:455-460.

32. Bayar A, Tuncay I, Atasoy N, et al. The effect of watching live arthroscopic views on postoperative anxiety of patients. *Knee Surg Sports Traumatol Arthrosc.* 2008;16:982-987.

33. Burks RT, Metcalf MH, Metcalf RW. Fifteen-year follow-up of arthroscopic partial meniscectomy. *Arthroscopy.* 1997;13:673-679.

34. Higuchi H, Kimura M, Shirakura K, et al. Factors affecting long-term results after arthroscopic partial meniscectomy. *Clin Orthop Relat Res.* 2000;(377):161-168.

35. Kirkley A, Griffin S, Whelan D. The development and validation of a quality of life-measurement tool for patients with meniscal pathology: the Western Ontario Meniscal Evaluation Tool (WOMET). *Clin J Sports Med.* 2007;17:349-356.

36. Englund M. The role of the meniscus in osteoarthritis genesis. *Med Clin North Am.* 2009;93:37-43.

37. Fabricant PD, Jokl P. Surgical outcomes after arthroscopic partial meniscectomy. *J Am Acad Orthop Surg.* 2007;15:647-653.

38. Englund M, Roos EM, Roos HP, Lohmander LS. Patient-relevant outcomes fourteen years after meniscectomy: influence of type of meniscal tear and size of resection. *Rheumatology (Oxford).* 2001;40:631-639.

39. Fauno P, Nielsen AB. Arthroscopic partial meniscectomy: a long-term follow-up. *Arthroscopy.* 1992;8:345-349.

40. Allum R. Complications of arthroscopy of the knee. *J Bone Joint Surg Br.* 2002;84:937-945.

41. DeLee J. Complications of arthroscopy and arthroscopic surgery: results of a national survey. *J Arthrosc Rel Surg.* 1985;1:214-220.

42. Small NC. Complications in arthroscopy: the knee and other joints, Committee on Complications of the Arthroscopy Association of North America. *Arthroscopy.* 1986;2:253-258.

43. Small NC. Complications in arthroscopic surgery performed by experienced arthroscopists. *Arthroscopy.* 1988;4:215-221.

44. Sherman OH, Fox JM, Snyder SJ, et al. Arthroscopy—"no-problem surgery." An analysis of complications in two thousand six hundred and forty cases. *J Bone Joint Surg Am.* 1986;68:256-265.

45. Mochida H, Kikuchi S. Injury to infrapatellar branch of saphenous nerve in arthroscopic knee surgery. *Clin Orthop Relat Res.* 1995;(320):88-94.

46. Rodeo SA, Sobel M, Weiland AJ. Deep peroneal-nerve injury as a result of arthroscopic meniscectomy. A case report and review of the literature. *J Bone Joint Surg Am.* 1993;75:1221-1224.

46a. Paul J, Kirchhoff C, Imhoff AB, Hinterwinner S: Infection after arthroscopy orthopade. 2008. Nov; 37(11):1050-2 PMID 1878 915.

47. D'Angelo GL, Ogilvie-Harris DJ. Septic arthritis following arthroscopy, with cost/benefit analysis of antibiotic prophylaxis. *Arthroscopy.* 1988; 4:10-14.

47a. Bert JM, Giannini D, Nace L. Antibiotic prophylaxis for arthroscopy of the knee: is it necessary? *Arthroscopy.* 2007;23:4-60.

48. Armstrong RW, Bolding F, Joseph R. Septic arthritis following arthroscopy: clinical syndromes and analysis of risk factors. *Arthroscopy.* 1992;8:213-223.

49. Berndt C, Ganko A, Whitehouse SL, Crawford RW. Heterotopic ossification within an arthroscopic portal after uneventful partial meniscectomy. *Knee.* 2008;15:416-418.

50. MacDessi SJ, Brophy RH, Bullough PG, et al. Subchondral fracture following arthroscopic knee surgery. A series of eight cases. *J Bone Joint Surg Am.* 2008;90:1007-1012.

SUGGESTED READINGS

Greis PE, Burks RT. Arthroscopic meniscectomy. In: McGinty J, ed. *Operative Arthroscopy*, 3rd ed. Lippincott Williams Wilkins: Philadelphia; 2002: 218-232.

Miller MD, Sekiya JK. Meniscal pathology. In: Miller MD, Sekiya JK, eds. *Core Knowledge in Orthopaedics: Sports Medicine.* St. Louis: Mosby Elsevier; 2006:27-41.

Volesky M, Johnson DL. The meniscus. In: Johnson DL, Pedowitz RA, eds. *Practical Orthopaedic Sports Medicine and Arthroscopy.* Philadelphia: Lippincott, Williams & Wilkins: 2006:657-672.

Meniscal Repair

Brian D. Shannon ● Peter R. Kurzweil

In 1885, Thomas Annandale performed the first meniscal repair.[1] Because of the lack of understanding regarding the role of the meniscus, this discovery went unheralded for many years. Over time, the major role that the menisci play in load distribution, shock absorption, secondary stabilization of the knee joint, and proprioception was better understood. The menisci transmit at least 50% of a compressive load with the knee in extension.[2] This increases to 85% in 90 degrees of flexion. Following a meniscectomy, the contact area is decreased by 50%, which increases the load per unit area and leads to subsequent degenerative changes in the knee. Removal of 15% to 34% of a meniscus can increase contact pressure more than 350%, so even partial meniscectomy can significantly alter joint biomechanics.[3]

As our knowledge of the essential role that the meniscus plays in proper knee function increased, preserving its function became increasingly important. Arthroscopic inside-out repair techniques gained popularity in the early 1980s.[4] Following that, outside-in procedures were developed to decrease the chance of neurovascular injury. Recently, all-inside methods are increasingly being performed because of ease of application, decreased operative times, and even lower risk to the neurovascular structures. These techniques have led to healing rates from 60% to 80% for isolated repairs and up to 90% with concomitant anterior cruciate ligament (ACL) reconstruction.[5]

The goal of this chapter is to provide a comprehensive overview of meniscal repair. Basic information about the menisci and their healing potential will be presented. We will review the process of proper patient selection, one of the most important aspects relating to success of the repair. Then, the different operative techniques will be presented in detail. Finally, the typical postoperative course, including rehabilitation, will be covered.

ANATOMY

The menisci are semilunar fibrocartilaginous structures that cover 50% of the medial and 70% of the lateral tibial plateaus.[6] In cross section, their superior surface is concave and the inferior surface is convex to facilitate congruency with the femoral and tibial articular surfaces. The medial meniscus is shaped like a "C" whereas the lateral meniscus more closely resembles an incomplete "O" that is open medially. The coronary ligaments anchor both menisci to the tibia. Additionally, the medial meniscus has extensive peripheral attachments to the capsule and deep medial collateral ligament (MCL). Because of fewer capsular attachments, the popliteal hiatus, and no link to the neighboring collateral ligament, the lateral meniscus is more mobile and can displace up to 1 cm with knee range of motion.[7] Its major connections to the posterior femur are through the ligaments of Humphrey and Wrisberg.

The solid microstructure of the menisci is 75% composed of collagen, with a 90% predominance of type I. The collagen is arranged in various patterns, but most of the fibers are aligned circumferentially.[8] The orientation of these fibers permits absorption of the hoop stresses generated during natural movement. Radially oriented fibers provide a link between the circumferential bundles and add strength to the overall construct.[9] Longitudinal or bucket handle meniscal tears disrupt these radial links between the circumferential collagen fibers. Repairing these tears may restore the biomechanical function of the native meniscus. Vertical mattress stitch configuration, which mimics the path of the radially oriented fibers, may secure more of the circumferential fibers and lead to greater repair strength more than other suture techniques.[10]

Thorough understanding of the meniscal microvasculature is necessary when considering repair of a tear because it plays a role in the potential for healing. Vessels from the superior and inferior branches of the medial and lateral genicular arteries perforate the menisci at the capsular attachments.[11] In the area of the popliteal hiatus, the lateral meniscus lacks this peripheral supply and is an area of relative avascularity. The entire meniscus has a blood supply at birth but by 9 months, the inner third is avascular.[12] By age 10, the menisci resemble those of an adult, with the outer 10% to 30% of the medial rim and 10% to 25% of the lateral rim vascularized. For clinical purposes, the menisci are often considered to have three zones, with the peripheral 3 mm considered vascular (red-red), more than 5 mm from the meniscocapsular junction, avascular (white-white), and between 3 and 5 mm, variable (red-white).[13]

PATIENT EVALUATION

History and Physical Examination

The diagnosis of a meniscal tear begins with a thorough initial evaluation in the office. Combining the patient's history, physical examination, and plain radiographs can lead to a sensitivity of 88% to 95%, specificity of 72% to 92%, and positive predictive value of 58% to 85% for meniscal injuries.[14] Meniscal tears in younger patients typically occur after an acute traumatic event, which often involves a twisting or hyperflexion mechanism. In the fourth decade and beyond, degenerative changes in the menisci often play a role in tears, so that less dramatic events, or even none at all, can results in a tear. Patients typically report pain, swelling, locking, catching, and giving out.

Physical examination begins with inspection of the knee for an effusion or focal joint line swelling, which may indicate a perimeniscal cyst. The presence of quadriceps atrophy may hint at the chronicity of the injury. One must determine whether range of motion loss is caused by a mechanical block. A bucket handle tear is a common cause for a locked knee. A complete ligamentous examination should be attempted to evaluate for concomitant pathology, although sometimes guarding from pain makes this impossible.

There are several tests described that focus directly on meniscal injuries. Unfortunately, no single physical examination finding can reliably predict the presence of a tear. A recent meta-analysis found a pooled sensitivity and specificity of 70% and 71% for McMurray's test, 60% and 70% for Apley's test, and 63% and 77% for joint line tenderness, respectively.[15] Despite these findings, the authors concluded that none of the tests could accurately diagnose a tear based on the heterogeneity of study results. They could not explain the wide variation seen between each individual study's results. Nevertheless, these tests are valuable to perform and help discern what is going on with the patient's knee.

Diagnostic Imaging

Radiographic evaluation begins with weight-bearing x-rays of the knee, if possible. Standard views should include anteroposterior (AP), lateral, patellofemoral, and 45-degree posteroanterior (PA) images. Although the menisci are not visualized on radiographs, they provide valuable information regarding knee alignment and other possible pathologic sources of knee pain, such as degenerative arthritis.

Magnetic resonance imaging (MRI) has become the gold standard for meniscal imaging, although one must take into account that up to 13% of asymptomatic patients younger than 45 and 39% older than 45 years may have a "positive" scan.[16] Benefits of MRI include providing additional information regarding associated injuries inside the knee, as well as tear location and configuration. A retrospective review following surgery for bucket handle meniscal tears has shown that whether a lesion was reparable or not could be accurately predicted 93% (26/28) of the time.[17] The criteria created for this study included rim width less than 4 mm, tear length more than 1 cm, and isosignals of the peripheral rim and inner fragment with the normal contralateral meniscus in the same knee, indicating a nondegenerative process. Typically, contrast is not necessary to image the menisci properly, but should be used in cases involving a prior repair or if more than 25% of the meniscus has previously been resected to evaluate for a re-tear.[18]

TREATMENT

Indications and Contraindications

Once a patient has been diagnosed with a symptomatic tear of the meniscus and surgery is indicated, a number of factors play a role when considering whether the tear in this particular patient can and should be repaired. We typically explain to patients that much like real estate, location is the most important factor in addressing reparability. Adequate vascularity is a requirement for healing, so tears in the peripheral red-red zone have the best chance of healing. Tear configuration is the second most important factor, because longitudinal and vertical tears have a higher rate of healing than radial, horizontal cleavage, or degenerative tears. The third factor is size, or length, of the tear. Usually, a tear must be at least 1 cm long to be considered for repair, because smaller tears may be inherently stable and heal without surgery or be asymptomatic.[19] Many of these factors are best judged arthroscopically. Acute tears also have a higher rate of healing than chronic injuries.[20]

Stability of the knee is another factor to consider when contemplating meniscal repair. Healing rates are less than 30% in an ACL-deficient knee that remains unreconstructed.[5] It has been shown in several studies that simultaneous ACL reconstruction enhances the success of meniscal healing.[21,22]

In general, many surgeons consider patients younger than 40 years for meniscal repair. Although some studies have shown that older patients can heal following repairs,[22] one has to weigh the risks and benefits versus a partial meniscectomy. Subjecting older patients to the risk of a possible second surgery if the tear doesn't heal, as well as the difficulties of rehabilitation, may be unnecessary, considering that they might do just as well with a meniscectomy. In addition, older people are more likely to have articular cartilage changes and tissues with poorer healing qualities, which can jeopardize the success of a repair.

Conservative Management

Nonsurgical treatment may be considered for a select group of tears. Partial or small (less than 5 mm) complete tears located in the peripheral third may heal without operative intervention. This should only be considered for acute traumatic tears. Chronic and degenerative lesions are less likely to improve without surgery. In addition, meniscal tears generally do not heal in ligamentously unstable knees and nonoperative management is typically avoided.

The protocol for conservative management is surgeon-dependent. It may involve a temporary restriction of weight bearing and immobilization. Following resolution of the effusion and pain from the acute injury, a rehabilitation protocol, including strengthening and range of motion, is generally instituted. The treating physician may consider restricting deep knee flexion for a period of time. If the symptoms return after resuming unrestricted activity, surgical intervention should be discussed.

Arthroscopic Technique

It is essential to have an extensive discussion with the patient prior to surgery that includes the risks and benefits of surgery. The need for compliance with the postoperative rehabilitation protocol, as well as the possibility that a repair may fail and require an additional procedure in the future, should be discussed. These factors may be unacceptable to patients and may lead them to opt for a meniscectomy instead of a repair. Patients should also be warned that not all tears are reparable and that the ultimate decision about treatment occurs during surgery. Hence, patients should be aware that there remains the possibility of a meniscectomy. Finally, it is important to address the potential need for additional incisions with a repair so that they are not a surprise postoperatively. This is typically brought up when educating patients about the possibility of neurovascular injury during meniscal repair.

Patient Positioning

We typically perform our knee arthroscopies under a general anesthetic and prefer this over regional or local anesthetic. In our experience, complete relaxation allows the surgeon to enjoy a few extra millimeters of joint opening, which permits better visualization and instrumentation in the medial and lateral compartments. We inject a local anesthetic with epinephrine around our incision sites after prepping the leg to assist with perioperative pain control and hemostasis. A femoral nerve block can also be considered to assist with pain management, but we typically do not use one routinely unless an ACL reconstruction is performed concomitantly. We apply a nonsterile tourniquet to the upper thigh of the operative extremity, but make every attempt during the procedure to minimize inflating it. It is essential to make sure that it is not engaged when assessing the vascularity of the tear site. Most procedures can be done without ever increasing the tourniquet pressure. Electrocautery is useful to help maintain hemostasis during the procedure.

We prefer to position the patient supine on the operating room table. A lateral thigh post permits valgus stressing of the knee to open the medial compartment. Work in the lateral compartment is accomplished with the patient in the figure-of-four position, resting the leg on the contralateral shin.

Diagnostic Arthroscopy

We prefer gravity inflow of lactated Ringer's solution to provide knee distention, and have found that a high-pressure pump can lead to extravasation of fluid into the surrounding soft tissues, which may contribute to increased postoperative swelling and pain. The cannula through which inflow is accomplished is placed in a standard anterolateral viewing portal. Using needle localization to make sure that the pathology can be reached, a medial working portal is established. We do not use a separate inflow-outflow portal.

Occasionally, it can be difficult to see the periphery of the posterior horn of the medial meniscus in tight knees. It is important not to force instruments into the compartment and risk scuffing of the articular cartilage. Usually, adjusting the knee angle, which is near full extension, and increasing the valgus load applied to the joint will open up the medial joint space sufficiently. Another option to aid visualization in this area is to use a 70-degree arthroscope through the intercondylar notch, although this is rarely needed in our experience. Posterolateral or posteromedial portals may also improve access to this area. In certain extremely tight knees, one may consider recessing the MCL by a "pie-crust" technique. We prefer to do this with a 14-gauge needle rather than a scalpel. Insert it into the joint through the MCL and, without removing it from the skin, repeatedly puncture the MCL multiple times while applying a valgus force. The joint space should slowly increase without creating a full-thickness iatrogenic tear of the ligament. If the knee joint opens excessively after this maneuver, we use a hinged knee brace postoperatively until the ligament tightens. When compared with the alternative of injury to the articular cartilage, the sequela of tearing the MCL seems to be fairly minor.

Meniscal Preparation

The meniscus tear site must be prepared properly prior to applying the fixation. We compare repairing the meniscus with treatment for nonunion of a bony fracture. Adequate blood flow to the area must be established, the two sides must be anatomically reduced, and stable fixation must be used to promote an environment conducive to healing. Failure at any of these stages can compromise the overall success.

First, fibrous tissue has to be removed from the meniscal edges to create surfaces conducive for healing. We typically accomplish this with a rasp, but one could also use a small motorized shaver. If a shaver is chosen, minimal or no suction should be used to avoid overly aggressive débridement.

There are multiple techniques to promote a vascular environment. Abrasion of the synovial fringes extending over the peripheral edges of the meniscus with a rasp can stimulate a proliferative response to enhance healing.[23] In a rabbit model, this has been shown to improve the mechanical properties of the healed meniscus significantly.[24] Another option is trephination of the peripheral meniscal rim. We prefer to do this by creating multiple perforations with an 18- or 20-gauge needle from outside-in. This technique creates conduits for vascular migration to the tear. It is important to minimize channel size to limit disruption of the collagen framework that provides the beneficial biomechanical properties of the meniscus.[25] Rotational flaps of vascular synovial pedicles have also been shown to aid meniscal healing in animal models, but are rarely used in humans because of difficulties applying this technique arthroscopically.[26]

Similar to an unstable fracture pattern, temporary fixation is used to hold the reduction before final fixation is inserted. With unstable meniscus tears, a probe is used to reduce and hold the inner portion to the peripheral side while a small needle is introduced from outside-in across the tear. The probe can then be removed and permanent fixation applied.

Fixation

It is important to achieve fixation that is perpendicular to the tear to maximize compressive forces across it. We find that this is usually best achieved by viewing through the ipsilateral portal and placing instrumentation through the contralateral portal. For fixation of posterior tears near the root, the surgeon may sometimes find it beneficial to switch portals and place the instruments through the ipsilateral side while being mindful of avoiding injury to the neurovascular structures. In addition, most devices used to place the fixation come in varying degrees of curvature to aid in proper placement.

Vertical mattress orientation of the sutures is preferred whenever possible. These have been shown to be superior biome-chanically to horizontal mattress and mulberry knot techniques.[27] The number of fixation points used depends on the length and stability of the tear. Most surgeons tend to space fixators or sutures 5 to 8 mm apart. It is important to range the knee several times after final fixation has been applied. If subsequent gapping or displacement is noted, additional fixation or alternate methods must be added.

The choice regarding which fixation technique to use varies based on tear size, configuration, and location, as well as surgeon preference (igs 1 to 6). It is also important to recognize that meniscal fixators cost significantly more than sutures. Typically, for tears located posteriorly, we prefer all-inside meniscal fixators to limit the risk of neurovascular injury. For anterior third tears, we typically use an outside-in technique. Once started, we often continue to use this technique into the middle third of the meniscus. It is not uncommon for us to achieve hybrid fixation with different techniques in the same tear.

Inside-Out Repair.   Inside-out repairs are best suited for middle or posterior tears. Medially, the saphenous nerve is at risk. With

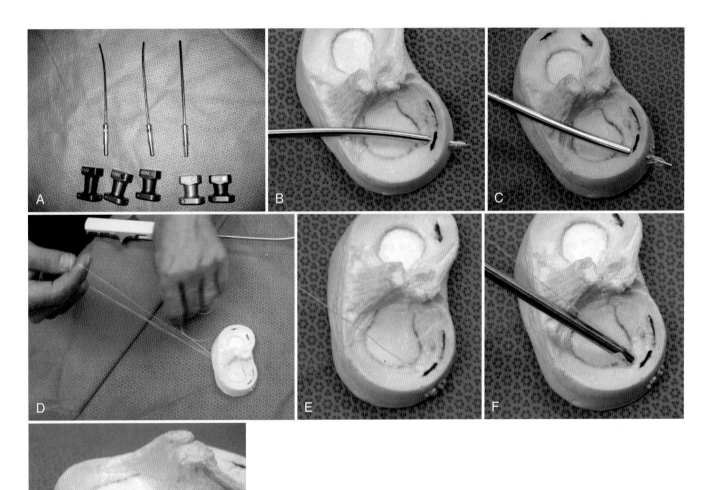

FIGURE 7-1 Biomet (Warsaw, Ind) MaxFire technique. **A,** Choose appropriate cannula and depth limiter. **B,** Deploy first anchor with the green lever. **C,** Retract green lever, reposition device, and deploy second anchor with red lever. **D,** Remove cannula and pull on loop until appropriate tension is achieved at repair site. **E,** Pull single strand to bring loop down to repair. **F,** Cut suture. **G,** Final view of repair.

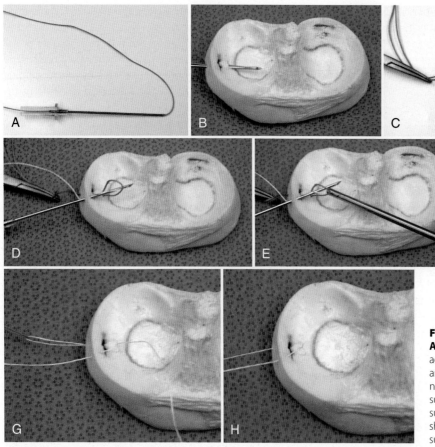

FIGURE 7-2 Outside-in spinal needle technique. **A,** Load suture into needle. **B,** Pass needle outside-in across tear. **C,** Withdraw needle, leaving intraarticular suture loop. **D,** Reload second suture into needle and pass across tear again. **E,** Pass second suture through loop and grasp it. **F,** Pull second suture out arthroscopic portal. **G,** Use first suture to shuttle second suture across tear. **H,** Tie second suture to complete the repair.

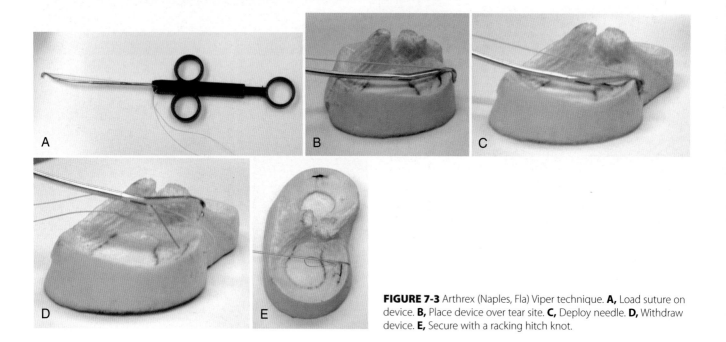

FIGURE 7-3 Arthrex (Naples, Fla) Viper technique. **A,** Load suture on device. **B,** Place device over tear site. **C,** Deploy needle. **D,** Withdraw device. **E,** Secure with a racking hitch knot.

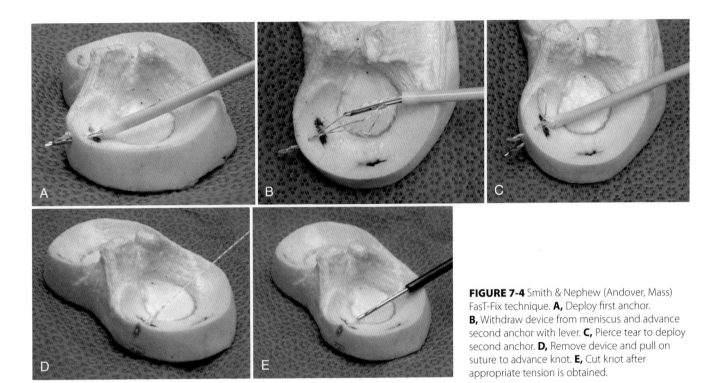

FIGURE 7-4 Smith & Nephew (Andover, Mass) FasT-Fix technique. **A,** Deploy first anchor. **B,** Withdraw device from meniscus and advance second anchor with lever. **C,** Pierce tear to deploy second anchor. **D,** Remove device and pull on suture to advance knot. **E,** Cut knot after appropriate tension is obtained.

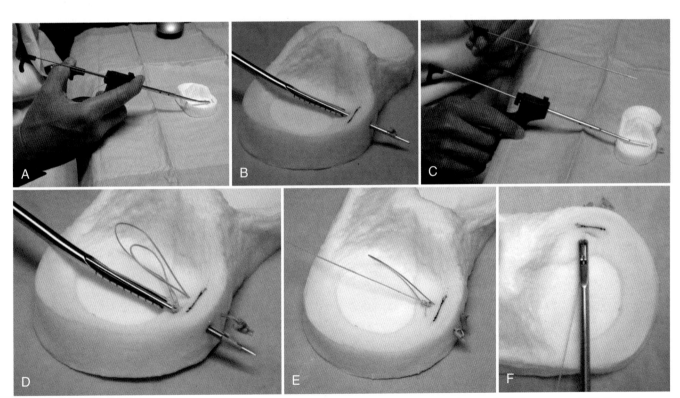

FIGURE 7-5 Arthrex (Naples, Fla) Meniscal Cinch technique. **A,** Hold device like a syringe. **B,** Deploy first needle. **C,** Remove needle. **D,** Reposition device and fire second needle. **E,** Pull on single strand. **F,** Cut suture once tensioned appropriately.

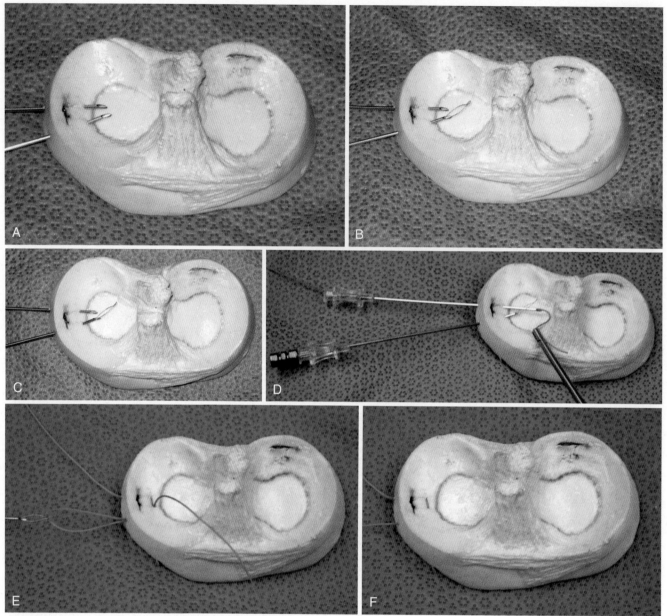

FIGURE 7-6 Smith & Nephew (Andover, Mass) Meniscus Mender II technique. **A,** Introduce both needles in desired position. **B,** Advance wire loop through needle. **C,** Advance suture through second needle after placing it through loop. **D,** Grasp suture and pull out through portal. **E,** Pull needle and wire loop out to shuttle suture across tear. **F,** Tie suture over capsule.

the arthroscope in the anterolateral portal, it is brought up to the medial tear to transilluminate the skin where the planned incision is to be made. One can visualize the saphenous vein in this manner, knowing that the nerve lies immediately posterior and therefore can be avoided. Flex the knee 90 degrees also to let the nerve slide posteriorly, away from the area that is being manipulated. A 4-cm incision is made in line with the posteromedial border of the tibia, just posterior to the MCL. Place one third of the incision proximally and two thirds distally to the joint line. Dissect carefully through the subcutaneous tissues. Incise the fascia anterior to the sartorius muscle. Retract it posteriorly, along with the semitendinosus. Anteriorly, you will see the superficial MCL. Develop the interval between the joint capsule and the medial head of the gastrocnemius bluntly with a finger. Place a

retractor or pediatric gynecologic speculum posteriorly to retract the gastrocnemius and semimembranosus.

The common peroneal nerve is at greatest risk laterally. Once again, flex the knee 90 degrees to let it drift posterior to the operative field. Make a 4-cm incision just posterior to the lateral collateral ligament. It should be centered just distally to the joint line, but should not extend beyond the level of the fibular head. This is the soft spot of the lateral knee, where posterolateral portals are made. After dissection through the subcutaneous tissues, identify the iliotibial band and biceps femoris. Retract the biceps posteriorly to protect the peroneal nerve. Elevate the lateral head of the gastrocnemius off the knee capsule and place a retractor or pediatric gynecologic speculum posteriorly.

The surgeon uses zone-specific cannulas to direct the sutures within the knee. These also aid in reducing slightly displaced tears while the sutures are passed. The cannula tips are fairly sharp to prevent slipping off the meniscus once placed; however, iatrogenic damage to the articular cartilage should be avoided as the cannulas are carefully inserted into the knee joint. Aim the cannula so that it is parallel or slightly inferior to the joint line. Use no. 2-0 non-absorbable sutures on double-armed flexible needles. Reusable Nitinol needles are also cost-effective. An assistant holds the gastrocnemius retractor while waiting to retrieve the sutures. Excellent communication is essential to pass each stitch safely. The surgeon lets the assistant know when he or she begins passing the suture. The assistant watches intently for the needle while making sure to keep herself or himself safely away from the surgical field to avoid an accidental stick. Once it is visible, the assistant notifies the surgeon to stop passing it and grabs it with a needle driver or mosquito clamp. If the needle is not visible after passing it 2 to 3 cm, the surgeon should reassess the situation to make sure that it is being directed in the proper orientation. Pass the second arm of the suture in a similar fashion. Cut off the needles and tag each pair of sutures with a clamp. Repeat this process as necessary at the desired points along the tear. On the lateral side, we try not to capture the popliteus tendon.

Once all the sutures have been placed, apply tension to them to assess the adequacy of the repair while visualizing and probing arthroscopically. If satisfied, then tie the stitches from posterior to anterior. Make sure to tension the construct adequately, but pulling too hard will either break the sutures or have them pull through the meniscus. The surgeon should try to visualize tying the knots over the capsule directly to avoid entrapping any vital structures.

Outside-In Repair. Although useful for tears in the anterior two thirds of the meniscus, it less useful for posterior third tears because of the inability to place sutures perpendicular to the tear. Typically, this technique permits a smaller incision than inside-out repairs. Sometimes, however, multiple passes through the meniscus are required until one is satisfied with placement; improper placement could damage the underlying collagen framework unnecessarily. The surgeon may initially consider intentionally passing the needle through the synovium superior to the meniscus to make sure that it has the proper orientation and location prior to perforating the meniscus itself.

One very simple and cost-effective technique was first described in 2004.[28] Preload an 18-gauge needle with a suture that is at least 40 cm long. Roughly 10 cm of the stitch should extend beyond the needle tip. Transilluminate the skin to help identify where the needle should be placed. Pierce both the inner and outer portions on the meniscus across the tear. The needle should be directed so that it comes out on the superior surface of the inner meniscal rim. Use an arthroscopic grasper through the ipsilateral portal to hold the loop inside the knee joint while withdrawing the needle. Pull the needle out away from the skin approximately 15 cm without unloading the suture, or the surgeon may choose to reload the needle with a second suture. Tag the two suture limbs coming from the skin. Reinsert the needle through the same track and perforate the superior portion of the peripheral rim only in a vertical mattress fashion. Direct the needle so that it passes through the suture loop held by the grasper. Use the grasper to grab the suture from the needle tip and pull it out the ipsilateral portal. Pull on the two sutures held by the tag clamp to shuttle the suture from the second needle insertion through the path from the first insertion. Remove the needle and repeat the process as necessary.

Regardless of the method, make a small incision once all the sutures have been passed. Spread bluntly down to the level of the capsule and tie the stitches down. Make sure not to entrap any vital structures. As an alternative, the surgeon could also make the incision initially at the start of the repair and subsequently pass the needles through it.

All-Inside Repair. A number of devices are on the market for all-inside repairs of meniscal tears. These have the benefit of less time needed to insert and the ability to be placed without the need of a surgical assistant. Also, accessory incisions may be avoided. Generally, these cost more than suture-based fixation methods.

The first generation of all-inside meniscal fixators consisted of rigid, bioabsorbable arrows, darts, and screws that could be placed across tears. Each device has a specific technique for insertion, but in general a curved cannula is used to place them in the proper location. After the tear is pierced with a trocar, the device is screwed or tapped into position. These fixators do not allow for the ability to tension the repair. In addition, several studies have demonstrated unacceptable failure rates and serious complications, including chondral scoring from the fixator's head, implant breakage, insertion difficulties, and postoperative joint line irritation from the devices.[29,30]

A second generation of suture-based meniscal fixators has emerged. These bioabsorbable implants incorporate dual anchors connected by a pretied, sliding, self-locking knot. The first anchor is deployed through the meniscus and capsule. Depending on the specific implant design, the second anchor is designed to sit on the meniscal surface or to be placed though the meniscus and capsule in another area. The sliding knot can be tensioned appropriately to compress the tear site. Care must be taken during insertion not to plunge too deeply through the capsule to avoid neurovascular injury.

Adjuncts to Repair

As noted, simultaneous ACL reconstruction has been shown to enhance the ability of the meniscus to heal. One theory is that the tear is bathed postoperatively in cytokines and growth factors from the bone marrow released during tunnel drilling and notchplasty.[19] This has led to the development of several methods to try and mimic this milieu. Intercondylar microfracture with an awl can simulate the environment created by a notchplasty, but the results have not been studied clinically.[31] A fibrin clot can be made with the patient's whole blood stirred in a container with a sintered glass rod. This should be placed in the tear prior to compressing it with the fixation. Studies have suggested that it may improve meniscal healing for red-white tears.[32] Platelet-rich plasma derived from whole-blood centrifugation provides growth factors in higher concentrations than fibrin clot and has shown promise in promoting healing elsewhere in the body, but has not been studied for meniscal repair.[19]

PEARLS & PITFALLS

1. Treat a meniscus tear like a bony nonunion.
2. Proper patient selection is essential to maximize the healing potential of a repair.
3. Make sure that the tourniquet is not inflated when assessing the vascularity of the tear.
4. Use temporary fixation to hold a tear in a reduced position.
5. Test the fixation to ensure that it is stable by having the patient flex and extend the knee.
6. Apply fixation perpendicular to the tear to maximize compression.
7. Avoid injuring the articular cartilage; "pie-crust" the MCL if necessary to obtain adequate exposure.
8. Use a vertical mattress suture configuration when possible.
9. Consider the use of adjunctive healing factors, such as platelet-rich plasma.
10. Strict adherence to the postoperative rehabilitation protocol will decrease the risk of failure.

Postoperative Rehabilitation Protocol

We do not follow an aggressive rehabilitation protocol postoperatively. The patient is toe-touch weight bearing for the first 2 weeks in a knee immobilizer. Sitting or supine range of motion exercises begin at week 3. Progressive weight bearing in the immobilizer is allowed during weeks 3 and 4. Unrestricted walking out of the brace starts after 4 weeks. We also encourage the use of a stationary bike at that time. We discourage squatting until the patient is 4 months postoperative to reduce forces applied to the repair while it is healing. Patients are allowed to return to cutting sports 6 months after surgery. When an ACL reconstruction is done at the same time, our rehabilitation protocol for the meniscal repair takes precedence.

CONCLUSIONS

The meniscus serves several essential functions in the normal knee. When injured, every effort should be made to preserve as much of the meniscus as possible. Certain types of tears are more amenable to repair than others. Historically, arthroscopically assisted suture repairs through an accessory incision are the gold standard for treatment and can provide excellent outcomes. However, there has been a recent trend toward less invasive all-inside implants because of their ease of insertion. Newer designs for the all-inside fixators have emerged, with lower complications and improved healing rates. In addition to the advances in implant design, there is evidence that adjuncts such as platelet-rich plasma may enhance the ability of the meniscus to heal. More research needs to be done in this area, but early data are promising. Overall, repair of the meniscus can be a satisfying procedure with a high chance of a successful outcome if it is performed correctly, with adherence to accepted indications.

REFERENCES

1. Annandale T. An operation for displaced semilunar cartilage. *Br J Med.* 1885;April 18:779.
2. Ahmed AM, Burke DL. In-vitro measurement of static pressure distribution in synovial joints. Part I: tibial surface of the knee. *J Biomech Eng.* 1983;105:216-225.
3. Seedholm BB, Hargreaves DJ. Transmission of the load in the knee joint with special reference to the role of the menisci. *Eng Med.* 1979;8:220.
4. Barber FA, McGarry JE. Meniscal repair techniques. *Sports Med Arthrosc Rev.* 2007;15:199-207.
5. Turman KA, Diduch DR. Meniscal repair:indications and techniques. *J Knee Surg.* 2008;21:154-162.
6. Rath E, Richmond JC. The menisci: basic science and advances in treatment. *Br J Sports Med.* 2000;34:252-257.
7. Scott WN, ed. *Surgery of the Knee,* 4th ed. Philadelphia: Elsevier; 2006:15-24.
8. Bullough PG, Munuera L, Murphy J, Weinstein AM. The strength of the menisci of the knee as it relates to their fine structure. *J Bone Joint Surg Br.* 1970;52:564-567.
9. McDevitt CA, Webber RJ. The ultrastructure and biochemistry of the meniscal cartilage. *Clin Orthop Relat Res.* 1990;(252):8-18.
10. Post MD, Akers MS, Vincent K. Load to failure of common meniscal repair techniques: effects of suture technique and suture material. *Arthroscopy.* 1997;13:731-736.
11. Arnoczky SP, Warren RF. Microvasculature of the human meniscus. *Am J Sports Med.* 1982;10:90-95.
12. Greis P, Bardana D, Holstrom M, Burks R. Meniscal injury. I. Basic science and evaluation. *J Am Acad Orthop Surg.* 2002;168-187.
13. DeHaven KE. Decision-making features in the treatment of meniscal lesions. *Clin Orthop Relat Res.* 1990;252:49-54.
14. Terry GC, Tagert BE, Young MJ. Reliability of the clinical assessment in predicting the cause of internal derangements of the knee. *Arthroscopy.* 1995;11:568-576.
15. Hegendus EJ, Cook C, Hasselblad V, et al. Physical examination tests for assessing a torn meniscus in the knee: a systematic review with meta-analysis. *J Orthop Sports Phys Ther.* 2007;37:541-550.
16. Boden SD, Davis DO, Dina TS, et al. A Prospective and blinded investigation of magnetic resonance imaging of the knee: abnormal findings in asymptomatic subjects. *Clin Orthop Relat Res.* 1992;282:177-185.
17. Thoreaux P, Rety F, Nourissat G, et al. Bucket handle meniscal lesion: magnetic resonance imaging criteria for reparability. *Arthroscopy.* 2006;9:954-961.
18. Magee T, Shapiro M, Rodriguez J, et al. MR arthrography of postoperative knee: for which patients is it useful? *Radiology.* 2003;229:159-163.
19. Scott WN, ed. *Surgery of the Knee,* 4th ed. Elsevier; 2006:481-490.
20. Rispoli DM, Miller MD. Options in meniscal repair. *Clin Sports Med.* 1999;18:77-91.
21. Cannon WD, Vittori JM. The incidence of healing in arthroscopic meniscal repairs in anterior cruciate ligament–reconstructed knees versus stable knees. *Am J Sports Med.* 1992;20:176-181.
22. Noyes FR, Barber-Westin SD. Arthroscopic repair of meniscus tears extending into the avascular zone with or without anterior cruciate ligament reconstruction in patients 40 years of age and older. *Arthroscopy.* 2000;16:822-829.
23. Ritchie JR, Miller MD, Bents RT, Smith DK. Meniscal repair in the goat model. The use of healing adjuncts and the role of magnetic resonance arthrography in repair evaluation. *Am J Sports Med.* 1998;26:278-284.
24. Okuda K, Ochi M, Uchio Y. Meniscal rasping for repair of meniscal tear in the avascular zone. *Arthroscopy.* 1999;15:281-286.
25. DeHaven KE, Arnoczky SP. Meniscal repair. Part I: basic science, indications for repair, and open repair. *J Bone Joint Surg* 1994;76:140-152.
26. Kobuna Y, Shirakura K, Niijima M. Meniscal repair using a flap of synovium. An experimental study in the dog. *Am J Knee Surg.* 1995;8:52-55.
27. Post WR, Akers SR, Kish V. Load to failure of common meniscal repair techniques: effects of suture technique and material. *Arthroscopy.* 1997;13:731-736.
28. Laupattarakasem W, Sumanont S, Kesprayura S, Kasemkijwattana C. Arthroscopic outside-in meniscal repair through a needle hole. *Arthroscopy.* 2004;20:654-657.
29. Kurzweil PR, Tifford CD, Ignacio EM. Unsatisfactory clinical results of meniscal repair using the meniscus arrow. *Arthroscopy.* 2005;21:905-907.
30. Lee GP, Diduch D. Deteriorating outcomes after meniscal repair using the meniscal arrow in knees undergoing concurrent anterior cruciate ligament reconstruction: increased failure rate with long-term follow-up. *Am J Sports Med.* 2005;33:1138-1141.
31. Freedman KB, Nho SJ, Cole BJ. Marrow-stimulating technique to augment meniscus repair. *Arthroscopy.* 2003;19:794-798.
32. McAndrews PT, Arnoczky SP. Meniscal repair enhancement techniques. *Clin Sports Med.* 1996;15:499-510.

Meniscal Transplantation

Nicole A. Friel ● Mark A. Slabaugh ● Brian J. Cole

Surgical treatment of meniscus lesions has changed significantly over time. Meniscal tears were traditionally treated with meniscal excision, but it became understood that loss of the meniscus alters the biologic and biomechanical environment of the knee.[1,2] The resulting degenerative changes in the involved compartment led us away from meniscus removal and toward meniscus preservation. Partial meniscectomy and meniscus repair procedures have become the standard of care. For patients for whom meniscal preservation is not an option, meniscal allograft transplantation can be done for a select subset of patients who have become symptomatic from their meniscal deficiency. This offers restoration of anatomic and biomechanical function.

With the advent of meniscal transplantation procedures, several techniques have evolved, including separate bone plugs on the anterior and posterior horns as well as bone bridges (keyhole, trough, dovetail, and bridge in slot variations). The bone bridge is almost always used for the lateral meniscus because of the close proximity between the anterior and posterior horns. The medial meniscus can be anchored with either plugs or a bridge, because the anatomy of the anterior horn is variable and the plugs may allow for minor modifications. We prefer the bridge in slot technique for lateral and medial menisci for a number of reasons, including its simplicity and secure bony fixation, ability to perform concomitant procedures easily, and the ability to maintain the native anterior and posterior meniscal horn attachments.

ANATOMY

The menisci are semilunar-shaped fibrocartilaginous structures that function in shock absorption,[3] load transmission,[4-6] secondary mechanical stability,[7,8] joint lubrication,[9] and nutrition.[10] Circumferentially oriented collagen fibers provide resistance to hoop stresses whereas radially oriented fibers hold the circumferential fibers together and provide resistance to shear.[11,12] The anterior and posterior horns attach to bone by interdigitating collagen fibers oriented to transmit load and shear optimally from the meniscus to the tibia.[13]

The menisci are composed of 74% water,[14] allowing for optimization in force transmission. The lateral meniscus carries 70% of the lateral compartment load, compared with 50% by the medial meniscus.[6,15] The menisci transmit 50% of the joint load when in knee extension and 90% when the knee is in flexion.[6,15] Loss of the meniscus, therefore, increases the load on the articular cartilage surfaces and facilitates the development of early degenerative changes. Loss of just 16% to 35% of the meniscal tissue can lead to a 350% increase in contact forces.[4] Clinical studies support meniscus preservation, because a greater size of meniscal resection is associated with a poor clinical outcome.[16-19]

PATIENT EVALUATION

History

Eliciting a thorough history is especially important because causative factors, associated injuries, and prior treatments can all affect the treatment plan. Often, patients report a specific knee injury with subsequent surgical treatment consisting of meniscectomy or meniscal repair. Patients usually describe a period of pain relief following the surgery but, over time, joint line pain and activity-related swelling ensue. Recent operative reports or photographs are useful to rule out arthritic changes, which would otherwise contraindicate meniscal transplantation. In a setting in which recent information is unavailable regarding the anatomy and pathology in the knee (e.g., from a recent arthroscopy), it might be prudent to consider a diagnostic arthroscopy to provide updated information for proper surgical planning.

Physical Examination

Examination often reveals full range of motion. Depending on recent activity, a joint effusion may be present. Joint line or femoral condyle tenderness is occasionally found. A thorough physical examination is essential to reveal malalignment, ligament deficiency, or articular cartilage lesions that would modify the treatment plan. These findings need to be addressed, either as a concurrent or staged procedure.

Diagnostic Imaging

A complete set of radiographs must be obtained to evaluate limb alignment and the degree of joint space narrowing and secondary osteoarthritic changes caused by a prior meniscectomy. In addition, a magnification marker or quarter should be placed on the cassette at the level of the joint line on two orthogonal views for meniscal sizing. Views include weight-bearing anteroposterior (AP) in full extension, weight-bearing posteroanterior (PA) in 45-degree-flexion, non–weight-bearing 45-degree-flexion, axial view of the patellofemoral joint, and a long leg mechanical axis view.

Magnetic resonance imaging (MRI) is usually reserved for challenging cases when certain questions are left unanswered. The extent of meniscectomy, status of the articular cartilage, and degree of subchondral edema in the involved compartment can all be assessed by MRI.

TREATMENT

Indications and Contraindications

The success of meniscal transplantation depends on careful selection of the ideal candidate. Typically, patients are relatively young (younger than 50 years) and often present with a history of prior total or subtotal meniscectomy with persistent pain localized to the meniscus-deficient compartment. The knee joint must be stable or stabilized and have normal alignment, with intact articular surfaces (grade I or II). Any grade III or IV lesions should be focal and require concomitant treatment.

Although not absolute contraindications, chondral defects, malalignment, or ligamentous instability all require consideration for concurrent or staged procedures to ensure that all joint pathology is addressed. In the past, full-thickness chondral defects were considered a contraindication; however, cartilage degeneration is not a significant risk factor for meniscal allograft failure.[20] Outcomes of many concurrent procedures, including meniscal transplantation with concurrent autologous chondrocyte implantation (ACI)[21,22] and osteochondral allograft[32] have shown excellent results in the carefully selected patient.

Concurrent or staged corrective osteotomy is indicated for patients with deviation toward the involved compartment. Axial malalignment can exert abnormal pressure on the newly placed graft, which can lead to loosening, overload, degeneration, and failure.[23-25]

Anterior cruciate ligament (ACL)–deficient patients who have had a prior medial meniscectomy may benefit from concomitant ACL reconstruction (ACLR) and meniscal transplantation. Many studies have shown that meniscectomized ACL-deficient knees lead to worsening degenerative changes. The more aggressive approach of combination ACLR and meniscal transplantation has good long-term follow-up as opposed to untreated (left alone) knees. In addition, the posterior horn of the medial meniscus is an important secondary stabilizer to anterior translation and may

be important in preventing secondary "stretch" of the ACL reconstructed knee.[7,26-28]

Contraindications for meniscal transplantation include diffuse arthritic changes, squaring or flattening of the femoral condyle or tibial plateau, significant osteophyte formation in the involved compartment, tibiofemoral subluxation, inflammatory arthritis, synovial disease, previous joint infection, skeletal immaturity, or marked obesity.

Conservative Management

Patients who have had a prior meniscectomy should have a trial of conservative treatment before consideration of operative measures. Activity modifications, anti-inflammatory medications, and occasionally injections can be recommended to help determine which patients can function without surgical intervention. More aggressive management of the relatively young patient following lateral meniscectomy might be considered, especially in female athletes with slight valgus who are at significant risk for the development of progressive lateral compartment arthritis.[29]

PEARLS & PITFALLS

- Patient selection for operative intervention is crucial. Patients must be able to understand the indications, activity limitations, and possible outcomes.
- Patients who are overweight or have unrealistic expectations regarding excessive postoperative function need to realize that the longevity of the meniscal graft is negatively affected by these two variables.

Arthroscopic Technique

Preoperative Planning

Allograft Sizing. The success of meniscal transplantation is dependent on careful size matching of the meniscus allograft to the native meniscus. Meniscal allografts are compartment- and size-specific. Anteroposterior and lateral preoperative radiographs with sizing markers are important for meniscal sizing (Figs. 8-1 and

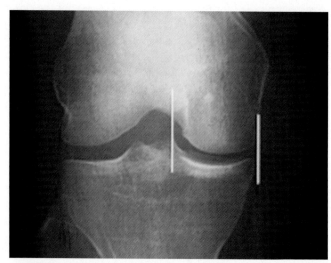

FIGURE 8-1 Preoperative AP radiograph, weight bearing. Note the slight medial compartment narrowing and sclerosis of the subchondral tibial plateau.

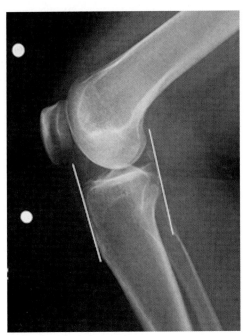

FIGURE 8-2 Preoperative lateral radiograph in flexion with sizing markers anteriorly, which allow the meniscus to be sized properly.

8-2). Allograft sizing is of significant importance, because oversized meniscal allografts lead to greater forces across the articular cartilage.[30] On the other hand, undersized allografts result in greater forces seen by the meniscal tissue.[30] The meniscus width is determined on the AP radiograph by measuring from the edge of the ipsilateral tibial spine to the edge of the tibial plateau. Meniscal length is determined on the lateral radiograph as determined by the AP dimension of the ipsilateral tibial plateau. These measurements, after correction for magnification, are multiplied by 0.8 for medial and 0.7 for lateral meniscus. Other methods using height and weight have been proposed, but are not routinely used.[31,32]

Meniscal Graft Processing and Preservation. Meniscal allografts are harvested using sterile surgical technique ideally within 24 hours after death and frozen to −80° C. Although other graft preservation methods are used, including secondary sterilization methods, fresh-frozen grafts remain the most commonly used allograft preservation method.[33-35]

Stringent donor selection is based on comprehensive medical and social history. The risk of disease transmission is further reduced by screening for human immunodeficiency virus (HIV), human T-cell lymphotropic virus (HTLV), hepatitis B and C, and syphilis. Blood cultures for aerobic and anaerobic bacteria, as well as lymph node sampling, may be performed. Graft processing, including débridement, ultrasonic-pulsatile washing, and use of ethanol to denature proteins, further lowers the risk of disease transmission.[36]

PEARLS & PITFALLS

- Be aware of the techniques used to sterilize the meniscal allograft; different companies use different proprietary sterilization techniques.

- Sizing of the meniscal allograft based on radiographs should be confirmed with the company representative prior to the day of surgery. The day of surgery is too late to find out that the graft is too small or large.

Anesthesia

Meniscal transplantation can be performed under regional, spinal, or general anesthesia based on surgeon and anesthesia preferences. Patient age, comorbidities, and adverse events with previous anesthesia are important in the decision-making process.

Positioning

The patient is positioned supine on a standard operating room table. A tourniquet is placed around the thigh, and the extremity is placed in a standard leg holder, allowing full knee flexion. It is important that the posterolateral or posteromedial corner be freely accessible for inside-out suturing of the meniscus.

Surgical Anatomy, Incisions, and Portals

Important surgical landmarks to be identified are the patella, patellar tendon, tibial plateau, and fibular head. Portals and incisions include inferomedial and inferolateral arthroscopy portals, an accessory outflow portal, a posterolateral or posteromedial incision, and a miniarthrotomy adjacent to or splitting the patellar tendon on the transplant side (Fig. 8-3).

Caution should be taken while making incisions because many structures are at risk, depending on the approach. These include the peroneal nerve and lateral collateral ligament with the posterolateral approach, the saphenous nerve and medial collateral ligament with the posteromedial approach, and the patellar tendon with the anterior miniarthrotomy. In addition, the posterior neurovascular bundle can be damaged during needle passage when suturing the meniscus in place, especially on the lateral side.

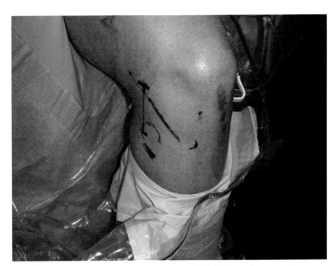

FIGURE 8-3 Intraoperative photograph of a left knee showing the lateral incisions in preparation for a lateral meniscal transplantation. The oblique mark shows the path of the iliotibial band. The head of the fibula is marked as well.

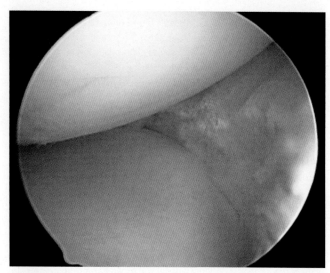

FIGURE 8-4 Intraoperative depiction of the anterior horn and body of a medial meniscus débridement in preparation for meniscal transplantation.

Examination Under Anesthesia and Diagnostic Arthroscopy

Examination under anesthesia evaluates range of motion and ligamentous instability. Diagnostic arthroscopy is completed to confirm the preoperative diagnosis and evaluate any changes in articular cartilage.

PEARLS&PITFALLS

- Diagnostic arthroscopy should confirm any arthrosis in the affected compartment; grade I or II cartilage damage is acceptable at the time of meniscal transplantation.
- Grade IV chondral damage should be treated with concomitant allografting of the femoral condyle.

Arthroscopic Preparation. Initially, the steps for medical and lateral meniscal transplantation are similar. The remaining meniscus is arthroscopically débrided to a 1- to 2-mm peripheral rim until punctate bleeding occurs (Fig. 8-4). The most anterior part of the meniscus can be excised with an no. 11 scalpel through the respective anterior portal. The anterior and posterior horn insertion sites should be maintained, because they are helpful markers during preparation of the slot. In addition, limited notchplasty along the posterior and inferior femoral condyle allows for improved visualization of the posterior horn during passage of the graft.

PEARLS&PITFALLS

- Resection of the femoral condyle at the notch can be performed to improve visualization for medial or lateral meniscal transplantation.
- Resection of the anterior horn is accomplished with a no. 11 blade or back biter.
- A no. 15 blade can also be used to resect the anterior meniscus because no. 11 blade tips often break if too much torque is placed on the knife.

Exposure. A miniarthrotomy is preformed directly adjacent to or through the patellar tendon on the affected side, in line with the patellar tendon fibers. To allow correct orientation of the slot and introduction of the graft, the arthrotomy is performed in line with the insertion sites of the anterior and posterior horns of the involved meniscus. Prior localization with a spinal needle to determine the proper trajectory is helpful to ensure proper incision location. The incision should extend approximately one-third above the joint line and two thirds below the joint line.

For lateral meniscal transplantations, a second posterolateral incision is made at the interval between the posterior edge of the iliotibial band and the anterior edge of the biceps femoris tendon. The gastrocnemius muscle-tendon junction is elevated off the posterior capsule at the joint line, and the meniscal retractor is placed anterior to the muscle. Proper retraction allows suture tying beneath these structures to minimize the chances of soft tissue tethering with flexion or extension.

For medial meniscal transplants, a second posteromedial incision is made, just anterior to the hamstrings tendons. The sartorial fascia is incised and the hamstrings tendons are retracted posteriorly. The interval is opened between the posteromedial aspect of the capsule just anterior to the gastrocnemius and semitendinosus tendons. Proper retraction facilitates retrieval and suturing of meniscal sutures.

PEARLS&PITFALLS

- Localization with a spinal needle helps determine the patellar incision and the proper trajectory of the meniscal bone slot.
- Incision should be at the joint line; an incision too inferior or superior will make it difficult to achieve the proper angles in subsequent steps.

Slot Preparaztion. Slot orientation follows the normal anatomy of the meniscal attachment sites. Electrocautery is used to establish a line connecting the center of the anterior and posterior horn attachment sites. Using this line as a guide, a 4-mm burr is used to make a straight anterior to posterior reference slot in the tibial plateau (Fig. 8-5). Slot height and width will equal the dimensions of the burr, and its alignment in the sagittal plane should parallel the slope on the tibial plateau. Slot measurements, including the AP length of the tibial plateau, are confirmed by placement of a depth gauge in the reference slot (Fig. 8-6). A drill guide is used to place a guide pin just distal and parallel to the reference slot (Figs. 8-7 and 8-8). The drill guide is advanced to but not through the posterior cortex. The pin is subsequently overreamed with a 7- or 8-mm cannulated drill bit (Fig. 8-9). A box cutter osteotome is then used to widen the trough to 7 to 8 mm and deepen it to 10 mm (Fig. 8-10). This is then refined with a 7- to 8-mm rasp to allow insertion of the bone bridge of the allograft. Final slot preparation is shown in Figure 8-11.

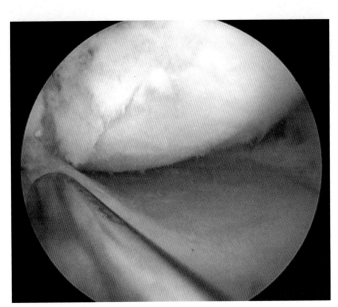

FIGURE 8-5 Intraoperative depiction of a 4-mm burr directly in line with the anterior and posterior horn of the medial meniscus. The burr will make a preliminary slot for measuring and placing the guide pin.

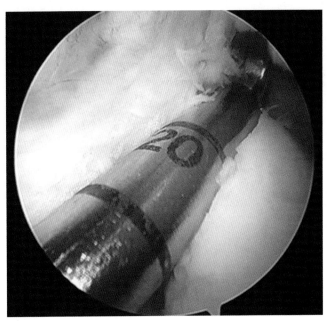

FIGURE 8-6 Intraoperative depiction of the depth gauge and guide pin placement.

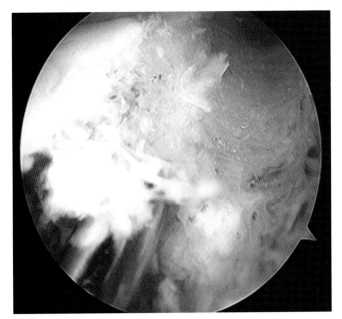

FIGURE 8-7 Intraoperative depiction of the burr slot with the guide pin inserted. Partial reaming has been performed to ensure that the trajectory and depth are appropriate prior to finishing reaming to the posterior cortex.

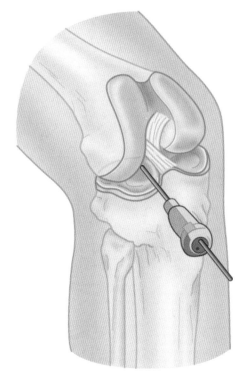

FIGURE 8-8 Schematic representation of a guide pin positioned in the superficial tibial plateau reference slot.

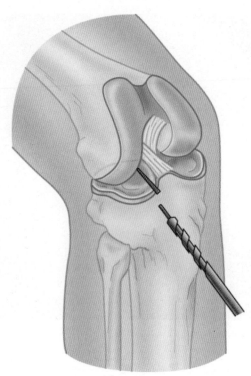

FIGURE 8-9 Schematic of a cannulated drill bit used to create the tibial tunnel over the pin placed through the guide just distal and parallel to the slot created by the burr.

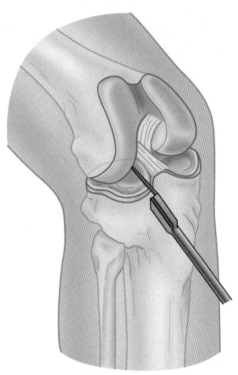

FIGURE 8-10 Schematic representation of the box cutter, which is impacted over the guide pin into the tibial tunnel to create a slot 7 to 8 mm wide all the way to the posterior cortex.

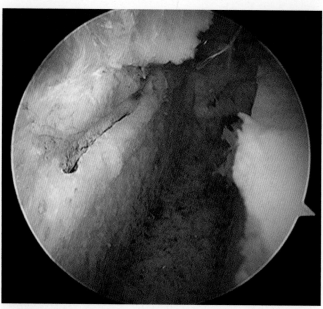

FIGURE 8-11 Intraoperative depiction of final slot preparation. The slot is 8 mm wide and extends to the posterior cortex.

PEARLS & PITFALLS

- Place the initial guide pin with the knee in flexion and do not penetrate the posterior cortex. Consider fluoroscopic guidance.
- Ensure that the box-cutting osteotome is in line with the prior burr cut.
- Use a curette to clear remaining bone from the slot.
- During initial burring for slot preparation in a medial meniscal transplantation, be aware of and avoid the ACL insertion. Approximately 25% of its insertion can be violated before concerns of instability arise.
- Do not violate the posterior cortex when reaming.

Meniscal Allograft Preparation. The meniscus allograft tissue arrives as a hemiplateau with an attached meniscus. All non-meniscal soft tissue is removed. Attachment sites of the meniscus are identified on the bone block, and the accessory attachments are débrided, leaving only true attachment sites (approximately 5 to 6 mm wide). The meniscus is then prepared to achieve the desired width and length, as determined by the slot preparation. The width of the bone bridge is intentionally undersized by 1 mm to facilitate graft passage into the slot and reduce inadvertent bridge fracture during placement. The bone bridge is then cut to a width of 7 mm and a height of 10 mm. Bone extending beyond the posterior horn attachment is removed so that the posterior wall of the bone bridge will be flush with the most posterior edge of the prepared slot. Bone extending to the anterior horn, however, should be preserved to maintain graft integrity and ease in graft insertion. A vertical mattress traction suture (0 polydioxanone [PDS]) is placed at the junction of the posterior horn and middle thirds of the meniscus (Fig. 8-12).

If the anterior horn attachment is larger (up to 9 mm wide), the attachment should be left intact and the width of the bone bridge should be increased accordingly in the area of the anterior horn insertion only. The remainder of the bone bridge should be

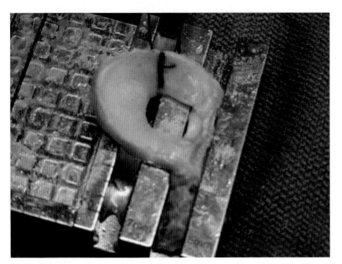

FIGURE 8-12 Final graft preparation shows that the meniscal horn attachment sites have been preserved and the bone bridge easily fits into an 8-mm slot. Also note the PDS suture at the posterior third junction of the meniscus.

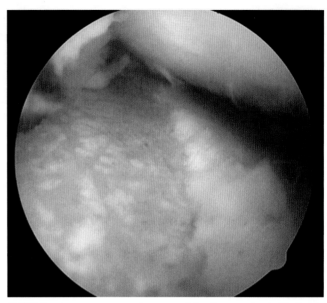

FIGURE 8-13 Intraoperative depiction of the slot completely filled with the bone bridge. This is held in place with a freer and fixed with an interference screw

the intended 7 mm. To accommodate the increased width, the corresponding area of the recipient slot should be widened.

PEARLS&PITFALLS

- All soft tissue should be removed from the meniscal graft and bone block to help with visualization during insertion.
- The word "TOP" is written on the superior portion of the meniscus to ensure that the graft has not flipped or rotated during insertion.
- Care must be taken to not damage the meniscal insertion sites when cutting the bone block.
- The bone block should be the same depth as the trough created to avoid a prominent bone block that needs to be burred down after insertion.

Meniscus Insertion and Fixation. Using a single-barrel, zone-specific meniscal repair cannula placed through the contralateral portal, a Nitinol suture-passing pin is placed through the capsule at the attachment site of the posterior middle third of the meniscus. The proximal end of the Nitinol pin is withdrawn from the anterior arthrotomy site, the allograft traction sutures are passed through the loop of the Nitinol pin, and the pin and traction sutures are withdrawn through the accessory incision. With the aid of the traction sutures, the meniscal allograft is pulled through into the joint through the anterior arthrotomy while the bone bridge is advanced into the tibial slot. The meniscus is manually reduced under the condyle with a finger placed through the arthrotomy. Appropriate varus or valgus stress is needed to open the ipsilateral compartment as well as flexion-extension aids in graft introduction and reduction.

Once the meniscus is reduced, the knee is cycled to ensure proper placement and capturing by the tibiofemoral articulation. A guidewire is inserted between the bone bridge and the medial eminence side of the slot. A tap is inserted over the guidewire to

create a path for the interference screw, with the bone bridge held in place manually (typically, a freer; Fig. 8-13). The bone bridge is then secured within the tibial slot with a 7 × 25-mm bioabsorbable cortical interference screw. This step is typically done in flexion under direct visualization.

Finally, the graft is attached to the capsule with eight to ten standard inside-out vertical mattress sutures (2-0 Ethibond) placed equally on the superior and inferior meniscal surfaces (Figs. 8-14 and 8-15). Sutures should be placed peripherally on the meniscus, because sutures placed in the middle or inner third of the meniscus can weaken the implant. For medial transplants, this fixation can be modified with the use of appropriate all-inside fixation devices placed most posteriorly and outside-in sutures placed most anteriorly.

PEARLS&PITFALLS

- If the slot is off slightly medially or laterally to the desired position, it is possible to realign the bone trough by placing the interference screw on the opposite side.
- Varus or valgus stress can open up the compartment to facilitate meniscal passage into the appropriate position.
- Meniscal stitches are started at the site of the traction sutures and placed sequentially anteriorly and posteriorly to ensure correct tension.
- At least 10 sutures are needed to secure the meniscus circumferentially.
- Too much pressure on the bone block during insertion can cause it to break. If this occurs, transosseous sutures are placed through the posterior and anterior bone blocks and passed through a drill whole made in the posterior and anterior central aspect of the tibial slot, facilitated by using an ACL guide. The sutures are retrieved from outside-in using a suture passer and tied over the anterior cortex to secure the two fragments of bone block.

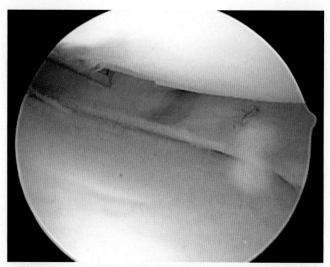

FIGURE 8-14 Intraoperative depiction of inside-outside meniscal repair. Note the vertical mattress orientation of the sutures. Sutures are placed alternatively on the inferior and superior surfaces.

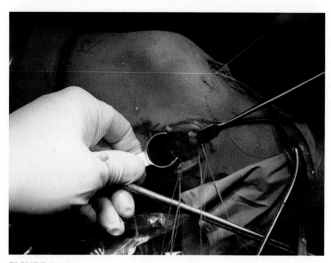

FIGURE 8-15 Intraoperative depiction of inside-outside meniscal repair of the transplant. A meniscal retractor is used to deflect the needles away from the posterior knee and out of the incision.

Closure. Standard closure of the arthrotomy and accessory portal incisions is performed.

Concurrent Procedures

Anterior Cruciate Ligament and Medial Meniscal Transplantation. In case of a concurrent ACL reconstruction, a soft tissue graft (hamstring autograft, Achilles allograft, tibialis anterior allograft, or hamstring allograft) is recommended, because this allows for a smaller diameter tibial tunnel. The ACL tibial tunnel is drilled as obliquely as possible, entering the medial aspect of the tibial footprint. Then, the femoral tunnel is drilled. Following tunnel placement, the meniscal slot should be prepared, as described earlier. Graft placement occurs in a sequential order—femoral fixation is completed first, followed by meniscal transplantation, and lastly tibial fixation of the ACL graft. The meniscus is secured with an interference screw between the ACL and the most lateral aspect of the

bridge. Tibial ACL fixation as the final step allows maximum separation of the tibiofemoral joint during meniscal transplantation.

> **PEARLS & PITFALLS**
>
> - Drill the tibial tunnel first before making the trough for the meniscal transplantation.
> - Soft tissue graft is preferred to make passing the graft easier with a meniscal transplant in place.
> - Notch the bone bridge at the site of ACL tibial tunnel to reduce intersection pressure of the ACL graft against the bone bridge.
> - With inadequate fixation from an interference screw, consider placing two transosseous sutures through the bone block anteriorly and posteriorly as described when the block inadvertently fractures during preparation or insertion. Remove a small segment of bone between the two bone blocks to accommodate the ACL as it courses from the tibia to the femur.

High Tibial Osteotomy and Medial Meniscal Transplantation. All aspects of the meniscal transplantation are performed first. Varus or valgus stresses are needed to place the meniscus graft and, if not completed first, could jeopardize fixation of the osteotomy. The open wedge osteotomy is performed as distally as possible, with the osteotomy wedge passing at least 1.5 cm below the bottom of the tibial slot.

> **PEARLS & PITFALLS**
>
> - Two Steinmann pins can be placed above the osteotomy site but below the slot to prevent propagation of the osteotomy into the slot.

Cartilage Restoration and Meniscal Transplantation. If ACI or osteochondral allografting is performed simultaneously, it is usually safer and easier to perform all steps of the meniscal transplantation and then proceed to the cartilage restoration procedure. Care should be taken, however, to avoid damage to the anterior horn of the transplanted meniscus with the arthrotomy and while placing osteochondral grafts.

> **PEARLS & PITFALLS**
>
> - Perform meniscal transplantation prior to the cartilage procedure. All the meniscal sutures except the anterior horn can be placed as noted above. The anterior horn can be stitched through the anterior arthrotomy at the end.
> - Avoid damage to the meniscus graft by flexing the knee and using a retractor while performing the cartilage procedure.

Postoperative Rehabilitation Protocol

Immediate partial weight-bearing is allowed in a hinged knee brace, with range of motion limited to 0 to 60 degrees of flexion for the first 2 weeks and to 90 degrees at 4 weeks. Non–weight-bearing flexion beyond 90 degrees is also allowed immediately. Progression to full weight bearing and range of motion as well as strengthening exercises are achieved at 4 weeks postoperatively. Squatting and pivoting are avoided

TABLE 8-1 Results of Meniscal Allograft Transplantation.

Study (Year)	No. of Patients	Follow-Up (yr)	Outcome
Rue et al (2008)[22]	31	3.1	80% with MTx + ACI completely or mostly satisfied; 71% with MTx + OA completely or mostly satisfied
Farr et al (2007)[21]	29	4.5	32/36 (89%) successful
von Lewinski (2007)[37]	5	20	Lysholm score of 74 points
Homman et al (2007)[38]	20	10	25% medial and 50% lateral failed; pain and Lysholm scores improved in 90%
Stone et al (2006)[20]	47	4.4	42/47 (89%) success
Kim and Bin (2006)[39]	14	4.8	92.9% survival
Sekiya and Ellingson (2006)[40]	32	3.3	96% had improvement in function and activity level
Verdonk et al (2006)[41]	31	12.1	90% satisfied with outcome; 18% failure rate
Cole et al (2006)[42]	45	2.8	41/45 (91%) successful; 77.5% completely or mostly satisfied
Verdonk et al (2005)[43]	100	7.2	74% 10-yr survival for medial; 70% 10-yr survival for lateral
Graf et al (2004)[44]	8	9.7	6/8 (75%) pleased with knee function and activity level
Sekiya et al (2003)[45]	28	2.8	86% normal or near-normal on IKDC examination; 26/28 (93%) "greatly improved" (21) or somewhat improved" (5)
Yoldas et al (2003)[46]	31	2.9	30/31 (97%) "greatly improved" (22) or somewhat improved" (8)
Van Arkel and de Boer (2002)[53]	57	5	Survival 76% for lateral, 50% for medial, 67% for combined
Ryu et al (2002)[48]	26	2.8	83% overall satisfaction
Wirth et al (2002)[49]	23	3 14	Lysholm score = 84 ± 12 at 3 yr; 75 ± 23 at 14 yr
Rath et al (2001)[50]	23	5.4	8/22 re-tears; 14/22 (64%) successful
Stollsteimer et al (2000)[51]	23	3.3	18/22 (82%) patients had improved pain
Cameron and Saha (1997)[23]	67	2.5	58/67 (87%) good to excellent results
Van Arkel and de Boer (1995)[47]	23	3	20/23 (87%) satisfactory results
Garrett (1993)[52]	43	2-7	35/43 (81%) successful

ACI, autologous chondrocyte implantation; MTx, meniscus transplant; OA, osteochondral allograft.

until 16 weeks, at which in-line running is permitted. Return to full activity is permitted after 6 months as long as strength is 80% that of the contralateral leg.

CONCLUSIONS

Meniscal allograft transplantation yields good to excellent results in almost 85% of patients (Table 8-1). Patients demonstrate significant decrease in pain, as well as an increase in activity. Long-term success is encouraging in well-selected patients but it is unknown whether meniscal transplantation is protective against the progression of degenerative changes.

REFERENCES

1. Allen PR, Denham RA, Swan AV. Late degenerative changes after meniscectomy. Factors affecting the knee after operation. *J Bone Joint Surg Br.* 1984;66:666-671.
2. Baratz ME, Fu FH, Mengato R. Meniscal tears: the effect of meniscectomy and of repair on intraarticular contact areas and stress in the human knee. A preliminary report. *Am J Sports Med.* 1986;14:270-275.
3. Voloshin AS, Wosk J. Shock absorption of meniscectomized and painful knees: a comparative in vivo study. *J Biomed Eng* 1983;5:157-161.
4. Seedhom BB, Hargreaves DJ. Transmission of load in the knee joint with special reference to the role of the menisci: part II. Experimental results, discussions, and conclusions. *Eng Med Biol.* 1979;8:220-228.
5. Seedhom BB, Dowson D, Wright V. Proceedings: functions of the menisci. A preliminary study. *Ann Rheum Dis.* 1974;33:111.
6. Walker PS, Erkman MJ. The role of the menisci in force transmission across the knee. *Clin Orthop Relat Res* 1975;(109):184-192.
7. Levy IM, Torzilli PA, Warren RF. The effect of medial meniscectomy on anterior-posterior motion of the knee. *J Bone Joint Surg Am.* 1982;64:883-888.
8. Markolf KL, Mensch JS, Amstutz HC. Stiffness and laxity of the knee—the contributions of the supporting structures. A quantitative in vitro study. *J Bone Joint Surg Am.* 1976;58:583-594.
9. MacConaill MA. The movements of bones and joints; the synovial fluid and its assistants. *J Bone Joint Surg Br.* 1950;32:244-252.
10. Renstrom P, Johnson RJ. Anatomy and biomechanics of the menisci. *Clin Sports Med.* 1990;9:523-538.
11. Bullough PG, Munuera L, Murphy J, et al. The strength of the menisci of the knee as it relates to their fine structure. *J Bone Joint Surg Br.* 1970;52:564-567.
12. McDevitt CA, Webber RJ. The ultrastructure and biochemistry of meniscal cartilage. *Clin Orthop Relat Res.* 1990;(252):8-18.
13. Gao J, Wei X, Messner K. Healing of the anterior attachment of the rabbit meniscus to bone. *Clin Orthop Relat Res.* 1998;(348):246-258.
14. Cole BJ, Carter TR, Rodeo SA. Allograft meniscal transplantation: background, techniques, and results. *Instr Course Lect.* 2003;52:383-396.

15. Ahmed AM, Burke DL. In-vitro measurement of static pressure distribution in synovial joints. Part I: tibial surface of the knee. *J Biomech Eng.* 1983;105:216-225.

16. Bonneux I, Vandekerckhove B. Arthroscopic partial lateral meniscectomy long-term results in athletes. *Acta Orthop Belg.* 2002;68:356-361.

17. Higuchi H, Kimura M, Shirakura K, et al. Factors affecting long-term results after arthroscopic partial meniscectomy. *Clin Orthop Relat Res.* 2000;(377):161-168.

18. Meredith DS, Losina E, Mahomed NN, et al. Factors predicting functional and radiographic outcomes after arthroscopic partial meniscectomy: a review of the literature. *Arthroscopy.* 2005;21:211-223.

19. Rockborn P, Gillquist J. Outcome of arthroscopic meniscectomy. A 13-year physical and radiographic follow-up of 43 patients under 23 years of age. *Acta Orthop Scand.* 1995;66:113-117.

20. Stone KR, Walgenbach AW, Turek TJ, et al. Meniscus allograft survival in patients with moderate to severe unicompartmental arthritis: a 2- to 7-year follow-up. *Arthroscopy.* 2006;22:469-478.

21. Farr J, Rawal A, Marberry KM. Concomitant meniscal allograft transplantation and autologous chondrocyte implantation: minimum 2-year follow-up. *Am J Sports Med.* 2007;35:1459-1466.

22. Rue JP, Yanke AB, Busam ML, et al. Prospective evaluation of concurrent meniscus transplantation and articular cartilage repair: minimum 2-year follow-up. *Am J Sports Med.* 2008;36:1770-1778.

23. Cameron JC, Saha S. Meniscal allograft transplantation for unicompartmental arthritis of the knee. *Clin Orthop Relat Res.* 1997;(337):164-171.

24. de Boer HH, Koudstaal J. Failed meniscus transplantation. A report of three cases. *Clin Orthop Relat Res.* 1994; (306):155-162.

25. Noyes FR, Barber-Westin SD, Rankin M. Meniscal transplantation in symptomatic patients less than fifty years old. *J Bone Joint Surg Am.* 2005;87(suppl 1):149-165.

26. Alford W, Cole BJ. Failed ACL reconstruction and meniscus deficiency. Background, indications and techniques for revision ACL reconstruction with allograft meniscus transplantation. *Sports Med Arthrosc Rev.* 2005;13:93-102.

27. Shelbourne KD, Gray T. Results of anterior cruciate ligament reconstruction based on meniscus and articular cartilage status at the time of surgery. Five- to fifteen-year evaluations. *Am J Sports Med.* 2000;28: 446-452.

28. Shoemaker SC, Markolf KL. The role of the meniscus in the anterior-posterior stability of the loaded anterior cruciate-deficient knee. Effects of partial versus total excision. *J Bone Joint Surg Am.* 1986;68: 71-79.

29. Alford JW, Lewis P, Kang RW, et al. Rapid progression of chondral disease in the lateral compartment of the knee following meniscectomy. *Arthroscopy.* 2005;21:1505-1509.

30. Dienst M, Greis PE, Ellis BJ, et al. Effect of lateral meniscal allograft sizing on contact mechanics of the lateral tibial plateau: an experimental study in human cadaveric knee joints. *Am J Sports Med.* 2007;35: 34-42.

31. Stone KR, Freyer A, Turek T, et al. Meniscal sizing based on gender, height, and weight. *Arthroscopy.* 2007;23:503-508.

32. Van Thiel G, Verma NN, McNickle AG, et al. Meniscal allograft size can be predicted by height, weight and gender. *Arthroscopy* 2009;25: 722-727.

33. Alford W, Cole BJ. The indications and technique for meniscal transplant. *Orthop Clin North Am.* 2005;36:469-484.

34. McNickle AG, Wang VM, Shewman EF, et al. Performance of a sterile meniscal allograft in an ovine model. *Clin Orthop Relat Res.* 2009;467: 1868-1876.

35. Rodeo SA. Meniscal allografts—where do we stand? *Am J Sports Med.* 2001;29:246-261.

36. Vangsness CT,Jr, Garcia IA, Mills CR, et al. Allograft transplantation in the knee: tissue regulation, procurement, processing, and sterilization. *Am J Sports Med.* 2003;31:474-481.

37. von Lewinski G, Milachowski KA, Weismeier K, et al. Twenty-year results of combined meniscal allograft transplantation, anterior cruciate ligament reconstruction and advancement of the medial collateral ligament. *Knee Surg Sports Traumatol Arthrosc.* 2007;15:1072-1082.

38. Hommen JP, Applegate GR, Del Pizzo W. Meniscus allograft transplantation: ten-year results of cryopreserved allografts. *Arthroscopy.* 2007;23: 388-393.

39. Kim JM, Bin SI. Meniscal allograft transplantation after total meniscectomy of torn discoid lateral meniscus. *Arthroscopy.* 2006;22:1344-1350.

40. Sekiya JK, Ellingson CI. Meniscal allograft transplantation. *J Am Acad Orthop Surg.* 2006;14:164-174.

41. Verdonk PC, Verstraete KL, Almqvist KF, et al. Meniscal allograft transplantation: long-term clinical results with radiological and magnetic resonance imaging correlations. *Knee Surg Sports Traumatol Arthrosc.* 2006;14:694-706.

42. Cole BJ, Dennis MG, Lee SJ, et al. Prospective evaluation of allograft meniscus transplantation: a minimum 2-year follow-up. *Am J Sports Med.* 2006;34:919-927.

43. Verdonk PC, Demurie A, Almqvist KF, et al. Transplantation of viable meniscal allograft. Survivorship analysis and clinical outcome of one hundred cases. *J Bone Joint Surg Am.* 2005;87:715-724.

44. Graf KW Jr, Sekiya JK, Wojtys EM, et al. Long-term results after combined medial meniscal allograft transplantation and anterior cruciate ligament reconstruction: minimum 8.5-year follow-up study. *Arthroscopy.* 2004;20:129-140.

45. Sekiya JK, Giffin JR, Irrgang JJ, et al. Clinical outcomes after combined meniscal allograft transplantation and anterior cruciate ligament reconstruction. *Am J Sports Med.* 2003;31:896-906.

46. Yoldas EA, Sekiya JK, Irrgang JJ, et al. Arthroscopically assisted meniscal allograft transplantation with and without combined anterior cruciate ligament reconstruction. *Knee Surg Sports Traumatol Arthrosc.* 2003; 11:173-182.

47. Van Arkel ER, de Boer HH. Human meniscal transplantation. Preliminary results at 2- to 5-year follow-up. *J Bone Joint Surg Br.* 1995;77: 589-595.

48. Ryu RK, Dunbar VWH, Morse GG. Meniscal allograft replacement: a 1-year to 6-year experience. *Arthroscopy.* 2002;18:989-994.

49. Wirth CJ, Peters G, Milachowski KA, et al. Long-term results of meniscal allograft transplantation. *Am J Sports Med.* 2002;30:174-181.

50. Rath E, Richmond JC, Yassir W, et al. Meniscal allograft transplantation. Two- to eight-year results. *Am J Sports Med.* 2001;29:410-414.

51. Stollsteimer GT, Shelton WR, Dukes A, et al. Meniscal allograft transplantation: a 1- to 5-year follow-up of 22 patients. *Arthroscopy.* 2000; 16:343-347.

52. Garrett JC. Meniscal transplantation: a review of 43 cases with two- to seven-year follow-up. *Sports Med Arthrosc Rev.* 1993;2:163-167.

53. Van Arkel ER, de Boer HH. Survival analysis of human meniscal transplantations. *J Bone Joint Surg Br.* 2002;84:227-231.

SUGGESTED READINGS

Packer JD, Rodeo SA. Meniscal allograft transplantation. *Clin Sports Med.* 2009; 28:259-283.

Verma NN, Kolb E, Cole BJ, et al. The effects of medial meniscal transplantation techniques on intra-articular contact pressures. *J Knee Surg.* 2008; 21:20-26.

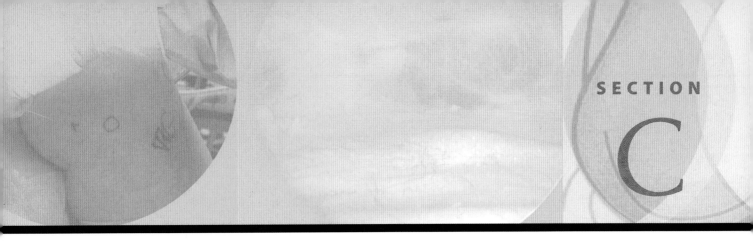

Patellar Techniques

Arthroscopic Evaluation and Diagnosis of the Patellofemoral Joint

Mark J. Lemos ● David W. Lemos ● Stephen E. Lemos

Historically, arthroscopy was used as a diagnostic modality. With the development of less invasive imaging technology (magnetic resonance imaging [MRI] and computed tomography [CT]), it is now rarely used as a purely diagnostic tool. Frequently, the exact cause of patellofemoral pain or maltracking is unknown and arthroscopy can help in the diagnosis and treatment of these problems. Causes of patellofemoral problems vary and include instability, maltracking, degenerative arthritis, and traumatic injury. With the advent of arthroscopy, orthopedic surgeons have added a significant tool to their diagnostic and therapeutic armamentarium.

In this chapter, we will focus on the following:

■ Preoperative assessment and classification of patellofemoral conditions
■ Patellofemoral arthroscopy—different techniques and tips; preferred technique
■ Specific pathologies (radiologic assessment, arthroscopic findings)—patellofemoral pain, chondromalacia, osteochondritis dissecans (OCD), instability, patellar maltracking

PATIENT EVALUATION

History and Physical Examination

History and physical examination continue to be the mainstay in the diagnosis of anterior knee pain. X-rays, CT, and MRI are all helpful imaging modalities to confirm possible diagnoses. Arthroscopy can also help in the confirmation and localization of patellofemoral lesions and in ruling out other pathologic lesions that may be responsible for the symptoms. However, it must also be mentioned that there are many pathologic lesions seen on arthroscopy that are asymptomatic. Primary complaints

by patients can be pain and/or instability caused by patellar dislocations, maltracking, overuse syndromes, tendinitis, localized trauma, saphenous neuritis, and apophysitis.

Patellofemoral pain usually presents as diffuse anterior knee pain. The pain generally worsens with activity and improves with rest. Most commonly, the onset is gradual and associated with physical activity. Chondral injury is usually worse during the activity and improves on stopping, whereas tendinitis improves with activity, but worsens in the period following activity. Also, tendinitis results in tenderness localized to the area of tendinitis (patellar tendon, quadriceps, iliotibial band).

Instability can result from pain-induced quadriceps inhibition secondary to meniscal pathology or ligamentous instability. This should be differentiated from patellofemoral instability. Patellar subluxation and dislocation can be differentiated from each other by weakness and effusion being prevalent with patellar dislocation. Only truly unstable subluxation results in abnormal motion of the patellofemoral joint. Crepitus and swelling are other common complaints indicating chondral injury.

Differentiating acute from chronic problems, the quality of the patient's pain, and what makes it better and worse all help the clinician make the diagnosis. Table 9-1 presents the major subjective differences when taking a history of a patient's problem with patellofemoral complaints.

The physical examination should be performed with the goal of systematically evaluating the entire lower extremity. Patellofemoral problems can stem from malalignment secondary to femoral anteversion, genu recurvatum, genu varum, genu valgum, tibial torsion, pes planus, or ligamentous laxity. The extensor mechanism should be evaluated, as well as patellar position, mobility, and tracking.

TABLE 9-1 Symptoms of Specific Patellofemoral Problems

Symptom	Chondral Injury	Tendinitis	Patellofemoral Arthrosis	Patellofemoral Instability
Pain worse	During activity	After activity	During activity	With subluxation
Popliteal pain	No	No	Yes	No
Nature of the pain	Mechanical	Localized to tendon	Ache	Sensation of abnormal motion of patellofemoral joint
Giving way	Yes	Yes	Yes	No
Weakness	Yes, 2 degrees to pain	Yes, 2 degrees to pain	Yes, 2 degrees to pain	Less consistent
Effusion	Small	No	Small	Large after patellar dislocations

Patellofemoral function and pathology are dependent on bony anatomy, lower limb alignment, and soft tissue restraints, including muscle function and ligamentous stability. Start with a general assessment of the patient's condition, ligamentous laxity, and overall posture. Perform a vascular examination of the lower extremities, including posterior tibial and dorsalis pedis pulses. A neurologic evaluation of sensation, motor strength, and reflexes should also be performed. Vascular and, more important, neurologic disorders can lead to patellofemoral problems that are not as easily treated and need to be identified to be managed appropriately.

Next, the examiner should evaluate the joints above and below the knee (hip along with the foot and ankle). It is easy to focus on the knee and patellofemoral joint. Examine all aspects of the knee prior to focusing on the suspected patellofemoral problem (Table 9-2).

Anatomy

The anatomical landmarks of the patellofemoral joint are the seven facets of the posterior patella (Fig. 9-1). The medial and lateral facets are each divided into roughly equal thirds and the seventh facet is the odd facet located on the extreme medial border of the patella. On the trochlear side, the patella articulates with the femoral joint surface on the medial and lateral sides of the trochlear groove. The contact area pressures vary in location and load depending on the level of flexion. The patellofemoral contact, load, and tracking are also affected by anatomical variants, as described by Wiberg and Baumgartl (Fig. 9-2). Also, anatomic abnormalities such as patella baja, patella alta, trochlear dysplasia, rotational alignment of the femur and tibia, foot alignment, tight lateral retinaculum, and vastus medialis strength also play a role in the tracking and articulating pressures and contact locations (Fig. 9-3).

TABLE 9-2 Physical Examination of the Patellofemoral Joint

Parameter	Features	Abnormal Findings
Observation	Alignment	Varus, valgus, patella (alta, baja, or squinting), decreased foot progression angle, pes planus (increased forefoot pronation)
Palpation	Knee joint	Effusion, tenderness, crepitus, pain with patellar compression on ROM
Range of motion (ROM)	Passive and active	Amount of ROM, limited end points, extensor lag
Special tests		
J sign	Centering of patella at >30 degrees of knee flexion	Significant lateral displacement of patella at terminal extension
Lateral pull test	Relax and contract quadriceps in extension	Lateral displacement of patella occurs with quadriceps contraction in full extension
Patellar glide test	Done at full extension and 20 degrees of flexion	Lateral → translation of > 50% of patella width is abnormal; if no hard end point, MPFL (53% of lateral stability) is out Medial → < 6 mm or < 30% patellar width is tight lateral retinaculum; >10 mm or >45% indicates hypermobile patella
Patellar tilt	Caused by adaptive shortening of lateral retinaculum; associated with increased lateral facet loading	Lateral border of patella cannot be elevated above medial border
Q angle measured at 20 to 30 degrees	Angle of ASIS-patella and patella-tibial tubercle	>15 degrees

ASIS, anterosuperior iliac spine.

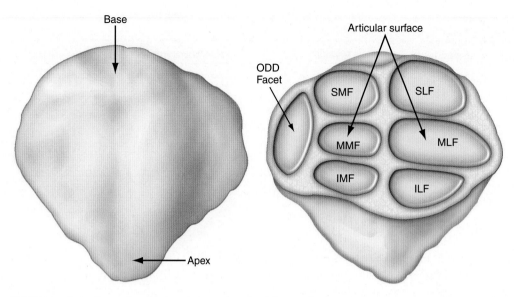

FIGURE 9-1 Seven facets described on the articular side of the patella. Illustrated are the superior medial facet (SMF), middle medial facet (MMF), inferior medial facet (IMF), superior lateral facet (SLF), middle lateral facet (MLF), inferior lateral facet (ILF), and odd facet.

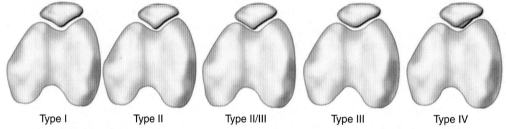

FIGURE 9-2 Anatomic variants of the patella as described by Wiberg and Baumgartl.[23] I. Equal medial and lateral facets which are both slightly concave (normal anatomy), II. Smaller medial than lateral facet, medial facet is flat or slightly convex, III. Very small medial facet which is convex, IV. Without a medial ridge or medial facet.

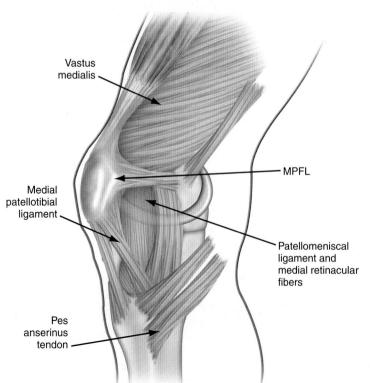

FIGURE 9-3 Anatomy of the medial aspect of the knee. The MPFL provides 53% of the restraint to lateral displacement of the patella. The patellomeniscal ligament and medial retinacular fibers are responsible for 22% of patellar restraint.

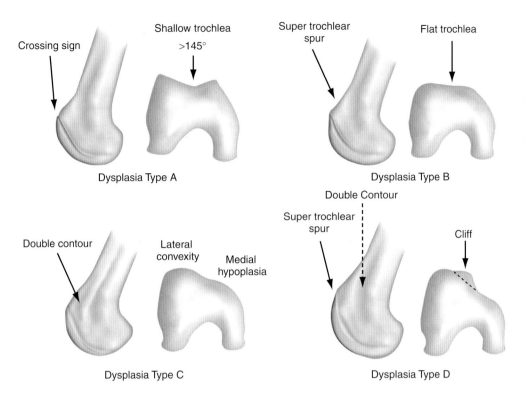

FIGURE 9-4 Trochlear dysplasia as described by Dejour. **Type A,** Shallow trochlea. Look for the crossing sign on the lateral x-ray. **Type B,** Flat trochlea. Look for trochlear spur on lateral x-ray. **Type C,** Lateral convexity and medial hypoplasia. Look for double contour on lateral. **Type D,** Cliff type; supratrochlear spur and double contour on lateral x-ray.

Alignment can also be assessed with the Q angle. As the knee angle changes the Q angle changes. It is largest with the knee in full extension. This has been proposed to be the reason for patellar subluxation/dislocation with the deforming force being greatest in the most unstable position. The foot-up model of the dynamic Q angle is based on the premise that increased foot pronation results in tibial internal rotation producing an inturned knee posture and "functional" valgus.

Anatomic variations responsible for patellofemoral problems vary, depending on the pathology. Excessive femoral anteversion, tibial torsion, patella alta, and shallow trochlea are all causes of patellar instability, and pain caused by instability (Fig. 9-4).

Diagnostic Imaging

Proper diagnostic imaging is very important in the diagnosis of the root cause of the problem. Patellofemoral pain versus instability can have similar causes. Limb alignment may be assessed on clinical examination. The first images that should be obtained because of availability and ease of use are x-rays. Obtaining standing anteroposterior (AP) lateral views, skyline views of the patellofemoral joint, and standing notch views help in assessing the bony anatomy of the knee. Standing long leg views are important to obtain to assess alignment. Long leg views can assess varus and valgus malalignment, and skyline views can assess patellofemoral cartilage thickness, gross patellar tracking, and whether there is increased patellar tilt. However, routine radiographs have been shown to identify fewer than 50% of osteochondral loose bodies.

When the patella does not engage in the trochlea by 15 to 20 degrees of knee flexion, patella alta may be present. Patella alta may be radiographically assessed in many ways. Laurin and

Merchant axial radiographs are obtained with the knee flexed 20 and 40 degrees, respectively (Fig. 9-5). These assess patellar tilt, but one tangential radiograph obtained at 30 degrees of flexion is sufficient in most cases. The x-ray beam is projected caudad at an angle of 30 degrees from the plane of the femur. A line is drawn along the lateral facet of the patella, and a second line is drawn between the condyles of the trochlea anteriorly. Normally, the angle between these two lines will be open laterally. However, if the lines are parallel or the angle opens medially, the patella is probably tilted.

Teitge and colleagues[1] have described a radiographic technique that can be helpful for diagnosing patellar instability. They obtained bilateral axial radiographs of the patellofemoral joints in anatomic position, with constant medial and lateral force applied to the patellae with an instrumented device, and then axial radiography was repeated. It was found that a 4-mm increase in medial or lateral patellar excursion compared with the patellar excursion on the asymptomatic knee correlated with patellar instability. Stress radiographs are helpful in identifying patients with congruity of the articular surfaces whose knees may subluxate or dislocate because of deficient ligamentous structures. Patients who are unable to relax the extensor mechanism because of pain or who have bilateral symptoms are not candidates for stress radiography.

Once x-rays have been evaluated, limb alignment may be further evaluated for rotational malalignment with an overlay alignment CT scan to measure femoral anteversion and tibial torsion. CT has been shown to be more sensitive than axial radiography in delineating patellar malalignment[2]; it allows axial cuts of the patellofemoral articulation at angles less than 20 degrees of knee flexion, which enhances the detection of subluxation as

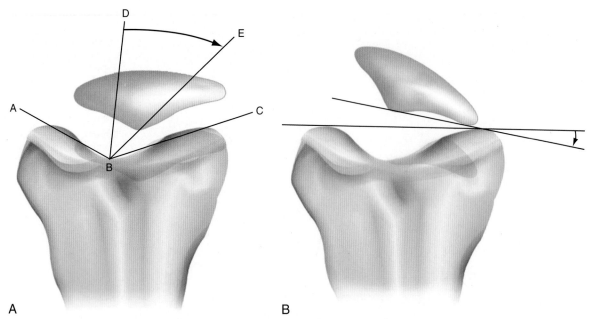

FIGURE 9-5 A, Diagram of the Merchant skyline radiographic view. The sulcus angle ABC is bisected by BD and line BE passes from the deepest point of the sulcus through the most posterior point on the ridge of the patella. The positive congruence angle DBE indicates lateral translation. **B,** The Laurin angle is negative, indicating patellar lateral tilt.

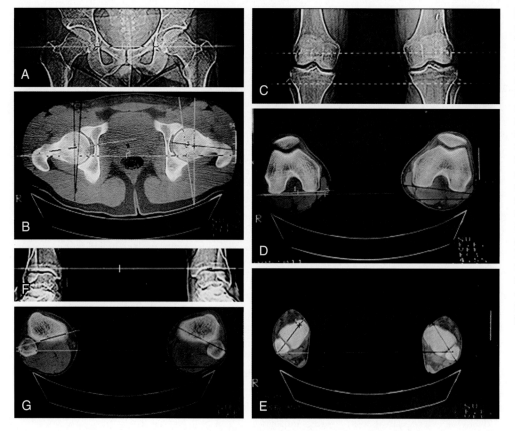

FIGURE 9-6 Top left, (A) Frontal scans of hips and (**B**) first transverse section. This should image the greater trochanter, femoral neck, femoral head, and acetabulum of both sides. **Right, (C)** Frontal scan of the knees and second and third transverse sections as seen on the frontal scan of the knees. (**D**) The second transverse section is made through the middle of the lateral condyle of the femur, below the lower pole of the patella. (**E**) The third section should image the tibial condyles and fibular head of both sides. **Lower left, (F)** Frontal scan of the ankles with the fourth reference line for the transverse section through the lower end of the tibia, which bisects the most distal area of the tibia. (**G**) The fourth transverse section should image the tibia and fibula on both sides.

the patella loses the stabilizing function of the lateral femoral condyle. Another role for CT is in identifying lateralization of the tibial tubercle, as measured by the distance between the tibial tubercle and the trochlear sulcus (Fig. 9-6). An axial CT image demonstrating the femoral trochlear groove is superimposed on an axial image of the tibial tubercle. A line is drawn on this superimposed image between the posterior margins of the femoral condyles. Two lines are drawn perpendicular to this line, one bisecting the femoral trochlear groove and the other bisecting the anterior tibial tuberosity. The distance between these two lines determines the extent of lateralization of the tibial tubercle. Values greater than 9 mm have been shown to identify patients with patellofemoral malalignment, with a specificity of 95% and a sensitivity of 85%.[3]

The mean tibial tuberosity-trochlear groove (TTTG) distance is 12 mm in the normal knee. However, in people with a history of patellar dislocation, it has been shown to be more than 20 mm (as measured by CT, with the knee extended) in 56% of individuals (Fig. 9-7).[4] There has been an association between trochlear and patellar dysplasia and patellofemoral arthritis. Of individuals with isolated patellofemoral osteoarthritis, 42% had a Wiberg type II patella.[5] The sulcus angle and TTTG distance have been shown to have the strongest correlations with patellar instability.[6]

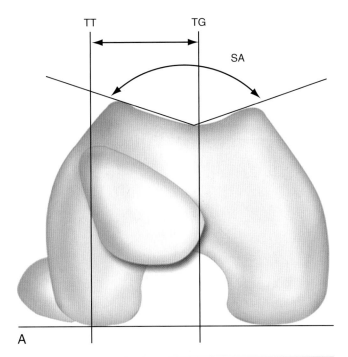

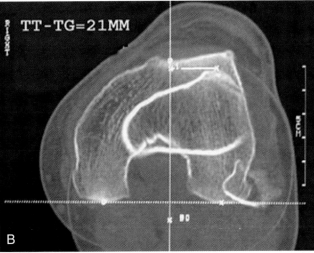

FIGURE 9-7 A, Diagram of TTTG distance. This also shows the sulcus angle (SA). **B,** The TTTG distance as measured by superimposing axial CT images of the tibial tubercle and the trochlear groove with the knee in extension.

A rotational CT scan is used to look at femoral anteversion and tibial torsion. Normal measurements for femoral anteversion vary widely and there is significant controversy regarding acceptable normal levels. The femoral anteversion range is 14 to 28 degrees, whereas the mean tibiofibular torsion range is 16 to 50 degrees.[7]

MRI is more effective at identifying articular-cartilage damage directly for large lesions or indirectly by changes in the underlying bone for smaller lesions. Sallay and associates[8] have used MRI to visualize the pathoanatomic features of patellar dislocations. They identified the essential lesion of patellar dislocations as a tear of the medial patellofemoral ligament (MPFL) off the femoral insertion. The location of the injury was confirmed by surgical exploration. Although other authors have identified avulsions of the MPFL from the patella with the use of MRI alone, this is an uncommon location for injury and may be overinterpreted on MRI studies of patients.

Joint Geometry

Stability of the patellofemoral joint is dependent on the shape of the trochlear groove and the steepness of the slope of the patellar facets. The trochlear groove was first analyzed radiographically by Merchant with the skyline radiographic view performed at 45 degrees of knee flexion. This assesses the patellar position within the groove. The congruence angle of Merchant[9] is used to identify lateral translation and the lateral patellar angle of Laurin is used to identify lateral tilt.[10]

The lateral facet of the patella is responsible for 60% of the load across the normal patellofemoral joint. As the knee flexes, the contact force on the patellofemoral joint increases. Conversely, as the knee moves toward full extension, the contact force decreases and the patella leaves the trochlear groove as it moves proximally. At this point, the patella is dependent on the soft tissues for lateral stability. Contact points on the femoral trochlea and patella change as the knee flexes more (Fig. 9-8).[11] The starting point of the patella is lateral, with a catching mechanism that moves the patella medially into the trochlear groove at initial flexion. The patella then tracks in the trochlear groove moving distally, laterally, and posteriorly in line with the groove orientation.

The amount of load across the patella increases with the degree of flexion, so that at 20 degrees the load across the patellofemoral joint is more proximal in the trochlear groove and more distal on the patella. The load across the patellofemoral joint increases with larger vector forces associated with increased knee flexion. The loads are larger more distally on the trochlea and, as noted, the lateral facet translates 60% of this load. The patellar surface that articulates with the femur changes from distal to proximal on the patella. Therefore, the larger loads seen on the patella are more proximal.[12] The forces have been estimated to increase to 20 times body weight with jumping, 7.6 times with deep squats, and 3.3 times with stairs.[13]

Therefore, abnormal loads resulting in cartilaginous damage are usually seen in the areas represented by higher flexion with chronic patellofemoral osteoarthritis (OA). Loads are also seen to be higher in knees with patella alta (Fig. 9-9). However, in cases of patellar instability and maltracking, the areas of pathologic

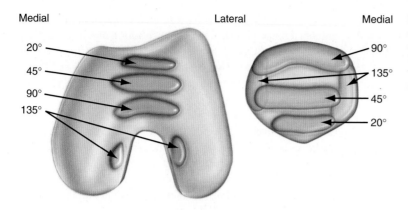

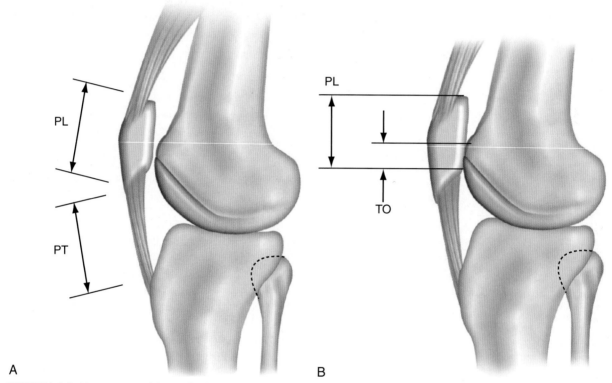

FIGURE 9-8 Knee flexion causes the patellofemoral joint contact area to move distally and posteriorly across the surface of the femur and proximally across the patella. However, in deep flexion, the patellar contact area changes to two separate areas as it bridges the femoral intercondylar notch.

FIGURE 9-9 A, Measurement of the Insall-Salvati ratio, which is the ratio of the patellar tendon length (PT) to the length of the patella (PL), as measured on a lateral knee xray. The PL/PT is normally 0.8 to 1.2. **B,** Measurement of the patellotrochlear index, which is a reflection of the functional height of the patella TO/PL It is used to examine for patella alta if the PL/PT ratio is negative.

findings represent the cause of the maltracking. A subluxating patella will be damaged with the dislocation and, more specifically, relocation of the patella, whereas a lateral tracking patella will have increased wear of the lateral facet and lateral trochlea.

Classification of Patellofemoral Disorders

A clinical classification of patellofemoral disorders was developed by Merchant[14] based on cause. The five major categories are trauma, patellofemoral dysplasia, idiopathic chondromalacia patella, osteochondritis dissecans, and synovial plicae. Also, pigmented villonodular synovitis (PVNS) can present as an asymptomatic finding, but can cause patellofemoral pain.[15] In this chapter, we will present examples of these different causes of patellofemoral problems and their arthroscopic presentations.

Holmes and Clancy[16] have proposed a clinical classification of anterior knee pathology that has three major classification classes: patellofemoral instability, patellofemoral pain with malalignment, and patellofemoral pain without malalignment (Box 9-1).

First, it is first important to characterize the primary complaint, instability versus pain. Second, what is the primary cause of the complaint? Once the differential diagnosis is narrowed down, diagnostic imaging can be used to work up the diagnosis. Finally, arthroscopy can be used to evaluate the cause and degree of the pathology further.

Box 9-1 Holmes-Clancy Clinical Classification of Anterior Knee Pathology

Patellofemoral Instability
- Subluxation or dislocation, single episode
- Subluxation or dislocation, recurrent
  Lateral subluxation or dislocation—normal functional Q angle; increased functional Q angle
- Femoral anteversion, external tibial torsion, genu valgum, foot hyperpronation
  Dysplastic trochlea
  Grossly inadequate medial stabilizers
  Patella alta
  Tight lateral retinaculum
  Medial subluxation or dislocation—iatrogenic
- Chronic dislocation patella—congenital, acquired
- Associated fractures
  Osteochondral
  Avulsion

Patellofemoral Pain With Malalignment
- Increased functional Q angle
  Femoral anteversion
  External tibial torsion
  Genu valgum
  Foot hyperpronation
- Tight lateral retinaculum (lateral patellar compression syndrome)
- Grossly inadequate medial stabilizers
- Patella alta
- Patella baja
- Dysplastic femoral trochlea

Patellofemoral Pain Without Malalignment
- Tight medial and lateral retinacular
- Plicae—medial, lateral, suprapatellar
- Osteochondritis dissecans
  Patella
  Femoral trochlea
- Traumatic patella
- Chondromalacia
- Fat pad syndrome
- Medial retinaculitis
- Patellofemoral osteoarthritis—post-traumatric, idiopathic
- Patellar tendinitis
- Quadriceps tendinitis
- Prepatellar bursitis
- Apophysitis—Osgood-Schlatter, Sinding-Larsen, Johanssen
- Symptomatic bipartite patella
- Other
  Quadriceps tendon rupture
  Patellar tendon rupture
  Patellar fracture
  Proximal tibial epiphysis (tubercle) fracture
  Contusion

TREATMENT

Arthroscopic Assessment of the Patellofemoral Joint

Arthroscopy can provide direct visualization of the patellofemoral joint and improve on the diagnostic accuracy of the cause of patellofemoral pain or instability. The patellofemoral chondral surfaces and medial and lateral restraints of the patella can be directly examined.

Position and Setup

The patient is placed supine on the operative table after anesthesia. A wide variety of anesthesia can be used—epidural, general, spinal, or local. Once the patient is under anesthesia, a physical examination should be performed, looking at range of motion, patella tracking, patella crepitus, and tightness of the lateral retinaculum, and a ligamentous examination of the knee should be carried out. Always compare the results with the contralateral knee. A leg holder should not be used, becaue it can interfere with use of the superior patellar portal in the examination of the patellofemoral joint. A tourniquet may or may not be placed.

Once the patient is prepped and draped, marks for the portals should be made. The superomedial portal is placed 2 cm above the superomedial pole of the patella, just medial to the central quadriceps tendon. This is a portal favored by Pidoriano and Fulkerson.[17]

However, Grana and coworkers[18] have found that viewing patellar tracking is equivalent from a superior or inferior portal. Nissen and colleagues[19] have favored the use of standard arthroscopic portals. The other three standard portals include the inferior lateral, inferior medial, and superior lateral portals. All portals can be used to maximize the visualization of the patellofemoral joint, as well as the rest of the knee joint. The use of the superomedial portal has the benefit of being less impaired if a post is used during arthroscopy compared with the superolateral portal. However, the superolateral portal may provide a better view of the lateral facet of the patella and the lateral side of the trochlea.

The evaluation of the patellofemoral joint should be divided into the assessment of joint surfaces and joint tracking.

Technique

As with any arthroscopic procedure of the knee, this is initiated with a thorough history and physical and imaging protocol. After this is carried out and determining that surgery is appropriate for an individual patient, many decisions are required. We find that the arthroscopic procedure performed for a patient with an isolated patellofemoral problem is often one of confirmation and/or exclusion of other diagnoses. By the time the patient and surgeon have decided an arthroscopic procedure should be performed, all nonoperative solutions have been exhausted. A decision to perform a specific procedure for the treatment of a problem, such as a medial patellofemoral ligament reconstruction for patellofemoral instability, has been made. Most surgeons prefer to perform a diagnostic arthroscopy prior to performing the definitive procedure that has been chosen.

Having confirmed with the patient in the preoperative holding area the procedure and knee that is being operated, on the patient is put on the operating room table in the supine position. After anesthesia has been induced, an examination of the uninvolved and involved knee is performed. Side to side differences are noted. Differences in the examination in the sleeping or anesthetized patient, compared with the awake patient, are also noted.

After examination, a tourniquet is applied to the leg prophylactically. We generally do not inflate the tourniquet unless necessary during the case for visualization purposes. Use of a leg holder versus a side post is left to the surgeon's preference. We use a side post that can be flipped down to allow complete access to the superior aspect of the knee for accessory portals (Fig. 9-10).

Initial evaluation after prepping and draping is performed through an inferior lateral patella portal (Fig. 9-11); care must be made to place this portal laterally enough away from the patella tendon and inferior enough from the patella so that easy manipulation up into the patellofemoral joint can be performed without injuring the articular cartilage. We prefer to perform the routine evaluation of the patellofemoral joint, medial gutter, medial compartment, lateral compartment, and intercondylar notch, perform the posterior examination, and then concentrate on the involved pathology in the patello-

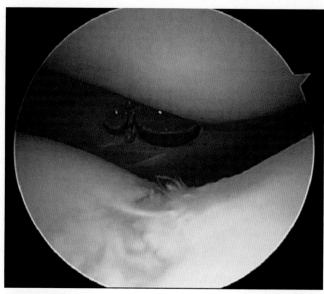

FIGURE 9-11 View of patellofemoral joint from the infralateral portal of the left knee.

femoral region. It is important to understand that fluid placed under pressure with a pump or gravity will affect normal mechanics within the knee. Also, the portals used can affect the patella and put it in a less than physiologic position when evaluating the knee. The superomedial portal can be useful in visualizing patellar tracking as well as looking at the angle of tilt of the patella (Fig. 9-12). The lateral facet should align with the trochlear groove by 20 to 25 degrees of knee flexion (Fig. 9-13) and the apex of the patella by 35 to 40 degrees of knee flexion (Fig. 9-14).

Grading of all articular cartilage lesions should be performed at this time, as well as sizing them and locating them geographi-

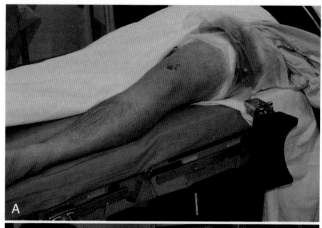

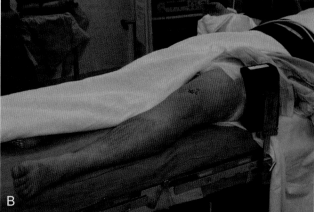

FIGURE 9-10 A, Leg with side post in down position. **B,** Leg with side post in up position.

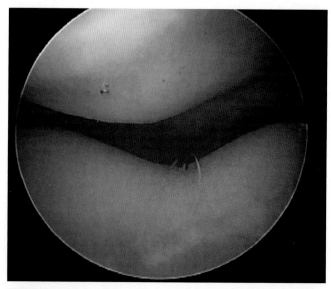

FIGURE 9-12 View of the patellofemoral joint from the superomedial portal of the left knee; patellar tilt with lateral subluxation at full extension.

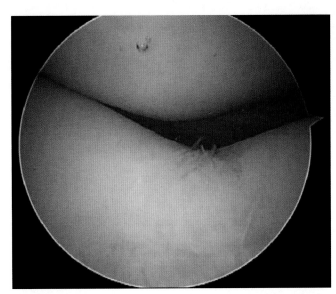

FIGURE 9-13 View of the patellofemoral joint from the superomedial portal of the left knee; patellar tilt with lateral subluxation at 20 degrees of flexion.

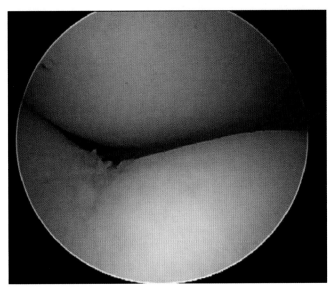

FIGURE 9-14 View from the superior medial portal of the left knee, with correction of patellar tilt; lateral subluxation at 40 to 50 degrees of flexion.

Evaluation of Joint Surfaces to Help Determine Treatment Options

Cartilage Lesions

The patellofemoral joint must first be assessed by the much less invasive techniques of x-ray evaluation using the sunrise view and the 30-degree bent knee lateral view and AP view of the knee. The most relevant x-ray is the sunrise view taken at 20 degrees of flexion. Kijowski and colleagues[20] have found that the most sensitive radiographic findings for degeneration of articular cartilage in the patellofemoral joint are marginal osteophytes. Joint space narrowing, subchondral sclerosis, and subchondral cysts were noted to be insensitive for osteoarthritis of the patellofemoral joint. MRI has also been used to assess the patellofemoral joint. Advantages include direct visualization; it is the most sensitive and specific diagnostic test available.

The patellofemoral joint surface may be examined directly with arthroscopy. Gomes and associates[21] have proposed a technique to assess the articular surface of the patella for cartilage breakdown more effectively. They used a Kirschner wire to maintain a 45-degree lateral tilt after a lateral retinacular release. However, a lateral retinacular release can be counterproductive and even devastating in some patients, specifically those with an already hypermobile patella. This technique, however, could be used to assist in some operative procedures to address chondral deficits.

If a patient has patellofemoral pain that presents as an articular type of pain, it may be treated conservatively, and often improves. However, if the pain persists for a prolonged follow-up period, it may then be necessary to assess the joint surfaces and treat the patient surgically. There has traditionally been a poor correlation between patellofemoral pain and patellofemoral cartilage lesions. Kettunen and coworkers,[22] however, have found that patients who had patellofemoral pain syndrome were more likely to have severe lesions of the patella or trochlear surfaces. These patients also had more functional limitations than patients with mild or no lesions. Assessment of the articular surface is done using the modified Outerbridge classification (Table 9-3).

Findings with patellofemoral arthroscopy may direct our understanding of the cause of patellofemoral pain. The location of pathologic lesions on the patella may help us determine whether the pain and lesions are secondary to malalignment, maltracking, or instability.

cally on the patella and trochlear groove. This should be documented by videography or drawings at the conclusion of the procedure, which can then be used by the surgeon and patient to plan definitive treatment if none has been done during the procedure.

Arthroscopy performed under local anesthesia can be beneficial in determining the cause of the patient's pain, specifically if it is not intra-articular. Most intra-articular pain generators will be anesthetized with the injection of the local anesthetic into the joint. This is not true, however, with extra-articular pain generators, and therefore potential differentiation can be performed at the time of arthroscopic evaluation.

TABLE 9-3 Modified Outerbridge Classification of the Articular Surface

Grade	Macroscopic Description
0	Normal
I	Softening or swelling
II	Fissuring or small erosions
III	Fragmentation, fissuring, deeper erosions, but not to subchondral bone
IV	Erosions down to subchondral bone

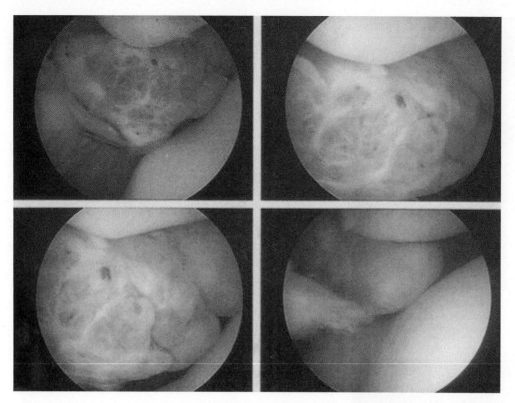

FIGURE 9-15 Example of PVNS in Patellafemoral joint. *(From Edwards MR, Tibrewal S. Patello-femoral joint pain due to unusual location of localized pigmented villonodular synovitis—a case report.* Knee. *2004;11:327-329.)*

If the cause of pain is secondary to instability, a significantly different pattern of wear is seen; this is often caused by the acute dislocation. The lesion is usually described as being located on the medial patella and lateral trochlea because of damage from the relocation of the patella within the trochlear groove.

Although the cartilaginous lesions are usually the cause of the pain, other causes of the pain and pathologic lesions are plicae, tight lateral retinaculum, synovitis, a released lateral retinaculum, or a torn or incompetent MPFL. The lateral retinaculum is an extension of the fibrous aponeurosis of the vastus lateralis muscle to the lateral patella. It is best seen with the arthroscope from the lateral infrapatellar portal.

The plicae are bands of remnant synovial tissue irritated by overuse or injury. They resemble a tendon and are usually found in the medial side of the knee at the level of the patella. The mechanism of the pain is thought to be that the plica gets caught between the patella and femur and causes a localized inflammation that results in patellofemoral pain.

Synovitis is usually seen as a diffuse inflammatory response, showing a red inflamed synovium. However, a patient can also have anterior knee pain from PVNS, which, although rare, has been reported.[15] In the one reported case, the PVNS was located in the patellofemoral joint (Fig. 9-15).

The MPFL is a thin structure found in the second layer on the medial side of the knee. It is responsible for 50% to 60% of the restraint of the patella from translating laterally out of the groove. An incompetent MPFL is usually caused by an acute injury. The MPFL normally appears to attach anteriorly at the superomedial border of the patella, where it blends with the tendon of the vastus medialis. Posteromedially, the MPFL attaches to the anterior aspect of the medial epicondyle of the femur. A tear is usually seen on the femoral side.

Medial instability is almost always caused by iatrogenic overrelease of the lateral retinaculum. In the past, this was overused as a method of treatment of lateral tracking because of the ease and speed of the procedure. The assumption was that the release of a tight lateral retinaculum would solve the patellar tracking problems. It is now believed that an isolated lateral release is almost never the answer in the treatment of patellofemoral pathology.

PEARLS&PITFALLS

PEARLS

- Arthroscopy is very sensitive and useful for evaluating the patellofemoral joint.
- the normal TT-TG distance is less than 12 mm.
- Use of a side post allows access to the leg from the superior medial portal.
- Superior portals (medial and lateral) allow unique visualization of the patella articulation with the femoral trochlea.
- An isolated lateral retinacular release is rarely indicated.

PITFALLS

- Many findings seen at arthroscopy may be asymptomatic.
- Obtaining the TT-TG distance requires specific CT software and is dependent on the radiologist's understanding of the measurement.
- Use of a leg holder inhibits the surgeon's ability to access the superior aspect of the knee.
- Superior lateral portals are difficult to use with a post and are at risk of developing fistulas.
- Medial subluxation can occur as a complication with a lateral release.

CONCLUSIONS

The diagnosis of patellofemoral problems requires a proper history and physical examination, as well as the use of radiography, CT, and MRI. However, arthroscopy of the patellofemoral joint is an important tool in the diagnosis of causes of patellofemoral pain and/or instability. Cartilaginous lesions, patellofemoral instability, and articular dysplasia can be assessed using this technique and, in some cases, surgical treatment can be directed and assisted by arthroscopy. It is important to remember that treatment should be based on arthroscopic findings in conjunction with clinical signs and symptoms.

REFERENCES

1. Teitge RA, Faerber W, Des Madryl P, et al. Stress radiographs of the patellofemoral joint. *J Bone Joint Surg Am*. 1996;78:193-203.
2. Inoue M, Shino K, Hirose H, et al. Subluxation of the patella: computed tomography analysis of patellofemoral congruence. *J Bone Joint Surg Am*. 1988;70:1331-1337.
3. Jones RB, Barlett EC, Vainright JR, et al. CT determination of tibial tubercle lateralization in patients presenting with anterior knee pain. *Skeletal Radiol*. 1995;24:505-509.
4. Steensen RN, Dopirak RM, McDonald WG. The anatomy and isometry of the medial patellofemoral ligament: implications for reconstruction. *Am J Sports Med*. 2004;32:1509-1513.
5. Smirk C, Morris H. The anatomy and reconstruction of the medial patellofemoral ligament. *Knee*. 2003;10:221-227.
6. Nomura E, Horiuchi Y, Kihara M. Medial patellofemoral ligament restraint in lateral patellar translation and reconstruction. *Knee*. 2000;7: 121-127.
7. Seber S, Hazer B, Köse N, et al. Rotational profile of the lower extremity and foot progression angle: computerized tomographic examination of 50 male adults. *Arch Orthop Trauma Surg*. 2000;120:255-258
8. Sallay PI, Poggi J, Speer KP, et al. Acute dislocation of the patella: a correlative pathoanatomic study. *Am J Sports Med*. 1996;24:52-60.
9. Merchant AC, Mercer RL, Jacobsen RH, et al. Roentgenographic analysis of patellofemoral congruence. *J Bone Joint Surg Am*.. 1974;56:1391-1396.
10. Laurin CA, Levesque HP, Dussault R, et al. The abnormal lateral patellofemoral angle: a diagnostic roentgenographic sign of recurrent patellar subluxation. *J Bone Joint Surg Am*. 1978;60:55-60.
11. Goodfellow J, Hungerford DS, Zindel M. Patello-femoral joint mechanics and pathology. 1. Functional anatomy of the patello-femoral joint. *J Bone Joint Surg Br*. 1976;58:287-290.
12. Amis AA. Current concepts on anatomy and biomechanics of patellar stability. *Sports Med Arthrosc*. 2007;15:48-56.
13. Hungerford DS, Barry M. Biomechanics of the patellofemoral joint. *Clin Orthop Relat Res*. 1979;(144):9-15.
14. Merchant AC. Classification of patellofemoral disorders. *Arthroscopy*. 1988;4:235-240.
15. Edwards MR, Tibrewal S. Patello-femoral joint pain due to unusual location of localized pigmented villonodular synovitis—a case report. *Knee*. 2004;11:327-329.
16. Holmes SW, WG Clancy. Clinical classification of patellofemoral pain and dysfunction. *J Orthop Sports Phys Ther*. 1998;28:299-306.
17. Pidoriano AJ, Fulkerson JP. Arthroscopy of the patellofemoral joint. *Clin Sports Med*. 1997;16:17-28.
18. Grana WA, Hinkley B, Hollingsworth S. Arthroscopic evaluation and treatment of patellar malalignment. *Clin Orthop Relat Res*. 1984;(186): 122-128.
19. Nissen CW, Cullen MC, Hewett TE, Noyes FR. Physical and arthroscopic examination techniques of the patellofemoral joint. *J Orthop Sports Phys Ther*. 1998;28:277-285.
20. Kijowski R, Blankenbaker D, Stanton P, et al. Correlation between radiographic findings of osteoarthritis and arthroscopic findings of articular cartilage degeneration within the patellofemoral joint. *Skeletal Radiol*. 2006;35:895-902.
21. Gomes JL, Marczyk LR, Ruthner RP. Arthroscopic exposure of the patellar articular surface. *Arthroscopy*. 2001;17:98-100.
22. Kettunen JA, Visuri T, Harilainen A, et al. Primary cartilage lesions and outcome among subjects with patellofemoral pain syndrome. *Knee Surg Sports Traumatol Arthrosc*. 2005;13:131-134.
23. Wiberg G, Baumgartl F: Klassification der patelleformen. In: Baumgartl ed. Das Kniegelenk, Berlin, Germany: Springer; 1964:276.

SUGGESTED READINGS

Colvin AC, West RV. Patellar instability. *J Bone Joint Surg Am*. 2008;90: 2751-2762.

Feller JA, Amis AA, Andrish JT, et al. Surgical biomechanics of the patellofemoral joint. *Arthroscopy*. 2007;23:542-553.

Nissen CW, Cullen MC, Hewett TE, Noyes FR. Physical and arthroscopic examination techniques of the patellofemoral joint. *J Orthop Sports Phys Ther*. 1998;28:277-285.

Arthroscopic Medial Plication for Patellar Instability

Jeffrey Halbrecht

The proper treatment of patellar instability requires a comprehensive understanding of patellofemoral anatomy and biomechanics, accurate physical examination skills, and appropriate imaging studies. Surgical options abound for this problem, but the patella is a sensitive structure, and inappropriate or overly aggressive procedures can have disastrous consequences. For patellar instability, I have found that less is more, and that arthroscopic realignment is the procedure of choice for the patient with routine instability that requires surgical intervention.

An acute dislocation of the patella may be described as a primary disruption of the patellofemoral relationship, where the patella is displaced out of the femoral sulcus. The direction of dislocation is most commonly lateral, although superior,[1] medial,[2] intra-articular,[1] and vertical intercondylar[3] have also been described. This chapter will deal only with the most common lateral patellar dislocation.

The incidence of acute dislocation of the patella is difficult to assess accurately, and has only been addressed in a few studies. McManus and colleagues[4] have reviewed the records of 94,875 pediatric visits to their emergency room over a 4-year period and found some evidence of patellar dislocation in 55 (0.05%), although only 33 (0.03%) could be proven to be acute dislocations. Cash and Hughston[5] reported treating 399 patients with this disorder over a 30-year period (13.3 patients/year). Castelyn and Handelberg[6] have reported an incidence of acute patellar dislocation of 2.44% in their series of knee injuries. More recently, Nietosvaara and associates[7] have reported an incidence of acute patellar dislocation in 43/100,000 adolescents/year (0.04%).

Most reports in the literature agree that acute patellar dislocation occurs in a young population, with an average age of approximately 20 years most commonly reported.[4,5] However, within this group, the incidence of redislocation appears to be significantly higher in patients who sustain their first dislocation at an earlier age.[4,8] Although earlier studies suggested that females appeared to be at a higher risk for both acute and recurrent dislocation.[8-10] more recent data suggest that the gender incidence may be equal.[11]

The natural history of acute dislocation has been addressed in a number of studies. Hawkins and coworkers[12] treated 20 patients conservatively (3 weeks of immobilization). At 40 months of average follow-up, 3 had redislocated (15 %), 4 had apprehension or complaints of instability (20%), and 15 had pain associated with patellofemoral (PF) crepitus. Remarkably, 100% were able to return to work and recreational sports. Cofield and Bryan[9] studied 48 patients with acute dislocations treated conservatively (closed reductions and immobilization for 1 to 6 weeks). Of these, 44% redislocated and 27% went on to require subsequent surgery. If subjective criteria are include, 52% were considered failures.

McManus and colleagues[4] reviewed 28 patients with acute dislocations; 21 were treated without surgery. Five patients redislocated and 11 were considered symptomatic. Cash and Hughston[5] have reported a redislocation rate of 20% to 43% among first-time dislocators treated with immobilization alone, with the rate depending on the presence of congenital predisposition (patellofemoral dysplasia). In a more recent study of 74 acute patellar dislocations, Atkin and assoociates[11] reported that 58% of patients were still symptomatic during strenuous activities at an early follow-up of 6 months.

Review of these studies suggests that the natural history of acute patellofemoral dislocation is that of a high percentage of redislocation (20% to 40%) and continued symptoms.

ANATOMY

The patella is the largest sesamoid bone in the human body[13] and, like other sesamoid bones, most likely evolved as a mechanism to protect the adjacent tendon (quadriceps in this case) from abrasion and to improve distribution of forces across the tendon.[14] In addition, the patella acts to improve the biomechanical leverage of the quadriceps during extension, acting as a fulcrum,[15] with its greatest effect seen at 20 degrees of flexion.[16]

Most animal species load the knee in a flexed position and have a well-stabilized patella maintained within the confines of the trochlea throughout the range of motion. Humans, on the other hand often load the knee near full extension, with the patella out of the confines of the trochlea and susceptible to instability. Interestingly, in great apes, the femoral diaphysis is straight and the trochlea is flat, with no elevation of the lateral trochlea ridge; however, the patella remains stable because the flexed angle of their knee. In humans, the distal femur evolved into an obliquity angle of 8 to 10 degrees, necessitating the development of a deeper trochlea sulcus, with an elevated lateral trochlear lip, to stabilize the patella.[17]

Patellar tracking is dependent on many anatomic factors. Static factors include bony anatomy and ligamentous structures. Dynamic factors include muscular interaction and change in anatomic relationships related to the range of motion of the knee. Static bony anatomy that contributes to PF stability includes the depth and shape of the trochlea, shape of the patella, femoral anteversion, and tibial rotation, along with the relative valgus alignment of the femoral-tibial articulation.

The Q angle is defined as the angle between the quadriceps mechanism and the patellar tendon, and is a helpful measure of patellar tracking. The greater the anatomic valgus, or the greater the external rotation present in the tibia, the larger the Q angle will be, resulting in a laterally directed force vector (Fig. 10-1). A normal Q angle is typically considered to be less than 15 degrees. Increased femoral anteversion will also result in a high Q angle by causing internal rotation of the femur relative to the tibia.

From full knee extension to approximately 20 degrees of flexion, the patella rests superior to the trochlea groove and is stabilized by a combination of ligamentous and muscular forces. Patellar stability at this point is determined by overall quadriceps tension, with medial-sided stability contributed by vastus medialis obliquus (VMO) contracture and medial patellofemoral ligament tension, whereas lateral stability is contributed by the lateral retinaculum. After approximately 25 degrees of flexion, the patella becomes engaged in the trochlear groove and stability is maintained by bony congruity with the trochlea.

Causative Factors

Disruption or distortion of any of these anatomic factors can result in patellofemoral instability.

Medial Patellofemoral Ligament Insufficiency

Numerous studies have shown that the medial patellofemoral ligament (MPFL) is the most important stabilizer of the patella to lateral translation. Hautamaa and associates[18] have shown in a cadaver biomechanical study that with serial sectioning the MPFL contributes 50% of the patellofemoral stability (Fig. 10-2).[19] In a similar study, Desio and coworkers[19] have shown that the MPFL contributes 60% of the stability, with the medial patellomeniscal ligament contributing an additional 13%. Clinical studies on pa-

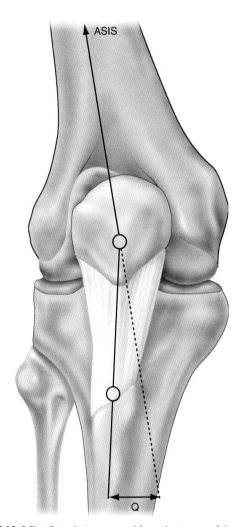

FIGURE 10-1 The Q angle is measured from the center of the patella to the anterior superior iliac spine (ASIS) superiorly and the tibial tubercle inferiorly. This measurement is a useful clinical method for evaluating patella alignment and tracking. An angle of more than 15 degrees is often considered abnormal. *(Modified from Halbrecht JL. Patella problems in athletes. In Johnson DJ, Pedowitz, RA, eds.* Practical Orthopaedic Sports Medicine and Arthroscopy. *Philadelphia: Lippincott, Williams & Wilkins, 2006:677-707.)*

tients with patellar dislocation also seem to confirm this finding, with both surgical and MRI evidence of disruption of the MPFL after patella dislocation.[20-22]

Trochlear Dysplasia

Trochlear dysplasia is thought to be a contributor to patellar instability, but is often difficult to measure accurately radiographically. Magnetic resonance imaging (MRI) is the most accurate method of measurement, with an MRI study showing a 100% sensitivity and a 96% specificity when a criteria of less than a 3-mm trochlear depth was used, measured 3 cm above the femorotibial articulation.[23] However, trochlear dysplasia is rare and, even when present, does not usually require direct treatment. In addition, patients with unilateral instability have trochlear dysplasia bilaterally, but only instability on the side where they have disrupted their MPFL. For rare cases of patella instability thought to be caused by severe trochlear dysplasia, several procedures have been described to deepen

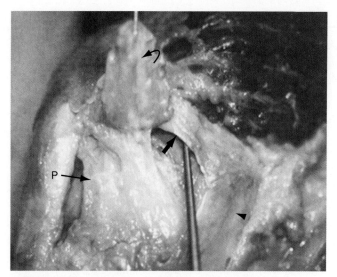

FIGURE 10-2 The medial patellofemoral ligament contributes more than 50% of the stability of the patella (P) to lateral dislocation, shown here in a cadaver dissection. The arrow next to P is on the patellomeniscal ligament. The curved arrow is on the patellotibial ligament, which has been reflected from the tibia. The large arrow points to the medial patellofemoral ligament, which is supported by a probe. The arrowhead is on the superficial medial collateral ligament. *(From Desio SM, Burks RT, Bachus KN. Soft tissue restraints to lateral patellar translation in the human knee. Am J Sports Med. 1998;26:59-65.)*

the trochlea (trochleoplasty), including osteotomy and elevation of the lateral trochlea with bone grafting[24] or undermining and deepening of the trochlea groove.[25] It is my experience that even in the presence of trochlear dysplasia, trochleoplasty is usually not necessary. The vast majority of cases of patellar instability can be managed with proximal soft tissue realignment, and occasionally with the addition of a tibial tubercle osteotomy.

Excessive Femoral Anteversion.   An increase in femoral anteversion will result in relative external rotation of the tibia. This will cause an increase in the Q angle and a tendency toward lateral tracking of the patella. Correction of patellar malalignment in this situation can theoretically be accomplished through a femoral osteotomy. However, because of the obvious invasiveness and risks, this procedure is very rarely recommended. As noted, treatment is directed at stabilization of the proximal soft tissues. If absolutely necessary, the relative external rotation of the tibia can be addressed by osteotomizing the tibial tubercle and moving it medially to decrease the Q angle. In my experience, this is necessary in less than 10% of cases.

Excessive Tibial External Rotation.   Excessive external rotation of the tibia can be a primary anatomic finding, rather than a result of femoral anteversion, and will also result in lateral displacement of the tibial tubercle and an increased Q angle. When this rotation is extreme, and the Q angle exceeds 20 degrees, consideration may be given to correcting this angle by osteotomy and medialization of the tubercle. However, in our experience, a proximal soft tissue alignment is still often quite successful. We reserve the addition of an osteotomy to cases with chondral damage to the lateral facet of the patella or lateral trochlea, where

elevation of the tubercle will unload the articular surface, or to those rare cases documented by CT or MRI as having a large offset between the tibial tuberosity and trochlear groove (tibial tuberosity–trochlear groove [TTTG] distance). This is more accurate than the clinical measurement of the Q angle and, in the rare case when the offset is more than 20 mm, I will consider an osteotomy of the tibial tubercle to correct the TTTG by moving the tubercle medially by 1 cm or more to obtain a TTTG distance closer to 10 to 15 mm.

Weak Vastus Medialis Obliquus.   The VMO is a distinct muscle grouping of the vastus medialis that has a distinct nerve supply[26] and whose fibers insert into the superomedial aspect of the patella at approximately 65 degrees to the longitudinal axis.[27] There can be anatomic variation on the insertion site to the patella. A more medial insertion results in a more medial stabilizing effect. A more superior insertion changes the force vector, providing less medial stabilizing force, and may be a contributor to lateral instability. Weakness of the VMO removes a significant dynamic stabilizing influence on the patella. Strengthening of this muscle is an important component of any rehabilitation program. The VMO contracts maximally in the terminal range of extension, and can be best strengthened with terminal, short-arc extension exercises.

PATIENT EVALUATION

History

The diagnosis of acute dislocation of the patella is not difficult if the patella is obviously dislocated at the time of presentation. However, if the patella spontaneously reduces, the diagnosis may be difficult. The patient will often report that the knee gave way or "popped out of place" during a twisting activity. The patient may give a history of previous subluxation episodes or a history of dislocation of the opposite knee. Patients with generalized hyperlaxity may also give a history of shoulder or ankle instability.

Understanding the mechanism of injury may be helpful in determining the diagnosis. Two mechanisms for acute lateral patellar dislocation have been proposed, direct and indirect. The indirect mechanism of injury results from a powerful quadriceps contracture against an internally rotated femur (externally rotated tibia) and usually involves a sudden twisting motion on a firmly planted foot, such as a sudden change of direction while playing soccer with cleats. The direct mechanism of dislocation involves a direct blow to the medial aspect of the patella, resulting from a fall or contact with another player during athletic activity. A combination of these two mechanisms may contribute to a single injury (Fig. 10-3).

Physical Examination

The first step in evaluating a patient for instability is to inspect the knee with the patient standing. Valgus alignment, foot pronation, and the presence of squinting patellae should be noted. The Q angle is an essential parameter for evaluating instability. It is measured from the anterosuperior iliac spine (ASIS) to the center of the patella, and from the center of the patella to the tibial tubercle. This angle should be evaluated in full extension as well as at 30 degrees of knee flexion and seated at 90 degrees. There is controversy regarding which evaluation is most

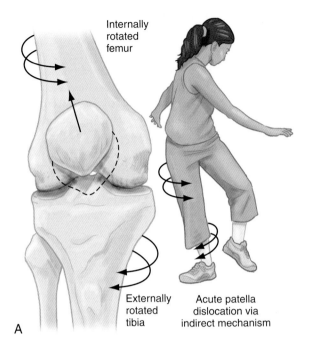

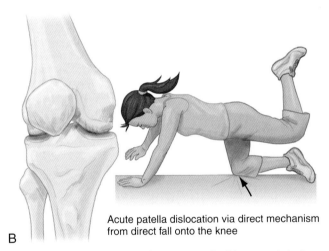

FIGURE 10-3 Two mechanisms for acute patella dislocation. **A,** Indirect mechanism. A powerful quadriceps contracture is imposed on an internally rotated femur (externally rotated tibia). **B,** Direct mechanism. Illustrated here is a direct blow to the medial aspect of patella, usually by a direct fall onto the knee. *(Modified from Halbrecht JL. Patella problems in athletes. In Johnson DJ, Pedowitz, RA, eds.* Practical Orthopaedic Sports Medicine and Arthroscopy. *Philadelphia: Lippincott, Williams & Wilkins, 2006:677-707.)*

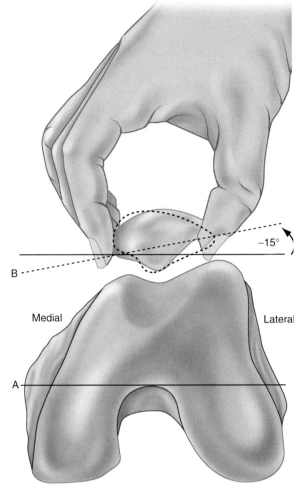

FIGURE 10-4 Positive patellar tilt test. **A,** This is defined as the inability to lift the lateral facet of the patella more than 15 degrees (or to neutral; **B**) and indicates a tight lateral retinaculum. *(Modified from Halbrecht JL. Patella problems in athletes. In Johnson DJ, Pedowitz, RA, eds.* Practical Orthopaedic Sports Medicine and Arthroscopy. *Philadelphia: Lippincott, Williams & Wilkins, 2006:677-707.)*

useful, and there has been significant intraobserver error reported.[28] In my practice, the 0- and 30-degree Q angles are most helpful.

The lateral retinaculum is then assessed for tightness, with the patient supine and the leg fully extended. If the examiner cannot lift the lateral edge of the patella 15 degrees, or to a neutral plane parallel to the examination table, the patellar tilt test is positive and indicates a tight lateral retinaculum. The examiner should also attempt to translate the patella medially. Movement of less than 15 mm, or one quadrant of the patellar width, indicates a tight lateral retinaculum (Fig. 10-4).

Laxity of the medial retinaculum (medial patellofemoral ligament) is then assessed by lateral translation of the patella and is compared with the opposite knee. The ability of the examiner manually to translate the patella laterally, more than 50% of the width of the patella, is a sign of instability, especially if this excursion is greater than the opposite knee. Subjective apprehension on the part of the patient with this maneuver indicates a positive apprehension test and also suggests instability.

The J sign is a dynamic test that demonstrates severe lateral translation of the patella with active terminal extension of the knee, and often is seen with more severe cases of instability, especially with a high-riding patella. The patient is asked to extend the knee actively against gravity. As the patella disengages from the trochlea, it jumps laterally, making an inverted J sign (Fig. 10-5).

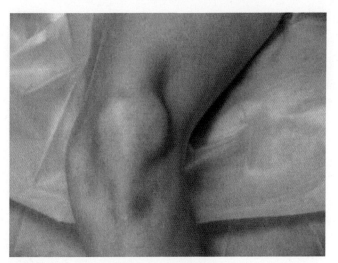

FIGURE 10-5 The J sign is an indication of significant lateral patellar tracking. It is demonstrated here as the patella jumps out laterally as the knee is actively extended, creating a an inverted letter J.

Acute Patellar Dislocation

When examining a first-time dislocator, confusion with an anterior cruciate ligament (ACL) tear is common. The patient will usually present with a large hemarthrosis that will be tender to palpation along the medial retinaculum. There may also be tenderness along the lateral trochlea and medial patella from direct contact and shearing forces during the relocation phase of the injury. Often, however, the pain may be diffuse, and the diagnosis will remain in doubt. Demonstration of a hemarthrosis by needle aspiration, associated with tenderness along the medial retinaculum and subjective apprehension with lateral translation of the patella, will help suggest the diagnosis. In the case of an osteochondral fracture, marrow fat globules may be evident in the knee aspirate.

Diagnostic Imaging

The standard evaluation of patients with PF symptoms will include an anteroposterior (AP), lateral and 45-degree tangential view of the patella (Merchant view; Fig. 10-6). The AP view is rarely help-

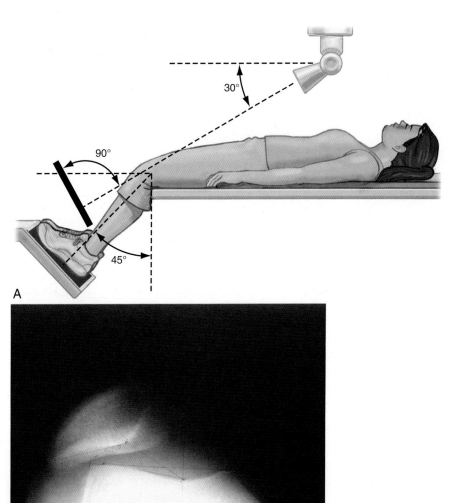

FIGURE 10-6 A, 45-degree patellofemoral view (Merchant view). This is extremely useful x-ray for evaluating the patellofemoral joint. **B,** Merchant view radiograph demonstrating lateral patellar tilt and translation. (**A** *modified from Halbrecht JL. Patella problems in athletes. In Johnson DJ, Pedowitz, RA, eds.* Practical Orthopaedic Sports Medicine and Arthroscopy. *Philadelphia: Lippincott, Williams & Wilkins, 2006:677-707.)*

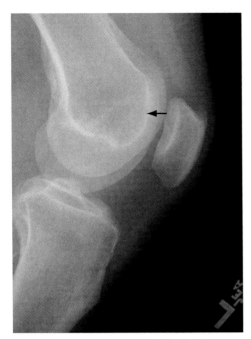

FIGURE 10-7 A true lateral x-ray can be helpful for determining trochlear depth (*arrow*).

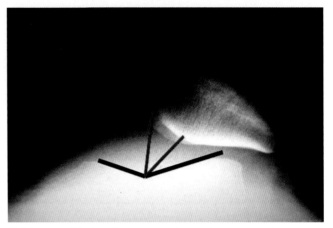

FIGURE 10-8 The Merchant view can be used to measure the congruence angle and patellar translation relative to the trochlear groove. In this patient with patellar instability, the values for both measurements were significantly abnormal. Red lines demonstrate abnormal congruence angle.

ful, but will reveal the presence of a bipartite patella or a patellar fracture. The lateral view is useful to identify loose bodies and patella alta or baja, and will reveal the presence of early degenerative changes with inferior or superior patella osteophytes. The lateral view will also reveal calcification or traction spurs associated with chronic patellar-quadriceps tendinitis, and will demonstrate irregularity of the tibial tubercle associated with Osgood-Schlatter disease. Trochlear depth and dysplasia may also be determined on the lateral view (Fig. 10-7),[29] although there is poor reproducibility and interobserver reliability.[30]

The Merchant view is useful to evaluate patellar alignment. Various measurements can be performed on this x-ray that are useful in assessing patellar tracking, including the congruence angle, tilt angle, and lateral translation (Fig. 10-8).

For acute dislocations that have spontaneously reduced, radiographs are often normal. However, the radiographs will be helpful if they reveal an osteochondral fracture fragment from the medial patellar facet or lateral trochlea. An avulsion fracture of the retinaculum off the medial border of the patella is even more diagnostic. Teitge[31] has suggested the use of an axial oblique view to visualize this avulsion better. The incidence of chondral and osteochondral fracture is up to 46% in patients with acute patellar dislocation,[32] although most of these are only visible by arthroscopic and MRI evaluation. Occasionally, the diagnosis of patellar dislocation can only be made by the demonstration of a torn medial retinaculum as seen by MRI (Fig. 10-9). In several studies, MRI was thought to be diagnostic in 81% to 87% of cases, whereas surgical evaluation was diagnostic in confirming a torn medial retinaculum in 94% to 100% of cases.[20-22]

MRI may also be useful to find subtle changes of chondromalacia in the patella and trochlea associated with the instability, or to observe chondral fractures and loose bodies. Computed tomography (CT) scanning can be useful to evaluate the patellofemoral joint in lesser degrees of flexion, when the standard 45-degree Merchant view does not demonstrate anticipated malalignment,[31,33] although I rarely order this study. Both MRI and CT scanning can be used to measure the TTTG distance; I prefer to use MRI, which provides similar information without radiation exposure, and also provides additional information about the status of the MPFL and cartilaginous structures (Fig. 10-10).

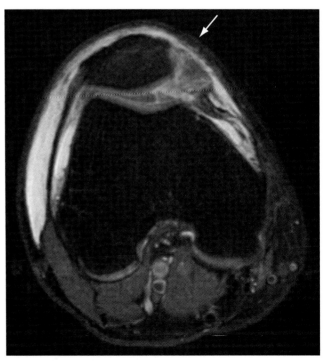

FIGURE 10-9 MRI can be useful to diagnose patellar instability, especially in acute cases in which disruption of the MPFL can be demonstrated (*arrow*).

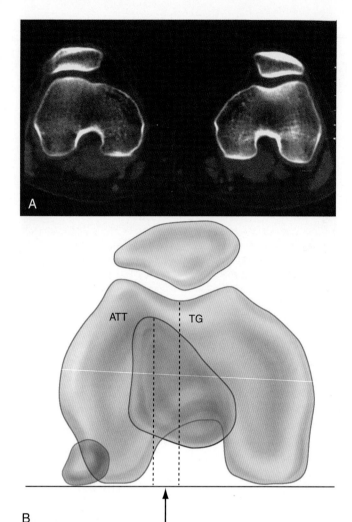

FIGURE 10-10 A, CT scanning is useful to evaluate patellar tracking in varying degrees of extension. **B,** It may be used as an objective way to measure the relationship of the tibial tuberosity (TT) to the trochlear groove (TG) to determine a true Q angle (using the TTTG distance).

TREATMENT

Conservative Management

The traditional treatment for a primary acute patellar dislocation has been nonoperative, although the exact method of treatment is controversial. Most literature studies recommend some type of immobilization followed by an aggressive rehabilitation program.[5,9,12] However the benefit of immobilization following patellar dislocation has not been proven, and results after immobilization and early range of motion appear to be the same.[5,9] Furthermore, there does not seem to be a correlation between the length of immobilization and results.[5,9,12]

Long-term results suggest that the natural history of nonoperative treatment of patellar instability is not as favorable as commonly thought. In a group of 20 patients with acute dislocations treated conservatively, Hawkins and coworkers[12] have reported a 20% incidence of ongoing instability and a 15% incidence of pain and crepitus. In their series of 48 patients with acute dislocations, Cofield and Bryan[9] reported a 44% incidence of redislocation; 27% of these patients went on to subsequent surgery and, taking

into account subjective criteria, 52% were considered failures. In 21 patients treated nonoperatively, McManus and colleagues[4] have reported 5 redislocations and 11 patients who remained symptomatic. Cash and Hughston[5] have reported a redislocation rate of 20% to 43%, depending on anatomic evidence of dysplasia predisposing to instability. In a more recent study, Fithian and associates[34] have shown that of 189 patients followed over a period of 2 to 5 years after an acute patellar dislocation, 17% of first-time dislocators and 49% of patients with a previous history of dislocation had recurrences. The risk for recurrence was higher in women.

Surgical Management

With the advent of less invasive methods of treatment, and with more critical reviews of the results of nonoperative treatment, more authors are recommending surgical treatment, even for acute patellar dislocation.[10,21,35,36] Relative indications for surgical treatment of a patellar dislocation include failure of conservative treatment, the presence of an osteochondral fracture (loose body), recurring instability, and significant residual subluxation on a postreduction Merchant view radiograph. Contraindications to the treatment of patients with patellas instability are rare, but would include patients with pain syndromes or reflex sympathetic dystrophy (RSD) that could be made worse with surgery. Care must also be taken with patients with unusual underlying pathology, such as Ehlers-Danlos syndrome, although I have successfully treated patients with such rare conditions as Charcot-Marie-Tooth disorder and nail patella syndrome.

Arthroscopic Technique

When surgery is selected as the treatment option, initial arthroscopic evaluation is routinely recommended to confirm the diagnosis and address any loose chondral or osteochondral fractures. The exact method of stabilization is controversial, and numerous procedures have been advocated, both open and arthroscopic.

Role of Lateral Release.   Various surgical techniques have been proposed to correct patellar instability. Lateral release alone has been described, although results have been mixed, with a high incidence of recurring instability.[37-39] Lateral release alone does not address the disrupted anatomy of the medial retinaculum and is not considered by most to be an effective treatment for true patellar instability or malalignment (subluxation).[40] I do not recommend isolated lateral release for patellar instability.

Role of Medial Retinacular Repair and Reefing.   When surgery is indicated for patellar instability, most recommend treatment for the disrupted medial retinacular structures and medial PF ligament, often called proximal soft tissue realignment. Complex surgical reconstruction of the medial structures, such as the extensive open reconstruction as described by Insall and colleagues,[41] have fallen out of favor, and minimally invasive open procedures for direct anatomic repair of the medial retinaculum and medial patellofemoral ligament have become the preferred method of repair.[36] Several arthroscopically assisted procedures have also been reported,[42-44] as well as an all- inside arthroscopic method,[45] which is my preferred technique at this time.

Whether to add a lateral release at the time of medial repair is controversial. Several authors routinely perform a lateral release at the time of medial repair,[36] whereas others have shown no advantage to adding a lateral release[22] or individualize the decision based on tightness of the lateral retinaculum.[32] My current recommendation is to base the decision on the tightness of the lateral retinaculum at the time of surgery, with a tendency toward recommending the lateral release if there is any doubt. An overly tight lateral retinaculum tethers the patella laterally, and will inhibit proper realignment despite medial reefing, especially in more chronic cases of recurring instability.

Distal bony realignment procedures are reserved for patients with severe cases of malalignment recurring instability and a high Q angle, or for patients who have failed previous proximal soft tissue realignment.

Arthroscopically Assisted Proximal Realignment

Initial recommendations for arthroscopic patellar realignment consisted primarily of arthroscopically assisted techniques using a medial incision. Yamamoto[44] has treated 30 acute patellar dislocations with arthroscopic lateral release, along with an arthroscopically assisted repair of the medial retinaculum. The transcutaneous passage of sutures through the retinaculum using a large curved needle was recommended, although the sutures were still tied through a medial skin incision. Only acute dislocations were treated. Reported results were excellent, with only one case of redislocation.

Small[43] reported a modified version of the Yamamoto technique, also using an arthroscopically assisted method and a small medial incision (Fig. 10-11). Patients with acute and recurrent dislocations were included, as well as those with malalignment and subluxation. Results were good to excellent in 92.5% of their 24 patients (27 knees), according to a subjective questionnaire. There were two recurrent subluxations, one reoperation for arthrofibrosis, and one superficial infection.

Henry and Pflum[42] have described an arthroscopically assisted technique using cannulated needles, but tied the sutures through a medial incision as well. No follow-up series or results were reported.

All-Arthroscopic Proximal Realignment:

A number of authors have described entirely arthroscopic proximal realignment procedures, with good results.[36,45-47] All these procedures have the advantage of eliminating any type of medial incision. The technique for arthroscopic realignment presented here is my preferred method of treatment for most patients with uncomplicated patellar instability.

Surgery is performed under general anesthesia with a thigh holder in place. A tourniquet is applied, but rarely inflated. Before plication, a healing response is created along the medial retinaculum by gently abrading the tissue with a rasp or shaving with a whisker blade (Fig. 10-12). Medial retinacular sutures are introduced percutaneously using an epidural needle (Tuohy needle; Teleflex Medical (Rusch), Deluth, Ga). An epidural needle is essential because the noncutting edge on the inner bevel of the tip prevents cutting or damaging the suture. The needle is placed adjacent to the patella and a no. 1 PDS suture is passed manually through the needle and retrieved arthroscopically through an accessory superolateral portal (Fig. 10-13). Although nonabsorbable braided suture could be used, I prefer an absorbable suture in this highly sensitive area to avoid postoperative irritation from permanent knots.

The needle is gently withdrawn from the retinaculum but not out of the skin. The needle is then redirected subcutaneously

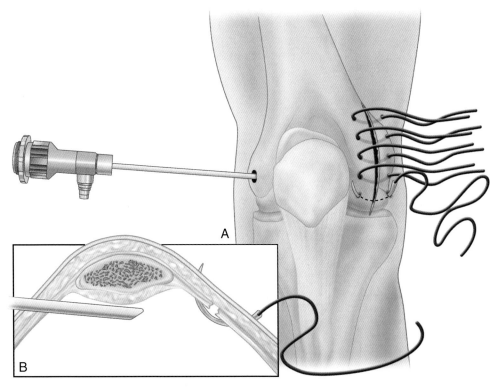

FIGURE 10-11 Arthroscopically assisted patellar realignment is performed by passing sutures percutaneously and then making an incision to tie the sutures. *(Modified from Halbrecht JL. Patella problems in athletes. In Johnson DJ, Pedowitz, RA, eds.* Practical Orthopaedic Sports Medicine and Arthroscopy. *Philadelphia: Lippincott, Williams & Wilkins, 2006:677-707.)*

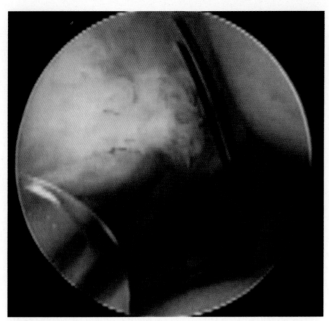

FIGURE 10-12 Arthroscopic view of medial retinacular abrasion with a shaver to stimulate a healing response prior to tying sutures.

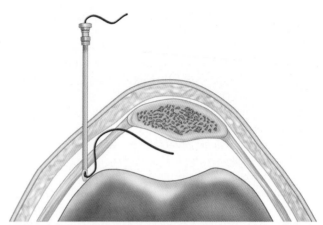

FIGURE 10-14 Second step of arthroscopic realignment. The needle is withdrawn to a subcutaneous depth, leaving the initial limb of suture within the needle. The needle is then reinserted 2 to 3 cm posteriorly, creating an internal loop of suture. *(Modified from Halbrecht JL. Patella problems in athletes. In Johnson DJ, Pedowitz, RA, eds. Practical Orthopaedic Sports Medicine and Arthroscopy. Philadelphia: Lippincott, Williams & Wilkins, 2006:677-707.)*

approximately 2 to 3 cm posteriorly and reinserted through the retinaculum (Fig. 10-14). This creates a loop of suture that is again retrieved through the same accessory portal. The needle is withdrawn completely and the process is repeated until four or five sutures are in place. The sutures are retrieved through an accessory proximal lateral portal and clamped for later imbrication of the medial retinaculum (Fig. 10-15). An arthroscopic lateral release is then performed with a standard electrocautery device. After the lateral release, the medial sutures are tied inside the joint from the proximal lateral or anteromedial portal using standard arthroscopic knot-tying techniques (Fig. 10-16).

Alignment and stability are checked and additional sutures added as necessary. I generally use four to six sutures. Occasionally, some dimpling of the skin will occur in the area of the sutures as the intra-articular knots are tied. The dimpling resolves with resorption of the sutures and postoperative rehabilitation,

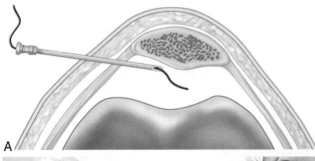

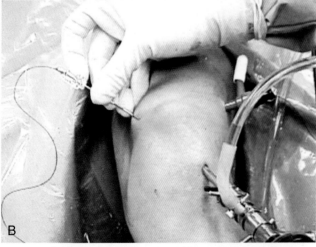

FIGURE 10-13 A, Schematic illustration of the initial step of arthroscopic patellar realignment by percutaneous passage of a suture through an epidural needle inserted adjacent to the patella. **B,** Arthroscopic view of needle insertion. *(A modified from Halbrecht JL. Patella problems in athletes. In Johnson DJ, Pedowitz, RA, eds. Practical Orthopaedic Sports Medicine and Arthroscopy. Philadelphia: Lippincott, Williams & Wilkins, 2006:677-707.)*

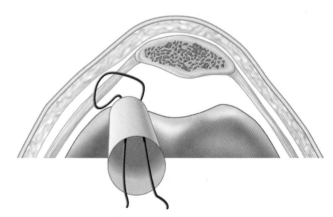

FIGURE 10-15 Both limbs of suture are retrieved and clamped for later tying. An average of four to six sutures is placed in a similar fashion for a typical case. Tying is performed after lateral retinacular release, if indicated. *(Modified from Halbrecht JL. Patella problems in athletes. In Johnson DJ, Pedowitz, RA, eds. Practical Orthopaedic Sports Medicine and Arthroscopy. Philadelphia: Lippincott, Williams & Wilkins, 2006:677-707.)*

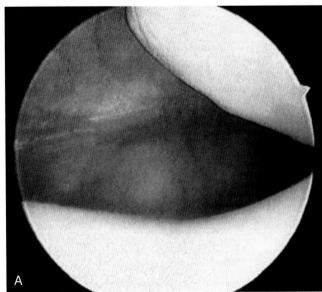

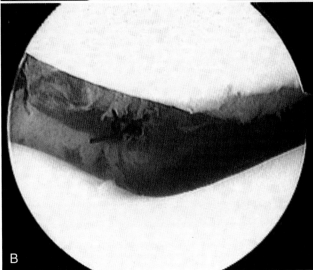

FIGURE 10-16 A, Preoperative arthroscopic view of lateral patellar instability. **B,** Postoperative arthroscopic view of centralized and stable patella after arthroscopic realignment.

and has not been a problem. However, if desired, the dimpling can be addressed intraoperatively by spreading gently in the subcutaneous tissues with a small scissor through the medial portal to release the subcutaneous tissue.

PEARLS

PEARLS

1. Use a beveled needle such as a Tuohy epidural needle to avoid damage to the sutures.
2. Take large bites of medial retinacular tissue (2 to 3 cm minimum).
3. Use an average of four to six sutures for a typical case.
4. Stimulate a healing response along the medial retinaculum before reefing using a whisker blade or a rasp.
5. Insert sutures before lateral release is performed to avoid extravasation.
6. Tie knots from the superolateral portal.

---

7. Initial puckering of the medial subcutaneous tissue may occur, but this resolves with rehabilitation.
8. Avoid stiffness postoperatively by allowing range of motion to begin at 1 week.
9. For rare patients with severely damaged native tissue as a result of previous surgery or unusual collagen disorders, consider reconstruction of the MPFL with graft (less than 5% of cases).
10. Distal realignment with a tibial tubercle osteotomy may rarely be added when the TTTG distance is more than 20 mm (less than 10% of cases)

Postoperative Management

Postoperative treatment involves a brace locked in full extension for 1 week, followed by range of motion and physical therapy for 2 to 3 months. Patients are instructed to begin quadriceps contractions and ankle pumps immediately postsurgery in the recovery room. After the first week, the brace is unlocked to enable patients to begin range of motion exercises, but bracing is continued for 3 more weeks until quadriceps strength returns. Patients are not allowed to flex past 90 degrees for 4 weeks, but may begin weight bearing immediately in the brace. Running is allowed at 3 months, followed by return to full twisting and impact sports between 4 and 6 months, depending on return of quadriceps strength.

Avoiding Complications

Complications are rare with this procedure, which is one of the attractive features of an entirely arthroscopic approach. Several technical pearls may be useful to mention. Some dimpling or bunching up of the subcutaneous tissue and skin may occur with this technique as tension is applied to the sutures, and the sutures are tied inside the joint. This will work itself free during rehabilitation, and has not been a problem in my experience. However, if the surgeon wishes to address this intraoperatively, a small dissecting scissor may be inserted through the medial portal and the skin freed from the sutures with gentle spreading of the scissor blades. Overtightening would be difficult to achieve with this technique, and I have yet to encounter this complication. This is also one of the advantages of an arthroscopic approach as opposed to an open reefing. Under arthroscopic guidance, one can titrate the medial reefing under direct vision by inserting as many sutures as necessary and taking as much of a bite of medial tissue as required to obtain a stable and neutral tracking patella. I typically take a 2- to 3-cm bite of tissue and use from four to six sutures.

Postoperative stiffness is possible, even with an arthroscopic approach to patellar realignment, and is a potentially devastating complication. This can be avoided by following the aggressive postoperative rehabilitation protocol outlined earlier. I have successfully avoided this complication using this technique and an accelerated rehabilitation program. It is essential to begin knee motion within 1 week of surgery.

Although I prefer an all-arthroscopic method of proximal realignment, open and arthroscopically assisted proximal realignment procedures can also be effective in preventing recurring instability. However, these procedures are more frequently accompanied by complications, including the risk of joint stiffness, scar tissue, and overcorrection. Medial PF reconstruction using a graft is reserved for rare cases of failed arthroscopic realignment, or patients with inadequate native tissue. I reserve distal realignment for patients with instability associated with significant arthrosis, or those rare patients with a TTTG distance of more than 20 mm on overlapped CT or MR imaging. In these patients, biomechanical unloading and bony realignment of the patellofemoral joint are indicated, in conjunction with a soft tissue arthroscopic realignment.

OUTCOMES

In a review of my 5-year results,[45] 93% of patients reported significant subjective improvement. The average Lysholm score improved from 41.5 to 79.3 ($P < .05$). Preoperative and postoperative radiographs were measured for congruence angle, lateral patellofemoral angle, and lateral patellar displacement, and all showed significant improvement postoperatively ($P < .05$; Fig. 10-17). There were no complications and no redislocations.

TABLE 10-1   Subjective Rating Score of Outcomes*

Symptom	Preoperative	Postoperative	*P* value
Pain	7.1	2.4	<.05
Swelling	6.0	0.8	<.05
Instability	8.2	0.8	<.05
Crepitus	6.6	2.5	<.05

*10, severe symptoms; 0, no symptoms.

Patients reported a significant improvement in pain, swelling, stair climbing, crepitus, and ability to return to sports ($P < .05$). Although the average Q angle in the study was 11 degrees, this procedure was successfully performed on patients with Q angles up to 20 degrees. None of the patients required a second operation for débridement of scar tissue or manipulation. All patients regained full range of motion as compared with the opposite side (Table 10-1).

CONCLUSIONS

I have now had over 10 years of follow-up on many patients, with continued good results. Arthroscopic realignment for patellar instability offers excellent results for stability and patient satisfaction, without the morbidity associated with more complex patellar realignment procedures. I continue to use this procedure as the main surgical treatment for most patients with lateral patellar instability.

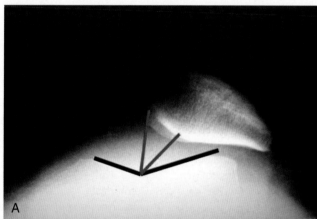

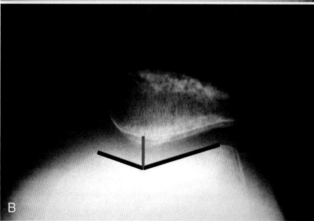

FIGURE 10-17 A, Preoperative Merchant view demonstrating significant patellar instability with increased tilt and lateral translation (*red lines,* increased congruence angle; *black lines* outline the trochlear groove [sulcus angle]). Lateral translation is evident by overhang of the patella over the lateral trochlear margin. **B,** Postoperative Merchant view of the same patient at 1 year following arthroscopic realignment, demonstrating central tracking (*red line* indicates an improved congruence angle to 0 degrees; *black lines* outline the trochlear groove [sulcus angle]). Translation has been eliminated.

REFERENCES

1. Friden T. A case of superior dislocation of the patella. *Acta Orthop Scand.* 1987;58:429-430.
2. Larson RL, Jones OC. Dislocations and ligamentous injuries of the knee. In: *Fractures in Adults.* 2nd ed. Philadelphia: Lippincott; 1984:.
3. Kaufman I, Habermann ET. Intercondylar vertical dislocation of the patella. A case report. *Bull Hosp Joint Dis.* 1973;34:222-225.
4. McManus MB, Rang M, Heslin J. Acute dislocation of the patella in children. *Clin Orthop Relat Res.* 1979;(139):88-91.
5. Cash JD, Hughston JC. Treatment of acute patella dislocation. *Am J Sports Med.* 1988;16:244-249.
6. Casteleyn PP, Handelberg F. Arthroscopy in the diagnosis of acute dislocation of the patella. *Acta Orthop Belg.* 1989;55:381-383.
7. Nietosvaara Y, Aalto K, Kallio PE. Acute patellar dislocation in children: incidence and associated osteochondral fractures. *J Pediatr Orthop.* 1994; 14:513-515.
8. Larsen E, Lauridsen F. Conservative treatment of patella dislocations: influence of evident factors on the tendency to redislocate and the therapeutic result. *Clin Orthop Relat Res.* 1982;171:131-136.
9. Cofield RH, Bryan RS. Acute dislocation of the patella: results of conservative treatment. *J Trauma.* 1977;17:526-531.
10. Vainionpaa S, Laasonen E, Silvenoinen T, et al. Acute dislocation of the patella. A prospective review of operative treatment. *J Bone Joint Surg Br.* 1990;72:366-369.
11. Atkin DM, Fithian DC, Marangi KS. et al. Characteristics of patients with primary acute lateral patellar dislocation and their recovery within the first 6 months of injury. *Am J Sports Med.* 2000;28:472-479.
12. Hawkins RJ, Bell RH, Anisette G. Acute patella dislocations: the natural history. *Am J Sports Med.* 1986;14:117-120.
13. Holingshead HW. *Anatomy for Surgeons.* 2nd ed. Vol 3. *The Back and Limbs.* Baltimore: Williams & Wilkins; 1990.
14. Dye SF. Patellofemoral anatomy. In: Fox JM, Del Pizzo W, eds. *The Patellofemoral Joint.* New York: McGraw-Hill; 1993:1-11.

15. Fu FH, Seel MJ, Berger R. Patellofemoral biomechanics. In: Fox JM, Del Pizzo W, eds. *The Patellofemoral Joint*. New York: McGraw-Hill; 1993: 49-51.

16. Perry J, Antonelli D, Ford W. Analysis of knee joint forces during flexed knee stance. *J Bone Joint Surg Am*. 1975;57:961-967.

17. Tardieu C, Dupont JY. The origin of femoral trochlear dysplasia: comparative anatomy, evolution and growth of the patellofemoral joint. *Rev Chir Orthop Reparatrice Appar Mot*. 2001;87:373-383.

18. Hautamaa PV, Fithian DC, Kaufmann KR, et al. Medial soft tissue restraints in lateral patellar instability and repair. *Clin Orthop Relat Res*. 1998;349:174-182.

19. Desio SM, Burks RT, Bachus KN. Soft tissue restraints to lateral patellar translation in the human knee. *Am J Sports Med*. 1998;26:59-65.

20. Nomura E. Classification of lesions of the medial patello-femoral ligament in patellar dislocation. *Int Orthop*. 1999;23:260-263.

21. Sanders TG, Morrison WB, Singleton BA, et al. Medial patellofemoral ligament injury following acute transient dislocation of the patella: MR findings with surgical correlation in 14 patients. *J Comput Assist Tomogr*. 2001;25:957-962.

22. Sallay PI, Poggi J, Speer KP, et al. Acute dislocation of the patella. A correlative pathoanatomic study. *Am J Sports Med*. 1996;24:52-60.

23. Pfirrmann CW, Zanetti M, Romero J, et al. Femoral trochlear dysplasia: MRI findings. *Radiology*. 2000;216:858-864.

24. Keene G, Marans HJ. Osteotomy for patellofemoral dysplasia. In: Fox JM, Del Pizzo W, eds. *The Patellofemoral Joint*. New York: McGraw Hill; 1993:169-176.

25. Peterson L, Karlsson J, Brittberg M. Patellar instability with recurrent dislocation due to patellofemoral dysplasia. Results after surgical treatment. *Bull Hosp Jt Dis Orthop Inst*. 1988;48:130-139.

26. Weinstabl R, Scharf W, Firbas W, et al. The extensor apparatus of the knee joint and its peripheral vasti. Anatomic investigation and clinical relevance. *Surg Radiol Anat*. 1989;11:17-22.

27. Huberti HH, Hayes WC, Stone JL, et al. Force ratios in the quadriceps tendon and ligamentum pateallae. *J Orthop Res*. 1984;2:49-54.

28. Greene CC, Edwards TB, Wade MR, et al. Reliability of the quadriceps angle measurement. *Am J Knee Surg*. 2001;14:97-103.

29. Grelsamer RP, Tedder JL. The lateral trochlear sign. Femoral trochlear dysplasia as seen on a lateral view roentgenograph. *Clin Orthop Relat Res*. 1992;281:159-162.

30. Remy F, Chantelo C, Folntaine C, et al. Inter-and intraobserver reproducibility in radiographic diagnosis and classification of femoral trochlear dysplasia. *Surg Radiol Anat*. 1998;20:285-289.

31. Teitge RA. Radiology of the Patellofemoral Joint. *Orthopedic Surgery Update Series*. Princeton, NJ: Continuing Professional Education Center; 1985.

32. Harilainen A, Myllynen P. Operative treatment in acute patella dislocation: radiologic predisposing factors, diagnosis and results. *Am J Knee Surg*. 1988;1:178-185.

33. Schutzer SF, Rambsy GR, Fulkerson JP. Computed tomographic classification of patellofemoral pain patients. *Orthop Clin North Am*. 1986;17:235-248.

34. Fithian DC, Paxton EW, Stone ML, et al. Epidemiology and natural history of acute patellar dislocation. *Am J Sports Med*. 2004;32:1114-1121.

35. Boring TH, O'Donoghue DH. Acute patella dislocation. Results of immediate surgical repair. *Clin Orthop Relat Res*. 1978;(136):182-185.

36. Ahmad CS, Stein BE, Matuz D, et al. Immediate surgical repair of the medial patellar stabilizers for acute patellar dislocation. A review of eight cases. *Am J Sports Med*. 2000;28:804-810.

37. Aglietti P, Pisaneschi A, De Biase P. [Lussazione recidivante di rotula: Tre tipi di trattamento chirurgico.] *G Ital Ortop Traumat*. 1992;13:25-36.

38. Dandy DJ, Griffiths D. Lateral release for recurrent dislocation of the patella. *J Bone Joint Surg Br*. 1989;71:121-125.

39. Sherman OH, Fox JM, Sperling H, et al. Patellar instability: Treatment by arthroscopic electrosurgical lateral release. *Arthroscopy*. 1987;3:152-160.

40. Fulkerson JP, Cautilli RA. Chronic patella instability: subluxation and dislocation. In: Fox JM, Del Pizzo W, eds. *The Patellofemoral Joint*. New York: McGraw-Hill; 1993:135-147.

41. Insall JN, Bullough PG, Burstein AH. Proximal tube realignment of the patella for chondromalacia patellae. *Clin Orthop Relat Res*. 1979;144:63-69.

42. Henry JE, Pflum FA Jr. Arthroscopic proximal patella realignment and stabilization. *Arthroscopy*. 1995;11:424-425.

43. Small NC. Arthroscopically assisted proximal extensor mechanism realignment of the knee. *Arthroscopy*. 1993;9:63-67.

44. Yamamoto RK. Arthroscopic repair of the medial retinaculum and capsule in acute patellar dislocations. *Arthroscopy*. 1986;2:125-131.

45. Halbrecht JL. Arthroscopic patella realignment: An all-inside technique. *Arthroscopy*. 2001;17:940-945.

46. Haspl M, Cicak N, Klobucar H, et al. Fully arthroscopic stabilization of the patella. *Arthroscopy*. 2002;18:E2.

47. Fukushima K, Horaguchi T, Okano T, et al. Patellar dislocation: arthroscopic patellar stabilization with suture anchors. *Arthroscopy*. 2004;20:761-764.

48. Halbrecht JL. Patella problems in athletes. In Johnson DJ, Pedowitz, RA, eds. *Practical Orthopaedic Sports Medicine and Arthroscopy*. Philadelphia: Lippincott, Williams & Wilkins: 2006:677-707.

SUGGESTED READING

Halbrecht JL. Mild patella instability: arthroscopic reconstruction. In: Fulkerson JP, ed. *Common Patellofemoral Problems*. Rosemont, IL: American Academy of Orthopaedic Surgeons; 2005:29-33.

Reconstruction of the Medial Patellofemoral Ligament

Matthew Stiebel ● Corey Edgar ● Anthony A. Schepsis

Recurrent lateral instability of the patella after traumatic patellar dislocation or subluxation usually requires attention to the medial soft tissue restraints for prevention of future pathologic lateral translation. Historically, procedures for addressing medial restraint insufficiency include reefing, vastus medialis obliquus (VMO) advancements, and nonanatomic tendon transfer procedures.[1,2] In addition to shortening or imbrication of the medial soft tissue restraints, several authors have described reconstructing or reinforcing the medial patellar structures with fascia lata, nylon, and even preserved skin.[3-6] Earlier proximal procedures for patellar instability can be summarized into two categories—advancement from structures above the patella or nonanatomic attachment from tendons anchored below the patella. Numerous earlier techniques of proximal VMO advancement and extensor mechanism equilibration have been summarized best by Ficat,[7] who described these proximal muscle transfers as a dynamic means of patellar control. Baker and colleagues[8] have summarized some of the early work of Galliazzi, with emphasis on a nonanatomic static semitendinosus tenodesis for the prevention of lateral subluxation.

In recent years, the medial patellofemoral ligament (MPFL), has been shown to be the primary soft tissue restraint against pathologic lateral translation of the patella. Therefore, restoration of this structure has been shown to be the most anatomic and physiologic approach for restoration of stability.

ANATOMY

The MPFL is a thickened band of retinacular tissue originating in the saddle area between the medial epicondyle and adductor tubercle and inserting on the proximal third of the medial border of the patella. Typically, the MPFL is approximately 55 mm long and is overlaid by the distal part of the VMO, with fibers merging into the deep aspect of the muscle.[9] Current techniques for addressing post-traumatic patellar instability have shifted focus to a restoration of the normal anatomy and the importance of the

MPFL. The primary restraints against lateral patellar mobility are passive.[10] The trochlea is the most important patellar stabilizer in normal knees beyond 20 degrees of flexion. If the patella is dislocating laterally, the medial restraints must be abnormally lax or deficient.

The MPFL has been shown to be the primary soft tissue restraint to lateral translation of the patella; it functions primarily in the first 30 degrees (before patellar engagement in the trochlea) and becomes lax in flexion.[6,10-13] Additionally, if the trochlear groove is deficient (dysplastic), the MPFL takes on an even greater role. The MPFL is believed always to sustain some form of injury during traumatic lateral dislocation of the patella. Logically, a repair or reconstruction of this structure should provide the most anatomic reproduction of normal patellar biomechanics. Even though other medial tissues, such as the medial patellotibial ligament, may contribute to patellar stability, addressing the primary static restraint to lateral patellar subluxation provides the most reproducible and reliable outcomes at present.[14] Reconstruction of the MPFL restores tracking to near-normal when the medial restraints are deficient. Current techniques for MPFL reconstruction differ from historical models and VMO advancement because of the emphasis on avoiding the creation of increased patellofemoral contact forces. VMO advancements and proximal reefings tend to tighten, therefore increasing the patellar joint contact forces in flexion. By anatomically reconstructing damaged normal anatomy, we attempt to correct patellar pathology without introducing a mechanism that will lead to medial facet overload and subsequent degenerative patellar disease.

PATIENT EVALUATION

History and Physical Examination

Success, as with any operation, relies mainly on proper patient selection. After an extensive history, the physical examination begins with examining the patient's standing leg alignment and gait.

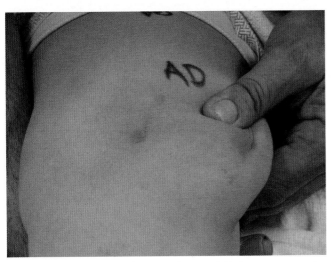

FIGURE 11-1 Lateral glide is measured at 0 and 30 degrees to asses the degree of laxity. This patient had a previous failed reefing procedure and the patella is completely dislocatable (4+ lateral glide).

A standing squat is helpful for demonstrating painful arc of motion and crepitus. We then have the patient flex and extend the knee while seated on the edge of the examination table to assess patellar tracking, specifically checking to see if the patella slides laterally with full extension, a J sign. Palpation of the patella with slight posterior pressure allows us to feel for crepitus and isolate the exact arc of pain better during active range of motion. With the patient supine, we assess lateral patellar translation, looking for abnormal increased glide. Specifically, we examine both knees at full extension and at 30 degrees of flexion (Fig. 11-1). We subdivide the patella into four quadrants and determine the extent (the number of quadrants) that the patella can be shifted laterally over the edge of the trochlea; MPFL patholaxity typically corresponds to 3+ to 4+ lateral glide at 30 degrees of flexion (Fig. 11-2). We also

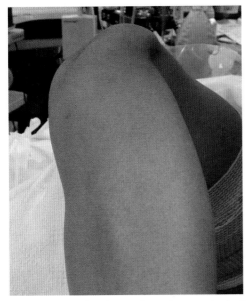

FIGURE 11-2 This shows that the patella can be completely dislocated at a high degree of flexion, indicating severe laxity and a high degree of dysplasia.

try to determine whether there is a hard or soft end point to translation, which can be helpful in determining whether there is any residual ligament function. Passive patellar tilt is examined to determine tightness of the lateral retinaculum. We have found the Sage sign, passive medial translation of the patella performed at 15 to 20 degrees of flexion, to be helpful in determining the need for lateral release. If the patella can be translated two quadrants or more, lateral release is not necessary, and may lead to debilitating medial instability if performed in this situation. In our practice, we often see patients with previously failed reefing procedures, previous lateral releases, and trochlear dysplasia, which may contribute to a more progressive laxity of medial restraints. In these cases, it is especially important to use the Fulkerson jump test to rule out iatrogenic medial patellar dislocations (postexcessive lateral release), which can present with the patient mistakenly reporting lateral dislocations.

Diagnostic Imaging

Standard imaging includes anteroposterior (AP) weight bearing, posteroanterior (PA) flexed weight bearing, a true lateral at 30 degrees of flexion to assess patellar height and trochlear dysplasia, and axial views (at 30, 60, and 90 degrees of flexion) to look at congruence and patellar rotation or tilt. Assessment of patellar height on the 30-degree lateral is performed using the Blackburn-Peel method, measured off the tibial plateau and articular surface of the patella, rather than the Insall-Salvati method. This eliminates the chance of misreading patella alta or infera, occasionally caused by a long nonarticular "nosed" portion of a patella, such as with a Cyrano-type morphology.[15] Trochlear dysplasia is also best assessed on the true lateral view, looking for the crossing sign and presence of a trochlear bump.

We routinely perform a calibrated computed tomography (CT) patellar tracking study with midaxial cuts from 0 to 60 degrees of knee flexion in 10-degree increments to assess patellar tracking from 0 to 60 degrees. This is the range in which stability occurs. The CT study also includes fixed-frame images from the trochlear groove to the tibial tubercle to measure tibial tuberosity-trochlear groove (TTTG) distance. From the CT cuts and Merchant view at 30 degrees, we can determine whether the patella is tilted. Normally, the patella will be centered in the trochlea; however, if the lateral facet is parallel to the anterior trochlea or if the angle formed by the lateral facet and the anterior trochlea is open medially, the patella is tilted. The congruence angle on a standard Merchant view should normally demonstrate that the patellar apex is medial to the bisected trochlea. The sulcus angle can be measured and should be 137 ± 6 degrees.[16] A higher measured angle helps us identify a flat, shallow, dysplastic trochlea. Finally, magnetic resonance imaging (MRI) can be helpful in determining the extent of chondral damage in the patellofemoral joint and the status of the soft tissue restraints, as well as ruling out other pathology. We prefer MR arthrography if advanced cartilage sequencing is not available.

This compilation of information is predicated on the understanding that patellofemoral problems are often multifactorial. Factors such as the presence of trochlear dysplasia, poor tissue quality, patellar cartilage damage, hip rotation, alignment, and status of the tibiofemoral joint may influence operative decisions.

As a stand-alone procedure, MPFL reconstruction is solely used for instability, whereas distal realignment surgery is better used to address tubercle malalignment with patellofemoral pain and/or instability. It is our experience that a Q angle more than 20 degrees at 30 degrees of flexion or a corresponding TTTG value more than 15 to 20 mm will bring the necessity of a distal osteotomy into serious consideration. In many cases, the presence of both scenarios may require a combined proximal and distal approach. Normal TTTG values, an increased lateral patellar glide, and a history of recurrent patellar dislocations following trauma suggest MPFL incompetence and the need for reconstruction.

TREATMENT

Indications and Contraindications

Our algorithm for deciding when to perform an MPFL reconstruction takes into account the amount of lateral laxity, degree of trochlear dysplasia, and quality of medial tissue structures. If the patient has a high degree of lateral patellar translation, some degree of trochlear dysplasia, and there is a suspicion of poor medial tissue restraints (or previous failed reefing or failed distal realignment), we proceed with MPFL reconstruction instead of depending on the quality of the medial soft tissues. Alternately, if there is less laxity, little to no dysplasia, and good medial tissue quality, we may perform a less invasive procedure, such as an arthroscopic or miniopen reefing of the medial structures. Relative but not absolute contraindications for MPFL reconstruction would include severe medial facet arthrosis, permanent tilt, subluxation with tubercle malalignment, or no true symptoms of instability. This is not an operation for pain or arthrosis.

Arthroscopic Technique

Graft Selection

We have used semitendinosus autograft in the past, but it is our current preference to use a semitendinosus allograft. Of note, in petite patients a gracilis tendon is often sufficient. We have found that the allograft performs just as well in this richly vascular, extra-articular environment. If an autograft is used , this is harvested though a separate incision over the pes anserine insertion. This tendon far exceeds the 200 N associated with native MPFL rupture in cadaver models; the doubled graft requires approximately 2000 N for rupture. It is also an order of magnitude stronger (150 N/ mm) than the average stiffness of the MPFL (12 N/mm).[10,17] The advantages of such a stiff graft include the resistance to stretching out over time and the ability to perform long term in high-demand situations, such as with trochlear dysplasia. The main disadvantage, however, is that it can place high compressive force on the patella if placed improperly or overtensioned. The graft is first doubled on itself on a standard graft preparation board. Next, a running baseball stitch (using no. 2 FiberWire [Arthrex, Naples, Fla] or comparable suture) for a distance of 25 mm is performed at each free end, creating a Y-shaped graft (Fig. 11-3). The doubled end is sutured for a distance of 25 mm and then sized (Fig. 11-4).

Arthroscopy is routinely carried out, assessing and addressing any chondral lesions and concomitant pathology. Lateral release is performed on an individual basis and can be done arthroscopically.

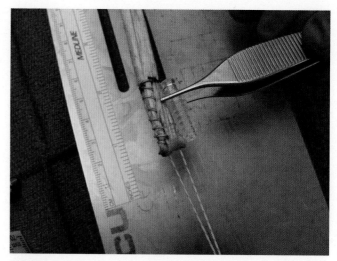

FIGURE 11-3 The doubled end of the graft is marked and sutured to a distance of 25 mm. This is the length of the biotenodesis screw to be used for femoral fixation, plus 2 mm.

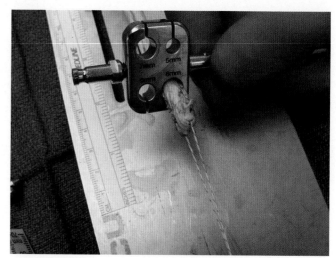

FIGURE 11-4 Only the first 3 cm of the doubled end of the tendon site needs to be sized after it has been

A two-incision approach is used; however, one long medial parapatellar incision could be used if a concomitant procedure such as cartilage restoration of the patella or trochlea is simultaneously performed. The first 3-cm longitudinal incision is made along the proximal medial border of the patella. Dissection is continued down subperiosteally along the proximal half of the medial patella border to the interval between layers 2 and 3 (between the MPFL and capsular layer; Fig. 11-5). This interval is bluntly developed medially toward the medial epicondyle using a curved Kelly clamp. The graft should always be placed extra-articularly (superficial) adjacent to the capsule. The second incision is made over the tip of the clamp as it overlies the saddle between the epicondyle and adductor tubercle (Figs. 11-6 and 11-7). The femoral attachment of the MPFL is identified using the landmarks of the medial epicondyle, medial collateral ligament (MCL), and adductor tubercle. The femoral attachment of the MPFL resides in the saddle between the adductor tubercle and medial epicondyle. The fascia is incised and a 2.4-mm guide pin (Bio-Tenodesis fixation set; Arthrex) is placed

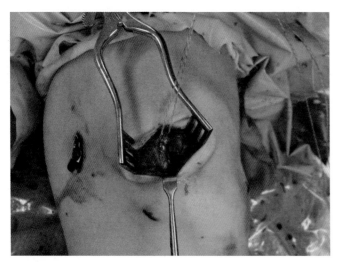

FIGURE 11-5 Dissection is carried down between layers 2 and 3 as a tag suture is placed in layers 1 and 2. sutured.

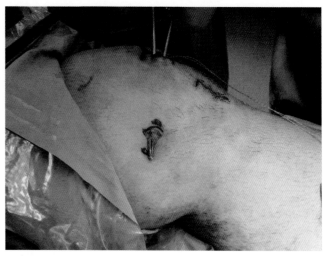

FIGURE 11-7 A C arm can also be used to identify the proper femoral attachment point (Schöttle's point), which is particularly helpful for obese patients in whom the landmarks are not palpable.

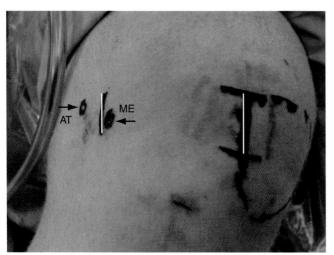

FIGURE 11-6 Two planned skin incisions. One longer utility incision can be used if other patellar procedures such as cartilage restoration are performed. AT, adductor tubercle; ME, medial epicondyle.

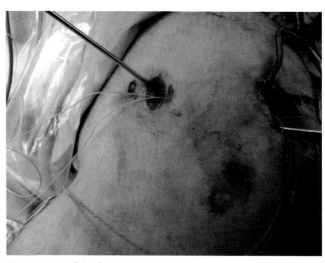

FIGURE 11-8 If the first guide pin placement is incorrect, it can be left as a reference while another pin is drilled.

just proximal and posterior to the epicondyle and distal and anterior to the adductor tubercle. A C arm can be helpful for identifying the correct pin placement properly, also known as Schöttle's point (Fig. 11-8).[18] A no. 2 suture is wrapped around this guide pin; the free ends are passed to the patellar incision with the clamp through the same MPFL–capsular interval layer and sutured into the patellar attachment site of the MPFL, which is along the proximal half of the medial patella. Note that the arms of the suture are at the proximal and distal extent of the patellar MPFL attachment footprint (Fig. 11-9). The suture is tied with all slackness removed, with the knee at 30 degrees of flexion. The knee is then placed through range of motion. The suture should become lax with increasing flexion and minimally change or slightly tighten in terminal extension (Fig. 11-10). The planned attachments sites and MPFL length should not overconstrain, overtension, or tilt the patella medially at any point during full range of motion.

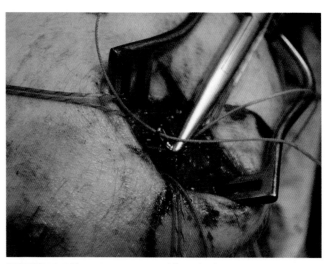

FIGURE 11-9 The sutures are passed from the femoral pin to the patellar capsule to simulate the role of the graft and assess length change characteristics through a range of motion.

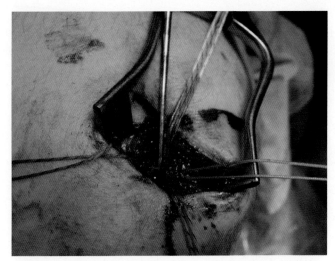

FIGURE 11-10 A probe is shown palpating the sutures through a range of motion. If the sutures tighten in flexion, the femoral guide pin must be moved distally.

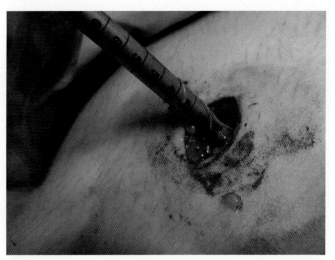

FIGURE 11-11 The femoral-sided dissection may put branches of the saphenous nerve at risk if not looked for.

The key to this operation is carefully determining the proper femoral attachment point.[18] The two factors most critical for preventing increased patellofemoral contact forces are determining the proper fixation point and avoiding graft overtensioning. The location of the femoral attachment site alters the graft distances (and therefore the graft tension) through knee range of motion much more than the patellar site as a result of the cam shape of the medial femoral condyle. This means that there is no true isometric point but rather an anisometric point, where the graft can have proper changes of length through a range of motion.[14] Even slight variations in position of the femoral attachment site can have major implications on the patellar tracking and contact forces.[19] If the suture does not exhibit the desired length changes during range of motion, the pin in the epicondyle must be repositioned. Usually, if there is excessive tightening in extension, the graft is too distal or posterior, and, if there is increased tension in flexion, the femoral point is too proximal or anterior. Distal-proximal variation has the greatest effect. Overconstraining not only causes abnormal contact forces on the medial facet of the patella, but also makes it more difficult to regain flexion in the postoperative rehabilitation. Our ultimate goal is to re-create a passive restraint to excessive lateral patellar displacement, specifically in extension and the early phases of flexion. It should re-create normal anatomy and therefore allow a normal degree of lateral patellar mobility, as compared with the contralateral knee. The graft should not be used forcefully to pull the patella medially, nor should it tighten in flexion when the patella engages the trochlea; This could result in loss of motion and markedly increased pressures on the medial facet.

Femoral Socket Preparation

When the appropriate femoral attachment site has been determined, a cannulated drill bit from the Bio-Tenodesis system is chosen that is 0.5 to 1 mm larger than the size of the doubled sutured end of the graft. The femoral socket is then drilled to a depth 2 mm longer than the designated screw size length, usually 25 mm (Fig. 11-11). In most cases, a 7- × 23-mm or

8- × 23-mm Bio-Tenodesis screw is used. The appropriately sized screw is loaded onto the Bio-Tenodesis driver. A no. 2 FiberWire suture loop or no. 2 FiberWire suture snare is passed through the center cannulation of the driver tip. The sutures from the graft are placed through the suture loop. The sutures extending from the graft are then pulled up into the center cannulation of the driver and secured as they exit the Bio-Tenodesis driver handle. The Bio-Tenodesis screwdriver tip (Bio-Tenodesis fixation set) is then advanced into the socket, pulling the graft into the socket with the screw in the posterior aspect of the socket and the tendon placed anteriorly (Fig. 11-12). The screw is then advanced into the socket until it is flush to the cortical bone rim. This technique allows for fixation into a closed socket, without requiring drilling through the opposite cortex.

Graft Length Selection and Patellar Fixation

We currently use a Bio-Suture Tak (Arthrex) reverse loop technique. Two doubly loaded 2.9- or 3.7-mm Bio-Suture Tak

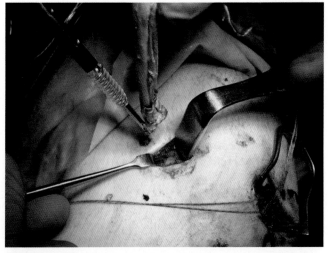

FIGURE 11-12 Drill a tunnel 0.5 mm larger than the measured graft and place the Bio-Tenodesis screw posterior to the graft.

anchors are reloaded in a loop-to-loop fashion with the FiberWire loop end rerouted through the suture anchor loop. This technique allows an easier method to fine tune graft tension and increase the surface area of tendon to bone contact. It involves removing the anchor from the insertion handle and removing both sutures from the eyelet. One of the sutures from the anchor is doubled on itself and the looped end is rethreaded through the eyelet. The second suture from the anchor is then passed through the loop of the first suture. It does not need to be rethreaded through the eyelet; it is captured in the loop of the first suture (Fig. 11-13). The four tails of the sutures are then passed back down the insertion handle using a passing wire so that the anchor can be reloaded onto the handle (Fig. 11-14). The suture anchors are placed in a trough, created with a small rongeur, in the medial edge of the patella (from the midwaist, superiorly) anterior to the articular cartilage, approximately 2 cm apart (Fig. 11-15). The two free arms

of the allograft tendon are brought through the developed soft tissue tunnel interval from the femoral attachment to the patella (Fig. 11-16). After pulling the sutures and graft tails through the soft tissue interval, the two free ends of the graft are pulled through the anchor suture loops (Fig. 11-17). One tail of the Y graft is through the midwaist loop and the other tail is through the proximal loop. The secondary suture loops from each anchor are then removed. The suture loops are temporarily cinched tight around the graft and held with hemostats (Fig. 11-18). The initial graft length is set at approximately 30 degrees of flexion, with both grafts pulled to length with slight tension and no laxity. The knee should be brought through a full range of motion, with the graft only slightly tightening between 30 and 0 degrees and becoming progressively lax in flexion. The graft tension should allow for identical lateral patellar translation as compared with the contralateral knee, or 1+ to 2+ lateral translation of the patella at

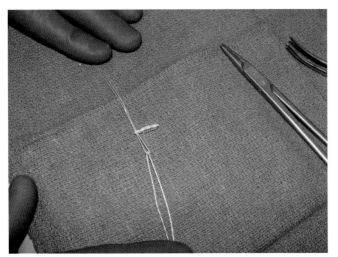

FIGURE 11-13 Reloading the anchor with a reverse loop means rethreading one of the anchor sutures through the eyelet while it is doubled (*blue suture*) and then passing the other suture (*tiger stripe*) through the loop of the first (*blue suture*).

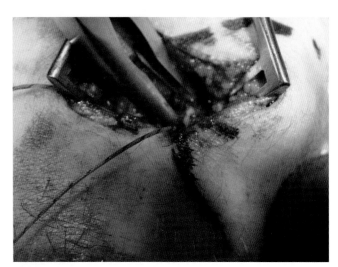

FIGURE 11-15 Trough being created with the rongeur. Another option is to use a light burring technique.

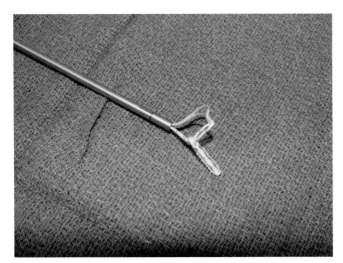

FIGURE 11-14 Rethreading all the suture ends back down the shaft of the anchor driver requires a thin, ~26-gauge wire or Prolene to reload the sutures in the insertion handle.

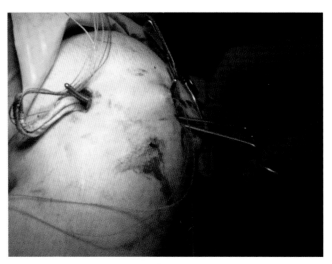

FIGURE 11-16 The distal free graft end is marked with a marker so that it does not get twisted when pulled under the tissue bridge and out though the patellar incision.

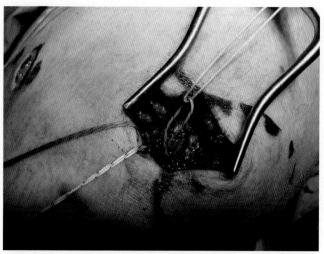

FIGURE 11-17 The reverse loaded anchor allows us to "cinch" the graft inside the tiger striped suture loop for tension adjustment and fixation—and then to discard the blue suture.

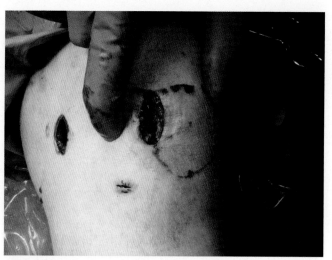

FIGURE 11-19 Normal physiologic glide. Avoid the impulse to overtension the graft.

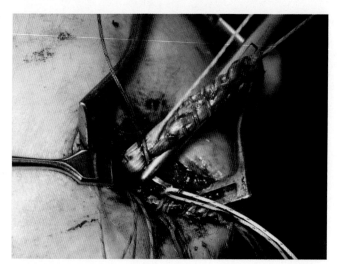

FIGURE 11-18 After the graft is passed though the looped suture (from the anchor) and tested for tension, the graft is marked; the free ends of the suture loops are passed through the tendon slightly medial to that point with a free needle and then tied.

0 and 30 degrees of knee flexion if the other side is affected (Fig. 11-19).

Once the ideal graft length is set, the locations of the suture loops are marked on the graft with a marking pen and the free ends of the sutures are passed through the tendon with a free needle and tied. The knee is taken through a range of motion and lateral patellar glide is rechecked during the final tensioning to avoid overtightening the graft. After tying the anchor suture loops, additional sutures can be added, further securing the graft to the soft tissue sleeve at the medial edge of the patella, and the remaining graft is passed back toward the femoral attachment and sutured to itself. We tie the sutures exiting the Bio-Tenodesis screw from the femoral attachment to the strands at the end of the graft tails as one final method of reinforcement against graft slippage. Layers 1 and 2 are reattached to the patellar periosteum or imbricated if more reinforcement is necessary.

PEARLS & PITFALLS

PEARLS

1. An allograft is just as effective as an autograft.
2. The femoral attachment of the MPFL resides in the saddle between the adductor tubercle and medial epicondyle, so the proximal posterior slope of the medial epicondyle is a good landmark to use for the femoral attachment.
3. Use fluoroscopy for identifying Schöttle's point in heavy patients, or even routinely.
4. Proper positioning of the femoral attachment is the key to successful surgery and requires testing in flexion and extension, with sutures attached to the patella. The suture is a good simulation of the graft before final socket preparation.
5. The contralateral knee should be tested to match medial and lateral patellar glide, if normal.
6. The anchors on the patella are reverse-loaded so that the graft may be pulled through the suture loops and easily tensioned on the patellar side.
7. Full range of motion should be easily obtained at the end of the procedure.
8. Be aggressive about regaining range of motion early.

PITFALLS

1. Avoid techniques that do not allow fine tuning of length and tension.
2. If the graft is fixed too proximally on the femur, it will tighten in flexion and may limit postoperative knee flexion.
3. Overconstraint of the MPFL will lead to premature patellofemoral arthrosis.
4. MPFL reconstruction is an instability procedure only; it is not an operation for pain.
5. Avoid large transverse tunnels through the patella, which can lead to fracture.
6. This procedure does not correct malalignment—that is, it is not meant to pull the patella into a centered location. This should be performed, if necessary, by adding a tubercle osteotomy, especially if the TTTG value of more than 20 mm and there is fixed lateral subluxation and/or rotation on the imaging studies.

COMPLICATIONS

Early complications range from the possibility of infection to deep venous thrombosis. We recommend use of compression stockings and aspirin prophylaxis. Late complications include a loss of knee range of motion, failure of fixation, recurrent instability, saphenous neuroma, pain at femoral or patellar fixation sites, and increased patellar pain and arthrosis caused by changes in joint forces. Usually, residual pain symptoms are mostly correlated with the status of the articular cartilage.

POSTOPERATIVE REHABILITATION PROTOCOL

A compressive soft dressing, antiembolism stockings, and a hinged knee brace, initially locked in extension, are applied. We encourage early aggressive range of motion and use a continuous passive range of motion machine beginning on postoperative day 2, with a goal of 120 degrees of flexion by 2 to 3 weeks postoperatively. Quadriceps isometrics are allowed. We allow weight bearing, as tolerated, with crutches and a knee brace locked in extension until the patient has good quadriceps control without lag. Standard patellofemoral proximal and core functional muscular exercises are performed throughout the postoperative period. Transition from a postoperative brace to a lateral buttress patellar stabilizing brace is encouraged as quadriceps control is regained, usually around week 6. We emphasize close monitoring of range of motion as essential to ensure that a full range of motion is achieved in the early postoperative setting. If distal realignment or articular cartilage procedures are performed concomitantly, the progression of exercises, range of motion, and weight bearing are modified accordingly.

After 6 weeks, progressive strengthening and functional exercises are continued postoperatively until full strength, endurance, and agility have been reestablished. Once all goals are met, activities are advanced through a functional progression program, with return to sports at 3 to 4 months. Patellofemoral bracing may be used according to patient and surgeon preference.

CONCLUSIONS

Although reconstruction of the medial patellofemoral ligament prevents recurrent dislocation of the patella, the biomechanics of the medial patellofemoral restraints are still not fully understood. Specifically, the role of the medial patellar meniscal ligament (MPML) and medial patellar tibial ligament (MPTL) are not completely understood. It has been shown that they are less important than the MPFL, but they may still have a role in patellar stability. The interaction of patella alta and trochlear dysplasia with MPFL reconstruction are other areas that warrant further investigation. Also, other authors have suggested alternative techniques for reconstruction. Instead of the reverse-loaded anchors, drill holes in the patella can be used for fixation,[20] the graft can be fixed into a closed patellar socket,[14] MPFL and MTFL ligaments can be reconstructed concurrently,[21] and other grafts such as the adductor longus can be used.[22]

REFERENCES

1. Hauser EW. Total tendon transplant for slipping patella. *Surg Gynecol Obstet.* 1938;66:199.
2. Insall J, Falvo KA, Wise DW. Chondromalacia patella. *J Bone Joint Surg Am.* 1976;58:1-8.
3. Bonvallent JM. Resultats de la reflection a la peau de l'aileron rotulien interne dans les luxatins recidivantes de la rotule. *Chirurgie.* 1973;99: 124-128.
4. Davis DK, Fithian DC. Techniques of medial retinacular repair and reconstruction. *Clin Orthop.* 2002;402:38-52.
5. Fulkerson JP. *Disorders of the Patellofemoral Joint.* 3rd ed. Baltimore: Williams and Wilkins; 1997.
6. Nomura E, Fujikawa T, et al. Anatomical study of the medial patellofemoral ligament. *Orthop Surg Suppl.* 1992;22:2-5.
7. Ficat P. *Pathologie Femoror-Patellaire.* Paris: Masson; 1970.
8. Baker RH, Carroll N, Dewar P, Hall J. Semitendinosus tenodesis for recurrent dislocation of the patella. 1972;54:103-109.
9. Amis, AA, Firer P, Mountney J, et al. Anatomy and biomechanics of the medial patellofemoral ligament. *Knee.* 2003;10:215-220.
10. Conlan T, Garth WP Jr, Lemons JE. Evaluation of the medial soft tissue restraints of the extensor mechanism of the knee. *J Bone Joint Surg Am.* 1993;75:682-693.
11. Burks RT, Desio SM, Bachus KN, et al. Biomechanical evaluation of lateral patellar dislocations. *Am J Knee Surg.* 1998;11:24-31.
12. Desio SM, Burks RT, Bachus KN. Soft tissue restraints to lateral patellar translation in the human knee. *Am J Sports Med.* 1998;26:59-65.
13. Hautamaa PV, Fithian DC, Kaufman KR, et al. Medial soft tissue restraints in lateral patellar instability and repair. *Clin Orthop Relat Res.* 1998;(349):174-182.
14. Farr J, Schepsis AA. Reconstruction of the medial patellofemoral ligament for recurrent patellar instability. *J Knee Surg.* 2006;19:307-316.
15. Grelsamer RP, Proctor CS, Bazos AN. Evaluation of patellar shape in the sagittal plane. A clinical analysis. *Am J Sports Med.* 1994;22:61-66.
16. Dejour H, Walch G, Nove-Josserand L, Guier C. Factors of patellar instability: an anatomic radiographic study. *Knee Surg Sports Traumatol Arthrosc.* 1994;2:19-26.
17. Hamner DL, Brown CH Jr, Steiner ME, et al. Hamstring tendon grafts for reconstruction of the anterior cruciate ligament: biomechanical evaluation of the use of multiple strands and tensioning techniques. *J Bone Joint Surg Am.* 1999;81:549-557.
18. Steensen RN, Dopirak RM, McDonald WG 3rd. The anatomy and isometry of the medial patellofemoral ligament: implications for reconstruction. *Am J Sports Med.* 2004;32:1509-1513.
19. Elias JJ, Cosgarea AJ. Tension in a reconstructed MPFL could overload medial patellofemoral cartilage: a computational analysis. *Am J Sports Med.* 2006;34:1478-1485.
20. Fithian DC, Paxton EW. Epidemiology and natural history of acute patellar dislocation. *Am J Sports Med.* 2004;32:1114-1121.
21. Drez D Jr, Edwards TB. Results of medial patellofemoral ligament reconstruction and treatment of patellar dislocation. *Arthroscopy.* 2001;17: 298-306.
22. Teitge RA, Spak RT. Lateral patellofemoral ligament reconstruction. *Arthroscopy.* 2004;20:998-1002.

SUGGESTED READING

Schöttle PB, Schmeling A, Rosenstiel N, et al. Radiographic landmarks for femoral tunnel placement in medial patellofemoral ligament reconstruction. *Am J Sports Med.* 2007;35:801-804.

Tibial Tubercle Transfer

John P. Fulkerson

The goal of patellofemoral stabilization surgery is central, tracking of the patella in the femoral trochlea. If stable tracking can be achieved using nonoperative means such as core stability physical therapy, and bracing, surgery should be avoided. The caregiver should also rule out retinacular[1,2] or articular[3,4] pain causing the knee to give way. A thorough history and examination,[5] using pain diagrams[6] as needed, is central to accurate diagnosis and appropriate surgical planning. Unfortunately, many patients with recurrent patellar instability require some form of stabilization to function adequately in work and daily life, particularly in more vigorous activities. This is particularly important because chronic lateral patellofemoral articular overload may eventually cause joint breakdown.[7] Debate continues regarding the evolution of trochlea dysplasia,[8,9] but it is likely that chronic lateral facet overload from lateral patellar tracking[10] may contribute to or cause deficiency of lateral trochlear containment of the patella.

It must be considered that balanced patellar tracking with optimal load distribution across the joint is best for patients and presumably minimizes risk of eventual cartilage deterioration and arthritis. Therefore, balanced tracking is of paramount importance. Multiple factors are involved in patellar tracking, including femoral version, tibial version, articular geometry, lower extremity kinematic function, muscle imbalance, foot and ankle mechanics, ligamentory balance of the knee, varies, valgus, body habitus, and posture. Some of these are correctable by nonoperative measures and should therefore be addressed before considering surgery.[11] Certainly, an articular lesion causing symptoms of giving way may be mistaken for patellar instability and should be treated appropriately, whether by simple débridement[12] or articular resurfacing.[13-18]

Procedures such as trochleoplasty and femoral and tibial derotation may be appropriate in rare patients but carry risks that many surgeons and patients find unacceptable. Therefore, traditional patellofemoral stabilization, using lateral release, medial retinacular restoration (medial patellofemoral ligament [MPFL] imbrication or reconstruction), and/or medial tibial tubercle transfer remain mainstays of patellofemoral stabilization. Lateral release[19-22] has been used widely in the past but has little relevance as an isolated procedure for patients with patellar instability[23] and can cause medial patellar instability[24] when used extensively or inappropriately.

The art of patellofemoral stabilization is to determine how best to achieve balanced patellar tracking with minimal long- and short-term risk. This is different for each patient and becomes more challenging as the degree of instability increases.

Restoration of patellofemoral balance by MPFL–medial capsule imbrication, often with release of a lateral retinaculum that has become adaptively tight, is desirable, particularly because it is known that the injured MPFL does heal,[25] albeit elongated, in most patients. Sometimes, a tendon graft needs to be added to ensure adequate medial retinacular–MPFL support of the patella,[26] but this should be done selectively, when less invasive surgery is judged to be insufficient. Many patients with less serious instability are happy to undergo a smaller procedure with the knowledge that another procedure might be needed in the future. This is occasionally preferable to the alternative risk of surgical complication from a more major surgical intervention. In any case, however, it is important to consider that the MPFL is an important restraint to lateral patellar instability[27-29]; be prepared to restore or reconstruct it selectively once adequate patellar tracking alignment had been ensured. Most important in this

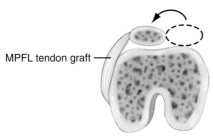

MPFL tendon graft

FIGURE 12-1 Pulling the patella from lateral to medial with an MPFL graft risks overloading the patellofemoral joint. Balance tracking first.

type of surgery is to avoid excessive patellofemoral joint loading, because the MPFL is a posteriorly oriented structure (Fig. 12-1). Tibial tubercle transfer is the best way to restore proper tracking of the patella in the trochlea in many cases, after which retinacular balance, including the MPFL, can be restored by imbrication or tendon graft reconstruction but without exerting force on the patella. Following tibial tubercle transfer balancing of the extensor mechanism, however, MPFL restoration is often unnecessary, because it usually adapts over time.

TREATMENT

Prerequisites

The patient must have exhausted all nonoperative options, including core stability, physical therapy, and bracing. The patient should lose weight, if necessary, and stop smoking before surgery.

Indications

In patients with more serious lateral patellar tracking, the medial-lateral distance[30] between the tibial tuberosity and trochlear groove (TTTG) is often 15 to 20 mm or more. A well-done axial radiograph at 45 degrees of knee flexion[31] and a precise lateral[32] radiograph are extremely important in determining the resting position of the patella with respect to the trochlea. The patient with prominent J tracking and disability related to serious lateral patellar tracking will often benefit most from medial transfer of the tibial tubercle.[33,34] This is a compensatory procedure that does not correct all the underlying structural problems; however, a medial tibial tubercle transfer yields functional stabilization of the patellofemoral joint quickly and without exerting a posteromedial pull vector on the patella. Tibial tubercle transfer yields balanced patellofemoral tracking, the possibility of immediate range of motion after surgery, and permanent stability when properly and accurately performed.

Tibial detrotation can accomplish this goal also but requires fibular head osteotomy and complete transection of the tibia. Tibial tubercle transfer alone, properly done, yields central patellar tracking without the risks involved with transtibial osteotomy and derotation.

Tibial tubercle transfer can also unload the distal patella by adding obliquity to the cut behind the tibial tubercle (anteromedial tibial tubercle transfer), thereby lifting up and unloading the distal and lateral patellar articulating surfaces. These are frequently fragmented and/or painful in the patient with chronic lateral patellar tracking.[35-40]

As the lateral and distal patella manifest evidence of degenerative cartilage related to excessive lateral pressure, anteromedial tibial tubercle transfer becomes more important for redistribution of contact forces on the patella and for enhanced stability and joint preservation. Long-term results of anteromedial tibial tubercle transfer have been very good in properly selected patients with lateral and distal patellar articular damage.[40,41] Medial patellofemoral ligament reconstruction is not as likely to help these patients and involves some risk of chronic pain if a fragmented distal medial patella receives added load following medial capsule ligamentous reconstruction.

Nonetheless, retinacular balancing in conjunction with tibial tubercle transfer can be helpful and sometimes necessary. In particular, when there is trochlear dysplasia,[42] supplemental MPFL advancement, imbrication, or reconstruction may help in achieving an optimal, balanced end result. The key here is achieving balanced tracking of the patella first (this often requires tibial tubercle transfer when there is an elevated TTTG distance, Q angle, and trochlea dysplasia) and then adjusting the retinacular-ligamentous peripatellar restraints. Note that retinacular restraints to pull the patella into place should not be used because of the risk of creating articular overload. Additionally, MPFL reconstruction must be done with exquisite attention to accuracy or articular excessive articular loading will likely occur.[43]

Tibial tubercle transfer also permits slight distalization of the extensor mechanism, which can be very helpful in re-establishing patellar tracking stability in the patient with patella alta. Slight tibial tubercle distalization at the time of medial or anteromedial tibial tubercle transfer may be appropriate for selected patients to further enhance stability.

In summary, medial, anteromedial, and/or distal tibial tubercle transfers are powerful and reliable surgical procedures in patellofemoral stabilization surgery. Determining when to use these procedures versus proximal reconstruction is based predominantly on the degree of lateral tracking, amount of patellofemoral dysplasia, and extent of articular breakdown that needs to be unloaded and/or balanced.

Arthroscopic Technique

After determining that the patient needs a tibial tubercle transfer, discuss options with the patient and be sure that he or she understands that you will do only what is necessary at the time of surgery. Perform an arthroscopy and consider the location of articular lesions in designing the osteotomy. Avoid adding load to any damaged, vulnerable joint surface by appropriate design of the osteotomy. Perform an arthroscopic lateral release, as needed, to correct patellar tilt or allow patellar immobilization medially.

Exsanguinate the extremity and inflate the tourniquet. Incise the skin longitudinally from the midpatellar tendon to about 5 cm distal to the tibial tubercle. Release the anterior tibialis muscle from the anterior tibia and reflect posteriorly all the way to the posterior tibia subperiosteally (Fig. 12-2). Dissect behind patellar tendon enough to expose 1cm above patellar tendon insertion.

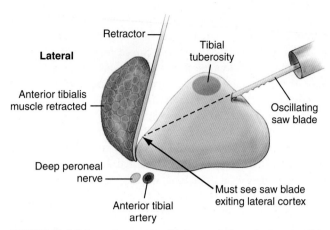

FIGURE 12-2 Release the anterior tibialis muscle from the anterior tibia and reflect posteriorly all the way to the posterior tibia subperiosteally.

Plan the osteotomy to provide a flat cut (tapered to anterior tibia distally) for pure medial tibial tubercle transfer (Elmslie-Trillat procedure; Fig. 12-3). Perform an oblique osteotomy from the anteromedial tibia, adjacent to the patellar tendon insertion (see Fig. 12-3) to achieve anteromedial tibial tubercle transfer (see Figs. 12-2 and 12-3A). Be sure of exposure and use an oscillating saw to make the cut, using a guide system as needed, but be sure that the cut is appropriate for the desired medial and anterior transposition of the tibial tubercle. Again, be sure to taper the osteotomy to the anterior tibia distally (Fig. 12-4).

Make the distal cut first and watch the saw blade at all times as it exits the tibial cortex laterally. Once this cut is completed to a level 1 cm above the medial patellar tendon insertion, make an oblique cut on the lateral side to connect the posterolateral extent of the lateral cut to above the patellar tendon. A final cut just above the patellar tendon connects the medial and lateral cuts and permits mobilization of the bone pedicle, which can then be moved medially (Elmslie-Trillat procedure) or anteromedially (Fulkerson procedure). Once the bone pedicle has been rotated to the desired position, often about 1 cm medially or anteromedially, depending on what is needed, check patellar tracking arthroscopically. Once tracking is optimal, lock the transferred tibial tubercle in its corrected position with two cortical lag screws into the posterior tibial cortex, obtain hemostasis, use drainage as needed, and close the skin only.

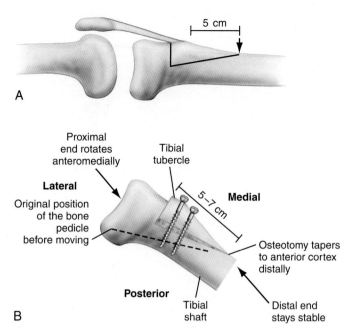

FIGURE 12-4 Lateral view of the patellofemoral joint. The osteotomy should be tapered to the anterior tibia distally.

Place the leg in a compressive wrap and knee immobilizer, use cryotherapy, and start the patient on range of motion exercises as soon as possible.

In the patient with documented patella alta, slight distalization of the tibial tubercle may be needed. This is not often necessary but is important in the patella alta patient to ensure proper timely entry of the patella into the trochlea. To accomplish distalization (usually no more than 5 to 8 mm), just enough to allow prompt entry of the patella into the trochlea arthroscopically at the initiation of flexion, remove about 1 cm of the distal tip of the bone pedicle, slide the pedicle distally the desired amount, and place an autogenous corticocancellous bone graft from the lateral metaphysis above the transferred pedicle. Then, secure the transferred bone pedicle, properly oriented, with two cortical lag screws into the posterior cortex. Another option is to make a proximal cut above the patellar tendon insertion, which is vertical and angled so that the tibial tubercle is forced slightly distally on medialization (Fig. 12-5). This technique is pertinent only when there is need for medialization at the time of tubercle distalization.

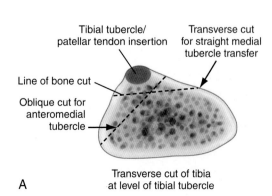

A

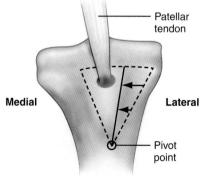

B Tibial tubercle rotated medially

FIGURE 12-3 Plan the osteotomy to provide a flat cut (tapered to anterior tibia distally) for pure medial tibial tubercle transfer (Elmslie-Trillat procedure). **A,** transverse cut. **B,** Tibial tubercle rotated medially.

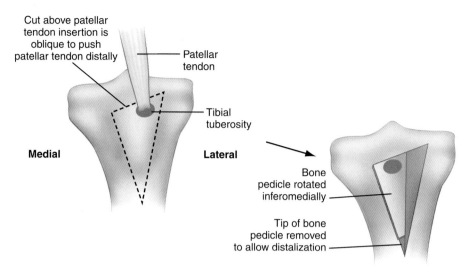

Cut above patellar
tendon insertion is
oblique to push
patellar tendon distally

Patellar
tendon

Tibial
tuberosity

Medial

Lateral

Bone
pedicle rotated
inferomedially

Tip of bone
pedicle removed
to allow distalization

FIGURE 12-5 Make the proximal cut above the patellar tendon insertion vertical and angled so that the tibial tubercle is forced slightly distally on medialization.

In the patient with patella baja, after making the proper cuts, remove bone as needed to allow the bone pedicle to slide proximally and securely against a proximal metaphyseal bone buttress. Be sure that all infrapatellar contracture is released and fully mobilized.

In cases of medial patellar instability related to previous excessive medial tibial tubercle transfer, a reverse tibial tubercle transfer can be appropriate. Again, be sure to release any contracture or tethering of the medial retinaculum distally.

Anterolateral tibial tubercle transfer (ALTTT) can be very effective in reversing a previous Hauser procedure. ALTTT can unload a worn out medial patellar articular surface. Anteromedial tibial tubercle transfer has been useful as an adjunct to articular resurfacing procedures and has been shown to be effective by Farr and associates.[35]

PEARLS & PITFALLS

PEARLS

1. Move the tibial tubercle only with accurate indications and for specific correction of alignment and articular unloading
2. Always taper the osteotomy toward the anterior tibial cortex distally
3. Always watch the saw blade as it exits bone under direct vision and follow it visually until done cutting.
4. For a steeper osteotomy, stay very close to the patellar tendon on the medial side to maximize the steepness of the angle and maximize anteriorization (offloading the distal patella)
5. Be sure to release any constraining scar or tight tissue laterally and in the fat pad region (particularly any contracture) at the time of the osteotomy.
6. Use the cortical lag screw technique. Do not use cancellous screws because they can be difficult to remove.
7. Start range of motion as soon as possible after surgery.
8. Delay running until 6 months postoperatively.

Postoperative Management

Compression, elevation, and cryotherapy are helpful for 1 to 2 weeks. After almost all tibial tubercle transfer procedures, knee range of motion should be started as soon as possible. Thus, fixation must be secure enough to permit this. Early motion out of the postoperative splint should encourage 90 degrees of flexion, once daily, by 2 to 3 weeks after surgery. Crutches should be used for 5 to 6 weeks with a gradual increase of weight bearing to full weight by 6 weeks. Most patients will then benefit from physical therapy to optimize motion, strength, proprioception, and return to optimal function.

REFERENCES

1. Fulkerson JP, Tennant R, Jaivin JS, Grunnet M. Histologic evidence of retinacular nerve injury associated with patellofemoral malalignment. *Clin Orthop Relat Res.* 1985;(197):196-205.
2. Biedert RM, Stauffer E, Friederich NF. Occurrence of free nerve endings in the soft tissue of the knee joint. A histologic investigation. *Am J Sports Med.* 1992;20:430-433.
3. Post WR. Anterior knee pain: diagnosis and treatment. *J Am Acad Orthop Surg.* 2005;13:534-543.
4. Post WR. Clinical evaluation of patients with patellofemoral disorders. *Arthroscopy.* 1999;15:841-851.
5. Fulkerson JP. Diagnosis and treatment of patients with patellofemoral pain. *Am J Sports Med.* 2002;30:447-456.
6. Post WR, Fulkerson J. Knee pain diagrams: correlation with physical examination findings in patients with anterior knee pain. *Arthroscopy.* 1994;10:618-623.
7. Ficat P. [The syndrome of lateral hyperpressure of the patella.] *Acta Orthop Belg.* 1978;44:65-76.
8. Dejour H, Walch G, Nove-Josserand L, Guier C. Factors of patellar instability: an anatomic radiographic study. *Knee Surg Sports Traumatol Arthrosc.* 1994;2:19-26.
9. Dejour H, Walch G, Neyret P, Adeleine P. [Dysplasia of the femoral trochlea.] *Rev Chir Orthop Reparatrice Appar Mot.* 1990;76:45-54.
10. Ostermeier S, Holst M, Hurschler C, et al. Dynamic measurement of patellofemoral kinematics and contact pressure after lateral retinacular release: an in vitro study. *Knee Surg Sports Traumatol Arthrosc.* 2007;15:547-554.
11. Ireland ML, Willson JD, Ballantyne BT, Davis IM. Hip strength in females with and without patellofemoral pain. *J Orthop Sports Phys Ther.* 2003;33:671-676.
12. Federico DJ, Reider B. Results of isolated patellar debridement for patellofemoral pain in patients with normal patellar alignment. *Am J Sports Med.* 1997;25:663-669.
13. Jones DG, Peterson L. Autologous chondrocyte implantation. *J Bone Joint Surg Am.* 2006;88:2502-2520.
14. Knutsen G, Drogset JO, Engebretsen L, et al. A randomized trial comparing autologous chondrocyte implantation with microfracture. Findings at five years. *J Bone Joint Surg Am.* 2007;89:2105-2112.
15. Knutsen G, Engebretsen L, Ludvigsen TC, et al. Autologous chondrocyte implantation compared with microfracture in the knee. A randomized trial. *J Bone Joint Surg Am.* 2004;86:455-464.

16. Lee G, Kelly MA. Isolated patellofemoral arthritis without malalignment. In: Fulkerson J, ed. *Common Patellofemoral Problems.* Rosemont, Ill: American Academy of Orthopaedic Surgeons; 2005:73-84.

17. Minas T. Autologous chondrocyte implantation for focal chondral defects of the knee. *Clin Orthop Relat Res.* 2001;(391 suppl):S349.

18. Saleh KJ, Arendt EA, Eldridge J, et al. Symposium. Operative treatment of patellofemoral arthritis. *J Bone Joint Surg Am.* 2005;87:659-671.

19. Lattermann C, Toth J, Bach BR Jr. The role of lateral retinacular release in the treatment of patellar instability. *Sports Med Arthrosc Rev.* 2007;15:57-60.

20. Ford DH, Post WR. Open or arthroscopic lateral release. Indications, techniques, and rehabilitation. *Clin Sports Med.* 1997;16:29-49.

21. Fulkerson JP, Schutzer SF, Ramsby GR, Bernstein RA. Computerized tomography of the patellofemoral joint before and after lateral release or realignment. *Arthroscopy.* 1987;3:19-24.

22. Panni AS, Tartarone M, Patricola A, et al. Long-term results of lateral retinacular release. *Arthroscopy.* 2005;21:526-531.

23. Fithian DC, Paxton EW, Post WR, Panni AS. Lateral retinacular release: a survey of the International Patellofemoral Study Group. *Arthroscopy.* 2004;20:463-468.

24. Hughston JC, Deese M. Medial subluxation of the patella as a complication of lateral retinacular release. *Am J Sports Med.* 1988;16:383-388.

25. Tom A, Fulkerson J. Restoration of native MPFL support after patella dislocation. *Sports Med Arthrosc Rev.* 2007;15:68-71.

26. Bicos J, Fulkerson JP, Amis A. Current concepts review: the medial patellofemoral ligament. *Am J Sports Med.* 2007;35:484-492.

27. Amis AA, Firer P, Mountney J, et al. Anatomy and biomechanics of the medial patellofemoral ligament. *Knee.* 2003;10:215-28.

28. Arendt EA, Fithian DC, Cohen E. Current concepts of lateral patella dislocation. *Clin Sports Med.* 2002;21:499-519.

29. Nomura E, Horiuchi Y, Kihara M. Medial patellofemoral ligament restraint in lateral patellar translation and reconstruction. *Knee.* 2000;7:121-127.

30. Goutallier D, Bernageau J, Lecudonnec B. [The measurement of the tibial tuberosity. Patella groove distance technique and results (*author's transl*)]. *Rev Chir Orthop Reparatrice Appar Mot.* 1978;64:423-428.

31. Merchant AC, Mercer RL, Jacobsen RH, Cool CR. Roentgenographic analysis of patellofemoral congruence. *J Bone Joint Surg Am.* 1974;56:1391-1396.

32. Malghem J, Maldague B. [Profile of the knee. Differential radiologic anatomy of the articular surfaces.] *J Radiol.* 1986;67:725-735.

33. Pritsch T, Haim A, Arbel, R, et al. Tailored tibial tubercle transfer for patellofemoral malalignment: analysis of clinical outcomes. *Knee Surg Sports Traumatol Arthrosc.* 2007;15:994-1002.

34. Trillat A, Dejour HL, Coutette A. Diagnostic et traitement des subluxations recidivantes de la rotule. *Rev Chir Orthop.* 1964;50:813-824.

35. Farr J, Schepsis A, Cole B, et al. Anteromedialization: review and technique. *J Knee Surg.* 2007;20:120-128.

36. Fulkerson JP. Anteromedialization of the tibial tuberosity for patellofemoral malalignment. *Clin Orthop Relat Res.* 1983;(177):176-181.

37. Fulkerson JP, Becker GJ, Meaney JA, et al. Anteromedial tibial tubercle transfer without bone graft. *Am J Sports Med.* 1990;18:490-496.

38. Fulkerson JP. Anteromedial tibial tubercle transfer. In: Jackson DW, ed. *Master Techniques in Orthopaedic Surgery: Reconstructive Knee Surgery,* Philadelphia: Lippincott, Williams & Wilkins; 2003:13-25.

39. Karamehmetoglu M, Ozturkmen Y, Azboy I, Caniklioglu M. [Fulkerson osteotomy for the treatment of chronic patellofemoral malalignment.] *Acta Orthop Traumatol Turc.* 2007;41:21-30.

40. Pidoriano AJ, Weinstein RN, Buuck DA, Fulkerson JP. Correlation of patellar articular lesions with results from anteromedial tibial tubercle transfer. *Am J Sports Med.* 1997;25:533-537.

41. Buuck D, Fulkerson J. Anteromedialization of the tibial tubercle: a 4- to 12-year follow-up. *Oper Tech Sports Med.* 2000;8:131-137.

42. Schottle PB, Scheffler SU, Schwarck A, Weiler A. Arthroscopic medial retinacular repair after patellar dislocation with and without underlying trochlear dysplasia: a preliminary report. *Arthroscopy.* 2006;22:1192-1198.

43. Elias JJ, Cosgarea AJ. Technical errors during medial patellofemoral ligament reconstruction could overload medial patellofemoral cartilage: a computational analysis. *Am J Sports Med.* 2006;34:1478-1485.

Arthritis and Cartilage Procedures

Degenerative Arthritis

Jack M. Bert

Significant controversy exists regarding the arthroscopic treatment of osteoarthritis (OA) of the knee. The indications for arthroscopic treatment of OA of the knee alone and in conjunction with other arthroscopic procedures will be reviewed.

Arthroscopic débridement for OA of the knee was initially reported by Burman and colleagues in 1934.[1] In 1941, Magnuson introduced the term "joint debridement."[2] During and after World War II, arthroscopy waned and the open Magnuson procedure, consisting of total synovectomy, osteophyte resection, cruciate ligament excision (if torn), and patellectomy became the treatment of choice for arthritis of the knee until the resurgence of arthroscopy in the early 1970s.[3]

ANATOMY

In 1743, William Hunter stated, "From Hippocrates to the present age, it is universally allowed that ulcerated cartilage is a troublesome thing and that once destroyed it is not repaired."[4] In 1849, Leidy confirmed this principle, stating that "a rupture of cartilage fragments is never united and that articular cartilage lacks regenerative power and the joint becomes filled with tough fibrous tissue."[5] As noted by Mankin, superficial lacerations of cartilage neither heal nor progress to more serious disorders if they are small lesions, but deep lacerations may be clearly visible years after injury.[6] When the subchondral bone is thus disrupted, interosseous blood vessels expose bone matrix growth factors, causing fibrin clot formation. Inflammation introduces new cells into the cartilage defect and these cells proliferate and begin matrix repair. The matrix of articular cartilage is a hyperhydrated tissue, with estimates of water content ranging as high as 80%; it contains type I collagen consisting of two alpha chains and one alpha-2 chain. It is this type I collagen that is formed when fibrous tissue regenerates when attempting to form normal hyaline articular cartilage.[7] Furthermore, mature repair tissue has a relatively low proteoglycan concentration. These reparative cells do not produce tissue with the unique composition, structure, and biochemical properties of normal articular cartilage.[8] After cartilage injury or during the progression of osteoarthritis, some chondrocytes proliferate but do not migrate through the matrix to enter the site of tissue injury. The repair tissue matrix, which is usually formed by undifferentiated cells containing primarily type I collagen, thus cannot restore normal articular cartilage properties. These reparative cells fail to organize the molecules that they produce to create a strong cohesive structure such as that of articular cartilage; rather, they produce other types of molecules that may interfere with the assembly of the cartilage matrix.

These alterations compromise the ability of cartilage to survive and function in the highly stressed mechanical environment found in load-bearing joints and may lead to further cartilage degeneration and osteoarthritis. Disruption of collagen cross-linking causes cartilage to lose its intrinsic tensile stiffness, strength, and shear stiffness, and this loss of proteoglycans and increased water content compromises its compressive and permeability properties.[9,10] A number of treatments have been attempted to stimulate repair or reformation of the articular surface of the knee joint. Arthroscopically, these treatments include marrow stimulation procedures, débridement and shaving of fibrillated cartilage, and joint lavage.

TREATMENT

Arthroscopic Technique

Marrow Stimulation Procedures

The concept of drilling through eburnated bone to stimulate reparative cartilage formation was originally described by Pridie in 1959 (Fig. 13-1).[11] Laboratory animal studies attempted to confirm these findings. Akeson and associates[12] drilled the subchondral bone of dog femoral heads and Mitchell and Shepard[13] drilled holes into the subchondral bone of rabbit knee joints. Both groups noted deterioration of the repair tissue within 1 year.

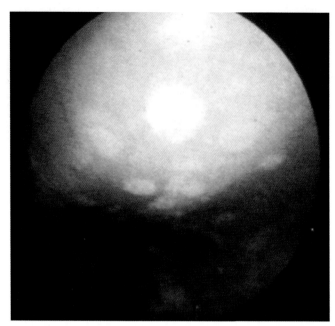

FIGURE 13-1 Fibrocartilage formation in medial femoral condylar drill holes (Pridie procedure).

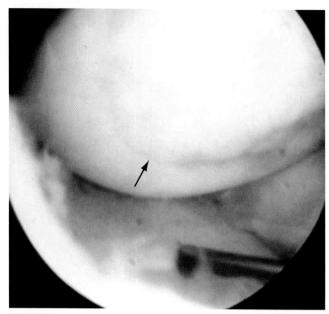

FIGURE 13-3 Arthroscopic view of a patient 4 years after abrasion arthroplasty showing resurfacing with fibrocartilage.

These experiments were the first to show that perforation of subchondral bone could stimulate repair of large areas of joint surface with fibrocartilaginous tissue, but the repair tissue lacked the proteoglycan concentration found in normal cartilage that was noted previously. Abrasion arthroplasty of grade IV eburnated chondral lesions using an arthroscopic burr to expose interosseus bleeding was introduced by Johnson[14] in 1981 (Fig. 13-2). The resulting hemorrhagic exudate formed a fibrin clot, allowing for fibrous repair tissue formation over the eburnated bone (Fig. 13-3). Only one of eight biopsy specimens showed any type II

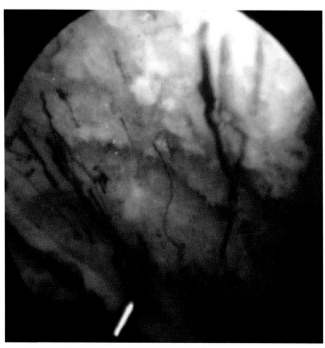

FIGURE 13-2 Abrasion arthroplasty showing bleeding bone.

collagen typical of hyaline cartilage at the time of arthroscopic review and biopsy, and the remainder had types I and III collagen. In a series of patients at our institution who had abrasion arthroplasty, at 5-year follow-up examinations, 15 had been converted to total knee replacement (TKR) and biopsies were obtained at the time of TKR. All patients had fibrocartilage and type I collagen on their biopsy specimens (Fig. 13-4). In this series of 126 patients who were treated for unicompartmental OA with abrasion arthroplasty plus débridement or arthroscopic débridement alone, only 51% had good to excellent results with abrasion arthroplasty at 5-year follow-up; 66% had good to excellent results with arthroscopic débridement alone.[15] Coventry and Bowman[16] have noted that formation of hyaline-like cartilage occurs in the unloaded medial compartment of several patients after valgus upper tibial osteotomy (Fig. 13-5). This finding was confirmed arthroscopically by Fujisawa and coworkers[17] 12 to 18 months after upper tibial osteotomies, which implies that regeneration of reparative cartilage can occur secondary to unloading of bone alone without additional surgery. Because adult articular cartilage does not heal and the regenerative tissue is not hyaline cartilage but fibrocartilage, it lacks normal amounts of proteoglycan. Thus, effective methods of repairing significant cartilage defects must provide cells that can migrate, proliferate, and differentiate in the chondral sites and produce and maintain a cartilage matrix. Furthermore, there must be a mechanical and biologic environment that promotes synthesis, assembly, and maintenance of articular cartilage matrix. This regenerative fibrocartilage has a difficult time transferring compressive loads and, therefore, cannot be expected to survive in an abnormal mechanical environment.[7-10]

Microfracture

Blevens and colleagues[18] have recommended the microfracture (MF) technique, in which they use an arthroscopic awl to create multiple perforations into the subchondral bone. They reported

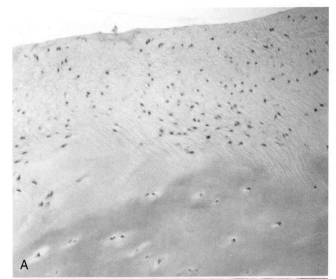

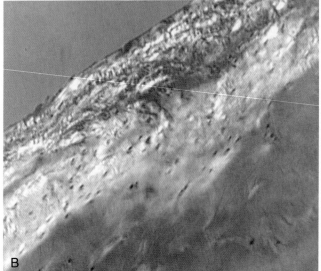

FIGURE 13-4 Electron microscopic view of regenerated fibrocartilage **(A)** with polarized light view **(B)** of same section showing the disorganized surface fibrocartilage compared to the hyaline cartilage cells beneath **(A, ×; B, ×).** *(Courtesy of Dr. Steven Arnoczky, Laboratory for Comparative Orthopedic Research, Michigan State University, East Lansing, Mich.)*

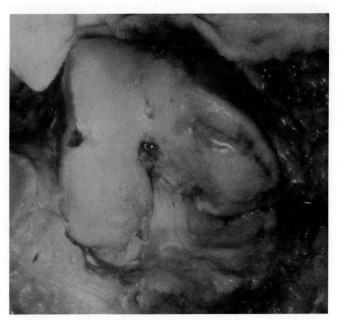

FIGURE 13-5 Valgus-producing upper tibial osteotomy showing formation of fibrocartilage on medial femoral condyle. *(Courtesy of Dr. Mark Coventry, Department of Orthopedics, Mayo Clinic, Rochester, Minn.)*

laginous repair tissue. They stated further that the "biochemical composition and durability of the presumed fibrocartilage repair tissue is unanswered." Clearly, there is no evidence that hyaline cartilage is regenerated by marrow stimulation.

Arthroscopic Débridement

Arthroscopic débridement as a treatment option for OA was reported by Sprague in 1981.[19] At 1-year follow-up, 74% of patients stated that their "knee was improved and more functional" than before surgery. The extent of arthritis, however, was not correlated clinically or roentgenographically with good success

266 patients between 1985 and 1990, with 3.7-year follow-up, using a grading system similar to that of the Outerbridge classification. After chondral surface débridement, the bone is perforated to a depth of 3 to 4 mm using an awl and the holes are placed approximately 4 to 5 mm apart in a full-thickness lesion with exposed subchondral bone (Fig. 13-6). Blood should be seen emanating from the microfracture holes after perforation is complete. A postoperative rehabilitation program was used to provide motion without applying high load stress to the treated chondral defect. Repeat arthroscopies were performed in 80 patients. In most chondral defects, subchondral bone was covered with cartilage of varying quality, and the term *hyaline-like* was introduced to describe the fibrocartilage surface. There was no evidence that hyaline cartilage was present at second-look arthroscopy, and the authors confirmed that the only type of tissue that was seen to regenerate over these surfaces was fibrocarti-

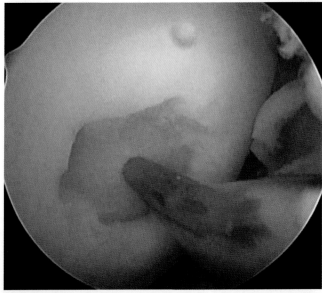

FIGURE 13-6 Intraoperative photo of femoral condyle. An awl is being used to begin the microfracture procedure.

rates. In the early to mid-1980s, some studies reported that the results of arthroscopic débridement were not correlated with age or extent of arthritis either roentgenographically or arthroscopically, with up to 11-year follow-up.[20,21] Gross and associates[22] and Ogilvie-Harris and Fitsialos[23] concluded in the early 1990s that OA severity was the best predictor of success after arthroscopic débridement, and that normally aligned knees with mild arthritis had the best results at 8-year follow-up. It is certainly not clear, however, that shaving a damaged articular cartilage relieves pain. Bentley[24] has reported that chondroplasty during arthrotomy produces unpredictable results, and only 25% of patients treated with patellar chondroplasty had satisfactory results beyond 1 year. In 1990, Timoney and coworkers[25] retrospectively reviewed 109 patients who had arthroscopic débridement for degenerative arthritis of the knee at 4.2-year follow-up. Using the Harris hip score (HHS), only 45% reported good results and 21% of the patients experienced worsened symptoms and subsequently had TKR. Moseley and colleagues,[26] in 1996, randomized 10 patients with osteoarthritis of the knee into a placebo group, an arthroscopic lavage group, and an arthroscopic débridement group. All 10 patients at 6 months reported improvement in their pain scores and satisfaction with their surgery, with the exception of one placebo patient, after their 6-month follow-up. This study was repeated in 2002[27] with a larger patient group at a VA hospital; 70% of these patients had moderate to severe OA. No significant differences were found among the three groups who had arthroscopy with débridement, arthroscopy with lavage, or placebo knee surgery. Of interest was that those patients who had positive magnetic resonance imaging (MRI) scans with meniscal tears were excluded from his study. It was concluded that there is no clear role for arthroscopy in knees with OA. Steadman and associates[28] recently reported a success rate of 71% using the WOMAC and Lysholm scoring system with 2-year follow-up results. Wai and coworkers[29] and Hawker and colleagues[30] have reported that up to 9.2% of patients had a TKR after 1 year and 18.4% had a TKR after 3 years subsequent to arthroscopic débridement. A number of studies have claimed that arthroscopic débridement and shaving help relieve the symptoms of osteoarthritis of the knee.[14,15,19-23,31] However, it is not clear why these patients improved and equally unclear as to why they stay improved for as long as 5 years postoperatively.

Alignment And Arthroscopic Débridement

Correlation of preoperative angular deformity with the results of arthroscopically débrided knees was originally reported by Salisbury and associates[31] in 1985. In patients with residual varus deformity, 32% noted improvement in pain at a minimum 1-year follow-up. Normal knee alignment was considered to be 1 to 7 degrees of femoral tibial valgus alignment preoperatively. Harwin[32] and Baumgartner[33] concluded that abnormal varus or valgus angulation was a statistically significant factor in predicting a failed result after arthroscopic irrigation and débridement. Similar findings were reported by Ogilvie-Harris and Fitsialos.[23] Those patients who have varus or significant valgus knee deformities with medial or lateral compartment disease, respectively, will have worse results than those with postoperative neutral or mild valgus alignment.

Arthroscopy And Tidal Lavage

In 1978, Bird and Ring[34] reported on a series of 14 patients who had arthroscopic lavage of the knee and 93% of patients improved by 1 week, but by 4 weeks only 50% had noted mild to moderate improvement. Jackson and colleagues[35] have reported on more than 207 patients with femoral tibial arthritic disease in the medial or lateral compartment who had lavage versus arthroscopic débridement with 2-year follow-ups in 1988. They found that débridement results in 68% improvement and lavage alone results in 45% symptomatic improvement. In 1991, Livesley and associates[36] compared osteoarthritic knees treated by arthroscopic lavage and physiotherapy with a control group treated by physiotherapy alone. The joint lavage group improved to a greater degree than the control group and the improvement lasted longer. in 1992, Ike and coworkers[37] compared a group of patients treated with standard medical treatment (nonsteroidal anti-inflammatory drugs, steroid injections, physical therapy, and analgesics) with those receiving tidal lavage in the office using local anesthesia. At 12 weeks, 62% of the tidal irrigation group patients and 36% of the medically managed patients were improved functionally and symptomatically. In 1993, Chang and colleagues[38] reported on two groups of patients, one that received arthroscopic surgery and débridement and the other needle joint lavage only. At 1 year, they concluded that the removal of soft tissue abnormalities via arthroscopic surgery does not generally improve pain and knee dysfunction associated with non–end-stage osteoarthritis any more than simple joint lavage, unless a meniscal tear was present.

Various explanations for symptomatic relief secondary to arthroscopic lavage have been postulated, such as removal of cartilage debris, crystals, and inflammatory factors. Temporary improvement in signs of inflammation may support the hypothesis that lavage removes inflammatory agents, although it is not clear what role these inflammatory agents contribute to pain.[39,40]

PEARLS&PITFALLS

PEARLS

- Cartilage does not have the capability of healing with regenerative hyaline cartilage. Therefore, care must be taken to avoid injury to the articular surface when performing arthroscopic procedures.
- Make certain when doing marrow stimulation that a well-circumscribed stable rim is created at the conclusion of the procedure.
- Arthroscopic débridement is indicated for the patient with mechanical symptoms, including locking, catching, giving way, or other findings indicative of a symptomatic torn meniscus, loose body, or chondral flap.

PITFALLS

- Avoid creating false expectations for the patient by explaining that the procedure being performed is temporary at best and has the potential to result in future surgery.
- Arthroscopic débridement is not indicated for arthritis when these signs are not present and will not be reimbursed for Medicare patients.

CONCLUSIONS

Arthroscopic débridement of the degenerative knee is a worthwhile procedure for younger patients and for older patients who desire symptomatic improvement and do not wish to risk the morbidity of a total knee replacement. Success rates for arthroscopic débridement vary between 50% and 67% depending on many factors, including patient age, degree of arthritis, activity level, and extent of follow-up. Arthroscopic lavage success rates vary between 45% and 51% and do not appear to have the same longevity of success as arthroscopic débridement. It is apparent from at least two studies comparing arthroscopic débridement with marrow stimulation in conjunction with débridement that marrow stimulation does not offer any greater benefit in the treatment of degenerative arthritis of the knee than débridement alone.[15,41]

There does not appear to be any advantage in performing arthroscopy in conjunction with upper tibial osteotomy compared with upper tibial osteotomy alone. The results are similar. Furthermore, the results of upper tibial osteotomy in conjunction with abrasion arthroplasty were identical to those in a similar series of patients who had upper tibial osteotomy alone.[42] Therefore, arthroscopic débridement or marrow stimulation in conjunction with upper tibial osteotomy (UTO) seems to be of limited value for improvement of symptoms compared with UTO alone. Furthermore, the prognostic value of the arthroscope in determining whether to proceed with UTO is of minimal value, as noted by Fujisawa and coworkers[17] and Keene and Dyreby.[43] They concluded there was no correlation in terms of prognosis and arthroscopic evaluation prior to UTO compared with the clinical results subsequent to UTO.

In 2002 and 2008, the American Academy of Orthopaedic Surgeons discussed the role of arthroscopy for OA of the knee.[44,45] It was concluded that there are clinical variables associated with improvement after arthroscopic débridement. These include preoperative mechanical symptoms, including locking, catching, or giving way, indicative of loose bodies, chondral flaps, and unstable meniscal tissue. Furthermore, on clinical examination, the patient should have medial joint line tenderness and a positive Steinmann test, indicating a symptomatic torn meniscus, as well as the presence of an unstable meniscal tear at the time of arthroscopy.[46] The arthroscope is therefore useful for the treatment of degenerative arthritis of the arthritic knee when these conditions are met.

REFERENCES

1. Burman M, Finkelstein H, Mayer L. Arthroscopy of the knee joint. *J Bone Joint Surg.* 1934;16:255.
2. Magnuson P. Joint debridement: Surgical treatment of degenerative arthritis. *Surg Gynecol Obstet.* 1941;73:1.
3. Isserlin LB. Joint debridement for osteoarthritis of the knee. *J Bone Joint Surg Br.* 1950;32:302-306.
4. Hunter W. On the structure and diseases of articulating cartilage. *Philos Trans R Soc Lond B Biol Sci.* 1743;9:267.
5. Leidy J. On the intimate structure and history of articular cartilage. *Am J Med Sci.* 1849;17:277.
6. Mankin HJ. Response of articular cartilage to mechanical injury. *J Bone Joint Surg Am.* 1982;64:460-466.
7. Buckwalter JA, Cruess R. Healing of musculoskeletal tissues. In: Rockwood CA, Green DP, Bucholz RW, eds. *Fractures in Adults.* 3rd ed. Philadelphia: JB Lippincott; 1991:181.

8. Mow VC, Rosenwasser MP. Articular cartilage: biomechanics. In: Woo SL, Buckwalter JA, eds. *Injury and Repair of the Musculoskeletal Soft Tissues.* Park Ridge, Ill: American Academy of Orthopaedic Surgeons; 1988:427.
9. Armstrong CG, Mow VC. Variations in the intrinsic mechanical properties of human articular cartilage with age: degeneration of water content. *J Bone Joint Surg Am.* 1982;64:88-94.
10. Woo SL-Y, Mow VC, Lai W. Biomechanical properties for articular cartilage. In Skalik R, Chein S, eds. *Handbook of Bioengineering.* New York: McGraw-Hill; 1987:41.
11. Pridie AH. The method of resurfacing osteoarthritic knee joints. *J Bone Joint Surg Br.* 1959;41:618.
12. Akeson WH, Miyashita C, Taylor TK, et al. Experimental cup arthroplasty of the canine hip. Extracellular matrix composition in cup arthroplasty. *J Bone Joint Surg Am.* 1969;51:149-164.
13. Mitchell N, Shepard N. Resurfacing of adult rabbit articular cartilage by multiple perforations of the subchondral bone. *J Bone Joint Surg Am.* 1976;58:230-233.
14. Johnson LL. Arthroscopic abrasion arthroplasty historical and pathologic perspective: present status. *J Arthrosc.* 1986;2:54-69.
15. Bert JM, Maschka K. The arthroscopic treatment of unicompartmental gonarthrosis: A five-year follow-up study of abrasion arthroplasty plus arthroscopic debridement and arthroscopic debridement alone. *Arthroscopy.* 1989;5:25-32.
16. Coventry MB, Bowman PW. Long-term results of upper tibial osteotomy for degenerative arthritis of the knee. *Acta Orthop Belg.* 1982;48:139-156.
17. Fujisawa Y, Masuhara K, Shiomi S. The effect of high tibial osteotomy in osteoarthritis of the knee: an arthroscopic study in 54 knee joints. *Orthop Clin North Am.* 1979;10:585-608.
18. Blevens FT, Steadman R, Rodrigo J, Silliman J. Treatment of articular cartilage defects in athletes: an analysis of functional outcome and lesion appearance. *J Orthop.* 1998;21:761-767.
19. Sprague NF III. Arthroscopic debridement for degenerative knee joint disease. *Clin Orthop Relat Res.* 1981;(160):118-123.
20. Jackson RW, Silver R, Marans R. The arthroscopic treatment of degenerative joint disease. *J Arthrosc.* 1986;2:11.
21. Shahriaree H, O'Connor RF, Nottage W. Seven years follow-up arthroscopic debridement of degenerative knee. *Filed View* 1982;1:1.
22. Gross DE, Brenner SL, Esformes I, Gross ML. The arthroscopic treatment of degenerative joint disease in the knee. *J Orthop.* 1991;14:1317-1321.
23. Ogilvie-Harris DJ, Fitsialos DP. Arthroscopic management of the degenerative knee. *J Arthrosc.* 1991;7:151-157.
24. Bentley G. The surgical treatment of chondromalacia of the patellae. *J Bone Joint Surg Am.* J Bone Joint Surg Br. 1978;60:74-81.
25. Timoney JM, Kneisl JS, Barrack RL, Alexander AH. Arthroscopy update #6. Arthroscopy in the osteoarthritic knee. Long-term follow-up. *Orthop Rev.* 1990;19:376-379.
26. Moseley JB Jr, Wray NP, Kuykendall D, et al. Arthroscopic treatment of osteoarthritis of the knee: a prospective, randomized, placebo-controlled trial. Results of a pilot study. *Am J Sports Med.* 1996;24:28-34.
27. Moseley B, O'Malley K, Petersen N, et al. A controlled trial of arthroscopic surgery for osteoarthritis of the knee. *N Engl J Med.* 2002;347:81-88.
28. Steadman R, Ramappa A, Maxwell B, Briggs K. An arthroscopic treatment regimen for osteoarthritis of the knee. *Arthroscopy.* 2007;23:948-955.
29. Wai E. Kreder J, Williams J. Arthroscpic debridement of the knee for osteoarthritis in patients fifty years of age or older: utilization and outcomes in the Province of Ontario. *J Bone Joint Surg Am.* 2002;84:17-22.
30. Hawker G, Guan J, Judge A, Dieppe P. Knee arthroscopyin England and Ontario: patterns of use, changes over time and relationship to total knee replacement. *J Bone Joint Surg Am.* 2008;90:2337-2345.
31. Salisbury RB, Nottage WM, Gardner D. The effect of alignment on results in arthroscopic debridement of the degenerative knee. *Clin Orthop Relat Res.* 1985;198:268-272.
32. Harwin S. Arthroscopic debridement for osteoarthritis of the knee: predictors of patient satisfaction. *Arthroscopy.* 1999;15:142-146.
33. Baumgartner M, Cannon W, Vittori J, et al. Arthroscopic debridement of the arthritic knee. *Clin Orthop Relat Res.* 1990; 253:197-202.
34. Bird HA, Ring EF. Therapeutic value of arthroscopy. *Ann Rheum Dis.* 37:78, 1978.
35. Jackson RW, Marans HJ, Silver RS. The arthroscopic treatment of degenerative arthritis of the knee. *J Bone Joint Surg Br.* 1988;70:332.

36. Livesley P, Doherty M, Needoff M, et al. Arthroscopic lavage of osteo-arthritic knees. *J Bone Joint Surg Br.* 1991;73:922-926.

37. Ike RW, Arnold WJ, Rothschild EW, Shaw HL. Tidal irrigation versus conservative medical management in patients with osteoarthritis of the knee: a prospective randomized study. Tidal Irrigation Cooperating Group. *J Rheumatol.* 1992;19:772-779.

38. Chang RW, Falconer J, Stulberg SD, et al. A randomized controlled trial of arthroscopic surgery versus closed-needle joint lavage for patients with osteoarthritis of the knee. *Arthritis Rheum.* 1993;36:289-296.

39. Dieppe PT, Muskinson BC, Willoughby DA. The inflammatory component of osteoarthritis. In Nuki ED, ed. *An Etiopathogenesis of Osteoarthritis.* London: Pitman Medical; 1980:117.

40. Goldenberg DL, Egan MS, Cohen AS. Inflammatory synovitis in degen-erative joint disease. *J Rheumatol.* 1982;9:204-209.

41. Rand J. Role of arthroscopy in osteoarthritis of the knee. *Arthroscopy.* 1991;7:358-363.

42. Fanelli GC, Rogers VP. High tibial valgus osteotomy combined with arthroscopic abrasion arthroplasty. *Contemp Orthop.* 1989;19:547.

43. Keene J, Dyreby JR Jr. High tibial osteotomy in the treatment of osteo-arthritis of the knee. The role of preoperative arthroscopy. *J Bone Joint Surg Am.* 1983;65:36-42.

44. American Academy of Orthopaedic Surgeons (AAOS). *Arthroscopic Sur-gery and Osteoarthritis of the Knee.* A Report for the Centers for Medicare and Medicaid Services. Coverage Analysis Group. December 2002. Available at: http://www.cms.hhs.gov/determinationprocess/downloads/id7a.pdf. Accessed January 14, 2010.

45. American Academy of Orthopaedic Surgeons (AAOS). *Treatment of Osteoarthritis of the Knee (Non-Arthroplasty).* Rosemont, Ill: American Academy of Orthopaedic Surgeons; December 2008.

46. Dervin G, Stiell I, Rody K, Grabowski J. The effect of arthroscopic de-bridement for osteoarthritis of the knee on health-related quality of life. *J Bone Joint Surg Am.* 2003;85;10-19.

Microfracture

Michael J. Medvecky ● Peter Yeh ● Peter Jokl

Articular cartilage lesions are a commonly encountered condition seen during arthroscopic surgery (Fig. 14-1)[1,2] and may be encountered incidentally in spite of improvements with magnetic resonance imaging (MRI). The limited repair capabilities of articular cartilage chondrocytes and the avascular nature of hyaline cartilage do not allow for any intrinsic healing capacity of full-thickness articular cartilage lesions that do not violate the subchondral bone.[3,4] Different techniques have been used in an attempt to create reparative or transfer cartilaginous tissue into the defect with the goal of improved pain relief, activity tolerance, and avoidance of long-term degenerative changes to the lesion or adjacent cartilage.[5] Multiple procedures have been used in the past several decades to promote reparative "regenerate" cartilaginous tissue ingrowth into the lesion.[6-8]

In the mid-1980s, Rodrigo and colleagues[9] and Steadman and associates[10] adapted the Pridie drilling technique by using an awl to create perforations within the subchondral bone layer. The technique was refined with the knowledge of the importance of the removal of the calcified cartilage layer, overlying the subchondral bone, to improve adherence to the subchondral bone.[11]

After penetration of the subchondral bone, bleeding from the bone marrow creates a fibrin clot within the defect. Marrow-derived pluripotential cells progressively differentiate into fibroblasts, osteoblasts, chondroblasts, and chondrocytes, without contribution from the adjacent articular cartilage. Shapiro and coworkers[12] have demonstrated after cellular labeling via autoradiography that the repopulation is mediated entirely by the proliferation and differentiation of mesenchymal cells from the bone marrow. The collagen matrix formed did not integrate into the adjacent native cartilage and this weak link is theorized to be the potential source of long-term repair tissue degradation. The repair tissue fibrocartilage is also primarily composed of type I collagen, which has decreased resilience and stiffness compared with the type II collagen seen in normal hyaline cartilage.

The risk of articular cartilage defect progression to degenerative arthritis is multifactorial and defect size may play a significant role in this process. A critical size of articular defect that is potentially damaging to adjacent cartilage is not known; the literature shows wide variability in defect size for which treatment had been indicated. Guettler and colleagues[13] have evaluated pressure readings from the peripheral rim of articular defects created at various sizes, ranging from 5 to 20 mm. Rim stress concentration was seen in defects of 10 mm and larger, suggesting this as a critical size defect, which may increase the risk of progressive deterioration of the adjacent cartilage.

TREATMENT

Indications and Contraindications

Indications

Microfracture treatment is ideally indicated as a first-line treatment of well-contained Outerbridge grade III or IV cartilage lesions less than 4 cm². Treatment of larger lesions has been described but most studies included lesions with a mean defect size of less than 4 cm².[14] Unstable chondral flaps that extend to the subchondral bone layer are also lesions amenable to this technique.

Secondary to its technical ease and limited surgical morbidity, microfracture marrow stimulation can be applied to cartilage lesions detected preoperatively by MRI or those found incidentally at the time of arthroscopic evaluation. We have also treated acute traumatic lesions in the polytrauma patient in the appropriate clinical setting (Fig. 14-2).

Patients sustaining acute, traumatic, chondral full-thickness lesions are best treated as soon as is practical logistically because duration of symptoms of less than 12 months has been associated with better postoperative outcome scores and improved microscopic repair cartilage grading.[15-17] Patients with chronic or

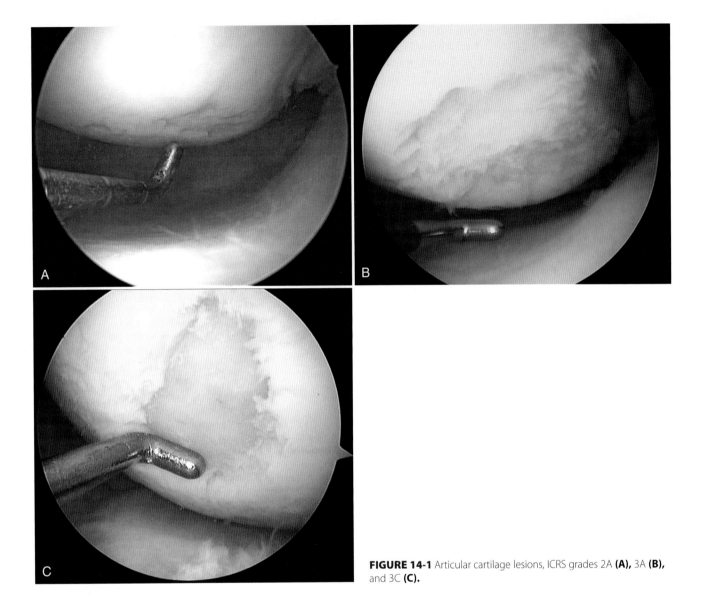

FIGURE 14-1 Articular cartilage lesions, ICRS grades 2A **(A)**, 3A **(B)**, and 3C **(C)**.

degenerative lesions are initially treated with nonsurgical measures, including activity modification, oral anti-inflammatory medication, physical therapy, dietary modifications, and weight loss, as well as potential articular injections such as corticosteroids or hyaluronic acid. Patients who fail nonoperative treatment are potential candidates for microfracture.

Age younger than 40 years, has been associated with better clinical outcome scores and better repair cartilage fills.[18,19] Increased body mass index has been demonstrated to be universally correlated with poor outcomes after microfracture treatment, with worst outcomes seen in those with a body mass index (BMI) more than 30 kg/m^2.[15]

These indications need to be compared with the limited knowledge we have concerning the natural history of nonoperative treatment of articular cartilage lesions and the lack of control groups in trials evaluating operative treatment of these lesions.[20] Some studies have demonstrated no difference in outcome for nonoperative management of these lesions compared with operative interventions.[21,22] Patient selection also needs to be consid-

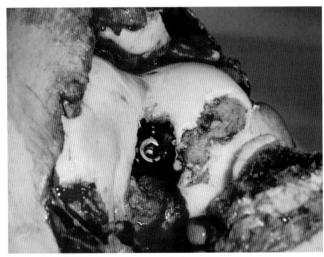

FIGURE 14-2 Microfracture also has applications for the treatment of acute traumatic lesions. This is evidenced by this patient with ipsilateral femoral shaft and patellar fractures and a traumatic chondral lesion of the lateral femoral condyle. (Note the retrograde femoral rod.)

ered in view of the intensive postoperative rehabilitation program that is usually prescribed following microfracture surgery. Weight-bearing limitations in the postoperative rehabilitation program result in the interruption of normal lifestyle and often induce disuse muscle atrophy.

Currently, the methodologic limitations of previous investigations do not allow us to make broad recommendations about differential indications based on an involved compartment. The Most studies fail to differentiate between patellofemoral and tibiofemoral lesions and there has yet to be a study that analyzed the patellofemoral joint in isolation.

When evaluating a patellofemoral lesion, we use radiographic measurement of the lateral patellofemoral and patellar tilt angles for patellar tilt and subluxation, respectively. This information, combined with MRI evaluation of lesion location, is used to decide whether lateral retinacular release should be considered with a lateral patellar facet lesion. We think that an anteromedialization (AMZ) may be considered for secondary or revision treatment in distal pole lesions but do not believe that the added morbidity is warranted in the first-line treatment of these lesions.

Chondral lesions on opposing surfaces (kissing lesions) present a unique clinical dilemma; little information is available to guide treatment. Well-contained lesions with opposing articular surfaces may need to be considered for microfracture treatment; however, any kissing lesions with one or both having a progressive transition to a full-thickness defect or opposing subchondral bone surface should be considered a degenerative lesion and contraindicated for microfracture.

Contraindications

Microfracture treatment is contraindicated for patients unwilling or unable to pursue the recommended postoperative activity modifications and associated rehabilitation protocols. Patient expectations must be discussed preoperatively in those with known acute articular cartilage lesions and patients undergoing treatment for degenerative lesions. The treatment requires a stable, perpendicular peripheral edge of articular cartilage and, therefore, is contraindicated in uncontained chondral lesions or lesions that gradually transition into a full-thickness defect.

Axial malalignment of more than 5 degrees for lesions in the tibiofemoral joint is an indication for simultaneous or staged corrective osteotomy (Fig. 14-3). Not only is joint malalignment detrimental to normal articular cartilage, but uncorrected malalignment can result in significantly increased contact pressure in the affected compartment, resulting in increased load and shear on the treated lesions.[23]

High-grade ligamentous instability will also result in increased shear force across the treated lesion and is a contraindication to microfracture treatment unless surgically treated simultaneously.[23]

Additional contraindications include generalized degenerative joint disease, inflammatory arthropathy, joint infection, and adjacent bony tumor. Meniscal deficiencies should be addressed prior to or at the time of microfracture.

Patient Evaluation Prior to Treatment

The evaluation of the patient for treatment of an articular cartilage lesion requires the assessment of a large number of variables.

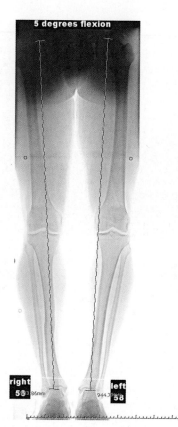

FIGURE 14-3 Weight-bearing standing x-rays are obtained for patients under consideration of treatment for articular cartilage disorders. This patient demonstrated asymmetrical genu varum; articular cartilage preservation surgery would be contraindicated prior to valgus producing osteotomy. WBL on right is ~45%; WBL on left is ~ 5%.

The history of present illness should include assessment of the mechanism of injury, with documentation of the acuity and cause of the lesion. Patients who have undergone previous nonsurgical and/or surgical treatment need to be questioned about the types of treatments and their response, because these will play a role in future treatment options. Patients previously having undergone surgical treatment should have a careful evaluation of their preoperative imaging, arthroscopic images, and operative reports. Articular cartilage lesions that have undergone previous treatment that violates the subchondral bone layer are unlikely to gain improvement via microfracture.

Concordant patient demographics that need consideration include age, prior medical and surgical history, occupation, and activity level, including recent activity level and activity goals. An assessment of the willingness to participate in a postoperative rehabilitation program is important if articular cartilage surgery restoration procedures are being considered.

Physical examination includes documentation of height and weight for determination of BMI. Standing alignment and gait assessment should be included in the examination. The varus thrust in stance phase or varus recurvatum gait would be consistent with a double- and triple-varus knee,[24] respectively, and should be considered contraindications to treatment of a medial compartment articular cartilage lesion, unless addressed prior to considering microfracture. Ligamentous integrity of the cruciate and collateral ligaments must be determined, because a deficiency results in abnormal knee translation and resultant excessive shear force on the articular cartilage. Assessment of residual loss of motion or muscular weakness is important because these may play a role in abnormal joint forces and resultant symptomatology. Previous incisions should be evaluated for neuroma formation.

Our radiologic evaluation includes weight-bearing images, including anteroposterior (AP), lateral, Rosenberg (posteroanterior taken at 45-degree flexion), and axial patellar views (Laurin) (Fig. 14-4). A full-length hip to ankle weight-bearing alignment film should also be obtained in the patient undergoing assessment of an articular cartilage lesion. The weight-bearing line (WBL) is measured by drawing a straight line from the center of the femoral head to the center of the tibiotalar joint.[25] The mechanical axis is measured by the angle created from a line drawn from the center of the femoral head to the midpoint between the tibial spines in comparison to a line from the center of the tibial spines to the center of the tibiotalar joint. Simultaneous or staged corrective osteotomy should be considered for patients who have greater than 5 degrees of tibiofemoral varus or valgus, based on the involved compartment. Patellofemoral alignment is evaluated via the axial patellar view and trochlear and patellar morphology seen by MRI.

MRI is useful for the preoperative assessment of the size, depth, and location of the articular cartilage lesion.[20,26,27] Several acquisition protocols have been recommended by the International Cartilage Repair Society (ICRS).[28] Spoiled gradient-recalled echo (SPGR) and fast spin-echo (FSE) techniques are the most accurate and widely used.[29,30] New pulse sequences and image acquisition methods are being investigated for improved diagnosis of articular cartilage abnormalities, disease progression, and biologic response

to treatment strategies.[29-31] The status of the ipsilateral meniscus is important to assess, particularly in a patient having undergone prior surgical treatment and partial meniscectomy. Adjacent and opposing articular surfaces also need to be carefully evaluated. The subchondral and metaphyseal bone are assessed for cyst formation, bone loss, or cavitation. Loss of osseous integrity or sphericity may play a role in impaired fibrocartilaginous ingrowth. The peripheral aspect of the lesion is also evaluated to determine whether there is containment of the lesion, because this is important to the success of microfracture treatment.

Treatment Options

Direct arthroscopic evaluation of articular cartilage lesions is considered the most accurate and reliable means of assessing chondral lesions in regard to size, depth, and location. The lesion size is measured with a calibrated probe. These variables are important in conjunction with preoperative imaging for determining the most appropriate treatment option to address the articular cartilage lesion. Many classification systems exist; the most recent Cartilage ICRS system (Fig. 14-5) uses predébridement and postdébridement measurements of lesion size. However, not included in this or other classification systems is documentation of the condition of the subchondral bone.

Historically, the Outerbridge system (Box 14-1) was the most commonly used classification system for articular cartilage lesions. A limitation of this classification is that the intermediate grades (grades II and III) are only differentiated based on size (more or less than 0.5 inch in diameter) and there is no quantification of the depth of the lesion. Lesions with exposure of subchondral bone are considered to be Outerbridge grade IV.[32,33]

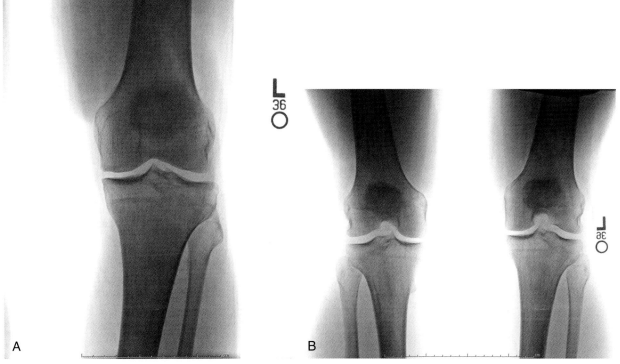

FIGURE 14-4 Radiographic evaluation includes weight-bearing AP and Rosenberg views demonstrating mild joint space narrowing on the AP view **(A)** but symmetrical joint space on the Rosenberg view **(B)**.

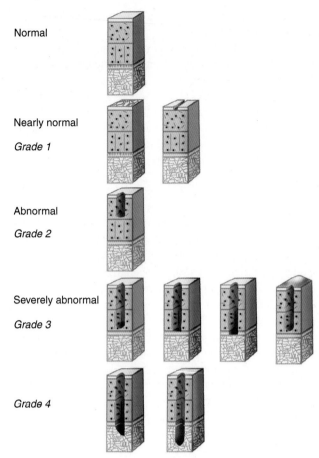

Normal

Nearly normal

Grade 1

Abnormal

Grade 2

Severely abnormal

Grade 3

Grade 4

FIGURE 14-5 ICRS articular cartilage grading system. Normal—grade 0= almost normal, grade 1A = superficial lesions and soft, grade 1B = and/or superficial fissures and cracks; abnormal—grade 2 = lesions extend <50% deep; severely abnormal—grade 3A = extend >50%, grade 3B = down to calcified layer, grade 3C = down to but not through subchondral bone, grade 3D = includes blisters, grade 4a = penetrating subchondral bone but not full diameter of defect, grade 4B = penetrating full diameter of defect.

Box 14-1 Outerbridge Classification

- Grade 0: normal cartilage
- Grade I: cartilage with softening and swelling
- Grade II: a partial-thickness defect with fissures on the surface that do not reach subchondral bone or exceed 1.5 cm in diameter
- Grade III: fissuring to the level of subchondral bone in an area with a diameter > 1.5 cm
- Grade IV: exposed subchondral bone

Arthroscopic Technique

We perform the microfracture procedure with the patient in the supine position using a well-padded pneumatic tourniquet on the patient's upper thigh, an arthroscopic leg holder, and general or regional anesthesia. A complete arthroscopic examination of the knee is performed using standard medial and lateral anterior portals. The articular surfaces are observed and palpated with an arthroscopic probe. The status and integrity of the menisci are also evaluated and documented. The ligamentous integrity of the

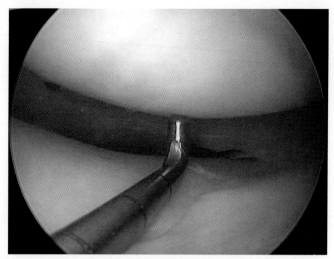

FIGURE 14-6 Arthroscopic gap test performed at 30 degrees flexion to verify functional integrity of the lateral collateral ligament.

knee is verified, particularly the lateral ligaments, using the arthroscopic gap test, with the knee positioned at 0 and 30 degrees of flexion (Fig. 14-6).

Accessory portals are occasionally used pending lesion location. If additional pathology is present that requires treatment, this is performed prior to the microfracture procedure to minimize the amount of time that the microfractured bone is exposed to elevated intra-articular fluid pressure and to allow for adequate clot formation.

The articular defect is assessed for size and location (Fig. 14-7). Associated articular flaps are removed and the margins are débrided back to a peripheral rim with edges perpendicular to the subchondral bone using a curette or arthroscopic knife (Fig. 14-8). Debris is evacuated with the arthroscopic shaver. After débridement, the size of the lesion is again measured with a calibrated probe and recorded. In addition, the arc of motion in which the lesion articulates with the opposing joint surface is recorded. The range of motion of contact will be used for planning the postoperative rehabilitation program (Fig. 14-9).

A curette is used to remove the calcified cartilage layer that is just superficial to the subchondral bone layer (Fig. 14-10). Débridement of this calcified cartilage layer has been shown to improve the bonding of the mesenchymal clot to the subchondral bone.[23,34] Care is also taken to avoid excessive débridement and subsequent thinning of the subchondral bone; this could stimulate subchondral bone overgrowth, with subsequent relative thinning of the overlying repair cartilage layer and, therefore, subsequent inferior biologic and biomechanical repair tissue quality.[15,35] Arthroscopic shaver use is minimized to avoid thinning of the subchondral bone.

Commercially available awls are used to create multiple perforations in the subchondral bone approximately 3 to 4 mm apart (Fig. 14-11).[10] The peripheral margin of the lesion is treated first, progressing toward the center of the lesion. Adequate spacing between the perforations is important to minimize the risk of subchondral bone collapse and subsequent cavitation. Perforation of the subchondral bone is performed with the awl tip aligned perpendicular to the subchondral bone layer. The knee is flexed or

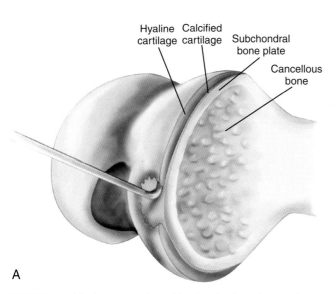

Hyaline   Calcified
cartilage cartilage   Subchondral
bone plate

Cancellous
bone

A

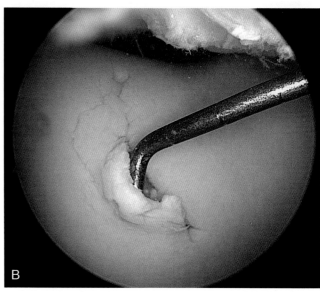

B

FIGURE 14-7 The lesion is evaluated for size, depth, and margin integrity. **A, B.** *(Adapted from Mithoefer K, Williams RJ 3rd, Warren RF, et al. The microfracture technique for the treatment of articular cartilage lesions in the knee. A prospective cohort study.* J Bone Joint Surg Am. *2005;87:1911-1920.)*

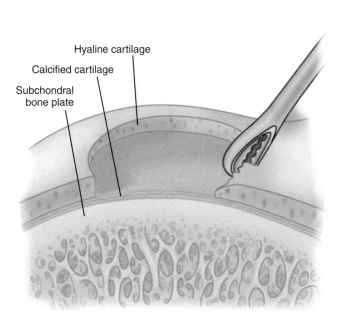

Hyaline cartilage

Calcified cartilage

Subchondral
bone plate

FIGURE 14-8 The margins are débrided to a peripheral rim with edges perpendicular to the subchondral bone using a curette or arthroscopic knife. *(Adapted from Mithoefer K, Williams RJ 3rd, Warren RF, et al. The microfracture technique for the treatment of articular cartilage lesions in the knee. A prospective cohort study.* J Bone Joint Surg Am. *2005;87:1911-1920.)*

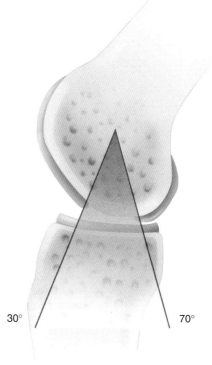

30°   70°

FIGURE 14-9 The lesion is evaluated for range of motion where it articulates with the opposing joint surface. This information is documented and used to guide the postoperative physical therapy program. *(Adapted from Mithoefer K, Williams RJ 3rd, Warren RF, et al. The microfracture technique for the treatment of articular cartilage lesions in the knee. A prospective cohort study.* J Bone Joint Surg Am. *2005;87:1911-1920.)*

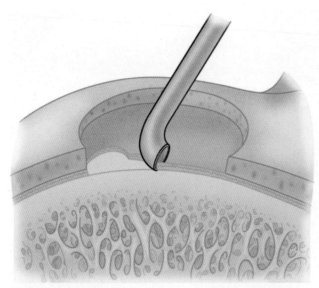

FIGURE 14-10 Careful débridement of the calcified cartilage layer is performed to avoid excessive thinning or cavitation, which can stimulate subchondral bone hypertrophy and subsequent thinning of the overlying repair cartilage layer. *(Adapted from Mithoefer K, Williams RJ 3rd, Warren RF, et al. The microfracture technique for the treatment of articular cartilage lesions in the knee. A prospective cohort study. J Bone Joint Surg Am. 2005;87:1911-1920.)*

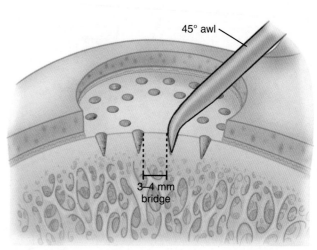

FIGURE 14-12 Initiation of the penetrations is performed at the peripheral edge of the lesion and progresses inward. Impaction at a perpendicular angle to the subchondral bone avoids skiving and disruption of a larger area of subchondral bone. *(Adapted from Mithoefer K, Williams RJ 3rd, Warren RF, et al. The microfracture technique for the treatment of articular cartilage lesions in the knee. A prospective cohort study. J Bone Joint Surg Am. 2005;87:1911-1920.)*

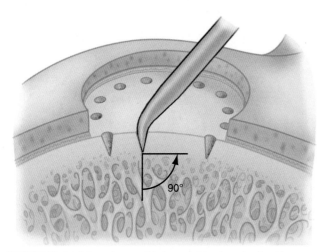

FIGURE 14-11 A 3- to 4-mm-wide bone bridge is maintained between perforations to maintain biomechanical integrity. *(Adapted from Mithoefer K, Williams RJ 3rd, Warren RF, et al. The microfracture technique for the treatment of articular cartilage lesions in the knee. A prospective cohort study. J Bone Joint Surg Am. 2005;87:1911-1920.)*

extended to optimize instrument positioning (Fig. 14-12). Microfracture awls are available in different tip angulations (30, 45, and 90 degrees) with the 30- or 45-degree awl used most commonly (Fig. 14-13). Care is taken to avoid skiving of the awl during impact. Skiving can create a large area of subchondral bone disruption or can break into an adjacent hole. Skiving can be avoided by toeing in the instrument tip and by impaction as close to perpendicular as possible by instrument angulation or knee position.

Patellar lesions more frequently require the use of the 90-degree awl. Patellar perforations are also more easily created by impacting the side of the handle rather than the end. Distal patellar pole lesions may also be more readily assessed via higher flexion angles and the 30-degree awl. Proximal pole lesions may be more readily accessed via suprapatellar accessory portals and the 90-degree awl. Counterpressure on the anterior aspect of the patella is needed for most patellar lesions. A mini-arthrotomy may be needed for patellar lesions if access is difficult to achieve.

Osseous debris is removed from the microfracture perforations with an arthroscopic shaver. Confirmation of adequate subchondral penetration is accomplished by observation of the release of blood and marrow fat droplets after lowering the arthroscopic intra-articular pump pressure. A drain is not used so as not to remove the mesenchymal clot and hematoma from within the joint (Fig. 14-14). Postoperative intraarticular anesthetic (1% lidocaine) is used without epinephrine. We have also more recently discontinued the use of bupivacaine secondary to reports of chondrotoxicity.[36-38] A compression dressing is used as well as cryotherapy for control of postoperative swelling and inflammation.

PEARLS & PITFALLS

PEARLS

- Careful patient selection is critical, including careful analysis of joint ligament stability and mechanical axis alignment.
- Better clinical outcome scores have been seen in the following patients:
  Younger than 40 years
  Symptom duration less than 12 months
  Lesion smaller than 4 cm²
  BMI less than 30 kg/m²
- There should be surgical creation of a well-shouldered, stable, perpendicular peripheral rim.

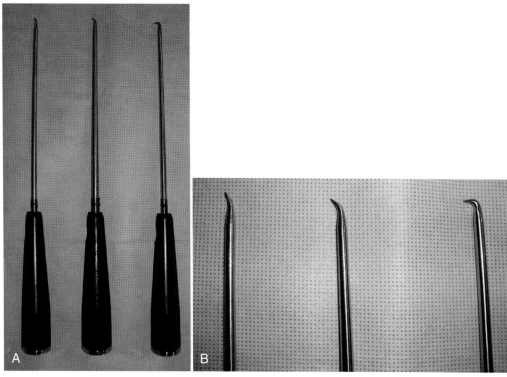

FIGURE 14-13 Microfracture awls are produced by several surgical companies and made in a variety of angles. They allow for controlled bone perforation and avoid heat necrosis that could occur with motorized drilling. **A,** ; **B,**

- Confirm sufficient penetration of the subchondral bone layer to allow access of pluripotential mesenchymal cells into the articular layer.
- Perform microfracture as the final procedure when addressing other joint pathology.

PITFALLS
- Avoid articular cartilage surgery in an unstable or malaligned knee.
- Avoid skiving, which can create cavitary defects on the subchondral bone.
- Carefully débride calcified cartilage layer but avoid thinning the subchondral bone.
- Premature weight bearing, particularly in tibiofemoral lesions, can lead to the displacement of the mesenchymal clot or may lessen the adherence to the subchondral bone or peripheral integration.

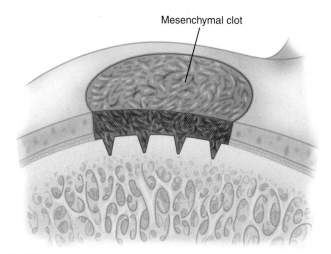

Mesenchymal clot

FIGURE 14-14 The arthroscopic pump pressure is lowered and release of marrow fat droplets and blood is verified. *(Adapted from Mithoefer K, Williams RJ 3rd, Warren RF, et al. The microfracture technique for the treatment of articular cartilage lesions in the knee. A prospective cohort study. J Bone Joint Surg Am. 2005;87:1911-1920.)*

POSTOPERATIVE REHABILITATION

Systematic analysis of the literature has demonstrated the variability of rehabilitation protocols after microfracture treatment.[14] Limited data exist on rehabilitation protocols after microfracture or the effect of continuous passive range of motion (CPM) and weight-bearing status. Basic science studies have demonstrated beneficial effects of continuous motion on cartilage nutrition, metabolism, and marrow stimulation procedures. In his animal model, Salter[9] has demonstrated improved metaplasia of repair tissue within created articular cartilage defects when CPM was used compared with those who did not undergo CPM. Rodrigo and associates[9] have also demonstrated an improved visual grad-

ing of cartilage repair tissue quality in those patients who used CPM compared with patients who were unable to comply with the postoperative CPM machine (55% vs. 85%). However, Marder and coworkers[39] have found no significant difference in outcome with or without the use of CPM or protective weight bearing in lesions smaller than 1 cm².

Tibiofemoral Lesions. Our postoperative weight-bearing protocol is predicated on lesion location. Patients with tibiofemoral lesions are advised to maintain foot-flat touchdown weight bearing (approximately 25%) for 6 to 8 weeks. CPM is initiated in the recovery room and its use is encouraged for 6 to 8 hours daily for approximately 6 weeks. The ROM initiated is typically from 0 to 60 degrees and is progressively increased in 10-degree increments until full passive ROM is achieved. The rate is set at one cycle/min but can be altered based on patient comfort. If a CPM unit is not covered by insurance carriers and is cost-prohibitive for patient rental, we instruct the patient to undergo approximately 500 cycles of passive ROM in three sessions daily. This is most easily performed by the patient in a closed-chain fashion doing rolling chair seated flexion (Fig. 14-15).

We usually encourage the patient to perform home exercises for the first 1 to 2 weeks after surgery, with an emphasis on rest, elevation, and cryotherapy to lessen the postsurgical effusion.[40]

Stationary bicycling without resistance and aquatic non–weight-bearing exercises may be initiated within 1 to 2 weeks post-operatively. Resistance exercises are started at approximately 8 weeks after surgery, avoiding the lesion contact ROM that was determined intra-operatively. Running, pivoting, and jumping exercises are restricted until approximately 6 to 8 months post-operatively, pending lesion site and location. Competitive level athletic activity is usually restricted until approximately 8 to 12 months postoperatively.

Patellar or Trochlear Lesion Microfracture.   The rehabilitation protocol following patellar or trochlear lesion microfracture differs from the above tibiofemoral protocol.[10,41,42] The patients are initiated at partial weight bearing in full extension using a knee immobilizer. They are progressed to full weight bearing more rapidly based on their quadriceps reactivation and control. However, ambulation is performed in the knee immobilizer to allow for limited flexion of less than 20 degrees. This is done to eliminate the shear force across the patellofemoral region that would occur with concentric and eccentric quadriceps contraction during ambulation. CPM is also used for patellofemoral lesions, initiated in low ranges of motion (0 to 20 degrees), progressing toward full motion without restriction.

The beneficial effects of joint motion on the healing of articular cartilage lesions are well documented. These include enhanced articular cartilage nutrition and metabolic activity and stimulation of pluripotential mesenchymal cells to differentiate into fibrocartilage. Pressure-dependent matrix flow from surrounding articular surfaces may influence chondrocyte metaplasia.[43]

Repair Cartilage Fill

Previous experimental studies using an equine model have demonstrated the volume of repaired tissue averaged approximately 64% (Fig. 14-16). A similar finding was seen by Mithoefer and

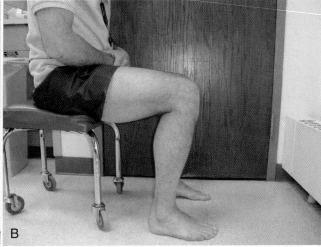

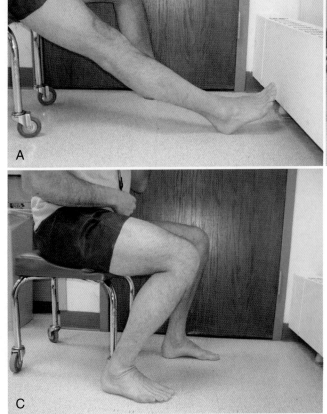

FIGURE 14-15 Rolling chair, closed-chain seated flexion to allow for controlled passive range of motion. **A,** ; **B,** ; **C,** .

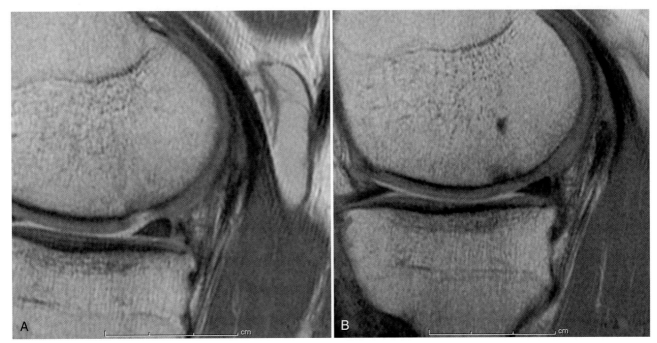

FIGURE 14-16 MRI sagittal proton density high-resolution images of medial femoral condyle full-thickness lesion. **A,** Patient with chronic anterior cruciate ligament–deficient knee. **B,** Image taken at 1-year follow-up demonstrates partial fill of defect, with apparent peripheral integration and no subchondral bone hypertrophy.

colleagues[15] in that most patients demonstrated a persistent depression of the defect; however, all patients with a fill volume of more than two thirds of the defect demonstrated significant improvement in knee function after the microfracture procedure. They also demonstrated persistent gaps between the native and repair cartilage in 92% of patients. This observation was also seen in previous clinical laboratory studies and in alternative articular cartilage repair strategies, including autologous chondrocyte implantation and mosaicplasty.[44,45] The failure of peripheral integration is thought to increase the shear stresses on the lesion, potentially leading to micromotion and degeneration.[12]

COMPLICATIONS

Complications related to the surgical procedure have been rarely reported.[9,44-48] Postoperative hemarthrosis or transient swelling is controlled with a postoperative RICE protocol (**r**est, **i**ce, **c**ompression, **e**levation).[8] We try to minimize the use of anti-inflammatory medication in the early postoperative course, if possible. We use active, passive, and pharmacologic adjuncts to minimize postoperative deep venous thrombosis (DVT) risk (e.g., muscle isometrics of the quadriceps, hamstrings, and gastrocnemius-soleus, compression stockings, and aspirin).[39, 44,45,47] Supplemental pharmacologic DVT prophylaxis is used on a patient-specific basis.

REFERENCES

1. Curl WW, Krome J, Gordon ES, et al. Cartilage injuries: a review of 31,516 knee arthroscopies. *Arthroscopy.* 1997;13:456-460.
2. Hjelle K, Solheim E, Strand T, et al. Articular cartilage defects in 1,000 knee arthroscopies. *Arthroscopy.* 2002;18:730-734.
3. Buckwalter JA. Evaluating methods of restoring cartilaginous articular surfaces. *Clin Orthop Relat Res.* 1999 (367 suppl):S224-238.
4. Buckwalter JA, Mankin HJ. Instructional Course Lectures, The American Academy of Orthopaedic Surgeons—Articular Cartilage. Part II: Degeneration and Osteoarthritis, Repair, Regeneration, and Transplantation. *J Bone Joint Surg Am.* 1997;79:612-632.
5. Magnussen RA, Dunn WR, Carey JL, Spindler KP. Treatment of focal articular cartilage defects in the knee: a systematic review. *Clin Orthop Relat Res.* 2008;(466):952-962.
6. Insall JN. The Pridie debridement operation for osteoarthritis of the knee. *Clin Orthop Relat Res.* 1974;(101):61-67.
7. Magnuson PB. The classic: joint debridement: surgical treatment of degenerative arthritis. *Clin Orthop Relat Res.* 1974;(101):4-12.
8. Pridie KH. A method of resurfacing osteoarthritic knee joints. *J Bone Joint Surg Br.* 1959;41:618-619.
9. Rodrigo JJ, Steadman JR, Silliman JJ, Fulstone HA. Improvement of full-thickness chondral defect healing in the human knee after debridement and microfracture using continuous passive motion. *Am J Knee Surg.* 1994;7:109-116.
10. Steadman JR, Rodkey WG, Rodrigo JJ. Microfracture: surgical technique and rehabilitation to treat chondral defects. *Clin Orthop Relat Res.* 2001;(391 suppl):S362-S369.
11. Frisbie DD, Morisset S, Ho CP, et al. Effects of calcified cartilage on healing of chondral defects treated with microfracture in horses. *Am J Sports Med.* 2006;34:1824-1831.
12. Shapiro F, Koide S, Glimcher MJ. Cell origin and differentiation in the repair of full-thickness defects of articular cartilage. *J Bone Joint Surg Am.* 1993;75:532-553.
13. Guettler JH, Demetropoulos CK, Yang KH, Jurist KA. Osteochondral defects in the human knee: influence of defect size on cartilage rim stress and load redistribution to surrounding cartilage. *Am J Sports Med.* 2004;32:1451-1458.
14. Mithoefer K, McAdams T, Williams RJ, et al. Clinical efficacy of the microfracture technique for articular cartilage repair in the knee: an evidence-based systematic analysis. *Am J Sports Med.* 2009;37:2053-2063.
15. Mithoefer K, Williams RJ 3rd, Warren RF, et al. The microfracture technique for the treatment of articular cartilage lesions in the knee. A prospective cohort study. *J Bone Joint Surg Am.* 2005;87:1911-1920.
16. Mithoefer K, Williams RJ 3rd, Warren RF, et al. Chondral resurfacing of articular cartilage defects in the knee with the microfracture technique. Surgical technique. *J Bone Joint Surg Am.* 2006;88(suppl 1):294-304.
17. Mithoefer K, Williams RJ 3rd, Warren RF, et al. High-impact athletics after knee articular cartilage repair: a prospective evaluation of the microfracture technique. *Am J Sports Med.* 2006;34:1413-1418.

18. Kreuz PC, Erggelet C, Steinwachs MR, et al. Is microfracture of chondral defects in the knee associated with different results in patients aged 40 years or younger? *Arthroscopy*. 2006;22:1180-1186.

19. Kreuz PC, Steinwachs MR, Erggelet C, et al. Results after microfracture of full-thickness chondral defects in different compartments in the knee. *Osteoarthritis Cartilage*. 2006;14:1119-1125.

20. McCauley TR, Disler DG. Magnetic resonance imaging of articular cartilage of the knee. *J Am Acad Orthop Surg*. 2001;9:2-8.

21. Messner K, Maletius W. The long-term prognosis for severe damage to weight-bearing cartilage in the knee: a 14-year clinical and radiographic follow-up in 28 young athletes. *Acta Orthop Scand*. 1996;67:165-168.

22. Shelbourne KD, Jari S, Gray T. Outcome of untreated traumatic articular cartilage defects of the knee: a natural history study. *J Bone Joint Surg Am*. 2003;85(suppl 2):8-16.

23. Frisbie DD, Oxford JT, Southwood L, et al. Early events in cartilage repair after subchondral bone microfracture. *Clin Orthop Relat Res*. 2003;(407): 215-227.

24. Noyes FR, Barber-Westin SD, Simon R. The role of high tibial osteotomy in the anterior cruciate ligament-deficient knee with varus alignment. In: DeLee JC, Miller MD, eds. *Orthopaedic Sports Medicine Principles and Practice*. 2nd ed. Philadelphia: WB Saunders; 2003:1900-1936.

25. Dugdale TW, Noyes FR, Styer D. Preoperative planning for high tibial osteotomy. The effect of lateral tibiofemoral separation and tibiofemoral length. *Clin Orthop Relat Res*. 1992 Jan 1992;(274):248-264.

26. Potter HG, Linklater JM, Allen AA, et al. Magnetic resonance imaging of articular cartilage in the knee. An evaluation with use of fast-spin-echo imaging. *J Bone Joint Surg Am*. 1998;80:1276-1284.

27. Sonin AH, Pensy RA, Mulligan ME, Hatem S. Grading articular cartilage of the knee using fast spin-echo proton density-weighted MR imaging without fat suppression. *AJR Am J Roentgenol*. 2002;179:1159-1166.

28. Brittberg M, Winalski CS. Evaluation of cartilage injuries and repair. *J Bone Joint Surg Am*. 2003;85(suppl 2):58-69.

29. Black BR, Chong le R, Potter HG. Cartilage imaging in sports medicine. *Sports Med Arthrosc*. 2009;17:68-80.

30. Recht MP, Goodwin DW, Winalski CS, White LM. MRI of articular cartilage: revisiting current status and future directions. *AJR Am J Roentgenol*. 2005;185:899-914.

31. Potter HG, Chong le R. Magnetic resonance imaging assessment of chondral lesions and repair. *J Bone Joint Surg Am*. 2009;91(suppl 1):126-131.

32. Noyes FR, Stabler CL. A system for grading articular cartilage lesions at arthroscopy. *Am J Sports Med*. 1989;17:505-513.

33. Outerbridge RE. The etiology of chondromalacia patellae. *J Bone Joint Surg Br*. 1961;43:752-757.

34. Frisbie DD, Trotter GW, Powers BE, et al. Arthroscopic subchondral bone plate microfracture technique augments healing of large chondral defects in the radial carpal bone and medial femoral condyle of horses. *Vet Surg*. 1999;28:242-255.

35. Brown WE, Potter HG, Marx RG, et al. Magnetic resonance imaging appearance of cartilage repair in the knee. *Clin Orthop Relat Res*. 2004 May 2004;(422):214-223.

36. Dragoo JL, Korotkova T, Kanwar R, Wood B. The effect of local anesthetics administered via pain pump on chondrocyte viability. *Am J Sports Med*. 2008;36:1484-1488.

37. Gomoll AH, Kang RW, Williams JM, et al. Chondrolysis after continuous intra-articular bupivacaine infusion: an experimental model investigating chondrotoxicity in the rabbit shoulder. *Arthroscopy*. 2006;22: 813-819.

38. Gomoll AH, Yanke AB, Kang RW, et al. Long-term effects of bupivacaine on cartilage in a rabbit shoulder model. *Am J Sports Med*. 2009;37: 72-77.

39. Marder RA, Hopkins G Jr, Timmerman LA. Arthroscopic microfracture of chondral defects of the knee: a comparison of two postoperative treatments. *Arthroscopy*. 2005;21:152-158.

40. Noyes FR, Berrios-Torres S, Barber-Westin SD, Heckmann TP. Prevention of permanent arthrofibrosis after anterior cruciate ligament reconstruction alone or combined with associated procedures: a prospective study in 443 knees. *Knee Surg Sports Traumatol Arthrosc*. 2000;8:196-206.

41. Solomon DJ, Williams RJ III, Warren RF. Marrow stimulation and microfracture for the repair of articular cartilage lesions. In: Williams RJ III, ed. *Cartilage Repair Strategies*. Totowa NJ: Humana; 2007:69-84.

42. Terry MA, Steadman JR, Rodkey WG, Briggs KK. Microfracture for chondral lesions. In: El Attrache NS, Harner CD, Mirzayan R, Sekiya JK, eds. *Surgical Techniques in Sports Medicine*. Philadelphia: Lippincott Williams & Wilkins; 2007:565-571.

43. Salter RB. The biologic concept of continuous passive motion of synovial joints. The first 18 years of basic research and its clinical application. *Clin Orthop Relat Res*. 1989;(242):12-25.

44. Knutsen G, Drogset JO, Engebretsen L, et al. A randomized trial comparing autologous chondrocyte implantation with microfracture. Findings at five years. *J Bone Joint Surg Am*. 2007;89:2105-2112.

45. Knutsen G, Engebretsen L, Ludvigsen TC, et al. Autologous chondrocyte implantation compared with microfracture in the knee. A randomized trial. *J Bone Joint Surg Am*. 2004;86:455-464.

46. Bae DK, Yoon KH, Song SJ. Cartilage healing after microfracture in osteoarthritic knees. *Arthroscopy*. 2006;22:367-374.

47. Gobbi A, Nunag P, Malinowski K. Treatment of full thickness chondral lesions of the knee with microfracture in a group of athletes. *Knee Surg Sports Traumatol Arthrosc*. 2005;13:213-221.

48. Gudas R, Kalesinskas RJ, Kimtys V, et al. A prospective randomized clinical study of mosaic osteochondral autologous transplantation versus microfracture for the treatment of osteochondral defects in the knee joint in young athletes. *Arthroscopy*. 2005;21:1066-1075.

Arthroscopic Osteochondral Transplantation

James Campbell Chow ● James C.Y. Chow ● Nick Frost

Successful treatment of articular cartilage lesions is a complex clinical issue. The mechanical demands placed on articular cartilage in the knee °require it to withstand shear and compressive loads. Additionally, the patients themselves are often demanding, wishing to continue an already active lifestyle. This is further complicated by the limited healing potential of articular cartilage. The clinical outcome of a focal cartilage defect is highly dependent on the size, depth, pattern, and location of the injury. Multiple grading schemes have been described in an effort to quantify this, and hopefully will steer effective clinical treatment. However, no general consensus exists regarding the treatment of these lesions, and controversy continues to surround this topic.

Techniques for marrow stimulation, such as abrasion arthroplasty, drilling, and microfracture, produce fibrocartilage rather than native hyaline cartilage. Good short- and midterm results have been reported by various authors. However, inconsistent long-term results have perpetuated the interest in finding alternative methods for treating full-thickness chondral lesions. These include autologous chondrocyte implantation, autologous osteochondral transplantation, fresh osteochondral allografting, and bulk allografting, as well as a whole host of synthetics, scaffolds and first-, second-, and third-generation cell-based technologies.[1-4] This chapter will focus on the COR system (DePuy Mitek; Raynham, Mass) for arthroscopic osteochondral transplantation.

The idea for the COR technique has its origins in an observation from anterior cruciate ligament (ACL) reconstruction that routine notchplasty is not associated with postoperative clinical sequelae. Because of this, the "notched" area (marginal cartilage in the lateral trochlear groove) of the knee can be used elsewhere, with minimal or no donor site morbidity. The design rationale for this technique is simple:

1. Do no harm. It is uncertain whether a deeply harvested plug can result in pathology of the surrounding subchondral bone.

Therefore, the designers limited the harvested bone to be no more than a routine ACL notchplasty (8 mm in depth).

2. Secure the plug. The most reproducible, simple, and robust method of fixation is that of a press fit.

3. Graft size is important. Working with different graft sizes, the designers found that a 4-mm-diameter plug is too fragile, leading to early failure. On the other extreme, an 8- to 10-mm-diameter plug is too large to be done easily arthroscopically. Experience has dictated that a 5.5-mm-diameter plug is ideal.

4. Reproducibility is important. The harvester is designed with a single horizontal tooth at the cutting edge. When tapped into place and twisted 720 degrees, it scores the bone at exactly an 8-mm depth. This reproducibly creates a graft exactly 8-mm deep.

5. Graft insertion must be controlled. A specially sized clear tube is designed to stabilize the graft during insertion, protecting the graft from "mushrooming," which is associated with graft cartilage damage, and ensuring that the graft is well-seated.

ANATOMY

Hyaline cartilage is has no nerve fibers and is avascular, deriving nutrition from its surrounding synovial fluid. Additionally, hyaline cartilage is composed mostly of matrix, with a relative paucity of live, active cellular material. Because of this, full-thickness articular cartilage defects have limited healing potential. When native healing of such defects occurs, fibrocartilage is formed in the defect. This is the goal of marrow-stimulating techniques, in which osseous bleeding at the defect initiates a cascade of fibrous scar healing. However, fibrocartilage is not as mechanically sound as hyaline cartilage under compressive or shear loads.

In adults, hyaline cartilage normally has a thickness of roughly 8 to 9 mm. As a person ages, the articular cartilage thins. The presence of pathology can accelerate this eroding process. To

THE EFFECT OF GRAPH HEIGHT MISMATCH ON CONTACT PRESSURES

FIGURE 15-1 The effect of graft height mismatch on contact pressures.

(1) Intact articular surface

(2) 4.5 mm dia. circular defect

(3) 4.5 mm dia. plug, 1.0 mm proud to adj. surface

(4) Plug 0.5 mm proud to adj. surface

(5) Plug flush with surface

(6) Plug sunk 0.5 mm

(7) Plug sunk 1.0 mm

A

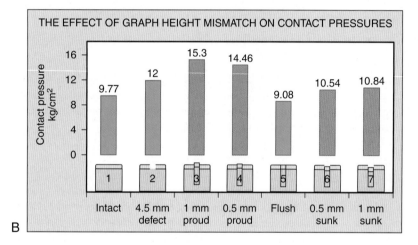

B

produce symptoms, articular cartilage must be thinned by more than 75% before subchondral nerve fibers can detect the change in contact surface pressure. However, overall size of the lesion also plays a role in this. A small chondral defect will not produce symptoms because the stress is distributed to the surrounding joint surface. Only when the cartilage defect becomes large enough, and thin enough will the patient become symptomatic.

To illustrate this point, Jason and Koh[5] have examined the contact pressures across an articular surface with respect to a focal defect and a grafted defect. Various graft height mismatches were modeled (Fig. 15-1), with the results shown in Table 15-1. Not surprisingly, plugs that were flush to their articular surfaces most closely resembled the contact pressure of the normal intact articular surface. However, plugs countersunk by 0.5 to 1.0 mm also closely mimicked the native pressures. Thus, filling a defect to a near-congruent articular surface can reproduce native articular-surfaced pressures. This is the foundation of autogenous osteochondral transplantation.

Autogenous osteochondral transplantation, or mosaicplasty, is a technique in which multiple smaller grafts are harvested from a less weight-bearing portion of the knee and transplanted to the clinically relevant defect. The use of several small grafts has several advantages: (1) it allows the surgeon to reconstruct the natural anatomic contour lost by the defect; (2) it provides some hyaline surface structure to the reconstruction; (3) it limits fibrous cartilage growth to the gaps between the grafts and defect border; (4) it reduces donor site morbidity; (5) it is relatively inexpensive; and (6) the entire reconstruction can be done in a single surgery.

Because small chondral defects will not produce symptoms, the goal of osteochondral transplantation is to decrease the size of large defects functionally to become less clinically significant.

TABLE 15-1   Effect of Graft Height Mismatch on Contact Pressures

Condition of Intra-articular Joint Surface	Contact Surface Pressure (kg/cm²)
Normal intact surface	9.77
Open 4.5-mm hole	12.00
Plug flush to the surface	9.08
Plug countersunk 0.5 mm to surface	10.54
Plug countersunk 1.0 mm to surface	10.84
Plug 0.5 mm proud to the surface	14.46
Plug 1.0 mm proud to the surface	15.30

PATIENT EVALUATION

History and Physical Examination

A history of an acute injury with a subsequent hemarthrosis can be found in focal chondral and osteochondral injuries. This has been reported to have as high as a 20% incidence in patients with no ligamentous instability. Often, patients can present with mechanical symptoms of locking, catching, pain, and recurrent effusions. Ligamentous and meniscal injury can present additional symptoms and challenges.[6-8]

A full thorough knee examination is necessary to determine the underlying pathology as well as any associated injuries.

Diagnostic Imaging

X-rays are required for effective evaluation and treatment of focal chondral defects. Anteroposterior and 30-degree postero-anterior weight-bearing radiographs are obtained to assess joint space narrowing with respect to the tibia and the distal and condylar surfaces of the femur. Non–weight-bearing lateral and Merchant view radiographs are helpful in assessing patellofemoral joint involvement, as well as irregularities not obvious on the weight-bearing views. If mechanical malalignment is suspected, standing long-leg alignment views are helpful.

Magnetic resonance imaging (MRI) can help delineate the size and pattern of the injury, as well as provide additional information about patients in whom x-rays fail to show more global involvement.

TREATMENT

Treatment should be tailored to various presenting factors. These include location and size of the lesion, age and weight of the patient, occupation, and type of sports involvement.

Indications and Contraindications

The COR system permits the arthroscopic harvesting of precisely sized articular cartilage–cancellous bone autografts from a suitable donor site, followed by the transplantation of these autografts to a precisely drilled defect site. The system can be used for open procedures if access to the defect or donor site is difficult. Indications for the procedure are single, full-thickness lesions at least 10 mm in diameter but not more than 35 mm in length or width. The depth of subchondral bone loss should not exceed 6 mm. Similar systems, although with some differences in design, are offered by the OATS system (Arthrex; Naples, Fla) and mosaicplasty (Smith and Nephew Endoscopy; Andover, Mass).

Indications for this procedure are as follows:

1. Physiologically young knee (not absolute chronologic age of the patient)
2. Focal defect 1 to 3 cm in diameter
3. Symptomatic defect
4. Good supporting bone
5. Healthy donor site
6. No associated articulating chondral defects (kissing lesions)

Contraindications include a history of degenerative joint disease or joint infection, intra-articular fracture, a diseased donor site, and multicompartment involvement. Additional physical contraindications relate to poor supporting bone at the recipient site, including a very large defect (more than 3 cm diameter), a deep defect (more than 6 mm deep), and extremely osteopenic subchondral bone stock. ACL disruption is not a contraindication, but concurrent ACL reconstruction is recommended in that case. Meniscal tears or prior surgeries on the lesion are not contraindications. No other area of significant chondral fibrillation or damage should be present. This technique is best performed on the femoral condyles and not on the tibial plateau.

Conservative Management

Conservative management has limited efficacy, and should be reserved for low-demand patients who wish to delay surgical intervention. Such management includes activity modification, nonsteroidal anti-inflammatory drugs, intra-articular injections, physical therapy, padded shoe orthoses, nutritional supplementation, and bracing.

Surgical Management

Other arthroscopic surgical options include lavage and débridement, chondroplasty, and microfracture. Open procedures include autologous chondrocyte implantation, open autologous osteochondral mosaicplasty, fresh osteochondral allografting and bulk allograft.

Arthroscopic Technique

Setup and Instrumentation

A spinal needle is used to determine portal placement to approximate an almost perpendicular approach to harvest and defect site. Of specific note, the senior author (JYCC) believes this to be a forgiving technique. A 10- to 20-degree arc off perpendicular can be tolerated well without clinical consequences. Excess prominences may be later trimmed with a bassinet. The number of bone grafts necessary for the grafting can be determined by using the harvester to score the site of the defect lightly.

Define the recipient sites, starting along the margin of the defect, to ensure a flush repair of the cartilage surface. Graft size should be limited to 6-mm-diameter grafts that are 8 mm deep. Smaller grafts are too fragile, whereas larger grafts may be too difficult to transplant arthroscopically and may increase donor site morbidity. A series of grafts can be arranged to optimize resurfacing of the defect. The original contour of the condylar surface can be easily re-created simply with this cluster of 6-mm grafts. If grafts longer than 8 mm are required to fill the defect, osteochondral transplantation is not indicated because of the lack of adequate supporting bone.

Preparation of the Defect Site

Débride loose fragments away from the cancellous bone bed with an oscillating shaver while avoiding generalized bone bleeding. Keeping in mind the number of grafts to be transplanted, position the Innovasive COR drill near a margin of the defect, as initially scored. Under arthroscopic vision, drill almost perpen-

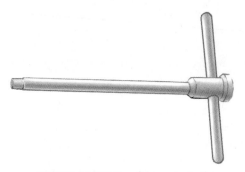

FIGURE 15-2 COR graft harvester tool.

dicularly until resistance is felt. Observe that the 8-mm drill stop is resting on the stable bone surrounding the repair site.

All holes may be drilled at once or osteochondral grafts may be implanted after each hole is drilled, maintaining a tight press fit. Care must be taken to ensure that a 1- to 2-mm bone bridge exists between recipient sites.

Harvesting COR Grafts

Insert the harvester (T-handled instrument) into the disposable cutter, screwing them together (Fig. 15-2). Advance the plunger through the lumen of the harvester, where it acts like an obturator to minimize soft tissue capture when passing the instruments into the joint. Once the assembly is properly positioned within the joint, replace the plunger with the anvil to minimize loss of fluid while harvesting grafts.

Position the cutter-harvester assembly on the non–weight-bearing donor site selected to provide the graft (Fig. 15-3). Ensure that the end of the cutter is almost perpendicular to the surface prior to taking the donor graft. In the knee, the superior and lateral aspects of the intercondylar notch may provide easiest arthroscopic access.

With a mallet, tap the anvil portion of this assembly into the bone 8 mm until it is fully seated at the cutter's depth stop. Rotate the T handle of the harvester clockwise a minimum of two complete revolutions. The cutter tooth undercuts the distal bone, scoring it to ensure precise harvesting of a donor plug. Supportive pressure must be maintained on the T handle during rotation to ensure control of plug depth. Remove the cartilage graft by gently twisting the T handle while withdrawing it from the joint.

Unscrew the harvester from the cutter. The bone graft will remain protected within the harvester tube until it is ready for transplantation into the defect site. If additional bone grafts are required to repair the defect, the cutter can be assembled onto another harvester and the process repeated until the appropriate number of grafts has been taken.

Cartilage Graft Implantation

Screw the delivery guide onto the harvester, which contains the first graft to be delivered. Place the tip of the plunger through the spacer ring into the proximal end of the harvester. Gently tap the plunger, advancing the bone graft beyond the tip of the deliver guide, as limited by the spacer ring. This 1- to 2-mm lead of bone assists in aligning the graft with the drill hole as it is inserted into the recipient site.

Position the graft over the drill hole. Withdraw the plunger from the harvester, removing the spacer ring. Gently reinsert the plunger, carefully pressing the plug to fit in the undersized drill hole, flush with the surrounding bone (Fig. 15-4). Excess prom-

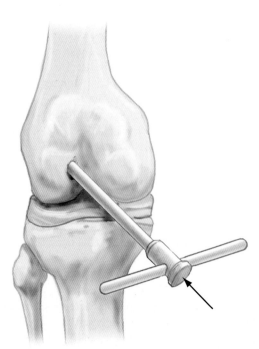

FIGURE 15-3 The graft is harvested from the non–weight-bearing ACL notch site.

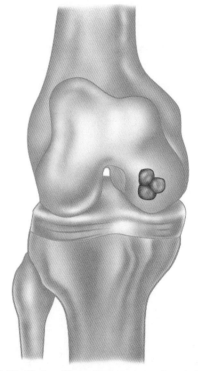

FIGURE 15-4 Defect filled with three osteochondral grafts.

inences may be trimmed with a basinet. Avoid impacting the graft to round off the corners, because this will mushroom the graft and damage the graft's integrity.

If the defect is deep or the decision is made to place a solitary graft (or grafts) away from the margin of the defect, the delivery guide may be partially unscrewed to reduce the insertion depth of the graft. This allows for a supportive press fit between the sides of the plug and drill hole while maintaining an elevated face on the cartilage graft.

PEARLS & PITFALLS

PEARLS

Recipient Site

1. Trim loose cartilage to a stable base at the periphery of the defect using the graft cutter tool.
2. Plan for the number and position of the grafts to be transplanted by using the harvester to score the defect.
3. There should be 1- to 2-mm osteochondral bridges remaining between recipient holes. To preserve the integrity of these bridges, holes should be drilled in an alternating fashion to sites of insertion of the donor plugs.
4. Prepare the recipient site prior to obtaining donor osteochondral grafts. This can allow immediate transfer of the donor graft to the defect. Donor graft size can also be adjusted if difficulty is encountered during the recipient site preparation.
5. Take note of the angle of flexion of the knee when drilling the recipient site graft holes. By using the same angle of knee flexion when inserting the grafts, it is easier to match the hole-graft trajectory.
6. The clear transfer tube is provided to allow complete visualization so that the graft can be inserted completely initially. Attempting to reseat the graft after a partial initial insertion without the supporting tube can increase the chances of mushrooming and graft damage.
7. When flexion of the knee is required to access a defect of the distal femoral condyle, the capsule and soft tissue will press against the defect under tension; this makes visualization with an arthroscope almost impossible. To alleviate this, an accessory portal can be used to introduce a lever arm tool (e.g., a joker) to retract the tissue away from the defect. An alternate method is to introduce Merseline tape (Ethicon; Somerville, NJ) around the tissues arthroscopically. Pulling directly on these tape loops creates a soft tissue intra-articular "tent" to aid in visualization.

Donor Site

1. The cutter tool must be turned 720 degrees (two full turns) to ensure complete shaping of the graft. Simple twisting of the cutter will free the graft from its donor site. Rocking is not necessary in the COR technique, and may damage the surrounding bone in the donor site.

PITFALLS

1. It is possible to have a graft-hole diameter mismatch when using holes and grafts of different diameters. Use of a single diameter for all grafts and holes can streamline the procedure and eliminate the possibility of this error.
2. To avoid damage to the adjacent subchondral bone during harvest, a maximum depth of 8 mm should be used during graft harvesting.

3. It is difficult to match the articular contour if the graft or recipient hole is made at an oblique angle. This may have an adverse effect on surrounding stresses at the defect, durability of the graft, and clinical outcomes. Both grafts and recipient holes must be harvested and inserted at a 90-degree angle to the articular surface.
4. If too much of the graft is presented outside the cannula prior to insertion, the graft will not be adequately supported and insertion forces may ruin the graft. To avoid this, we recommend leaving the graft only 1 mm proud from the cannula, thus aiding in graft alignment while still protecting the integrity of the construct during press fit.
5. If toggling of the drill occurs while creating the recipient hole, an oversized hole can be made. This situation can be salvaged by redrilling the hole with a larger drill and using the next size larger donor plug (e.g., step up from 6 to 8 mm).

Postoperative Rehabilitation

Full weight bearing as tolerated without restrictions is the typical postoperative management. Range of motion is encouraged to promote joint health. Crutches and pain control are discontinued when the patient feels ready, often within the first week postoperatively.

OUTCOMES

Patient selection is paramount to success of this technique. Because of the relatively narrow indications listed above, the senior author's experience (JCYC) includes only 40 cases from 1996 to May 2009. This includes 23 women and 17 men, ranging in age from 20 to 75 years (mean, 50.5 years). The defects ranged from 1.5 to 3 cm in diameter, with the exception of one case.

Patient follow-up results have been monitored. In 1999, 3-year results showed 86% with good to excellent results. In 2001, the 5-year results showed 76% with good to excellent results. In 2008, at 13 years, 74% of the patients still had good to excellent results. Repeat x-rays and MRI scans were obtained for asymptomatic patients who agreed to participate in this study (Fig. 15-5). In only one MRI was there a persistent bone graft margin, indicating the possibility of delayed incorporation, at 4 years and 7 months postoperatively. The patient was asymptomatic with a congruent articular surface (Fig. 15-6). The significance of this finding is uncertain, but it may not be related to clinical sequelae.

One patient had a 4-cm defect (outside of our recommended defect size), necessitating the transplantation of four graft plugs (Fig. 15-7). In this particular case, the patient was young and wished to undergo osteochondral transplantation as a final effort to temporize the necessity for a knee replacement. The patient was well-informed and accepted a potentially high risk of failure prior to surgery. Ultimately, this patient returned pain-free to playing baseball with his children (see Fig. 15-7C).

Second-look arthroscopy was performed in one case. This patient had a medial femoral osteochondral transplantation graft in August 1997. Two years later, the patient returned with persistent pain and repeat arthroscopy was performed (Fig. 15-8). On second look, the original graft site showed excellent gross congruity, incorporation, and no signs of failure. A new, full-thickness defect

Text continued on p. 142.

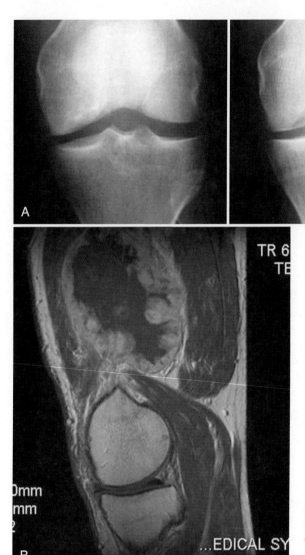

FIGURE 15-5 A, Sample radiographs at preoperative evaluation, 2 months postoperatively, and 5 years postoperatively. Maintenance of joint line congruity can be seen in these standard weight-bearing AP views of the knee in identical positions. **B,** MRI scan of left knee 9 years after medial femoral condyle osteochondral transplantation. Joint congruity and chondral surface remain intact.

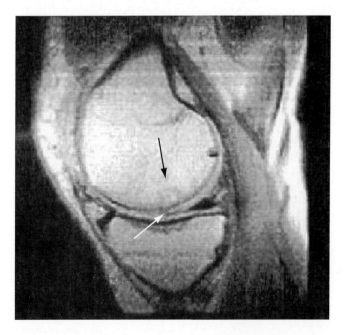

FIGURE 15-6 Persistent bone graft margin (*black arrow*) with congruency at the articular surface (*white arrow*).

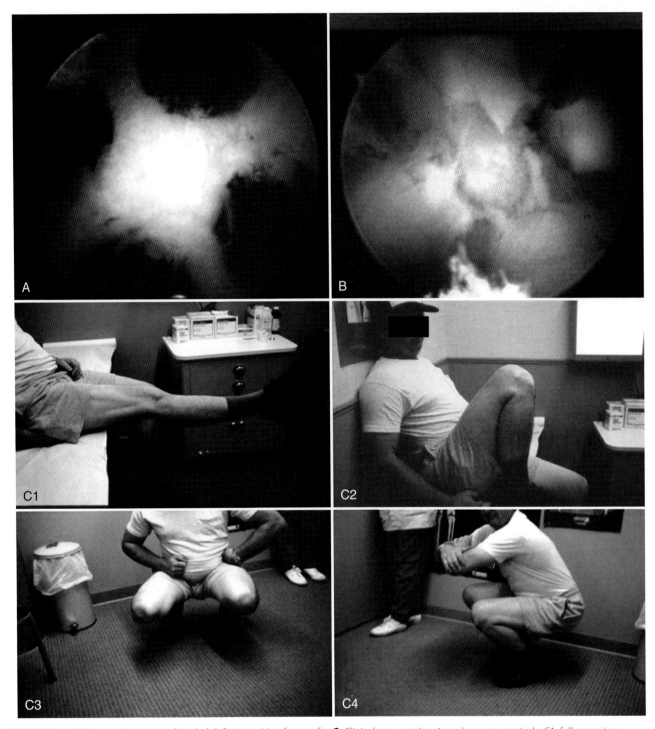

FIGURE 15-7 A, B, Large 4-cm osteochondral defect requiring four grafts. **C,** Clinical presentation 4 weeks postoperatively. C1, full extension; C2, full flexion; C3, full squat, frontal view; C4, full squat, side view.

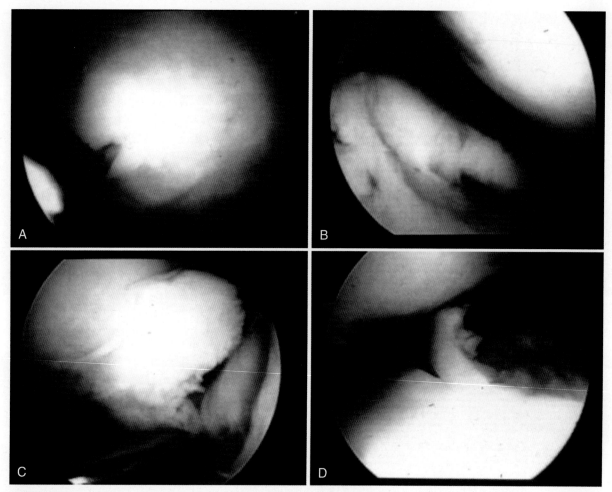

FIGURE 15-8 Second-look arthroscopy, 2 years post–osteochondral transplantation. **A,** Full congruent incorporation of the graft on the medial femoral condyle. A new lateral tibial defect is present. **B,** Defect on lateral tibial joint surface not seen during placement of original graft. **C,** Loose cartilage fragment from lateral femoral condyle. **D,** View of loose fragment from the defect of the lateral tibial joint surface with the scope placed anteromedially.

was present in the tibia of the opposite compartment. This patient ultimately had a total knee arthroplasty in 1999.

Although difficult to prove, it is possible that osteochondral transplantation may slow the development of arthritis in the absence of mechanical or systemic pathology. Anecdotally, an 85-year -old female patient presented for left total knee arthroplasty. She had received an osteochondral transplant in her right knee 10 years earlier. The comparison x-ray of both knees shown in Figure 15-9 reveals a remarkable difference.

CONCLUSIONS

Osteochondral defects treated by marrow stimulation techniques have resulted in inconsistent long-term results. This has perpetuated the interest in finding alternative methods of treating full-thickness chondral lesions. These include autologous chondrocyte implantation, autologous osteochondral transplantation, fresh osteochondral allografting and bulk allograft, and a number of synthetics, scaffolds and first-, second-, and third-generation cell-based technologies.

The goal of osteochondral transplantation is twofold: (1) to remove the pathology of the osteochondral defect's cartilage, subchondral bone, and interface; and (2) to replace the defect new graft to decrease the defects surrounding forces. Although there is no nerve fiber or blood supply in the bone plug graft, there is an assumption that the existing joint fluid will allow the cartilage cells to survive. This is further supported by the fact that the plug is harvested and inserted within a short period of time. The bone plug fills in the defect and allows the live hyaline cartilage cells to help fill the graft. If the graft is placed correctly, it will decrease the size of the lesion and direct pressure to the contact surface of the subchondral bone, thus relieving the symptoms. Also, because the bone plug lacks nerve fibers and blood supply, there is no sensitivity at the graft-harvested site.

Full-thickness defects smaller than 1 cm in diameter are not thought to be appropriate for treatment with this technique. They do not seem to be clinically troublesome and do well when left alone. It follows that a smaller defect—only 6 mm in diameter (COR technique donor site)—in an area that is not load

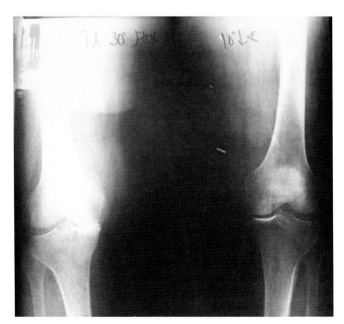

FIGURE 15-9 Bilateral view 10 years post–osteochondral transplantation. The joint line is maintained in the operative knee and terminal arthritis is present in the contralateral knee.

bearing and does not affect the patellofemoral articulation should also be well tolerated. These defects fill in without additional bone grafting and are covered with fibrocartilaginous scar, much like the area between donor plugs and the adjacent intact hyaline cartilage.

Overall, experience indicates that the primary goal of osteochondral transplantation is not to reproduce a normal anatomic, physiologic, or biomechanical knee joint surface. The goal of this procedure is simply to decrease the patient's clinical sequelae regarding the defect being treated. This may be related to decreasing the effective size of the defect, and thus decreasing the biomechanical shear and compressive forces surrounding these defects. This is illustrated by Jason and Koh's research on force transmissions surrounding peridefect- and periplug-related contact pressures (see Fig. 15-1 and Table 1).[5] Because of this phenomenon, this is a forgiving technique and the angle of graft insertion can be 10 to 20 degrees off of perpendicular without clinical consequences. The senior author speculates that the remodeling potential of the narrow fibrocartilage in the inter-graft space may make this possible. This is supported with our second-look arthroscopy findings (Fig. 15-8), and the good to excellent clinical results may be highly related to patient selection.

Arthroscopic osteochondral transplantation is an acceptable option for treating full-thickness osteochondral defects in appropriately selected patients. The arthroscopic technique is straightforward, with a low incidence of complications. The intergraft areas fill in, creating a homogenous appearance. The ability to manage these conditions arthroscopically at the time of discovery offers the advantage of convenience, a single procedure, and cost savings.

REFERENCES

1. McNickle AG, Provencher MT, Cole BJ. Overview of existing cartilage repair technology. *Sports Med Arthrosc.* 2008;16:196-201.
2. Kerker JT, Leo AJ, Sgaglione NA. Cartilage repair: synthetics and scaffolds: basic science, surgical techniques, and clinical outcomes. *Sports Med Arthrosc.* 2008;16:208-216.
3. Sgaglione NA. Biologic approaches to articular cartilage surgery: future trends. *Orthop Clin North Am.* 2005;36:485-495.
4. Sgaglione N, Miniaci A, Gillogly S, et al. Update on advanced surgical techniques in the treatment of traumatic focal articular cartilage lesions of the knee. *Arthroscopy.* 2002;18:9-32.
5. Jason L, Koh MD. The effect of graft height mismatch on contact pressures following osteochondral grafting. *Am J Sports Med.* 2004;32:317-320.
6. Areon A, Loken S, Heir S, et al. Articular cartilage lesions in 993 consecutive knee arthroscopies. *Am J Sports Med.* 2004;32:211-215.
7. Hjelle K, Solheim E, Strand T. Articular cartilage defects in 1,000 knee arthroscopies. *Arthroscopy.* 2002;18:730-734.
8. Noyes FR, Bassett RW, Grood ES, et al. Arthroscopy in acute traumatic hemarthrosis of the knee. *J Bone Joint Surg Am.* 1980;62:687-695.
9. Ferkel RD, Zanotti RM, Komenda GA, et al. Arthroscopic treatment of chronic osteochondral lesions of the talus: long-term results. *Am J Sports Med.* 2008;36:1750-1762.
10. Sgaglione NA. The future of cartilage restoration. *J Knee Surg.* 2004;17:235-243.
11. Kon E, Delcogliano M, Filardo G, et al. Second-generation issues in cartilage repair. *Sports Med Arthrosc.* 2008;16:221-229.
12. Coons DA, Barber FA. Arthroscopic osteochondral autografting. *Orthop Clin North Am.* 2005;36:447-458.
13. Marcacci M, Kon E, Delcogliano M, et al. Arthroscopic autologous osteochondral grafting for cartilage defects of the knee: prospective study results at a minimum 7-year follow-up. *Am J Sports Med.* 2007;35:2014-2021.
14. Magnussen RA, Dunn WR, Carey JL, Spindler KP. Treatment of focal articular cartilage defects in the knee: a systematic review. *Clin Orthop Relat Res.* 2008;(466):952-962.
15. Cain EL, Clancy WG. Treatment algorithm for osteochondral injuries of the knee. *Clin Sports Med.* 2001;20:321-342.
16. Koulalis D, Di Benedetto P, Citak M, et al. Comparative study of navigated versus freehand osteochondral graft transplantation of the knee. *Am J Sports Med.* 2009;37:803-807.
17. Hangody L, Vásárhelyi G, Hangody LR, et al. Autologous osteochondral grafting—technique and long-term results. *Injury.* 2008;39(suppl 1):S32-9.
18. Hangody L, Füles P. Autologous osteochondral mosaicplasty for the treatment of full-thickness defects of weight-bearing joints: ten years of experimental and clinical experience. *J Bone Joint Surg Am.* 2003;85(suppl 2):25-32.
19. Hangody L, Feczkó P, Bartha L, et al. Mosaicplasty for the treatment of articular defects of the knee and ankle. *Clin Orthop Relat Res.* 2001;(391 suppl):S328-S336.
20. Kircher J, Patzer T, Magosch P, et al. Osteochondral autologous transplantation for the treatment of full-thickness cartilage defects of the shoulder: results at nine years. *J Bone Joint Surg Br.* 2009;91:499-503.
21. Patil S, Butcher W, D'Lima DD, et al. Effect of osteochondral graft insertion forces on chondrocyte viability. *Am J Sports Med.* 2008;36:1726-1732.
22. Barber FA, Chow JCY, Chow JCC. Autogenous osteochondral transplantation. In: Chow JCY, ed. *Advanced Arthroscopy.* New York: Springer-Verlag; 2000:573-579.
23. Chow JCY , Hantes ME, Houle JB, Zalavras CG Arthroscopic autogenous osteochondral transplantation for treating knee cartilage defects: a 2 to 5 year follow-up study. *Arthroscopy.* 2004;20:681-690
24. Brittberg M, Lindahl A, Nilsson, et al. Treatment of deep cartilage defects in the knee with autologous chondrocyte transplantation. *N Engl J Med.* 1994;331:889-895.
25. Stedman JR, Briggs K, Rodrigo J, et al. Outcomes of microfracture for traumatic chondral defects of the knee: average 11-year follow-up. *Arthroscopy.* 2003;19:477-484.
26. Alford J, Cole B. Cartilage restoration, part 1: basic science, historical perspective, patient evaluation, and treatment options. *Am J Sports Med.* 2005;33:295-306.
27. Alford J, Cole B. Cartilage restoration, part 2: techniques, outcomes, and future directions. *Am J Sports Med.* 2005;33:443-460.

28. Sgaglione N. The biological treatment of focal articular cartilage lesions in the knee: future trends? *Arthroscopy*. 2003;19:154-160.

29. Brown W, Potter H. Magnetic resonance imaging appearance of cartilage repair in the knee. *Clin Orthop Relat Res*. 2004;(422):214-223.

30. Sgaglione N. Decision making and approach to articular cartilage surgery. *Sports Med Arthrosc Rev*. 2003;11:192-201.

31. O'Driscoll S. The healing and regeneration of articular cartilage. *J Bone Joint Surg Am*. 1998;80:1795-1807.

32. Barber A, Chow J. Arthroscopic osteochondral transplantation: histologic results. *Arthroscopy*. 2001;17:832-835.

33. Horas U, Pelinkovic D, Aigner T. Autologous chondrocyte implantation and osteochondral cylinder transplantation in cartilage repair of the knee joint: a prospective comparative trial. *J Bone Joint Surg Am*. 2003; 85:185-192.

Allograft Osteochondral Transplantation

Thomas R. Carter

The treatment of chondral defects presents a formidable challenge. A variety of treatment methods are available, but all have shortcomings.[1] Osteochondral allografts have been used for the treatment of chondral lesions for more than 20 years.[2] They have the advantage of providing true articular cartilage rather than hyaline-like cartilage or fibrocartilage. They are particularly valuable when treating large defects and those with bone loss because they are not limited by size, depth, or shape of the lesion.

BASIC SCIENCE

Although the efficacy of osteochondral allografts has been shown for many years, disease transmission continues to be the area of greatest concern.[3] Unfortunately, methods used to sterilize tissue have significant detrimental effects on osteochondral allografts.[4] Sterilization methods not only devitalize all the chondrocytes, but also have negative effects on the material properties of the graft. Fortunately, the risk of disease transmission is slight if the tissue is retrieved, handled, and processed in strict accordance with standardized guidelines of the American Association of Tissue Banks (AATB).[5]

Grafts are harvested within 24 hours of the donor's death to minimize contamination and maintain chondrocyte viability. The grafts are then processed in a clean room environment and thoroughly lavaged to remove blood components, which are the main source of pathogens and immunologic sensitization. After cultures are obtained, the grafts are treated with several antimicrobials and subsequently stored at 4° C until used.

The initial clinical series reported using grafts within 1 week from procurement because it was found that the sooner the graft is implanted, the greater the chance of chondrocyte survival.[6,7] Although the minimum chondrocyte viability for graft success is unknown, it is clear that this play a vital role in graft integrity.[8] However, disease testing and safety precautions have resulted in

tissue banks generally not releasing grafts for use until about 3 weeks. Fortunately, current storage methods are able to maintain 80% cell viability at 4 weeks.[9,10] In addition, the biomechanical properties of the graft are not statistically affected at that time.[11,12] However, more recent testing has shown that in commercially available grafts, a large percentage of the viable cells do not exhibit full function.[13]

Because of the limitations of fresh grafts with regard to storage and assurance of sterility, other methods of preservation, including freeze drying and fresh-frozen methods, have been evaluated.[14] Unfortunately, fresh-frozen grafts have no viable chondrocytes. Freeze drying not only destroys all cells but also alters the graft's material properties.[15]

Host immune response is another area of concern with allograft transplantation. It is well known that musculoskeletal allografts are capable of inducing cell-mediated and humeral immune responses in the host.[16,17] The predominant mechanism is cell-mediated, and by reducing the number of allogenic cells, the immune response would therefore be reduced. The primary source of allograft cells is the blood and bone marrow elements. The immune load is significantly reduced by removing them during graft processing,.

Chondrocytes can also evoke an immune response and matching the surface antigens has been presented as one method to reduce the load further. However, the limited number of osteochondral allografts available would make it extremely difficult to match the donor to the recipient. Fortunately, any host sensitization has not precluded favorable results. It has been suggested that because chondrocytes are embedded in the dense matrix, which acts as a barrier, intact grafts are considered immunologically privileged. However, there is a consensus that patients with autoimmune disease or inflammatory arthropathies are not appropriate candidates for osteochondral allografts. Although it may be implemented, the morbidity associated with immunosuppression does not justify its use.

PATIENT EVALUATION

History and Physical Examination

Candidates for osteochondral allografts for focal defects typically fall into three categories—osteochondritis dissecans (OCD), post-traumatic lesions, and revision surgery.[18-20]

Making the diagnosis of OCD by history can be difficult. Most patients with OCD have nonspecific joint pain that is insidious in onset. It is usually aggravated with activity and resolves with rest. In the pediatric population, it can often be overlooked and considered to be growing pains. Intermittent swelling may also occur if early symptoms are ignored. As the disease progresses, it may be associated with mechanical symptoms, such as catching and locking and subsequent feeling a loose body. Post-traumatic lesions and revision surgery have an obvious cause to raise awareness of articular cartilage injury. However, the symptoms are typically the same as those of OCD.

Physical examination findings may very widely. In early stages of OCD, the examination may be unremarkable. With any lesion, swelling may be present, ranging from a subtle swelling to a frank effusion. One must remember that any knee swelling in the younger patient without obvious cause should raise the suspicion of OCD, especially in a very active individual.

Pain on deep palpation of the involved area may be present. If the lesion has become partially detached, pain with clicking or popping can be found at a distinct range of pain. If the lesion has become completely separated, mechanical symptoms of a loose body may be seen. Quadriceps atrophy may be present; knowing the degree of atrophy may be helpful if the duration of symptoms is unclear.

Diagnostic Imaging

Image techniques are important not only for diagnosis, but also for treatment planning. Most osteochondral lesions can be seen on plain radiographs and should be the starting point. The initial series should include standing anteroposterior with the leg in full extension, 45-degree weight-bearing posteroanterior (PA; tunnel), lateral, and patellar sunrise views. Typically, a magnification marker is placed on the tunnel and lateral views and used as a reference if graft size matching is needed. Most OCD lesions occur on the lateral aspect of the medial femoral condyle and are most clearly seen on the tunnel view. Lateral femoral OCD lesions tend to be more posterior and are thus not always as obvious.

Plain radiographs are also used for comparison and serial following of the lesions during healing and deterioration. Standing full length films should be obtained once the diagnosis of a chondral lesion is confirmed to evaluate the mechanical axis.

Magnetic resonance imaging (MRI) is the gold standard for evaluating osteochondral and chondral lesions. If the diagnosis is in question, MRI is very sensitive for excluding or confirming pathology. If a defect is seen on plain films, MRI is recommended to determine the extent of the lesion and integrity of the articular cartilage. For example, if fluid is present behind the lesion, this indicates an unstable fragment and the need for surgery.

Bone scans (technetium bone scintigraphy) have been used to determine the extent of activity within the lesion and monitor progress of healing. However, their use has declined because of the advantages of MRI.

TREATMENT

Indications and Contraindications

Because of the risk of infection, limited availability, and cost, as well as consideration of other available treatment options, osteochondral allografts are typically reserved for chondral lesions that are 2 cm^2 or larger. The cause of the defect, patient age and activity level, concurrent pathology, and rehabilitation requirements are other variables that need to be considered when evaluating a potential candidate.

With regard to cause, isolated OCD and traumatic lesions have the best outcomes. Defects in the presence of diffuse degenerative changes or inflammatory arthropathies are contraindicated. Treatment of lesions secondary to avascular necrosis (AVN) may be appropriate, but only if the involvement is not progressive and the cause is understood. In addition, lesions limited to one joint surface (unipolar) fare much better than those on opposing surfaces (bipolar or kissing lesions).

When evaluating the knee, one must look beyond just the lesion. Ligament instability, absence of the meniscus, and limb malalignment have negative effects on outcome. Ligament reconstruction and meniscal allograft transplantation need to be performed concurrently or in a staged capacity. With respect to the mechanical axis, there is general agreement that if it passes through the involved compartment, realignment should be performed. However, there it is also general agreed that the degree of correction does not need to be as much as when performing an osteotomy for an arthritic knee. Typically, the aim is to pass the mechanical axis through the opposite tibial spine.

Patient age is of some debate, with most reporting an upper age limit of 40 to 45 years; it is thought that these lesions are associated with degenerative changes. However, others have implanted grafts in patients 60 years of age or older. The cause of the lesion is vital when dealing with the age factor. In the uncommon case of a mature patient with an isolated lesion and no other pathology, age alone should not be considered a contraindication. Older patients with low activity demands may be better suited for joint arthroplasty. Other relative contraindications include obesity (body mass index [BMI] >30 kg/m^2), smoking, and chronic steroid use. Although sometimes taken for granted, patient expectations also need to be strongly considered. For example, it is not uncommon for patients with large lesions to regard the procedure as one that will enable them to return to unrestricted activities. Patients need to understand that high-impact activities such as distance running and contact sports should be avoided.

Conservative Management

Focal chondral defects are a common finding and can have a significant effect on limiting a patient's activities and quality of life.[21,22] Symptomatic lesions can be treated nonoperatively with modification of activities, anti-inflammatories, viscosupplementation, and rehabilitation. Although these can be of benefit, many patients continue to be symptomatic.

Surgical Treatment

Several surgical options are available in addition to osteochondral allografts, but each has its advantages and disadvantages. The simplest is débridement-chondroplasty, but the benefits are commonly short-lived. Microfracture is technically easy to perform, with limited morbidity, but results in fibrocartilage filling the defect.[23,24] As a result, the outcomes deteriorate after a few years, and lesions larger than a few centimeters do poorly. Autogenous osteochondral transfer has the benefit of improving normal articular cartilage and being able to fill bone deficiencies.[25,26] However, donor availability is limited and it is recommended for lesions smaller than 2 to 2.5 cm². Autologous chondrocyte implantation (ACI) is often discussed as an alternative to osteochondral allografts. It can also treat large lesions and is recommended for lesions up to 16 cm².[27] However, it results in hyaline-like cartilage and should not be used by itself for defects more than 6 to 8 mm deep. In addition, it is technically challenging, with many published studies having a re-operation rate of 30%.

Surgical Technique

After the patient is found to meet the criteria for an osteochondral allograft, the next step is to obtain a graft (Fig. 16-1) The tissue bank used should be AATB certified to minimize the risk of infection and obtain a graft of high quality. The upper age limit of the donor of a graft is unclear. However, many surgeons recommend that the donor be younger than 35 to 40 years because of concern about tissue quality, with degenerative changes being present in older donors. Size and contour of the graft to match the recipient is another factor to be considered when selecting a graft.

Several methods can be used in an effort to match the graft and host. MRI and computed tomography (CT) scans can be used for the greatest accuracy, but plain radiographs are typically sufficient. Most commonly used are 45-degree PA and lateral views, with a magnification marker to evaluate the need for any size adjustment.

When the graft is obtained, it should be opened and inspected at the beginning of the procedure. However, because there can be a significant time delay from when the graft is requested to when it is obtained, diagnostic arthroscopy should first be performed if

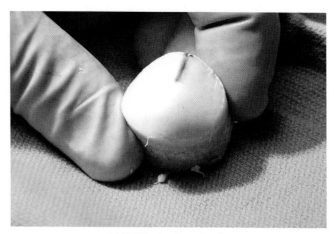

FIGURE 16-2 Dowel graft.

there is any question of change in knee pathology. Once the graft has been opened, it should be maintained in the storage solution until it is prepared. As noted, this decreases the chance of chondrocyte death, which can occur if the graft is in saline solution or exposed to the air.

The graft can be prepared using a dowel or shell configuration.[28,29] Dowel grafts are cylindrical plugs, often compared with the smaller autologous osteochondral autografts, and are prepared with commercially available instrumentation (Fig. 16-2). Shell grafts are manually prepared with osteotomes, saws, and rongeurs to match the defect (Fig. 16-3). Because dowel grafts are less time consuming to prepare, are easier to match, and are often press-fit, they are usually the method of choice for femoral and patellar defects. Shell grafts are generally reserved for massive grafts and those not amenable to dowel grafts. These would include tibial plateau grafts and posterior femoral condyle lesions, which cannot be reached at a 90-degree angle to the surface needed to prepare dowel grafts. In addition, if the meniscus is not intact, the tibial plateau allograft should include the meniscus. If the host meniscus is normal, the meniscus and its horn attachment are left intact.

The principles are the same for dowel and shell grafts. Femoral lesions can often be exposed through a miniarthrotomy, but more extensive lesions may require the exposure used for joint arthroplasty. The lesion is débrided to a vascular base to enable the graft to heal. Grafts were usually 1-cm thick or more but, with the development of dowel grafts and better fixation methods, the thickness is typically 6 to 8 mm. Basically, there should be enough bone to have the graft incorporate to the host, but not so little that the graft is unstable. If the base is not vascular at a short depth, it is extended until bleeding occurs. However, tibial plateau grafts should be at least 1 cm to have sufficient bone to enable graft fixation with screws or other means.

The initial step with the dowel method is to measure the defect using cannulated sizing cylinders (Fig. 16-4). Several systems are available, with most having cylinders in 5-mm increments ranging from 15 to 35 mm. The smallest cylinder that encompasses the defect should be selected. It is then stabilized perpendicular to the surface and a guide pin drilled through the cannulated cylinder and advanced until it is secure in the bone. Because the guide pin is used as a reference for subsequent drilling, it is crucial to have the

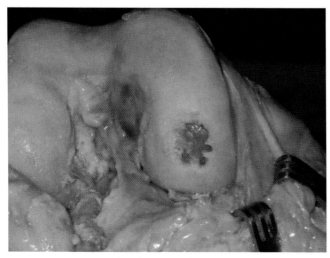

FIGURE 16-1 Osteochondral lesion of the lateral femoral condyle.

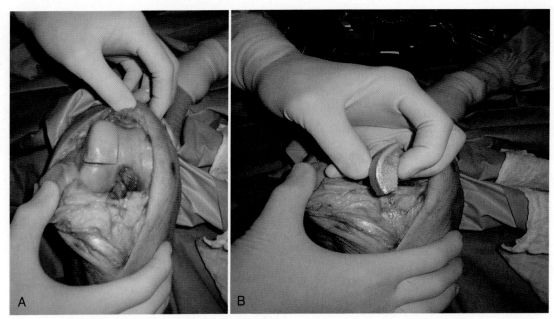

FIGURE 16-3 A, Shell graft after placement in recipient site. **B,** Lateral view of shell graft.

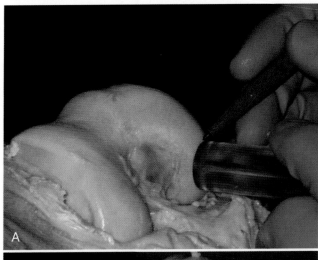

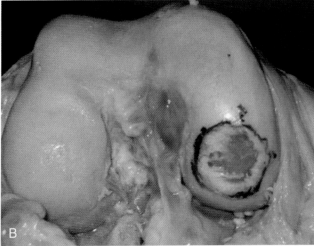

FIGURE 16-4 A, Cylindrical template used to determine size of defect. **B,** Smallest size found to encompass lesion is 2.5 cm.

pin at 90 degrees to the surface. Any tilt will result in the recipient site being oblique and increase the difficulty in matching the graft.

Before reaming, a scoring instrument of the same diameter is placed over the pin and manually twisted to cut through the outer border of the articular cartilage. Its purpose is to decrease the risk of the reamer damaging the normal articular cartilage. The reamer is advanced to a depth of 6 mm (Fig. 16-5) but, if needed, reaming can continue until a bleeding base is present. Irrigation should be performed during the use of any powered instrumentation to minimize the risk of thermal necrosis. A cannulated tamp is used to compress the bottom of the defect to ensure a firm base and limit the risk of collapse. The guide pin is removed and the four quadrants of the recipient site are measured to help determine the donor graft thickness.

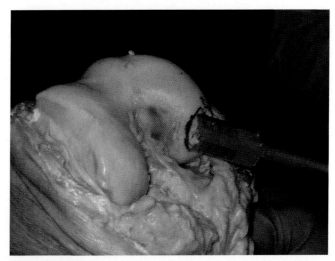

FIGURE 16-5 Cannulated reamer used to prepare recipient site to appropriate size and depth.

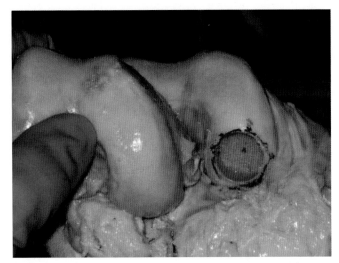

FIGURE 16-6 Recipient site completed and allograft evaluated for matching donor site.

Although the graft can be prepared at the same time as the host site, it is recommended that it not be completed until the recipient site has been prepared. Although it may save time, it is much easier to make adjustments to the graft than to the host.

The allograft preparation starts by evaluation of the optimal harvest site (Fig. 16-6). The sizing cylinder is used to mark the area in the same manner as the defect. In addition, a marking pen is used to identify the 12 o'clock position of the graft to ensure correct orientation so it can be identified.[30] The graft is then set in the cutting jig (Fig. 16-7). The entire graft may be set into the device, but it is prudent to take the time to cut the base of the graft so that it can be secured in a position that ensures that the coring device is 90 degrees to the articular cartilage. As noted, oblique cuts can result in a graft that may be difficult to place and could result in a plug with variable thickness of articular cartilage.

With the graft correctly positioned, the cylindrical core reamer, with its inserted extruding rod, is used to harvest the plug. The plug is removed and marked at its four quadrants to match the recipient site (Fig. 16-8). The articular side of the graft is held in the grasping clamp, with the four marks flush with the surface of the clamp (Fig. 16-9). An oscillating saw is then used to cut the graft to the measured length.

The bone tamp should again be used at the recipient site prior to inserting the graft. Occasionally, the borders of the site expand just enough to impede graft placement. If the initial positioning is difficult, an arthroscopic rasp can be used to round the bottom millimeter of the bone. Caution is needed so as not to remove excess bone, which can affect the stability of the graft. Optimally, the graft should be inserted with firm finger pressure. A tamp can be gently used to assist the insertion, but forceful pressure could damage the graft.[31] If the graft is proud by as little as 1 mm, shear forces can result in articular damage and affect the stability of the graft.[32,33] By contrast, if the graft is countersunk more than 1 mm, it will serve only as a bone filler. If there is insufficient bone, wafers of bone can be cut from the graft excess and used to make up the difference. If

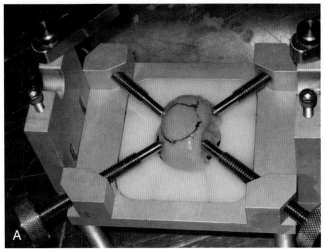

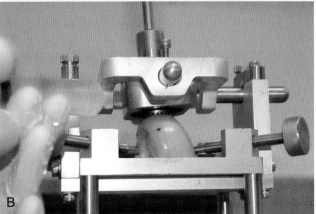

FIGURE 16-7 A, Allograft placed in cutting jig. The dowel articular surface is parallel to the base. **B,** Graft in cutting jig. the coring device is at 90 degrees to the articular surface.

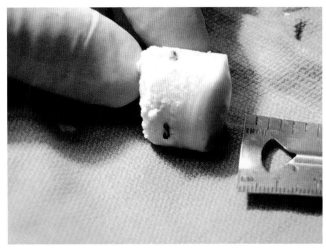

FIGURE 16-8 Harvested plug, marked to match recipient site.

the graft is difficult to remove, one should not forcefully try to pry the graft out. A threaded K wire can be drilled in the graft for ease of removal.

If the graft is press-fit accurately, it will not require additional fixation (Fig. 16-10). If there is any question of stability, such as a graft that is not more than 75% to 80% contained, one should

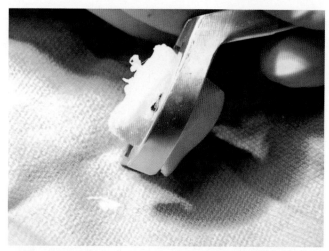

FIGURE 16-9 Grasping clamp with marks flush to surface of clamp.

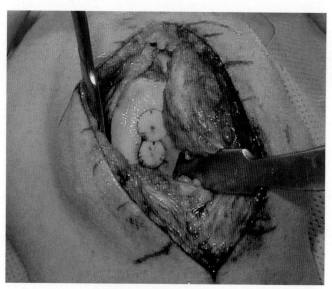

FIGURE 16-11 Double plug.

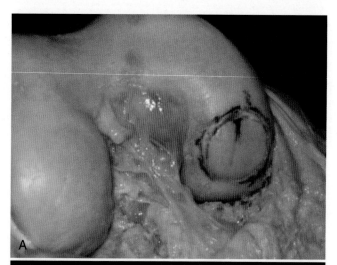

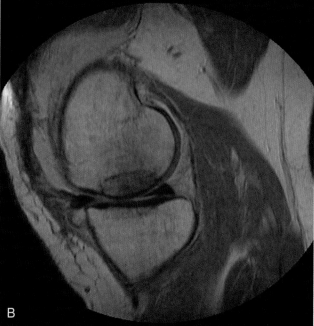

FIGURE 16-10 A, Final appearance of dowel graft secured with press fit. **B,** MRI scan of completed graft.

not hesitate to supplement fixation. Various methods have been used, but recently developed very small, compressive bioabsorbable screws are favored.

If a lesion is not circular or larger than 35 mm, multiple plugs can be used (Fig. 16-11). They are a placed in the same manner as multiple autogenous osteochondral grafts. The grafts abut each other, and attention to detail is needed to reproduce the nature curve of the surface.

If additional procedures are to be performed (e.g., meniscal allograft implantation and/or osteotomy), these are usually done at the same time as the osteochondral allograft. If the surgeon prefers to stage the procedures, the osteotomy should be done first.

Historically, there has been some debate as to when an osteotomy should be performed. However, with the less demanding techniques, there has been a shift to lower the threshold for performing an osteotomy. Conversely, the degree of correction is less than the goal when completing an osteotomy for osteoarthritis. Transferring the mechanical axis to the opposite tibial spine is commonly used as the goal. If an osteotomy is done, it should be performed on the bone opposite the allograft to avoid vascular insult.

PEARLS&PITFALLS

PEARLS
- Inspect the graft for size, shape, and quality before induction of anesthesia.
- When preparing the recipient site, always err by using a smaller size to avoid damage to normal articular cartilage. If needed, the site can always be enlarged.
- Make certain that all cuts involving the articular cartilage are perpendicular to the surface to optimize graft match and uniform thickness of the cartilage.
- When obtaining the graft, cut it several millimeters longer than the final donor length. The excess can be used to fill the recipient site if needed; it already matches the width of the plug.

- If the lesion is not circular or square, it is often better to use two smaller grafts that one large graft, which would require removal of normal articular cartilage.

PITFALLS

- The recipient should only be reamed to a depth of a 5 to 6 mm before checking the base for vascular supply. Initially, reaming to 8 mm or more may result in the unnecessary removal of host bone.
- If the graft is difficult to insert, make certain that all edges of the recipient site are cleared of debris and the end of graft is smooth, because forceful insertion will result in graft damage and cell death.
- A graft that is more than 1 mm oblique at the surface should be removed and the base adjusted to fit flush. If one attempts just to lever the graft to change its position, the tissue frequently becomes damaged; this often results in loss of press-fit fixation.

Postoperative Rehabilitation

The postoperative treatment is dependent on several variables, including the size, location, and stability of the graft, as well as additional procedures performed. It is common practice to use continuous passive motion for 6 to 8 hours daily for the initial 4 to 6 weeks, with only toe-touch weight bearing during this time. For large grafts, such as tibial plateaus, weight bearing may be limited for as long as 12 weeks. Ultimately, progression of weight bearing is decided by radiographic evidence that the graft has maintained proper position and the bone is incorporating. Activities such as swimming and low-resistance stationary bicycling are often permitted at 4 to 6 weeks. Low-impact activities with strengthening, including proprioceptive training, are gradually progressed after full weight bearing. Recreational sports are typically permitted at 4 to 6 months postoperatively. There is disagreement as to whether patients treated for OCD or well-contained isolated lesions should be active in high-impact activities or sports. However, there is general agreement that in salvage cases, these types of activities should be avoided.

OUTCOMES

Osteochondral allograft success for treating chondral lesions has been well documented in the orthopedic literature. In addition, the follow-up of these studies is of longer duration than that for the other biologic procedures. There have been several published reports, but the University of Toronto and University of California at San Diego have had the most experience.

The University of Toronto began its osteochondral allograft program in 1972 and reported the results of their first 100 patients in 1985.[34] These patients encompassed a wide variety of pathology and had variable outcomes. However, it was found that using shell grafts for post-traumatic lesions resulted in a 75% success rate (36 of 48). They subsequently published their intermediate and long-term results using grafts for post-traumatic knee lesions. Of the 126 knees in 122 patients treated, 108 (86%) were successful.[35] The average follow-up was 7.5 years (range, 2 to 22 years), with a survivorship of 95% at 5 years, 85% at 10 years, and

74% at 15 years for femoral condyle grafts. For tibial plateau grafts, the survivorship was 95% at 5 years, 80% at 10 years, and 65% at 15 years.[36] In 2008, the University of Toronto reported their findings from a critical analysis of the 69 known failures treated at their institution.[37] They found that the grafts that failed early (less than 1 year) lacked viable chondrocytes and cartilage matrix staining. The importance of proper graft handling and timely implantation to maintain chondrocyte viability and graft quality was stressed. Analyses also showed a trend toward better survivorship with adjunct meniscal allograft transplantation and realignment osteotomies. Finally, the importance of mechanical stability and fixation was evident. It was found that graft instability leads to nonunion and continued remodeling at the host-graft interface.

The University of California at San Diego (UCSD) instituted their use of osteochondral allografts in 1983. In 1999, they published the results of 211 patients treated for defects secondary to OCD, trauma, or AVN.[38] The mean follow-up was 52 months (range, 12 to 186 months). Good to excellent results were reported in 177 of 211 patients (84%). Analyses of the treated knee lesions showed success in 116 of 125 (93%) femoral, 26 of 40 (65%) tibiofemoral, and 35 of 46 (76%) patellofemoral grafts. Uncorrected ligamentous instability, limb malalignment, and bipolar lesions were found to be associated with increased failure rates. In 2007, UCSD published their experience of treating OCD lesions with osteochondral allografts.[39] In 64 patients, 66 knees were treated, with a mean allograft size of 7.5 cm^2. The mean follow-up was 7.7 years (range, 2 to 22 years). Only one patient was lost to follow-up. Of the remaining 65 knees, 47 (72%) were rated good to excellent, 7 (11%) were rated fair, and 1 (2%) was rated poor. An additional 10 patients(15%) underwent reoperation.

CONCLUSIONS

Osteochondral allografts have proven application for treating chondral and osteochondral lesions. They provide true hyaline cartilage, are not limited by shape or size, and have the longest proven efficacy of any current treatment options. The disadvantages are possible disease transmission, immunogenicity, limited availability, and cost. At present, these allografts should be considered when treating chondral lesions larger than 2 cm^2; they constitute one of the preferred methods for treating these lesions when bone loss is more than 4 to 5 mm.

REFERENCES

1. Sgaglione NA, Miniaci A, Gillogly SD, et al. Update on advanced surgical techniques in the treatment of traumatic focal articular cartilage lesions in the knee. *Arthroscopy.* 2002;18:9-32.
2. Gortz S, Bugbee WD. Fresh osteochondral allograft processing and clinical application. *J Knee Surg.* 2006;19:231-240.
3. Tomford WW. Current concepts review. Transmission of disease through transplantation of musculoskeletal allografts. *J Bone Joint Surg Am.* 1995; 11;1742-1754.
4. Asselmier MA, Caspari RB, Bottenfield S. A review of allograft processing and sterilization techniques and their role in transmission of human immunodeficiency virus. *Am J Sports Med.* 1993;21;170-175.
5. Pearson K, Dock N, Brubaker S, eds. *Standards for Tissue Banking.* 12 ed. McLean, Va: American Association of Tissue Banks, 2008.
6. Czitrom AA, Keating S, Gross AE. The viability of articular cartilage in fresh osteochondral allografts after clinical transplantation. *J Bone Joint Surg Am.* 1990;72:574-581.

7. Maury AC, Safir O, Las Heras F, et al. Twenty-five year chondrocyte viability in fresh osteochondral allograft. *J Bone Joint Surg Am.* 2007; 89:159-165.

8. Oakeshott RD, Farine Pritzker KP, et al. A clinical and histologic analysis of failed fresh osteochondral allografts. *Clin Orthop Relat Res.* 1988; 80:1795-1812.

9. Allen R, Robertson C, Pennock A, et al. Analysis of stored osteochondral allografts at the time of surgical transplantation. *Am J Sports Med.* 2005;33:1479-1484.

10. Ball ST, Amiel D, Wlliams SK, et al. The effects of storage on fresh human osteochondral allografts. *Clin Orthop Relat Res.* 2004;(418):246-252.

11. Pearsall A, Tucker J, Hester R, et al. Chondrocyte viability in refrigerated osteochondral allografts used for transplantation within the knee. *Am J Sports Med.* 2004;32:25-31.

12. Williams RJ III, Dreese JC, Chen CT. Chondrocyte survival and material properties of hypothermically stored cartilage. An evaluation of tissue used for osteochondral allograft transplantation. *Am J Sports Med.* 2004; 32:132-139.

13. Lightfoot A, Martin J, Amendola A. Fluorescent viability stains overestimate chondrocyte viability in osteoarticular allografts. *Am J Sports Med.* 2007;35:1817-1823.

14. Gortz S, Bugbee WD. Allografts in articular cartilage repair. *Instr Course Lect.* 2007;56:469-480.

15. Malinin T, Temple HT, Buck BE. Transplantation of osteochondral allografts after cold storage. *J Bone Joint Surg Am.* 2006;88:762-770.

16. Phipatankul W, VandeVord P, Teitge R, et al. Immune response in patients receiving fresh osteochondral allografts. *Am J Orthop (Belle Mead NJ).* 2004;33:345-348.

17. Rodrigo JJ, Schnaser AM, Reynolds HM Jr, et al. Inhibition of the immune response to experimental fresh osteochondral allografts. *Clin Orthop Relat Res.* 1989;(243):235-253.

18. Aubin PP, Cheah HK, Davis AM, et al. Long-term follow-up of fresh femoral osteochondral allografts for posttraumatic knee defects. *Clin Orthop Relat Res.* 2001;(391 suppl):S318-S327.

19. Garrett JC. Fresh osteochondral allografts for treatment of articular cartilage defects in osteochondritis dessicans of the lateral femoral condyle in adults. *Clin Orthop Relat Res.* 1994;(303):33-37.

20. Spak R, Teitge R. Fresh osteochondral allografts for patellofemoral arthritis. Long-term follow-up. *Clin Orthop Relat Res.* 2006;444:193-200.

21. Aroen A, Loken S, Heir S, et al. Articular cartilage lesions in 993 consecutive knee arthroscopies. *Am J Sports Med.* 2004;32:211-215.

22. Curl WW, Krome J, Gordon E, et al. Cartilage injuries. A review of 31,516 knee arthroscopies. *Arthroscopy.* 1997;13:456-460.

23. Mithoefer K, Williams RJ III, Warren RF, et al. Chondral resurfacing of articular cartilage defects in the knee with the microfracture technique. Surgical technique. *J Bone Joint Surg Am.* 2006;88(suppl 1);294-304.

24. Steadman JR, Briggs KK, Rodrigo JJ, et al. Outcomes of microfracture for traumatic chondral defects of the knee. Average 11-year follow-up. *Arthroscopy.* 2003;19:477-484.

25. Bobic V, Carter T. Osteochondral autologous graft transfer. *Oper Tech Sports Med.* 2000;8:168-178.

26. Hangody L, Füles P. Autologous osteochondral mosaicplasty for the treatment of full thickness defects of weight bearing joints: ten years of experimental and clinical experience. *J Bone Joint Surg Am.* 2003; 85(suppl 2):25-32.

27. Peterson L, Brittberg M, Kiviranta I, et al. Autologous chondrocyte transplantation; biomechanics and long-term durability. *Am J Sports Med.* 2002;30:2-12.

28. Convery FR, Akeson WH, Meyers MH. The operative technique of fresh osteochondral allografting. *Oper Tech Orthop.* 1997;7:340-344.

29. Jamali AA, Emmerson BC, Chung C, et al. Fresh osteochondral allografts. *Clin Orthop Relat Res.* 2005;(437):176-185.

30. Below S, Arnocsky S, Dodds J, et al. The split-line pattern of the distal femur. A consideration in the orientation of autologous artilage grafts. *Arthroscopy.* 2002;18:613-617.

31. Bozazjani BH, Chen AC, Bae WC, et al. Effects of impact on chondrocyte viability during insertion of human osteochondral grafts. *J Bone Joint Surg Am.* 2006;88:1934-1943.

32. Huang FS, Simonian PT, Norman AG, et al. Effects of small incongruities in a sheep model of osteochondral autografts. *Am J Sports Med.* 2004;32:1842-1848.

33. Koh JL, Wirsing K, Lautenschlager E, et al. The effect of graft height mismatch on contact pressure following osteochondral grafting. A biomechanical study. *Am J Sports Med.* 2004;32:317-320.

34. McDermott AG, Langer F, Pritzker KP, et al. Fresh small-fragment osteochondral allografts. Long-term follow-up study on first 100 cases. *Clin Orthop Relat Res.* 1985;(197):96-102.

35. Gross AE, Shasha N, Aubin P. Long-term follow-up of the use of fresh osteochondral allografts for posttraumatic knee defects. *Clin Orthop Relat Res.* 2005;(435):79-87.

36. Shasha N, Krywulak S, Backstein D, et al. Long-term follow-up of fresh tibial osteochondral allografts for failed tibial plateau fractures. *J Bone Joint Surg Am.* 2003;85(suppl 2):33-39.

37. Gross AE, Ont O, Kim W, et al. Fresh osteochondral allografts for posttraumatic knee defects. Long-term follow-up. *Clin Orthop Relat Res.* 2008; (466):1863-1870.

38. Bugbee WD, Convery FR. Osteochondral allograft transplantation. *Clin Sports Med.* 1999;18:67-75.

39. Emmerson BC, Jamali A, Bugbee WD. Fresh osteochondral allografting in the treatment of osteochondritis dissecans of the femoral condyle. *Am J Sports Med.* 2007;35:907-914.

Approach to Chondral Damage in the Patellofemoral Joint

Jason Koh

Chondral defects of the patellofemoral joint are the most common type of articular cartilage defect found in the knee.[1] They also comprise a significant portion of most isolated grade IV articular cartilage defects in the knee joint. These lesions may be found incidentally but also may be a common source of pain and discomfort in the knee.[2] Trochlear articular cartilage defects can be symptomatic. The approach to this joint can be complex and may require a combination of arthroscopic and open surgical techniques, up to and including arthroplasty, which is beyond the scope of this chapter.[3,4] I shall primarily discuss arthroscopic techniques for chondral defects.

ANATOMY AND PATHOANATOMY

The patellofemoral joint of the knee is a complex articulation, with multiple facets on the patella and a complex, saddle-shaped trochlear groove.[5-7] The articular cartilage on the patella itself is the thickest articular cartilage in the body, measuring up to 7 mm thick on the medial facet. Chondral defects on the patella may be have several causes, including degeneration, direct trauma, malalignment, and patellar instability.[8-10] The mechanics of the patellofemoral joint are complex and are determined by a number of factors, including neuromuscular coordination, geometry of the trochlea, overall alignment of the extensor mechanism, including the quadriceps tendon, trochlear groove, and tibial tubercle, and soft tissue restraints such as the medial patellofemoral ligament.[3,11-13] These restraints help guide patellofemoral motion and often determine whether articular cartilage damage occurs and is symptomatic. For example, excessive patellar malalignment with a laterally tilted and subluxated patella can contribute to excessive articular cartilage wear on the lateral facet of the patella.[14,15] Direct trauma to the patella, such as from a dashboard-type injury, in which a flexed knee contacts the dashboard, may result in a central articular cartilage damage to the patella or trochlea.[16-19]

In addition, many central articular cartilage defects are noted in young athletic individuals. These often have a linear fissure in the center of the trochlea. This reflects the significant forces placed on the patellofemoral joint during activities of daily living and other forms of physical exertion. For example, the joint reaction forces on the patellofemoral joint during stair climbing are up to two to four times body weight, and jumping can create forces up to six to eight times body weight.[20-25] These loads can result in failure of the underlying articular cartilage and subchondral bone.

PATIENT EVALUATION

History and Physical Examination

Patients with symptomatic articular cartilage lesions of the patellofemoral joint generally complain of anterior knee pain, particularly when ascending or descending stairs or after sitting.[4] Occasionally, patients may complain of crepitus or a symptomatic click as the knee goes into flexion or extension. Elements of the history to obtain from the patient also include known or suspected rheumatologic disease, history of trauma to the knee from a direct blow, history of patellar instability, activity level of the patient, recent changes in activity level, timing of the injury, and whether the pain is acute or chronic. In patients who have already sought previous treatment, it is important to identify the nature of treatment, including physical therapy, bracing, and taping and any previous surgery. Complaints of recurrent or consistent effusions should also be identified. Knee pain diagrams often provide relevant clinical information.[26]

Physical examination should combine static and dynamic evaluation. The presence or absence of any effusion should be noted and the knee should be carefully palpated and evaluated for ligamentous and patellar instability. At 30 degrees of knee flexion, the patella will typically translate laterally approximately 9 mm and have a relatively firm end point because of the check rein of the medial patellofemoral ligament.[27] The patella should also translate medially 7 mm and the lateral patellar retinaculum should allow the patella to be tilted to a neutral position, where the anterior surface of the patella is parallel to the ground while the patient is supine. Quadriceps development, particularly that of the vastus medialis obliquus muscle, should be assessed.[4] Extensor alignment including femoral version, Q angle, and tibial rotation can provide insights into patellar tracking.

A specific evaluation of the articular cartilage of the patellofemoral joint should be performed. The knee should go through an active range of flexion and extension and the presence of any significant crepitus should be assessed. I prefer to perform this examination with the patient lying supine, with the hip flexed to 90 degrees and the knee actively flexed and extended against gravity. In my clinical practice, this has been found to identify and elicit patellofemoral or articular cartilage complaints more precisely than while the patient is sitting. This also allows an assessment of hamstring tightness, which may contribute to patellofemoral symptoms. Another specific test to assess for chondral defects in the patellofemoral joint is the Clark patellar compression test. Two fingers of the examiner are held at the top of the patella to stabilize it in the trochlea with the knee extended, and the patient is asked to activate the quadriceps mechanism. This tightens the quadriceps and forces the patella into the patellofemoral joint; it is positive if pain is elicited. In addition, the medial and lateral facets of the patella can sometimes be directly palpated for tenderness. However, unlike many parts of the femoral tibial articulation, the central trochlea usually cannot be directly assessed by palpation.

The Q angle with the knee extended is of limited benefit. The Q angle with knee flexed to 30 degrees is a more accurate representation of the actual location of the patella and the trochlea groove compared with the location of the tibial tubercle.

Dynamic examination of the knee should be performed as well. Abnormalities of gait should be identified.[28] Evaluation of knee stability and identification of pain or crepitus while doing a step-up or step-down maneuver may help elicit specific complaints. A single leg squat test may also elicit pain and will allow evaluation of relative knee valgus or internal rotation, which can increase patellofemoral forces.

Diagnostic Imaging

Radiography

An anteroposterior (AP) radiograph can provide information about the existence of a bipartite patella. The relative location of the patella to the trochlear groove and tibial tubercle can be determined as a secondary bony density on the proximal tibia.

A true lateral view with overlapping femoral condyles, with less than 5% displacement, can provide valuable information regarding the relative patellar height. This can be assessed using various ratios, including the Insall-Salvati index and Blackburne-Peel method (Fig. 17-1)—the articular surface

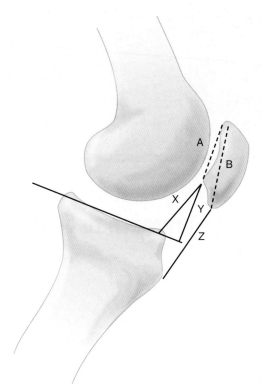

FIGURE 17-1 Methods of measuring patellar height. Normal for all ratios 1:1(± 0.2)—Blackburne-Peel (most reliable), A:Y; Caton, A:X; Insall-Salvati, B:Z. *(Adapted from Merchant AC. Patellofemoral imaging.* Clin Orthop Relat Res. *2001;(389):15-21.)*

length compared with the distance from its inferior margin to the tibial plateau. This technique has been demonstrated to be the most reliable. A true lateral view can also yield information about the degree of trochlear dysplasia. The trochlear groove can be identified on the lateral x-rays, on which a dense white line of the trochlea should not intersect vvthe bone of the lateral femoral condyle (Fig. 17-2). A sunrise or Merchant view at 45 degrees of flexion can give indicate patellar tracking within the trochlea and the presence of lateral patellar tilt or subluxation. A number of measurements have been described; however, I agree with Merchant that "(f)or most patients, it is quicker and just as good to eyeball the film rather than spend time drawing lines and calculating measurements."[29]

Magnetic Resonance Imaging

Magnetic resonance imaging (MRI) is currently the best modality to image articular cartilage defects.[30,31] Appropriate articular cartilage sequences and thin cuts often reveal articular cartilage damage, such as chondromalacia, chondral flaps, or delamination. In addition, it can also identify areas of underlying subchondral bony edema. MRI is also useful to assess abnormalities of soft tissue that may be contributing to underlying chondral damage or patellofemoral pain, such as synovitis, lesions of the medial patellofemoral ligament, tendinopathy, and articular cartilage loose bodies. MRI can also be used to perform measurements of tibial tubercle to trochlear groove distance. This can indicate conditions that could lead to patellar instability and subsequent articular cartilage damage.

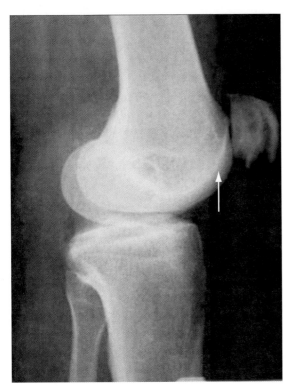

FIGURE 17-2 Lateral radiograph demonstrating trochlear dysplasia. The *arrow* shows the trochlear groove. Note how it starts after the curve of the femoral condyle.

TREATMENT

Treatment options for chondral lesions of the patellofemoral joint can be conservative or surgical. Many patients have symptoms of patellofemoral pain. Diagnostic imaging studies other than plain radiography may not be clinically indicated.

Conservative Management

In most cases, initial management should consist of physical therapy for quadriceps strengthening, with or without patellar bracing, relative rest, and appropriate analgesic medications, including acetaminophen or nonsteroidal anti-inflammatory drugs (NSAIDs). Patients with symptomatic patellofemoral pain may have been previously shown to have substantial weakness of quadriceps muscle activity and, specifically, weakness of the vastus medialis obliquus.[32]

Arthroscopic Technique

Surgical approaches to symptomatic chondral defects of the patellofemoral joint can vary, ranging from arthroscopic débridement to articular cartilage transplantation techniques and realignment techniques. In this chapter, the focus will be limited to the arthroscopic treatment of these lesions. However, the treating physician should be aware that open surgical techniques may be critically important in the treatment of these disorders, particularly in the case of gross malalignment, to provide increased stability or unload a damaged area of articular cartilage.

Arthroscopic surgical techniques for the patellofemoral joint vary from simple débridement to microfracture procedures and osteochondral autograft transplantation. In addition, in rare cases,

arthroscopic lateral release or medial plication can assist in the realignment of soft tissues affecting the patellofemoral joint and patellar tracking. However, isolated lateral release has extremely limited application and may result in medial instability.[4,33]

Arthroscopic chondroplasty should consist of débridement of unstable articular cartilage flaps to a stable margin. These flaps can be a source of pain and discomfort. Patients may experience a click at a specific degree of knee flexion or significant crepitus. Such delaminations often occur at the calcified cartilage layer and can easily progress. I recommend the use of mechanical débridement[2,34] with an arthroscopic shaver to remove these flaps rather than electrocautery or radiofrequency devices, because there is a concern for adjacent articular cartilage damage caused by the heat produced by the electrocautery.[35,36] Technical recommendations for the mechanical débridement of grade II or III chondromalacia include the use of a small-radius (3.5- to 4.5-mm), high-speed, smooth-edged shaver. Arthroscopic portal placement may need to be adjusted distally to allow instruments access to the undersurface of the patella. Typically, in cases in which there is significant grade III or crabmeat-type chondromalacia, the noncutting part of the shaver blade is placed at the base of the articular cartilage surface so that the fronds can be sharply amputated at their base (Fig. 17-3). The irregular strands and rough surface can lead to symptomatic crepitus and recurrent effusions in the joint. If there are full-thickness articular cartilage flaps, it is sometimes easier to amputate them sharply at their base by using an arthroscopic Beaver blade. Occasionally, it is useful to use a curved shaver to access the undersurface of the patella.

A microfracture procedure for chondral defects of the patellofemoral joint is typically less successful than microfracture involving the femoral condyles.[37] The lesion is typically prepared by débriding unstable articular cartilage edges until a very sharply defined margin of the defect is created. The calcified cartilage layer in the bed of the defect must be removed. This is

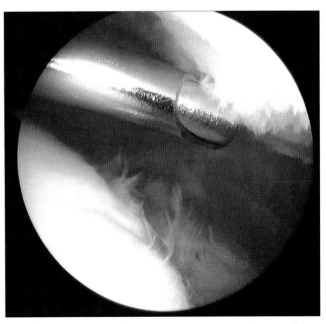

FIGURE 17-3 Arthroscopic chondroplasty with shaver blade parallel to surface. Note that noncutting part of blade is at base of the fronds.

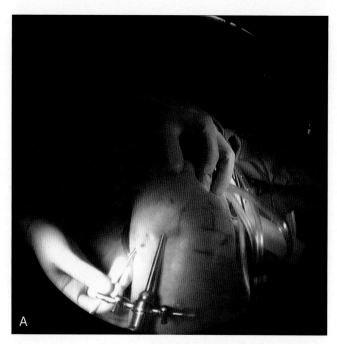

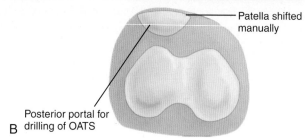

Patella shifted manually

Posterior portal for
B   drilling of OATS

FIGURE 17-4 A, B, Posterior portal for perpendicular patellar drilling for the osteochondral allograft procedure.

sometimes easier to perform by using sharp curettes or an arthroscopic Beaver blade to scrape away the calcified cartilage layer. Multiple perforations are then made in the bone, starting at the periphery and separated by approximately 3 to 4 mm. This can be done with a sharp awl or K wire or drill bit. Particularly on the patella, drilling rather than an awl may be preferred because the underlying subchondral bone is thick, and it can be difficult to stabilize both the patella and awl enough to allow adequate perforation of the underlying bone. If an awl is chosen, a 90-degree angle may be helpful to avoid skiving.[38] Drilling can be performed by using accessory nontraditional portals located more posteriorly than the standard medial inferior lateral or proximal superior lateral portals (Fig. 17-4).

Osteochondral Autograft Transplantation

Osteochondral autograft transplantation has been demonstrated in some studies to be effective in the patellofemoral joint.[8,10,39,40] With relatively larger defects. there is difficulty in reproducing the saddle-shaped geometry of the trochlear articulation. In addition, the articular cartilage thickness of the patella is typically not replicated by the use of osteochondral plugs harvested from the femoral condyle. Despite this, the results for osteochondral autograft transplantation for this area are relatively good, and is my preferred technique for significant articular cartilage lesions

of the patellofemoral joint, in particular for those involving damage to or cystic changes of the subchondral bone.

With arthroscopically performed osteochondral autograft transplantation, it is critical to have appropriate orientation of grafting and harvesting tools. Ideally, these should be perpendicular to the articular cartilage surface. Therefore, a considerable amount of time is spent in using a spinal needle as a localizer to identify the appropriate trajectory for the orientation of harvesting and grafting equipment. Accessory portals may need to be created to perform this procedure.

Typically, the area of the defect is débrided and the margins of the defect identified. After appropriate identification of the perpendicular orientation to the articular cartilage defect, the sizing tools are placed arthroscopically through the appropriate portal to determine the circumference of the defect (Fig. 17-5A) and the number of appropriate osteochondral autograft transplant plugs that will be needed to fill in the defect. In the case of articular cartilage defects on the patella it may be extremely difficult to use standard arthroscopic portals to achieve a perpendicular location to the patella. The spinal needle can be used to identify the appropriate trajectory and orientation of a portal. I have used a more posterior nonstandard portal.

Graft harvest can be performed from several areas of the knee, including the lateral edge of the trochlea, distal femur just proximal to the sulcus terminalis, or and intercondylar notch. Whichever donor site it chosen, it is essential that the harvest be performed with the instruments as perpendicular as possible to the articular cartilage surface to maintain the appropriate alignment of the graft after implantation. If this is done arthroscopically, it is critical that appropriate visualization be achieved. This may require the débridement of the fat pad or retraction of soft tissues through an accessory portal or by use of a percutaneously placed spinal needle or suture as a retractor. An osteochondral plug at least 8 mm long (typically 10 to 12 mm) is obtained using a tubular chisel. The plug is removed from the joint and measured at its four quadrants for length and assessment of any slope of the surface. A plug with a diameter of 6 to 11 mm is harvested.

The defect site is then prepared. This can be done by using a perpendicularly placed tubular chisel or a drilling system to create the bony socket for the osteochondral plug. Particularly for patellar defects, it is recommended that a drill system be used because the bone of the patella is extremely hard and the patella has minimal stability. This can be done by one of two techniques. A guide pin is placed perpendicular to the surface, followed by appropriate reaming over the guide pin. The second method is to use a specially designed drill guide with a flat tip and a retrograde drilling technique. With this method, a retro drill pin is passed anterior to posterior through the patella; the cutter tip is flipped and the drill bit attached within the joint to drill a socket in a retrograde fashion (see Fig. 17-5B and C). The patella typically has to be subluxated manually, either medially or laterally, so that instruments will not damage the adjacent femoral articular cartilage.

After the appropriate socket has been created, a calibrated measuring rod is placed within the socket to provide more precise measurement of the socket in the various quadrants. The donor plug is then appropriately rotated to the correct orienta-

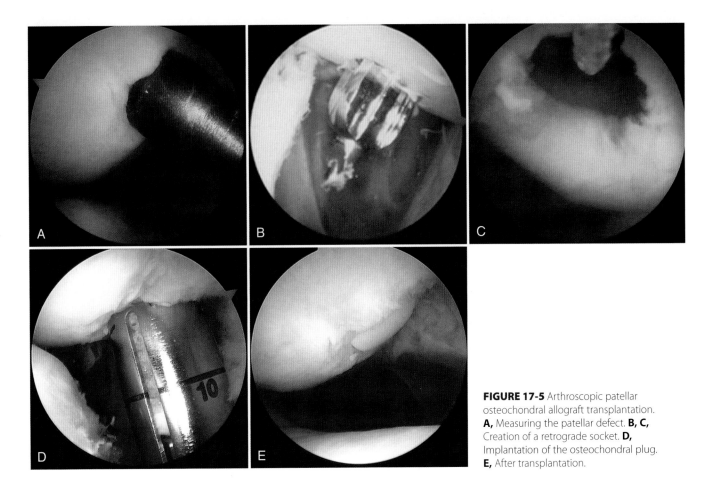

FIGURE 17-5 Arthroscopic patellar osteochondral allograft transplantation. **A,** Measuring the patellar defect. **B, C,** Creation of a retrograde socket. **D,** Implantation of the osteochondral plug. **E,** After transplantation.

tion to minimize any incongruities and gently delivered into the prepared socket using a press-fit technique (see Fig. 17-5D).

A unique approach to the patellar side involves placement of a small microsuture anchor into the bony plug. A passing suture can be placed through the retrograde pinhole and used to shuttle the sutures from the suture anchor in the plug to pull the osteochondral plug into the patellar socket. The graft can be then secured into the socket by securing the sutures, which can be done by creation of a mulberry knot or by a small anchor used to create an interference fit.

It is critical to have congruency of the articular surface. If perfect congruency cannot be achieved, it is preferable to have the donor cartilage slightly countersunk with respect to the adjacent articular cartilage (see Fig. 17-5E).[41]

PEARLS & PITFALLS

PEARLS

1. Use a spinal needle as a guide to where arthroscopic portals can be placed to address the articular cartilage defect.
2. Take advantage of the fact that the patella is mobile. If necessary, slightly deflate the joint and subluxate the patella to bring the chondral damage to the instrument.
3. An arthroscopic knife can help create sharp margins and amputate unstable articular cartilage flaps without causing further delamination.
4. A calcified cartilage layer can be removed by scraping with the tip of an arthroscopic knife.

PITFALLS

1. It is important to understand the causes of the articular cartilage lesion. If there is malalignment of the patellofemoral joint, this must be addressed for the most successful outcome.
2. Microfracture procedures for the patellofemoral joint typically have less satisfactory results compared with those of the femoral condyles.
3. The subchondral bone of the patella is extremely hard and thick; it can be difficult for microfracture awls or osteochondral autograft transfer (OAT) chisels to prepare the defect. Drilling is preferable.
4. Standard arthroscopic peripatellar portals may not be in the appropriate positions to address the chondral defects. If necessary, accessory portals may need to be created.

Postoperative Rehabilitation

Following arthroscopic chondroplasty of the patella, patients may undergo immediate weight bearing. If a simple débridement has been performed, the knee can go through a full range of motion, with normal weight bearing. However, if a microfracture or osteochondral autograft transplant has been performed, weight bearing with the knee in a flexed position may unduly load the treated areas. Weight bearing can be permitted with the knee in full extension. However, weight bearing while the knee is flexed should be strictly limited during the first 4 to 6 weeks following the procedure.[38] Continuous passive motion may enhance the articular cartilage repair and there are some limited data suggesting that the use of hyaluronic acid may also enhance the articular cartilage repair.

Following 4 to 6 weeks of limited weight bearing on the flexed knee, activities can be gradually progressed, depending on the patient's function and pain. It is estimated that for most patients, it will be approximately 6 months before they can resume normal sports activities and that maximum medical improvement may require up to 12 to 18 months of recovery.

REFERENCES

1. Curl WW, Krome J, Gordon ES, et al. Cartilage injuries: a review of 31,516 knee arthroscopies. *Arthroscopy.* 1997;13:456-460.
2. Levy AS, Lohnes J, Sculley S. et al. Chondral delamination of the knee in soccer players. *Am J Sports Med.* 1996;24:634-639.
3. Fulkerson JP. The effects of medialization and anteromedialization of the tibial tubercle on patellofemoral mechanics and kinematics. *Am J Sports Med.* 2007;35:147.
4. Fulkerson JP. Diagnosis and treatment of patients with patellofemoral pain. *Am J Sports Med.* 2002;30:447-456.
5. Feller JA, Amis AA, Andrish JT. et al. Surgical biomechanics of the patellofemoral joint. *Arthroscopy.* 2007;23:542-553.
6. Senavongse W, Amis AA. The effects of articular, retinacular, or muscular deficiencies on patellofemoral joint stability. *J Bone Joint Surg Br.* 2005;87:577-582.
7. Shih YF, Bull AM, Amis AA. The cartilaginous and osseous geometry of the femoral trochlear groove. *Knee Surg Sports Traumatol Arthrosc.* 2004;12:300-306.
8. Jakob RP, Franz T, Gautier E, Mainil-Varlet P. Autologous osteochondral grafting in the knee: indication, results, reflections. *Clin Orthop Relat Res.* 2002;(401):170-184.
9. Nomura E, Inoue M, Kurimura M. Chondral and osteochondral injuries associated with acute patellar dislocation. *Arthroscopy.* 2003;19:717-721.
10. Nho SJ, Foo LF, Green DM. et al. Magnetic resonance imaging and clinical evaluation of patellar resurfacing with press-fit osteochondral autograft plugs. *Am J Sports Med.* 2008;36:1101-1109.
11. Amis AA. Current concepts on anatomy and biomechanics of patellar stability. *Sports Med Arthrosc.* 2007;15:48-56.
12. Farahmand F, Naghi Tahmasbi M, Amis AA. The contribution of the medial retinaculum and quadriceps muscles to patellar lateral stability—an in-vitro study. *Knee.* 2004;11:89-94.
13. Merican AM, Kondo E, Amis AA. The effect on patellofemoral joint stability of selective cutting of lateral retinacular and capsular structures. *J Biomech.* 2009;42:291-296.
14. Hunter DJ, Zhang YQ, Niu JB. et al. Patella malalignment, pain and patellofemoral progression: the Health ABC Study. *Osteoarthritis Cartilage.* 2007;15:1120-1127.
15. Kalichman L, Zhu Y, Zhang Y. et al. The association between patella alignment and knee pain and function: an MRI study in persons with symptomatic knee osteoarthritis. *Osteoarthritis Cartilage.* 2007;15:1235-1240.
16. Atkinson PJ, Haut RC. Injuries produced by blunt trauma to the human patellofemoral joint vary with flexion angle of the knee. *J Orthop Res.* 2001;19:827-833.
17. Buckwalter JA, Martin JA, Olmstead M. et al. Osteochondral repair of primate knee femoral and patellar articular surfaces: implications for preventing post-traumatic osteoarthritis. *Iowa Orthop J.* 2003;23:66-74.
18. Gobbi A, Kon E, Berruto M. et al. Patellofemoral full-thickness chondral defects treated with Hyalograft-C: a clinical, arthroscopic, histologic review. *Am J Sports Med.* 2006;34:1763-1773.
19. Hjelle K, Solheim E, Strand T. et al. Articular cartilage defects in 1,000 knee arthroscopies. *Arthroscopy.* 2002;8:730-734.
20. Crossley KM, Cowan SM, Bennell KL, McConnell J. Knee flexion during stair ambulation is altered in individuals with patellofemoral pain. *J Orthop Res.* 2004;22:267-274.
21. Hungerford DS, Barry M. Biomechanics of the patellofemoral joint. *Clin Orthop Relat Res.* 1979;(144):9-15.
22. Mason JJ, Leszko F, Johnson T, Komistek RD. Patellofemoral joint forces. *J Biomech.* 2008;41:2337-2348.
23. Powers CM, Ward SR, Chen YJ. et al. Effect of bracing on patellofemoral joint stress while ascending and descending stairs. *Clin J Sports Med.* 2004;14:206-214.
24. Powers CM, Ward SR, Chen YJ. et al. The effect of bracing on patellofemoral joint stress during free and fast walking. *Am J Sports Med.* 2004;32:224-231.
25. Reilly DT, Martens M. Experimental analysis of the quadriceps muscle force and patellofemoral joint reaction force for various activities. *Acta Orthop Scand.* 1972;43:126-137.
26. Post WR, Fulkerson J. Knee pain diagrams: correlation with physical examination findings in patients with anterior knee pain. *Arthroscopy.* 1994;10:618-623.
27. Fithian DC, Mishra DK, Balen PF. et al. Instrumented measurement of patellar mobility. *Am J Sports Med.* 1995;23:607-615.
28. Heino Brechter J, Powers CM. Patellofemoral stress during walking in persons with and without patellofemoral pain. *Med Sci Sports Exerc.* 2002;34:1582-1593.
29. Merchant AC. Patellofemoral imaging. *Clin Orthop Relat Res.* 2001;(389):15-21.
30. Potter HG, Linklater JM, Allen AA, et al. Magnetic resonance imaging of articular cartilage in the knee. An evaluation with use of fast-spin-echo imaging. *J Bone Joint Surg Am.* 1998;80:1276-1284.
31. Shindle MK, Foo LF, Kelly BT. et al. Magnetic resonance imaging of cartilage in the athlete: current techniques and spectrum of disease. *J Bone Joint Surg Am.* 2006;88(suppl 4):27-46.
32. Makhsous M, Lin F, Koh JL. et al. In vivo and noninvasive load sharing among the vasti in patellar malalignment. *Med Sci Sports Exerc.* 2004;36:1768-1775.
33. Fithian DC, Paxton EW, Post WR. et al. Lateral retinacular release: a survey of the International Patellofemoral Study Group. *Arthroscopy.* 2004;20:463-468.
34. Federico DJ, Reider B. Results of isolated patellar debridement for patellofemoral pain in patients with normal patellar alignment. *Am J Sports Med.* 1997;25:663-669.
35. Edwards RB 3rd, Lu Y, Uthamanthil RK, Bogdanske JJ. et al. Comparison of mechanical debridement and radiofrequency energy for chondroplasty in an in vivo equine model of partial thickness cartilage injury. *Osteoarthritis Cartilage.* 2007;15:169-178.
36. Ryan A, Bertone AL, Kaeding CC. et al. The effects of radiofrequency energy treatment on chondrocytes and matrix of fibrillated articular cartilage. *Am J Sports Med.* 2003;31:386-391.
37. Mithoefer K, Williams RJ 3rd, Warren RF, et al. The microfracture technique for the treatment of articular cartilage lesions in the knee. A prospective cohort study. *J Bone Joint Surg Am.* 2005;87:1911-1920.
38. Mithoefer K, Williams RJ 3rd, Warren RF. et al. Chondral resurfacing of articular cartilage defects in the knee with the microfracture technique. Surgical technique. *J Bone Joint Surg Am.* 2006;88(suppl 1):294-304.
39. Hangody L, Fules P. Autologous osteochondral mosaicplasty for the treatment of full-thickness defects of weight-bearing joints: ten years of experimental and clinical experience. *J Bone Joint Surg Am.* 2003;85(suppl 2):25-32.
40. Gudas R, Kalesinskas RJ, Kimtys V. et al. A prospective randomized clinical study of mosaic osteochondral autologous transplantation versus microfracture for the treatment of osteochondral defects in the knee joint in young athletes. *Arthroscopy.* 2005;21:1066-1075.
41. Koh JL, Wirsing K, Lautenschlager E, Zhang LO. The effect of graft height mismatch on contact pressure following osteochondral grafting: a biomechanical study. *Am J Sports Med.* 2004;32:317-320.

Chondrocyte Transplantation Techniques

Kai Mithoefer • Bert R. Mandelbaum

Developing concepts and methods that can restore hyaline articular cartilage has been the goal of researchers and clinicians for centuries.[1] In 1994, Brittberg and coworkers[2] reported on the first successful use of autologous chondrocytes in human subjects with full-thickness articular cartilage lesions of the knee using a two-step implantation technique. Since its first description, chondrocyte transplantation has been performed in more than 15,000 patients worldwide and many research studies have clinically validated this surgical technique as a reliable method for biologic restoration of hyaline-like articular cartilage.[3-13] Based on the evolution and better understanding of the treatment of articular cartilage defects and cell-based implantation techniques in recent years, this demanding surgical technique has undergone several technical modifications. These recent developments can help reduce patient morbidity and technique-specific complications. Chondrocyte implantation techniques continue to evolve using modern tissue engineering technologies.

PATIENT EVALUATION

History

Obtaining a thorough history in patients with chondral defects presents a critical first step in the treatment process and selection of patients who are appropriate candidates for chondrocyte implantation. Patients with articular cartilage defects typically present with a spectrum of mechanical symptoms from the defect. Symptoms from cartilage defects are usually nonspecific and can mimic other forms of knee pathology, such as meniscal tears. Pain with weight bearing is usually present with impact activities. Cartilage defects of the femoral condyles often produce point tenderness over the femoral condyle rather than the joint line. Catching and locking sensations can occur from cartilage flaps or larger defects. Joint effusion is frequently reported, particularly after demanding impact activities. Defects of the patella or troch-

lea usually lead to pain when ambulating stairs, driving a car, getting out of a chair, or assuming a squatting position. Symptoms of patellar instability may be reported. Articular cartilage defects may present acutely after joint trauma such as knee ligament tears or chronically. Patients considered for chondrocyte transplantation techniques may have undergone prior cartilage repair procedures and a detailed evaluation of the prior surgical procedures should be performed. The time since the initial injury, as well as the types of previous surgeries, should be recorded because these factors have been shown to affect the outcome after chondrocyte implantation.

Physical Examination

Physical examination includes evaluation of gait pattern and lower extremity alignment. Hip, knee, and ankle range of motion should be assessed and any joint effusion noted. Because articular cartilage lesions are frequently found in patients with acute hemarthrosis, acute or chronic ligamentous instability, patellar dislocation or maltracking, or lower extremity malalignment, these factors should be routinely evaluated. Depending on defect location and size, mechanical symptoms may or may not be present and may overlap with meniscal tests. The patient's body mass index (BMI) should be assessed because it has been shown to correlate with functional outcome after articular cartilage repair.

Diagnostic Imaging

Plain radiographs, including weight-bearing anteroposterior (AP) and lateral views, Rosenberg and tunnel views, long-leg films, and Merchant views, can help identify osteochondral lesions, joint space narrowing, patellar maltracking, or lower extremity malalignment. Cartilage-sensitive magnetic resonance imaging (MRI) presents a sensitive, specific, and accurate tool for noninvasive diagnosis of articular cartilage injury.[14,15] Images should be obtained in three planes; using fast spin-echo imaging with a repetition time (TR) of 3500 to 5000 msec and moderate echo time (TE) provides high contrast resolution among articular cartilage, subchondral bone, and joint fluid. Cartilage-sensitive MRI provides useful information about meniscal and ligamentous status, subchondral bone, lesion size, and depth Because of the pathologic changes in the surrounding cartilage, the final size of the defect intraoperatively is usually larger than the defect size measured on preoperative MRI. In addition to its use for preoperative diagnosis, cartilage-sensitive MRI can be helpful for postoperative evaluation of cartilage repair. Routine postoperative MRI is recommended to evaluate the cartilage repair tissue and detect potential complications, such as graft hypertrophy. If available, newer technologies, such as T2 mapping, delayed gadolinium-enhanced MRI of cartilage (dGEMRIC), and T1 rho relaxation mapping, can be used to obtain additional details about cartilage morphology pre- and postoperatively.[15]

Preoperative Planning and Counseling

Based on the history, physical examination, and radiologic information, the indication for autologous chondrocyte transplantation or adjuvant procedures is discussed with the patient. In-depth preoperative patient counseling is critically important to determine the patient's demands, assess his or her ability to comply with the postoperative rehabilitation protocol, and create realistic expectations and goals for postoperative knee function and activity level.

TREATMENT

Indications and Contraindications

Chondrocyte implantation is indicated for symptomatic, high-grade chondral and osteochondral defects of the knee in active patients who are physiologically too young for arthroplasty. This technique can be successfully used as a first-line treatment of femoral condylar, trochlear, and patellar lesions larger than 2 cm^2, or used as a revision technique for failed prior cartilage repair procedures.[8,11-13] The technique can be successfully used for isolated, multiple, and kissing cartilage defects. Prerequisites for successful autologous chondrocyte transplantation include adequate range of motion, appropriate axial alignment or patellar tracking, ligamentous stability, and the ability to comply with the postoperative rehabilitation protocol. Adjuvant procedures may be indicated to correct coexisting knee pathology; these can be performed simultaneously with chondrocyte transplantation without negative effects of the complex procedures on the postoperative functional outcome and activity level.

Absolute contraindications for autologous chondrocyte transplantation include generalized osteoarthritis, inflammatory arthropathies, and joint sepsis. Patients unable to comply with the postoperative rehabilitation and weight-bearing protocols should also not be treated with this technique. A body mass index (BMI) more than 30 kg/m^2 has been associated with limited improvement after knee articular cartilage repair and presents a relative contraindication. Patients with severe meniscal deficiency should be considered for meniscal allograft transplantation at the time of chondrocyte transplantation.

Arthroscopic Technique

Autologous chondrocyte transplantation of the knee is carried out as a two-stage procedure.

Stage 1: Chondrocyte Harvest

Step 1. Arthroscopic Evaluation.   The first stage involves a thorough diagnostic arthroscopy. In addition to identification of the known articular cartilage defect, the meniscal and ligamentous status is evaluated and the entire articular cartilage is inspected to rule out any additional cartilage defects. Partial meniscectomy or meniscal repair can be performed at the time of this arthroscopy because it minimally affects the course after the initial arthroscopy and can decrease operative time during the second-stage procedure. However, surgical treatment of meniscal deficiency or ligamentous pathology should be performed simultaneously with autologous chondrocyte implantation to avoid repetitive operative joint trauma and prolonged rehabilitation. During the first-stage arthroscopy, the cartilage defect is identified and existing cartilage flaps are débrided back to a stable and healthy peripheral margin. Following thorough débridement, the size of the articular cartilage lesion is measured and its containment documented. The knee is taken through a full range of motion and the arc of motion during which the lesion articulates with the opposing joint surface is carefully recorded (Fig. 18-1). The opposing joint surface should always be carefully inspected for the presence of a kissing lesion or signs of low grade cartilage injury.

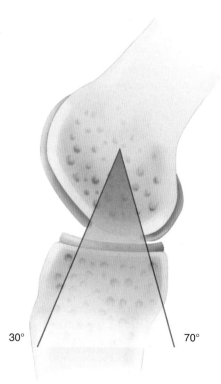

30°   70°

FIGURE 18-1 The exact location and range of articulation of the defect are noted carefully to facilitate postoperative rehabilitation in the nonloading safe zone.

Step 2. Chondrocyte Harvesting.   Following initial arthroscopic evaluation, chondrocyte graft harvesting of 200 to 300 mg of normal articular cartilage is obtained from a lesser weight-bearing area of the injured knee, generally the medial or lateral superior ridge of the femoral condyle or intercondylar notch. The intercondylar notch is preferred for patellofemoral lesions. Using cartilage that has been débrided from the cartilage defect as graft is not recommended because chondrocyte quality from this area has been shown to be inferior. Graft procurement is done best with an angled or ring curette. The grafted cartilage tissue is sent for standardized commercial isolation and culturing of chondrocytes. Implantation of cultured chondrocytes is performed after 2 to 4 weeks when a sufficient number of cells has been obtained for the size of the defect (range, 4 to 12 million cells). Chondrocyte viability is routinely tested and should be more than 95% before implantation.

Stage 2: Chondrocyte Implantation

Step 1. Addressing Concomitant Pathology.   Malalignment, ligamentous instability, and/or meniscal injury and deficiency are known to contribute to the development of articular cartilage lesions and surgically addressing these concomitant pathologies is critical for an effective and durable articular cartilage repair.[11-13] Concomitant ligament reconstruction, meniscal allograft, or osteotomy should be performed before autologous chondrocyte implantation. Isolated or combined adjuvant procedures, including anterior cruciate ligament (ACL) reconstruction, high tibial osteotomy, or meniscal allograft and repair do not negatively affect postoperative activity levels after autologous chondrocyte transplantation.[9] Simultaneous rather than staged adjuvant procedures avoid prolonged rehabilitation, promote postoperative activity, and provide a significant cost benefit.

Step 2. Chondrocyte Implantation.   Chondrocyte implantation is performed using a parapatellar arthrotomy in a tourniquet-controlled bloodless field. The cartilage defect is again débrided back to a healthy cartilage margin and the calcified cartilage is carefully débrided without violating the subchondral bone using a ring curette (Fig. 18-2A). If bleeding is encountered, hemostasis of the defect bed can be achieved by application of thrombin or fibrin glue. Intralesional osteophytes can be débrided using a 4-mm burr without compromising the subchondral bone. A template of the defect is created with sterile aluminum foil or paper and then used to harvest an appropriately sized periosteal flap from the proximal medial border of the tibia. When using periosteum, the tissue patch should be slightly larger than the defect because of a tendency of the periosteum to contract. Any adherent fatty or connective tissue needs to be carefully removed to minimize the potential for graft hypertrophy. The periosteal flap is then sutured flush to the articular cartilage defect using interrupted 6-0 Vicryl sutures (Ethicon; Somerville, NJ), with the cambium layer facing into the defect (see Fig. 18-2B). As an alternative to the periosteum, a type I or III collagen membrane can be used to cover the defect (Fig. 18-3). This allows for smaller incisions, reduces patient morbidity, and minimizes the potential for graft hypertrophy. The rim of the periosteal flap or collagen membrane is sealed watertight with fibrin glue (Tisseel; Baxter; Deerfield, Ill) except for one corner, where the implanted chondrocytes are injected into the defect. Following cell injection, the remaining corner of the periosteal flap is secured with sutures and sealed with fibrin glue. If a tourniquet was used, it should be released and meticulous hemostasis should be obtained. Drains are not normally used so as to avoid injury to the periosteal cover or fibrin seal of the defect from direct abrasion by the drain during postoperative joint mobilization. A compression dressing is placed and cryotherapy used routinely. Bracing is not necessary for isolated chondrocyte transplantations but may be used if simultaneous adjuvant procedures require postoperative protection.

Deep Chondral or Osteochondral Defects

In patients with lesions deeper than 1 cm, autologous bone grafting should be performed in combination with autologous chondrocyte implantation (ACI). Implantation of chondrocytes in these cases is performed using the sandwich technique. The os-

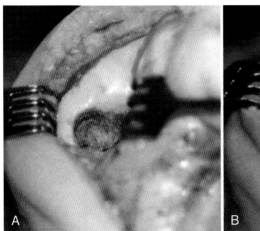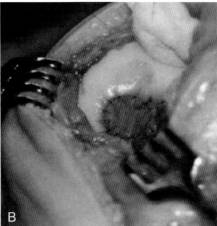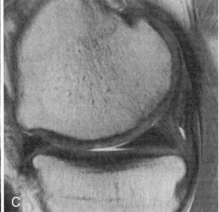

FIGURE 18-2 A, Articular cartilage defect of the femoral condyle before implantation. **B,** Cartilage defect after coverage with periosteum. **C,** Cartilage-sensitive MRI scan at 36 months postoperatively.

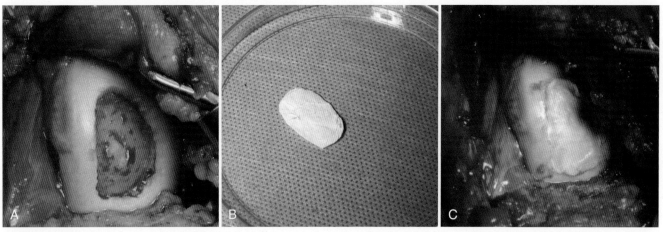

FIGURE 18-3 A, Cartilage defect of femoral condyle. **B,** Collagen membrane shaped to the contour of the defect. **C,** Collagen membrane covering the defect

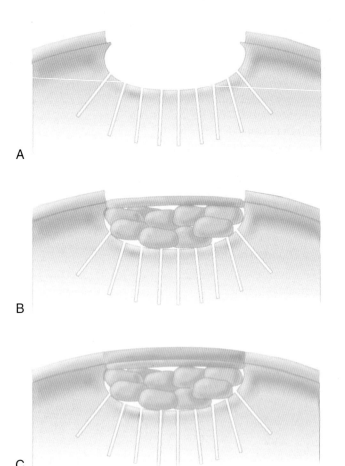

FIGURE 18-4 Stepwise description of the sandwich technique of autologous chondrocyte transplantation for deep osteochondral defects. **A,** The defect is débrided to stable chondral and bony margins and the bony base is drilled to facilitate bony healing. Bone grafting of the defect to the level of the subchondral bone plate is then performed. **B,** The bone graft is covered with the first periosteal patch placed with the cambium layer facing into the defect and sealed with fibrin glue. **C,** The second periosteal patch is sutured to the cartilage margin and the chondrocyte cell suspension is injected between the periosteal patches. *(Adapted from Mandelbaum BR, Gerhardt MB, Peterson L. Autologous chondrocyte implantation of the talus. Arthroscopy. 2003;19(suppl 1):129-37).*

seous defect is filled with cancellous bone graft from the iliac crest or proximal tibia to the level of the subchondral plate. One periosteal flap or collagen membrane sized for the defect is then anchored with the facing toward the joint using fibrin glue applied between the patch and bone graft. A second sized periosteal flap or membrane is then placed facing into the defect and secured to the surrounding cartilage with interrupted 6-0 Vicryl sutures. The rim is again sealed with fibrin glue and the cultured chondrocytes are implanted between the two periosteal flaps or collagen membranes (sandwich technique; Fig. 18-4).

PEARLS & PITFALLS

PEARLS

1. Assess for and address concomitant joint pathology (e.g., alignment, instability, meniscal pathology).
2. Avoid staging adjuvant procedures to reduce prolonged rehabilitation and facilitate return to activity.
3. Record the location and articulation of defect to facilitate postoperative rehabilitation in a safe zone.
4. Substituting periosteum with collagen membrane or matrix-associated chondrocyte implantation (MACI) can reduce invasiveness and the risk for graft hypertrophy.
5. The sandwich technique is useful for deep chondral and osteochondral defects.
6. An accelerated postoperative weight-bearing protocol can help promote postoperative function.

PITFALLS

1. Failure to recognize and treat concomitant joint pathology can be problematic.
2. There is a limited success rate for tibial defects and kissing lesions.
3. Avoid exercising through pain and effusion during rehabilitation.
4. Graft delamination from failure to treat symptomatic graft hypertrophy can occur.

Postoperative Rehabilitation Protocol

Postoperative management varies, depending on the lesion location, size, and concomitant procedures. Rehabilitation is based on the biology of the cartilage repair tissue. During the initial proliferation phase (0 to 4 weeks), the developing repair cartilage tissue requires protection and weight bearing is avoided in tibio-femoral defects. Patients with patellofemoral cartilage lesions immediately start weight bearing in a knee brace locked in full extension. Continuous passive motion (CPM) used for 6 hours/day for 4 weeks should be implemented. Closed kinetic chain exercises such as stationary biking are allowed at 2 weeks; limited arc-strengthening exercises are initiated with range of motion modifications based on the location of the lesion and patellar contact pattern observed at the time of surgery. In the second matrix production phase (4 to 8 weeks), weight bearing is advanced by 25% per week depending on lesion size, location, and the patient's symptoms. Pain and swelling indicate too rapid progression of rehabilitative exercises and should be reduced. The third maturation phase is characterized by low-impact ac-tivities and advanced based on the patient's symptoms. Running is usually allowed at about 6 to 8 months after chondrocyte transplantation while cutting and pivoting exercises are avoided until 8 to 10 months postoperatively. Early weight bearing has been shown to promote postoperative function.[18] Magnetic reso-nance imaging (MRI) is recommended before return to high-impact pivoting activities (see Fig. 18-2C).

COMPLICATIONS

Complications after chondrocyte transplantation include stiffness and adhesions in up to 10% of patients. Graft hypertrophy is seen in 25% to 63% of postoperative MRI images but has been described as clinically symptomatic in only 13% to 15%.[2-15] Symptomatic hypertrophy can be effectively treated by ar-throscopic chondroplasty. Hypertrophy may lead to partial de-tachment or graft delamination. Substituting the periosteum with collagen membranes or second-generation MACI effectively re-duces the risk for periosteal hypertrophy.[19,20] Graft failure has been described in 6% to 7% of patients. Grafts usually fail be-tween 12 and 24 months after surgery and frequently show central degeneration. Treatment with revision chondrocyte im-plantation has been shown to be effective in many cases.[13] All patients with graft failure should be carefully evaluated for the presence of subtle instability, axial malalignment, or patellar mal-tracking, which have been shown to lead to lower success rates after autologous chondrocyte transplantation.

OUTCOMES

Autologous chondrocyte transplantation has been successfully used for hyaline-like restoration of full-thickness articular carti-lage lesions in the knee with long-term durability of functional improvement of up to 11 years.[11,12] Good to excellent results were found in 92% of isolated femoral condyle lesions, 89% of osteochondritis dissecans, 75% of femoral condyle lesions with concomitant anterior cruciate ligament reconstruction, 67% of patients with multiple lesions, and 65% of patellar lesions.[2-13] Return to sport is possible in 33% to 96% of patients, with the best return rates in competitive and adolescent athletes. Patients with single lesions, younger age, and short preoperative intervals have the best results.[9,10] Accelerated weight bearing can improve

long-term functional results.[18] Correcting axial malalignment, patellar maltracking, and ligamentous laxity is critical for the functional improvement.

CONCLUSIONS

Limitations of this technique include its invasiveness, long post-operative rehabilitation, and periosteal hypertrophy, which may lead to acute graft delamination. This cartilage repair technique provides significant functional improvement with high return rates to demanding sports and excellent durability, even under high athletic demands in primary and revision settings.

Scaffold-associated second-generation autologous cartilage transplantation techniques use three-dimensional biodegradable scaffolds to support the chondrocytes temporarily until they are replaced by matrix components synthesized from the implanted cells. MACI has been used with promising results in Europe and Australia but is not yet routinely available in the United States.[19,20] The use of the biomatrix seeded with chondrocytes reduces surgi-cal invasiveness and has the theoretic advantages of less chondro-cyte leakage, more homogeneous chondrocyte distribution, and less graft hypertrophy. Arthroscopic MACI has been described, with improvement of knee function in up to 90% (Fig. 18-5).

Future developments are aimed at improving cellular matrix production by using more productive characterized chondro-cytes with more sophisticated bioactive scaffolds that include growth factors and stimulate a more natural spatial distribution of chondrocytes within the repair cartilage.[21-23] Other promising future approaches include identification and selective expansion of specific chondrocytes subpopulations capable of producing more hyaline-like repair cartilage tissue and implantation of neo-cartilage tissue produced in specifically designed bioreactors.[24]

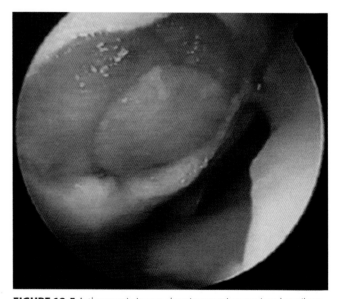

FIGURE 18-5 Arthroscopic image showing matrix-associated cartilage implant (MACI, Hyalograft C; Fidia Advanced Biopolymers; Abano Terme, Italy) following arthroscopic placement. *(From Kon E, Gobbi A, Filardo G, et al. Arthroscopic second-generation autologous chondrocyte implantation compared with microfracture for chondral lesions of the knee. Prospective nonrandomized study at 5 years. Am J Sports Med. 2009;37:33-41).*

REFERENCES

1. Mandelbaum BT, Browne JE, Fu F, et al. Articular cartilage lesions of the knee. *Am J Sports Med.* 2000;26: 853-861.
2. Brittberg M, Lindahl A, Nilsson A, et al. Treatment of deep cartilage defects in the knee with autologous chondrocyte transplantation. *N Engl J Med.* 1994;331:889-895.
3. Bentley G, Biant LC, Carrington RW, et al. A prospective, randomised comparison of autologous chondrocyte implantation versus mosaicplasty for osteochondral defects in the knee. *J Bone Joint Surg Br.* 2003; 85:223-230.
4. Fu F, Zurakowski D, Browne, et al. Autologous chondrocyte implantation versus debridement for treatment of full-thickness chondral defects of the knee: an observational cohort study with 3-year follow-up. *Am J Sports Med.* 2005;33:1658-1666.
5. Horas U, Pelinkovic D, Aigner T. Autologous chondrocyte implantation and osteochondral cylinder transplantation in cartilage repair of the knee joint: A prospective comparative trial. *J Bone Joint Surg Am.* 2003; 85:185-192.
6. Knutsen G, Drogset JO, Engebertson L, et al. A randomized trial comparing autologous chondrocyte implantation with microfracture. Findings at five years. *J Bone Joint Surg Am.* 2007;89:2105-2112.
7. Knutsen, G, Engebretsen L, Ludvigsen TC, et al. Autologous chrondrocyte implantation compared with microfracture in the knee. *J Bone Joint Surg Am.* 2004;86: 455-464.
8. Mandelbaum B, Browne JE, Fu F, et al. Treatment outcomes of autologous chondrocyte transplantation for full-thickness articular cartilage defects of the trochlea. *Am J Sports Med.* 2007;35:915-921.
9. Mithöfer K, Peterson L, Mandelbaum BR, Minas T. Articular cartilage repair in soccer players with autologous chondrocyte transplantation: functional outcome and return to competition. *Am J Sports Med.* 2005; 33:1639-1646.
10. Mithöfer K, Minas T, Peterson L, et al. Functional outcome of articular cartilage repair in adolescent athletes. *Am J Sports Med.* 2005;33: 1147-1153.
11. Peterson L, Minas T, Brittberg M, et al. Two- to 9-year outcome after autologous chondrocyte transplantation of the knee. *Clin Orthop Relat Res.* 2000;(374):212-234.
12. Peterson L, Brittberg M, Kiviranta I, et al. Autologous chondrocyte transplantation. Biomechanics and long-term durability. *Am J Sports Med.* 2002;30:2-12.
13. Zaslav K, Cole BJ, Brewster R, et al. A Prospective study of autologous chondrocyte transplantation in patients with failed prior treatment for articular cartilage defect of the knee. Results of the study of the treatment of articular repair (STAR) clinical trial. *Am J Sports Med.* 2009; 37:42-55.
14. Brown WE, Potter HG, Marx RG, et al. Magnetic resonance imaging appearance of cartilage repair in the knee. *Clin Orthop Relat Res.* 2004; (422):214-223.
15. Potter HG, Chong LR. Magnetic resonance imaging assessment of chondral lesions and repair. *J Bone Joint Surg Am.* 2009;91(suppl 1):126-31.
16. Mithoefer K, Williams RJ, Potter HG, et al. The microfracture technique for treatment of articular cartilage lesions in the knee: a prospective cohort study. *J Bone Joint Surg Am.* 2005;87:1911-1920.
17. Hambly K, Bobic V, Wondrasch B, et al. Autologous chondrocyte implantation postoperative care and rehabilitation: science and practice. *Am J Sports Med.* 2006;34:1020-1038.
18. Kreuz PC, Steinwachs M, Erggelet C, et al. Importance of sports in cartilage regeneration after autologous chondrocyte implantation. *Am J Sports Med.* 2007;35:1261-68.
19. Bartlett W, Skinner JA, Gooding CR, et al. Autologous chondrocyte implantation versus matrix-induced autologous chondrocyte implantation for osteochondral defects of the knee: a prospective, randomized study. *J Bone Joint Surg Br.* 2005;87:640-645.
20. Kon E, Gobbi A, Filardo G, et al. Arthroscopic second-generation autologous chondrocyte implantation compared with microfracture for chondral lesions of the knee. Prospective nonrandomized study at 5 years. *Am J Sports Med.* 2009;37:33-41.
21. Saris DBF, Vanlauwe J, Victor J, et al. Comparison of characterized chondrocyte implantation versus microfracture in the treatment of symptomatic cartilage defects of the knee: results after three years. Paper presented at: Proceedings of the 8th World Congress of the International Cartilage Repair Society; May 23-26, 2009; Miami.
22. Saris DBF, Vanlauwe J, Victor J, et al. Characterized chondrocyte implantation results in better structural repair when treating symptomatic cartilage defects of the knee in a randomized controlled trial versus microfracture. *Am J Sports Med.* 2008;36:235-246.
23. Mithoefer K, McAdams T, Scopp J, Mandelbaum B. Emerging options for treatment of articular cartilage injury in the athlete. *Clin Sports Med.* 2009;28:25-40.
24. Crawford D, Heveran C, Cannon D, et al. An autologous cartilage tissue implant NeoCart for treatment of grade III chondral injury to the distal femur: prospective clinical safety trial at 2 years. *Am J Sports Med.* 2009; 37:1334-1343.

Proximal Tibial Osteotomy

Annunziato Amendola ● Eugenio Savarese ● Armando Gabrielli

High tibial osteotomy (HTO) is a surgical procedure used to change the mechanical weight-bearing axis and alter the loads carried through the knee. Conventional indications for HTO are medial compartment osteoarthritis and varus malalignment of the knee causing pain and dysfunction, but the indications for HTO have expanded with concomitant cartilage regeneration procedures and meniscal transplantation. Knee instability has been considered a contraindication; however, today the indications for HTO include patients with chronic ligament deficiencies and malalignment, because this procedure can change not only the coronal but also the sagittal plane of the knee, improving stability. In addition, despite good long-term results with total knee arthroplasty, there remains a significant concern regarding the longevity of these prostheses, particularly in younger patients. In contrast, osteotomy provides an alternative that preserves the knee joint, which, when appropriately performed, should not compromise later arthroplasty should this be necessary. The reported results of proximal tibial osteotomy vary considerably across the literature, but in general the procedure provides good relief of pain and restoration of function in approximately 80% to 90 % of patients at 5 years and 50% to 65 % at 10 years.[1] Most authors who have analyzed these results have found that success is directly related to ideal patient selection and achieving optimal alignment.[2] Accurate preoperative assessment and surgical technique are therefore essential to achieve a satisfactory outcome. This chapter will discuss the importance of alignment, clinic evaluation, radiographic assessment, indications and contraindications, techniques, and special situations regarding proximal tibial osteotomy.

ANATOMY

Importance of Alignment

The tibia has a coronal and sagittal plane, and it is mandatory to consider both in every situation. The normal anatomic axis (coronal plane) of the knee has a range from 5 to 7 degrees. In varus knees (malalignment in the coronal plane), degeneration of the articular cartilage tends to progress because of deviation of the mechanical axis.[3] In the normal knee, the medial posterior tibial slope (sagittal plane) is usually 9 to 11 degrees and the lateral posterior tibial slope is generally 6 to 11 degrees; however, a wide range of values have been reported in various studies.[4,5] The sagittal plane of the knee has often been ignored but its changes cause important modifications in the biomechanics of the knee and in joint stability. Decreased posterior tibial slope causes posterior tibia translation and helps the anterior cruciate ligament (ACL)–deficient knee. In contrast, increased tibial slope causes anterior tibial translation and helps the posterior cruciate ligament (PCL)–deficient knee. Some studies[6,7] have demonstrated that the correction of the alignment is associated with the regeneration of articular cartilage that seemed apparently normal.

PATIENT EVALUATION

Perhaps the most important part of achieving success with proximal tibial osteotomy is selection of the appropriate patient.

History and Physical Examination

A thorough clinical assessment requires a detailed history and physical examination. Specific analysis of this information will help determine whether a patient is likely to benefit from osteotomy. Important aspects of a patient's general history include age, occupation, activity level, and medical and surgical history. Particularly significant are the expectations that the patient has for activity postoperatively. The patient may have noticed an increasing deformity or a static long-term malalignment. Pain history should focus on the site and severity, as well as aggravating and relieving factors. A history of locking, catching, or instability may indicate a mechanical source of symptoms, and the specific details of each of these symptoms should be sought to determine

whether other procedures, such as arthroscopy, may be beneficial as an adjunct to osteotomy. Lower limb alignment should be assessed at each level, and the gait should be observed for any abnormalities, particularly a thrust in the direction of the deformity, indicating a significant dynamic component. Presence of deformity in all three planes should be assessed, particularly rotational deformity, because this is more difficult to assess later radiographically. Whether a deformity is fixed or correctable should be determined. The prresence of an effusion is determined and location of tenderness should be recorded carefully. Range of motion is measured, particularly looking for a flexion contracture and the amount of flexion comfortably achieved. Good mobility of the knee is a prerequisite, with no less then 110 degrees of flexion and no more than 10 degrees of extension loss. Patellar tracking and the presence of crepitus is to be noted, although the status of the patellofemoral joint is not determinate of indication. Ligaments are examined, including the ACL, AMC, PCL, medial cruciate ligament (MCL), and lateral cruciate ligament (LCL). Adjacent joints are examined and assessment of neurovascular function is essential.

Diagnostic Imaging

In 1992, Dugdale and colleagues[8] proposed a flow chart for the radiologic evaluation of a patient with a varus of the knee, which was later modified by Noyes and associates.[9] They stated that the patient should get stress x-rays if physical examination reveals any of the following: positive varus stress test, increased varus during thrust, increased tibial external rotation at 30 degrees of knee flexion, or varus recurvatum during standing or walking. If the x-rays are positive, the patient should get supine, full-length anteroposterior (AP) x-rays of both legs to evaluate the alignment. If the physical examination reveals none of these, the patient should get full-length double-stance AP x-rays of both legs. If a varus deformity is absent, they suggested that the patient undergo a soft tissue reconstruction; if this deformity is present, it is important to evaluate whether a lateral joint line opening is associated. If this is the case, the patient should get stress x-rays; if not the case, two methods to evaluate the amount of correction to perform during surgery could be used (see later). Since this study, many other reports have been published for radiographic evaluation of the alignment of the lower limb. We believe that the following imaging studies with (standard and stress x-rays) be obtained for these patients.

Standard X-Ray Evaluation

A full-length, double-stance AP x-ray is mandatory to evaluate femorotibial alignment (Fig. 19-1), as described by Moreland and coworkers.[10] An AP x-ray is taken from the hips to the ankles with the patient standing and the patellae looking forward using a suitable cassette to filter the x-ray beam gradually for proper visualization of both hips and ankles.

Dugdale and colleagues[8] have proposed two methods to quantify the amount of correction to perform if a malalignment is present. In both methods, a line along the tibial plateau and its intersection with the desired mechanical axis of the lower extremity is marked (in this chapter this point is called P for simplicity). A line is traced from the center of the femoral head to

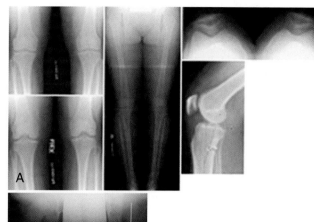

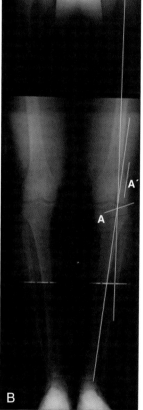

FIGURE 19-1 Standard radiographic assessment of the knee. **A,** Standing AP view and posteroanterior view in 30 degrees of knee flexion (*left*); bilateral standing long-leg anteroposterior view from hip to ankle (*center*); Merchant and lateral views (*right*). **B,** Standing AP view of both limbs to calculate correction required. See text for details.

P and a line is traced from the center of the tibiotalar joint to P. In the first method, the angle formed at the intersection between these two lines represents the amount of correction required. In the second method, the radiographic film is cut along the osteotomy line and along a vertical line that converges with the first. Leaving a 2-mm hinge at the medial tibial margin, the distal part of the film is rotated until the femoral head, P, and the tibiotalar joint are along the same line. The overlapping wedge margin is the amount of correction to perform. It was also demonstrated that if lateral and/or posterolateral soft tissue structures are insufficient, for every increase of 1 mm in the lateral joint line width, there is 1 degree of added varus. Supine X-rays are important to eliminate the added varus because of the deficiency of the lateral and/or posterolateral structures and to evaluate the actual amount of correction to perform. It was also shown that after HTO, the mechanical axis of the lower extremity is translated laterally—

3 to 4 mm for each degree of valgus correction—and this value depends on the height of the patient. We essentially use the same technique as described earlier to estimate the correction required.

The bilateral long-leg standing view is used (see Fig. 19-1B) to calculate the desired location of the new mechanical axis. If the two intersection lines are drawn from the center of the hip and from the center of the ankle, through the lateral tibial spine or 62% of the joint, bringing these two lines together will create the new mechanical axis. The osteotomy is drawn (line A) and measured and transposed to the two intersecting lines (line A′); the amount of opening measured at that point is the amount of correction required.

A lateral x-ray view is used to evaluate posterior tibial slope. A number of methods have been reported to quantify its value. Dejour and Bonnin[4] have recommended tracing a line along the proximal tibial anatomic axis (PTAA) and a line along the tibial plateau; the angle between these two lines is tibial slope. Moore and Harvey,[11] in 1974, described the tibial plateau angle. They recommended tracing a line along the anterior tibial cortex (ATC) and a line along the medial tibial plateau; the angle between these two lines is tibial slope.

Brazier and associates[5] have proposed three other methods:

1. Trace a line along the posterior tibial cortex (PTC) and a line is traced along the medial tibial plateau; the angle between these two lines is tibial slope.
2. Trace a line along the proximal fibular anatomic axis (PFAA) and a line along the medial tibial plateau; the angle between these two lines is tibial slope.
3. Trace a line along the fibular shaft axis (FSA) and a line along the medial tibial plateau; the angle between these two lines is tibial slope.

They compared these three techniques and stated that the most reliable are the PTAA and PTC methods.

Cullù and coworkers[12] have compared the various methods and found higher values for the same patients using the method described by Moore and Harvey[11] and lower values with the PFAA method.[5] We recommend using the line along the articular surface of the medial tibial plateau and the anatomic axis (PTAA) for assessing the posterior slope, because it is simple and reproducible.

Stress X-Ray

The lateral stress view, according to the Telos method, was first described by Jacobsen in 1976.[13] The patient lies in the lateral decubitus position with the knee flexed at 90 degrees and is encouraged to relax. The heel is fixed to a stand and the arm of the Telos GA II device (Telos; Weterstadt, Germany) applies a posterior force to the tibia. In this position, a lateral x-ray is taken. The test is then performed with the knee at 25 degrees of flexion.[13] This method is important in chronic PCL-deficient knees to evaluate anterior and posterior tibial translation with regard to the femur. It is also useful to detect a fixed posterior tibial subluxation, as described by Strobel and colleagues[14] in 2002; they found it to be present in 44% of patients with a PCL lesion.

The lateral stress view using the kneeling method[15] also measures posterior subluxation. The patient kneels on a bench with the knee in 90 degreesof flexion; the bench supports the lower legs only up to the tibial tubercle. A lateral x-ray is taken.

In addition, a lateral stress view with hamstring contraction was described by Chassaing and associates[16] in 1995. The patient lies in the lateral decubitus or seated position, with the knee at 90 degrees of flexion and the heel fixed to a stand. A lateral x-ray is taken while the patient contracts the hamstring for at least 10 seconds.[17]

Finally, a lateral stress view is obtained according to the gravity method described by Stäubli and Jakob in 1990.[18] The patient lies in the supine position with the hip and the knee at 90 degrees of flexion, supported by an assistant, with the leg in neutral rotation. In this position, a lateral x-ray is taken.

The axial stress view described by Puddu and coworkers[19] in 2000. The patient lies in the supine position, with both knees at 70 degrees of flexion, the feet plantigrade in moderate plantar flexion, and the tibia in neutral rotation. The x-ray beam is directed parallel to the longitudinal patellar axis from distal to proximal and the distance between the anterior tibial profile and the center of the femoral groove is measured. The side to side difference is the amount of posterior instability.

Jung and colleagues, in 2006,[17] compared these five methods, focusing on posterior translation, side to side difference, condylar rotation, time to perform the test, and pain during the test. Considering all these factors, they stated that the most effective methods are with the Telos device at 90 degrees of knee flexion and the kneeling method, even if they are painful and time-consuming procedures. The Telos procedure is the most expensive but the most reliable for detecting a posterior tibial subluxation.

Magnetic Resonance Imaging

Magnetic resonance imaging (MRI) is useful to evaluate the meniscal, articular cartilage, and soft tissue (ligamentous) status of the knee. In addition, with compartment overload, there may be subchondral edema, indicating the need for unloading that compartment. Traumatic subchondral bone lesions[20] can easily be detected.

TREATMENT

Indications And Contraindications

Proper patient selection is fundamental for satisfactory postoperative results. In general, having the knee joint in good condition will result in a more predictable outcome. Naudie and associates[1] have concluded that younger patients who have excellent knee range of motion (ROM), higher functional demand, and a lower grade of osteoarthritis (OA) will have better outcomes, and that the survival of the HTO will be much longer than in more advanced knees.

Indications

- Varus knee with mild to moderate medial compartment osteoarthritis
- Varus knee with associated medial cartilage defects (i.e., osteochondritis dissecans, osteonecrosis)

- Varus knee associated with a medial meniscal transplantation
- Varus knee with associated instability (ACL, PCL, PLC) and evidence of medial compartment overload or lateral or posterolateral thrust
- Mild valgus deformity (may be corrected on the tibial side)
- Age, activity level, status of the patellofemoral joint, gender of patient, body mass index (BMI)—relevant factors

Contraindications

- Extreme deformity associated with a fixed subluxation of the tibia
- Severe lateral or tricompartmental OA
- Fixed flexion contracture, more than 10 to 15 degrees
- Inflammatory disease
- Severe osteoporosis
- Severe patellofemoral osteoarthritis,[20] age, high BMI—relative contraindications

Arthroscopic Technique

Proximal tibial osteotomy can be used to correct the varus knee associated with pain and functional impairment. The correction could be acute or gradual, depending on the amount and complexity of deformity. Acute correction techniques include the following:

- Lateral closing wedge osteotomy
- Medial opening wedge osteotomy
- Dome osteotomy (rarely done)

Gradual correction is obtained by external fixation.

Lateral Closing Wedge Osteotomy (Acute Correction)

Jackson[21] in 1958 and Wardle[22] in 1962 described the earliest techniques of proximal tibial valgus osteotomies with a lateral closing wedge, but it was popularized by Coventry[23] and Insall and coworkers.[24] The goal is correction of alignment, as noted, which is achieved by removing a laterally based wedge of bone and closing the resultant defect. The main cited advantages of this procedure over the opening wedge technique are avoidance of the need for a bone graft, a more stable construct postoperatively allowing earlier weight bearing, and ta heoretically decreased risk of nonunion. The disadvantages of this procedure include the following: (1) difficulty in predicting the amount of correction in the coronal and sagittal planes; (2) inability to adjust the correction intraoperatively; (3) the requirement for two bone cuts; (4) violation of proximal tibiofibular joint or fibular head; and (5) palsy of the external popliteal sciatic nerve. The proximal anteromedial tibial cortex, viewed in cross section, has an oblique or triangular shape and forms an angle of 45 ± 6 degrees with the posterior margin of the tibia; the lateral tibial cortex, however, is almost perpendicular to the posterior margin of the tibia. Because of the same anatomic features, a lateral closing wedge osteotomy causes small decreases in the posterior tibial slope. However, Amendola and colleagues[25] have demonstrated that a lateral closing wedge HTO causes a decrease in the posterior tibial slope (Fig. 19-2).

The technique described here is used at our institution when a lateral closing wedge osteotomy is indicated. All patients

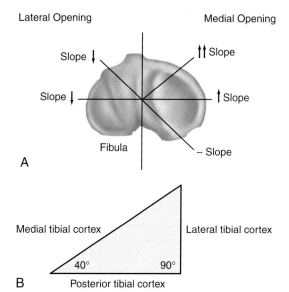

FIGURE 19-2 A, Cross section of the tibia seen from above. Note the different angles between the medial and posterior cortices and between the lateral and posterior cortices. **B,** A closing wedge HTO causes a decrease in posterior tibial slope; an opening wedge HTO causes an increase in posterior tibial slope.

should receive a prophylactic preoperative dose of intravenous antibiotics. The patient lies in a supine position on the radiolucent operating table; the leg is draped in a sterile fashion. Setup should allow radiographic visualization of the lower limb from hips to ankles, with the fluoroscope coming in from the contralateral side. A lateral support is placed to allow the knee to rest unsupported at 90 degreesof flexion, the position used during most of the procedure. A marking pen is used to outline the fibular head, lateral joint line, patellar tendon, and tibial tubercle. The leg is raised and a tourniquet is inflated. Arthroscopy is performed to treat mechanical symptoms, evaluate articular cartilage and menisci, and occasionally to confirm the indication for HTO.[9] We use an L-shaped skin incision with the vertical limb along the lateral edge of the tibial tubercle and the horizontal limb parallel and 1cm distal to the lateral joint line, taken posteriorly to the anterior aspect of fibular head. Dissection is carried down to expose the fascia of the anterior compartment, which is incised along the anterolateral crest of the tibia, leaving a 5-mm cuff for later closure. A Cobb elevator is used to elevate the muscle from the anterolateral surface of the tibia and the iliotibial tract is elevated from Gerdy's tubercle proximally. The common peroneal nerve is not routinely exposed but is palpated and protected throughout the procedure.

A number of methods for treatment of the proximal tibiofibular joint have been described, including joint excision or disruption, fibular osteotomy, and excision of the fibular head. We prefer to disrupt the joint but preserve the fibular head. The proximal tibiofibular joint is exposed, the anterior capsule incised, and a curved osteotome is directed posteromedially to disrupt this articulation and mobilize the fibula so as not to impede later correction. A Z-shaped retractor is placed through this joint along the posterior

aspect of the tibia to protect posterior soft tissues. It is critical that this retractor be placed directly against bone along the posterior cortex to protect the neurovascular structures.

The lateral edge of the patellar tendon is identified and a second Z retractor is placed underneath it to protect it during the osteotomy. In this way, the proximal tibia is exposed from the tibial tubercle to the posterolateral cortex and is therefore prepared for the osteotomy. In removing a laterally based wedge, an angular cutting guide can be used or a specific-sized wedge can be removed. The angled cutting jig system (Guidant) was initially described by Hofmann and colleagues[27]; it allows for easier use of preoperative calculations and should increase the accuracy of the resultant correction. With this system, the initial step involves making two 3.5-mm drill holes parallel to and approximately 1 cm distal to the joint line, across to but not through the medial cortex. A line drawn between these two holes should match the posterior slope of the tibia and the position is checked in both planes with the fluoroscope. These holes are the site of the final proximal fixation and serve as the reference for the remainder of the cuts. Two temporary pins are placed in these holes and a third hole is then drilled distal to these through the medial cortex; this allows measurement of the tibial width to guide for depth of the saw cut. Using the jig, the proximal cut of the osteotomy is performed using a calibrated saw blade to a depth 10 mm less than the measured tibial width. The first jig is removed and a second jig is used, which has a blade that lies in the first saw cut to its full depth and has angled cutting slots at 2-degree increments. The second saw cut is made through the chosen angled slot, with the jig controlling the depth of the saw cut by its position.

In making these cuts, it is important to check the position of the anterior and posterior retractors to ensure soft tissue protection and to cut the anterior and posterior cortices fully, to within 1 cm of the medial cortex. The wedge can then be removed. If initial wedge removal is incomplete, it is important to ensure complete removal of the entire wedge using a combination of curettes, rongeurs, and osteotomes before closing the osteotomy; otherwise, there is a significant risk of intra-articular fracture. It is also important to ensure that the wedge is complete to 1 cm from the medial cortex or there is a chance of the hinge opening medially, making the osteotomy unstable and potentially leading to overcorrection.

A three-holed L-shaped plate is fixed to the proximal fragment using two 6.5-mm cancellous screws through the previously drilled holes. A unicortical drill hole is then made distal to the plate in the lateral cortex; this serves as an anchoring point for a compression clamp, which is applied to the distal hole of the plate. Using this clamp, the osteotomy is closed slowly, at approximately 1 mm/min, allowing for plastic deformation of the intact medial hinge and thus a stable construct. Under fluoroscopic control, the final result is checked before the plate is secured with three 4.5-mm cortical screws distally. A drain is placed against the bone and closure is completed in layers. Fascial closure is interrupted and should attempt to cover the plate as much as possible without undue tension.

Medial Opening Wedge Osteotomy (Acute Correction)

Open wedge osteotomy has not been used as long as the lateral closing wedge osteotomy. It was first described by Hernigou and coworkers[26] although this technique had been used since 1951 by Debeyre. At the beginning of the 1990s, Puddu[28] developed a plate (Puddu plate, Arthrex spacer plate; Arthrex; Naples, Fla), which supports osteotomy surfaces internally by metal spacers (wedges) to prevent further collapse and that has metal blocks (spacer teeth). In 2000, Fowler and colleagues[29] modified Puddu's open wedge osteotomy technique. The most recent modification is lower profile and is a six-hole spacer plate (ContourLock HTO plate; Arthrex). The TomoFix plate (internal plate fixator, plate fixator, or rigid plate fixation; Synthes; West Chester, Pa) was developed by Lobenhoffer and colleagues.[30] In addition, a C plate or T plate can be used.

The theoretical advantages of opening wedge over closing wedge osteotomy include the restoration of anatomy with the addition of bone to the diseased medial side, the ability to achieve predictable correction in the coronal and sagittal planes, the ability to adjust correction intraoperatively, the requirement for only one bone cut, avoidance of proximal tibiofibular joint disruption and invasion of the lateral compartment, and the relative ease of combining it with other procedures, such as ACL reconstruction. The disadvantages of this procedure include the creation of a defect that requires bone graft with attendant harvest morbidity and a theoretic higher risk of nonunion, as well as the longer period of restricted weight bearing postoperatively.

Medial opening wedge osteotomy has been the preferred technique in our institution for the last 10 years for these reasons. All patients should receive a prophylactic preoperative dose of intravenous antibiotics; general endotracheal anesthesia is preferred because it allows the surgeon to get a bone block from the iliac crest, if needed. The patient lies in a supine position on the radiolucent operating table and the leg is draped in a sterile fashion; if a bone block is needed, the ipsilateral iliac crest is similarly draped. Setup should allow radiographic visualization of the lower limb from hips to ankles, different from the closing wedge osteotomy in which the fluoroscope is coming from the ipsilateral side. A lateral support is placed to allow the knee to rest unsupported at 90 degrees of flexion, the position used for much of the procedure. A marking pen is used to outline the fibular head, lateral joint line, patellar tendon, and tibial tubercle. The leg is raised and tourniquet is inflated.

Arthroscopy is performed as indicated, as with the closing wedge technique. A vertical incision is made just behind the pes anserine, between the medial border of the patellar tendon and the posterior border of the tibia. the sartorius fascia is cut to visualize the hamstring tendons. Under fluoroscopic control, a guide wire is positioned medially to laterally. The wire is placed at the level of the superior aspect of the tibial tubercle anteromedially, at about 1.5 cm below the lateral articular margin of the tibia. A cortical osteotomy is performed with an oscillating saw, inferiorly to the guide wire, and it is continued with an osteotome under fluoroscopic control (Fig. 19-3). When the osteotomy is completed, the medial tibia is opened with a wedge of a suitable width (Fig. 19-4). It is important to make the cut parallel to the joint surface in the sagittal plane, with the apex of the osteotomy at the proximal tibiofibular joint, to obviate the need for disrupting this articulation.

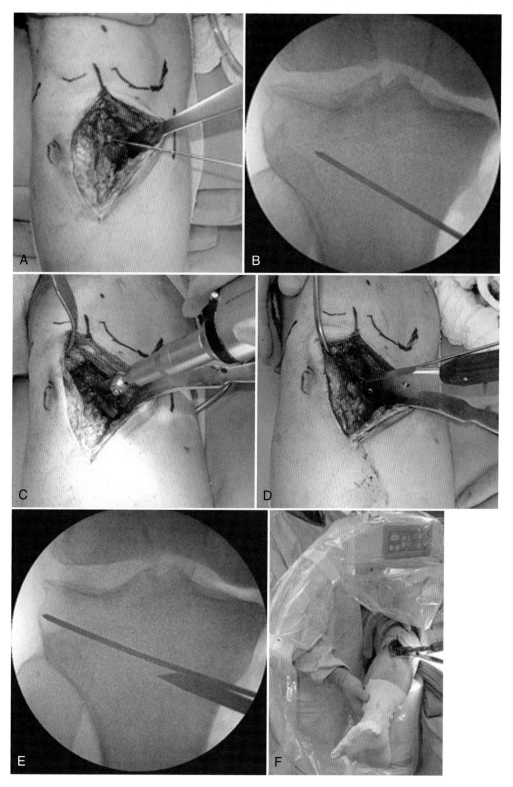

FIGURE 19-3 A, B, Under fluoroscopic control, a guide wire is positioned medially to laterally. The wire is placed at the level of the superior aspect of the tibial tubercle anteromedially. **C,** A cortical osteotomy is performed with an oscillating saw, inferior to the guide wire. **D, E, F,** It will be continued with an osteotome under fluoroscopic control.

Wedges have a graduated scale to quantify the angular correction achieved.[9] The position of the wedge is important to correct the deformity on the sagittal plane; the proximal anteromedial tibial cortex, viewed in cross section, has an oblique or triangular shape and forms an angle of 45± 6 degrees with the posterior margin of the tibia. However, the lateral tibial cortex is almost perpendicular to the posterior margin of the tibia. Because of these anatomic features, a wedge placed anteriorly causes an increase in posterior tibial slope, whereas a posterior wedge tends to decrease the posterior tibial slope slightly.[31]

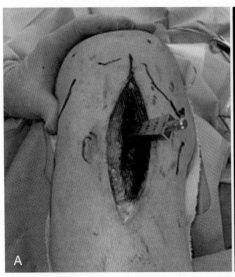
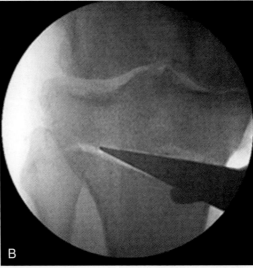

FIGURE 19-4 A, B, When the osteotomy is completed, the medial tibia is opened with a wedge of a suitable width. The position of the wedge is important to correct the deformity in the sagittal plane; a wedge placed anteriorly causes an increase in the posterior tibial slope, whereas a posterior wedge tends to decrease the posterior tibial slope slightly.

Anterior and posterior gaps of the osteotomy are then measured with a ruler, which is important to calculate the amount of increase in posterior tibial slope. If the anteromedial gap is half of the posteromedial gap, the slope will not change; for each millimeter of increase of the anterior gap, the posterior tibial slope will increase by 2 degrees. An image intensifier and alignment rod are used to control coronal and sagittal alignment during axial loading of the joint (Fig. 19-5). If the anterior gap is more

than 1 cm, it is better to perform an osteotomy to lift up the tibial tubercle of the same amount to avoid patella infera (patella baja). When the correction in the two planes is achieved, the osteotomy is stabilized with a plate with four holes (Arthrex), with two 6.5-mm proximal cancellous screws and two 4.5-mm distal cortical screws (Fig. 19-6). Generally, to fill the osteotomy gap, a carefully shaped allograft bone block from a donor is used (Fig. 19-7). Under fluoroscopic contro,l the final result is

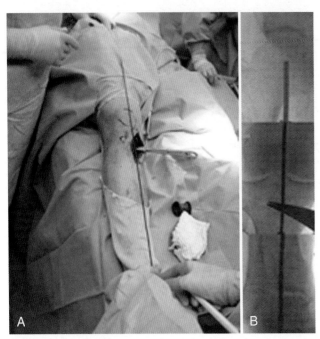

FIGURE 19-5 A, B, An image intensifier and an alignment rod are used to control coronal and sagittal alignment during axial loading of the joint.

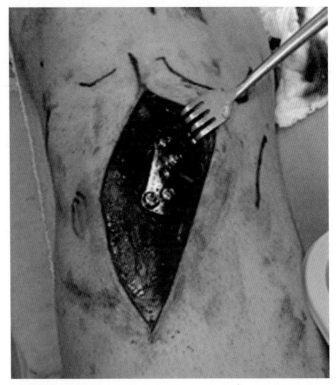

FIGURE 19-6 The osteotomy is stabilized with a plate with four holes (Arthex) with two 6.5-mm proximal cancellous screws and two 4.5-mm distal cortical screws.

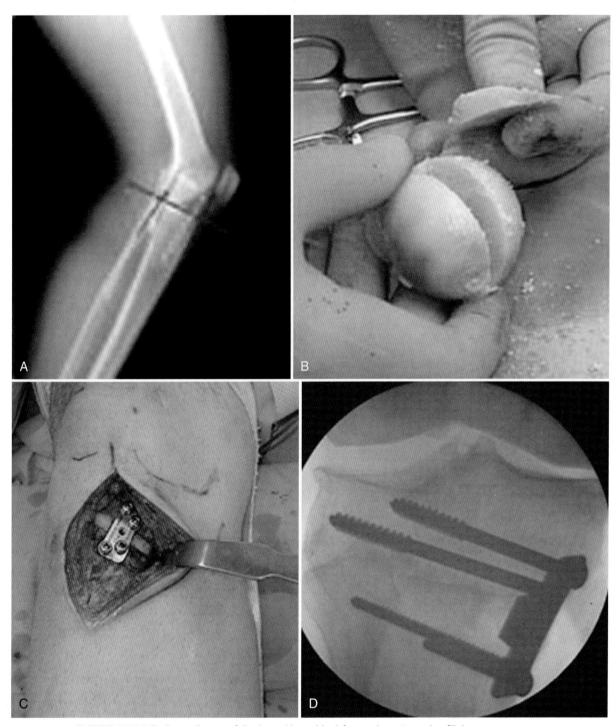

FIGURE 19-7 A-D, Generally a carefully shaped bone block from a donor is used to fill the osteotomy gap.

checked before the tourniquet is deflated; hemostasis and skin suturing are then performed.[9]

PEARLS&PITFALLS

1. The key to success of realignment osteotomy is patient selection—clinical and radiographic signs of overload, knee condition, and patient expectations.

2. The success of any soft tissue procedure around the knee (e.g., articular cartilage resurfacing, meniscal transplantation) is dependent on reducing the mechanical overload if the mechanical axis lies within that compartment.

3. Preoperative planning is essential to avoid overcorrection or undercorrection—bilateral standing x-rays, intraoperative examination and fluoroscopy; check and recheck.

4. During the procedure, it is imperative to assess the effect of the osteotomy on the posterior (lateral) tibial slope; with osteotomy for OA or resurfacing procedures, the slope should remain unchanged.

5. With a closing wedge osteotomy, the tendency is to decrease the tibial slope; this must be kept in mind to remove less bone anteriorly than posteriorly, and to make sure that the wedge is closed posteriorly (usually the fibula may prevent this).

6. With an opening wedge osteotomy, the tendency is to increase slope. To avoid this, subperiosteal posteromedial relase is essential; the opening wedge must be closed more anteriorly than posteriorly and at least half as wide anteriorly than posteriorly (or less).

Postoperative Management

Postoperative management is the same for both techniques described. The patient will use a hinged brace for 6 to 8 weeks, with partial weight bearing during this time, using crutches. Radiographs are taken at the 6- to 8-week mark and, if early healing of the osteotomy is evident, the brace is discontinued and the patient progressed to weight bearing as tolerated. A second radiograph is obtained at the 3-month mark; if the osteotomy is united, the activity level can be increased as tolerated. A long-leg alignment film is taken at 6 months to assess the accuracy of the correction.

External Fixation (Gradual Correction)

Use of an external fixator to achieve a gradual correction has been advocated by some for f large deformities, and good results have been reported with this technique.[32] There are potential advantages with this technique. First, large corrections may be technically impossible with standard closing or opening wedge techniques because of excessive bone removal compromising fixation and creating deformity in the closed wedge technique, or excessive soft tissue tension in the opening wedge technique. External fixators also allow constant manipulation of the alignment during the healing process to optimize alignment.[32] Circular external fixators also allow easy manipulation of angular and translational correction in all three planes, as required.

Special Situations with High Tibial Osteotomy

Cartilage Resurfacing Procedures

The ability of HTO to stimulate articular cartilage reparation with fibrocartilage has been reported by many authors.[33] The use of cartilage resurfacing techniques in association with HTO has the rationale of trying to achieve better cartilage regeneration and potentially better outcomes. Articular cartilage defects can be managed by marrow stimulation (e.g., subchondral drilling, abrasion arthroplasty, microfracture), autologous cultured chondrocyte implantation, osteochondral autograft transplantation (e.g., mosaicoplasty), or autogenous periosteal grafts.[34]

The most commonly performed procedures reported in the literature are abrasion arthroplasty, microfractures, and the implantation of autologous chondrocytes. Some have demonstrated that autologous chondrocyte implantation is a management option for chondral defects, but this is contraindicated in the presence of tibiofemoral malalignment, which would impose mechanical overload to the repair tissue. For this reason, in patients with concurrent chondral defects and varus knee malalignment, we recommend correcting the malalignment with a proximal tibial osteotomy plus arthroscopic autologous chondrocyte implantation.[35] Some researchers have agreed that the degenerative knee can be treated by using a chondral resurfacing procedure, such as microfracture or abrasion arthroplasty, will improve results obtained with an osteotomy alone.[36] Akizuki and colleagues,[36] in a prospective study, compared the cartilage regeneration in osteoarthritic knees treated with HTO alone and HTO plus abrasion arthroplasty. At approximately 12 months after arthroscopy, they observed better regeneration in the abrasion arthroplasty group. They did not find any significant clinical difference between the two groups at 2 to 9 years of follow-up.

Matsunaga and associates[37] have compared patients with medial knee OA treated with proximal lateral closing wedge tibial osteotomy alone, osteotomy plus microfracture, and osteotomy plus abrasion arthroplasty. They observed that the repair of the cartilage was better in the abrasion arthroplasty group than in the other two groups at 1 year after surgery. No difference in the clinical outcome was found among the three groups at 5 years after surgery. In conclusion, all these techniques demonstrated the ability to stimulate cartilage regeneration better than osteotomy alone, but the clinical benefit has still to be demonstrated.

Meniscal Transplantation

Generally, meniscectomy results in joint overload and osteoarthritis in the long term. The use of meniscal transplantation has been popularized and described in many studies and reviews. The association of an osteotomy with meniscal transplantation proposes to relieve pain in a compromised medial compartment and protect the transplanted tissue from overload, improving its long-term viability.[38]

The indications for unloading the compartment undergoing meniscal transplantation with an osteotomy remain author- and surgeon-dependent. Our indications and preferred techniques are as follows. We do not compare the alignment with the unaffected knee because we believe that is mandatory to protect the graft. Usually, the correction needed is small, unless a congenital deformity is present. Although overcorrection in osteoarthritic knees yields better result, it should be avoided in this case and the target should be a knee with an alignment as normal as possible.

Medial meniscus transplantation is indicated when the mechanical axis lies within that compartment on double-limb

standing x-rays. The preferred technique is opening wedge HTO to correct the mechanical axis to the lateral tibial spine (do not overcorrect). Lateral meniscus transplantation is also indicated when the mechanical axis lies within that compartment on double-limb standing x-rays. The preferred technique is opening wedge distal lateral femoral osteotomy to correct the mechanical axis just to the medial tibial spine (do not overcorrect). Better results were reported when meniscal transplantation was associated with the osteotomy than with medial meniscal transplantation without osteotomy.[39]

In conclusion, it seems logical that protecting the transplanted tissue from overloading, or at least changing the original loads that led to its failure, is a necessity. However, but the long-term clinical benefit has still to be demonstrated.

Ligament Instability

Traditionally, knee instability has been considered a contraindication. Currently however, the indications for HTO include patients with chronic ligament deficiencies and malalignment, because this procedure can change not only the coronal but also the sagittal plane of the knee. The sagittal plane modification has a significant impact on biomechanics and joint stability. Decreased posterior tibial slope causes posterior tibia translation and helps the ACL-deficient knee. Conversely, increased tibial slope causes anterior tibial translation and helps the PCL-deficient knee (Fig. 19-8). A medial opening wedge HTO increases posterior tibial slope if the plate is placed anteromedially but does not change the posterior tibial slope if the plate is placed posteromedially. A lateral closing wedge HTO that has equal anterior and posterior gaps along the lateral tibial cortex would have little effect on posterior tibial slope. Some have noted that soft tissue techniques alone, without correction of the alignment, often have poor results because a bone deformity overstresses them.[40] Furthermore, soft tissue destruction causes a decrease in neuromuscular joint control, which over time can worsen the malalignment.[41] Some studies[26] have found satisfying results after HTO in monocompartmental knee OA and varus alignment, but there are few studies about the results of HTO in the unstable knee.[42,43] Rupture of the ACL, if untreated, leads to chronic anterior knee instability. Recurrent nonphysiologic translation-rotation movements of the unstable knee cause increased stress for menisci and cartilage, which often results in meniscal tears and medial cartilage degeneration. However, the problem of the combination of painful unicompartmental degeneration and symptomatic instability cannot be addressed by osteotomy or ACL reconstruction alone. There is no agreement in the literature about which patients require one and which require both procedures, and whether they are to be performed staged or simultaneously.[9,44]

Generally, the most common indication for simultaneous HTO and ACL replacement is anterior knee instability (chronic) in symptomatic varus malalignment. If malalignment is constitutional and no medial symptoms are present, osteotomy in addition to ACL replacement should only be performed if there is considerable meniscal loss and varus angulation is significant. The extent of unicompartmental joint degeneration should be mild. Usually, patients who are considered for the combined

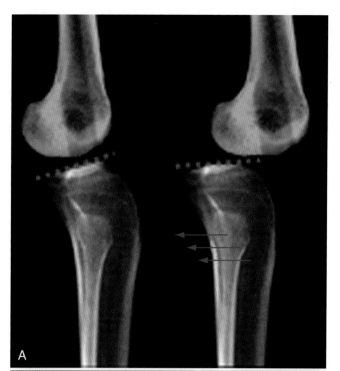

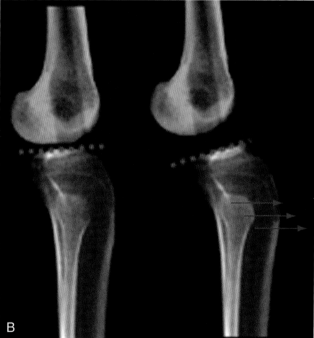

FIGURE 19-8 A, A decrease in posterior tibial slope causes posterior tibial translation and helps the ACL-deficient knee. **B,** An increase in tibial slope causes anterior tibial translation and helps the PCL-deficient knee.

HTO and cruciate ligament reconstruction procedures is younger than 40 years. However, there is no absolute contraindication for the simultaneous procedure in older patients. Factors more important than age in the diagnostic assessment include the patients' level of activity and extent of the medial degenerative changes. For example, if degeneration is advanced and the primary complaint is pain rather than instability, only HTO should be performed because in advanced osteoarthritis, tight joint play may even worsen the symptoms. In this case, a staged procedure,

with HTO initially followed by ACL reconstruction if instability problems persist, may be considered.

In conclusion, chronic knee instability in varus malaligned knees with mild unicompartmental degeneration can effectively be treated by simultaneous HTO and cruciate ligament reconstruction, especially in younger patients. Patients with a varus of the knee and posterolateral instability often present the so-called hyperextension varus thrust gait; during the gait cycle, the knee with posterolateral instability tends to go in varus and hyperextend, with an increase in adduction and a decrease in abduction moments. For the treatment of a PCL- or PLC-deficient knee associated with varus malalignment to improve function and stability, recent studies on the biomechanics of the knee after HTO suggest performing this procedure before soft tissue reconstruction, because soft tissue procedures alone often give poor results. The patient should be evaluated 6 to 8 months later and, if the knee is still unstable, soft tissue reconstruction should be performed. We believe that evaluation of the deformity is essential for the treatment of complex knee instability. Before performing any type of soft tissue surgery, correct bone alignment should be determined in the coronal and sagittal planes.

CONCLUSIONS

Proximal tibial osteotomy can be used to correct varus and valgus deformities in the management of isolated medial or lateral compartment osteoarthritis. There are a number of operative techniques described to achieve this goal and the relative merits of each have been outlined. Whatever the technique used, critical to the success of the procedure are the selection of the appropriate patient and the attainment of a precise correction without complications. If these goals are met, proximal tibial osteotomy should provide long-term relief of pain and restoration of function.

REFERENCES

1. Naudie D, Bourne RB, Rorabeck CH, Bourne TJ. The Insall Award. Survivorship of the high tibial valgus osteotomy. A 10- to -22-year followup study. *Clin Orthop Relat Res*. 1999:18-27.
2. Yasuda K, Majima T, Tsuchida T, Kaneda K. A ten- to 15-year follow-up observation of high tibial osteotomy in medial compartment osteoarthrosis. *Clin Orthop Relat Res*. 1992;(282):186-195.
3. Phisitkul P, Wolf BR, Amendola A. Role of high tibial and distal femoral osteotomies in the treatment of lateral-posterolateral and medial instabilities of the knee. *Sports Med Arthrosc Rev*. 2006;14:96-104.
4. Dejour H, Bonnin. Tibial translation after anterior cruciate ligament rupture. Two radiological tests compared. *J Bone Joint Surg Br*. 1994;76:745-749.
5. Brazier J, Migaud H, Gougeon F, et al. Evaluation of methods for radiographic measurement of the tibial slope. A study of 83 healthy knees. *Rev Chir Orthop Reparatrice Appar Mot*. 1996;82:195-200.
6. Odenbring S, Egund N, Lindstrand A, et al. Cartilage regeneration after proximal tibial osteotomy for medial gonarthrosis. An arthroscopic, roentgenographic, and histologic study. *Clin Orthop Relat Res*. 1992;(277):210-216.
7. Agneskirchner JD, Hurschler C, Stukenborg-Colsman C, et al. Effect of high tibial flexion osteotomy on cartilage pressure and joint kinematics: a biomechanical study in human cadaveric knees. Winner of the AGA-DonJoy Award 2004. *Arch Orthop Trauma Surg*. 2004;124:575-584.
8. Dugdale TW, Noyes FR, Styer D. Preoperative planning for high tibial osteotomy. The effect of lateral tibiofemoral separation and tibiofemoral length. *Clin Orthop Relat Res*. 1992;274:248-264.
9. Noyes FR, Barber-Westin SD, Hewett TE. High tibial osteotomy and ligament reconstruction for varus angulated anterior cruciate ligament-deficient knees. *Am J Sports Med*. 2000;28:282-296.
10. Moreland JR, Bassett LW, Hanker GJ. Radiographic analysis of the axial alignment of the lower extremity. *J Bone Joint Surg Am*. 1987;69:745-749.
11. Moore TM, Harvey JP Jr. Roentgenographic measurement of tibial-plateau depression due to fracture. *J Bone Joint Surg Am*. 1974;56:155-160.
12. Cullù E, Aydogdu S, Alparslan B, Sur H. Tibial slope changes following dome-type high tibial osteotomy. *Knee Surg Sports Traumatol Arthrosc*. 2005;13:38-43.
13. Jacobsen K. Stress radiographical measurement of the anteroposterior, medial and lateral stability of the knee joint. *Acta Orthop Scand*. 1976;47:335-344.
14. Strobel MJ, Weiler A, Schulz MS, et al. Fixed posterior subluxation in posterior cruciate ligament-deficient knees: diagnosis and treatment of a new clinical sign. *Am J Sports Med*. 2002;30:32-38.
15. Louisia S, Siebold R, Canty J, Bartlett RJ. Assessment of posterior stability in total knee replacement by stress radiographs: prospective comparison of two different types of mobile bearing implants. *Knee Surg Sports Traumatol Arthrosc*. 2005;6:476-482.
16. Chassaing VDF, Touzard R, et al. Etude radiologique du L.C.P. à 90 de flexion. *Rev Chir Orthop*.1995;81:35-38.
17. Jung TM, Reinhardt C, Scheffler SU, Weiler A. Stress radiography to measure posterior cruciate ligament insufficiency: a comparison of five different techniques. *Knee Surg Sports Traumatol Arthrosc*. 2006;14:1116-1121.
18. Stäubli HU, Jakob RP. Posterior instability of the knee extension. A clinical and stress radiographic analysis of acute injuries of the posterior cruciate ligament. *J Bone Joint Surg Br*.1990;2:225-230.
19. Puddu G, Gianni E, Chambat P, De Paulis F. The axial view in evaluating tibial translation in cases of insufficiency of the posterior cruciate ligament. *Arthroscopy*. 2000;16:217-220.
20. Puddu G, Cipolla M, Cerullo G, et al. Osteotomies: the surgical treatment of the valgus knee. *Sports Med Arthrosc*. 2007;15:15-22.
21. Jackson JP. Osteotomy for osteroarthritis of the knee. Proceedings of the Sheffield Regional Orthopaedic Club. *J Bone Joint Surg Br*. 1958;40:826.
22. Wardle EN. Osteotomy of the tibia and fibula. *Surg Gynecol Obstet*. 1962;115:61-64.
23. Coventry MB. Upper tibial osteotomy. *Clin Orthop Relat Res*. 1984;(182):46-52.
24. Insall J, Shoji H, Mayer V. High tibial osteotomy. A five-year evaluation. *J Bone Joint Surg Am*. 1974;56:1397-405.
25. Amendola A, Rorabeck CH, Bourne RB, Apyan PM. Total knee arthroplasty following high tibial osteotomy for osteoarthritis. *J Arthroplasty*. 1989;4(suppl):S11-S17.
26. Hernigou P, Medevielle D, Debeyre J, Goutallier D. Proximal tibial osteotomy for osteoarthritis with varus deformity. A ten- to thirteen-year follow-up study. *J Bone Joint Surg Am*. 1987;69:332-354.
27. Hofmann AA, Wyatt RW, Beck SW. High tibial osteotomy. Use of an osteotomy jig, rigid fixation, and early motion versus conventional surgical technique and cast immobilization. *Clin Orthop Relat Res*. 1991;(271):212-217.
28. Puddu G. High tibial osteotomy. The arthritic knee in the young athlete, SYM 15. Paper presented at: 11th ESSKA 2000 Congress and 4th World Congress on Sports Trauma; 2004; Athens.
29. Fowler PJ, Tan JL, Brown GA. Medial opening wedge high tibial osteotomy: how I do it? *Oper Tech Sports Med*. 2000;1:32-38.
30. Lobenhoffer P, De Simoni C, Staubli AE. Open-wedge high tibial osteotomy with rigid plate fixation. *Tech Knee Surg*. 2002;1:93-105.
31. Rodner CM, Adams DJ, Diaz-Doran V, et al. Medial opening wedge tibial osteotomy and the sagittal plane: the effect of increasing tibial slope on tibiofemoral contact pressure. *Am J Sports Med*. 2006;34:1431-1441.
32. Magyar G, Ahl TL, Vibe P, et al. Open-wedge osteotomy by hemicallotasis or the closed-wedge technique for osteoarthritis of the knee. A randomised study of 50 operations. *J Bone Joint Surg Br*. 1999;81:444-8.
33. Amendola A. Panarella L. High tibial osteotomy for the treatment of unicompartmental arthritis of the knee. *Orthop Clin North Am*. 2005;36:497-504.
34. Peterson L, Brittberg M, Kiviranta I, et al. Autologous chondrocyte transplantation. Biomechanics and long-term durability. *Am J Sports Med*. 2002;30:2-12.
35. Alford JW, Cole BJ. Cartilage restoration, part 2: techniques, outcomes, and future directions. *Am J Sports Med*. 2005;33:443-60.

36. Akizuki S, Yasukawa Y, Takizawa T. Does arthroscopic abrasion arthroplasty promote cartilage regeneration in osteoarthritic knees with eburnation? A prospective study of high tibial osteotomy with abrasion arthroplasty versus high tibial osteotomy alone. *Arthroscopy.* 1997;13:9-17.

37. Matsunaga D, Akizuki S, Takizawa T, et al. Repair of articular cartilage and clinical outcome after osteotomy with microfracture or abrasion arthroplasty for medial gonarthrosis. *Knee.* 2007;14:465-471.

38. Cameron JC, Saha S. Meniscal allograft transplantation for unicompartmental arthritis of the knee. *Clin Orthop Relat Res.* 1997;(337):164-171.

39. Annunziato A. Knee osteotomy and meniscal transplantation: indications, technical considerations and results. *Sports Med Arthrosc Rev.* 2007; 15:32-38.

40. Christel P. Basic principles for surgical reconstruction of the PCL in chronic posterior knee instability. *Knee Surg Sports Traumatol Arthrosc.* 2003;11:289-296.

41. Lephart SM, Pincivero DM, Rozzi SL. Proprioception of the ankle and knee. *Sports Med.* 1998;25:149-155..

42. Fowler PJ, Kirkley A, Roe J. Osteotomy of the proximal tibia in the treatment of chronic anterior cruciate ligament insufficiency. *J Bone Joint Surg Br.* 1994;76(suppl):26.

43. Naudie DD, Amendola A, Fowler PJ. Opening wedge high tibial osteotomy for symptomatic hyperextension-varus thrust. *Am J Sports Med.* 1994;32:60-70.

44. Williams RJ 3rd, Wickiewicz TL, Warren RF. Management of unicompartmental arthritis in the anterior cruciate ligament-deficient knee. *Am J Sports Med.* 2000;28:749-760.

Ligamentous Procedures

Anterior Cruciate Ligament Repair

Walter Shelton

Anterior cruciate ligament (ACL) repair is not a new idea, having first been reported by the Mayo Robinson in 1885.[1] Prior to 1970, little emphasis was given to repairing the ACL. Most techniques centered on repairing extra-articular structures with the idea that a competent ACL was not required for normal knee function. Conservative treatment of ACL tears resulted in poor healing rates and a high incidence of instability.[2,3] Primary repair alone did not improve results.[4-6] Reasons for this lack of healing potential were thought to be lack of blood clot formation, insufficient blood supply, differences in intrinsic cell migration, impaired growth factor ability, and the effect of synovial fluid on cell morphology.[7,8]

In the 1970s, Marshall and colleagues[9] increased interest in repairing ACL tears; their technique used primary suture repair. Good results with the repair of proximal tears were obtained. Two randomized studies[2,3] have shown no difference in functional outcomes between repair and conservative treatment with about one third in each group having residual instability. Subsequent focus centered on reconstruction of the torn ACL rather than repair.[10] With better understanding of ACL anatomy, including ligamentous function and insertion footprint anatomy, interest in repair of the ACL has resurfaced. Recent basic science research[11-15] looking at growth factors, gene therapy, and tissue-friendly scaffolds has shown promise for future progress in ACL repair.

ANATOMY

The ACL has been described anatomically in two bundles, one anterior medial (AM) and one posterior lateral (PL; Fig. 20-1). Whereas the primary function of the larger anterior medial bundle is to resist anterior translation of the tibia on the femur,

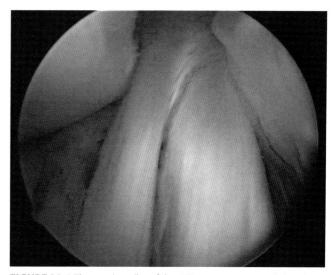

FIGURE 20-1 The two bundles of the ACL, one anterior medial and one posterior lateral.

the posterior lateral bundle also resists abnormal anterior lateral rotation of the tibia on the femur.

The ACL is actually made up of many ligamentous fibers, each attaching a specific point on the tibia to a specific point on the femur. As the knee moves back and forth from flexion to extension, there is a cascade of tightening and loosening of these fibers. The anterior medial bundle fibers become tight toward higher degrees of flexion and the posterior lateral fibers become more taught in extension.

This attention to multiple ligamentous fiber attachment sites has led to the concept of ACL femoral and tibial footprints (Fig. 20-2). A goal of preserving or reconstructing attachment sites

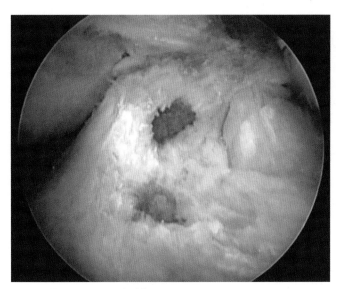

FIGURE 20-2 ACL tibial footprint. *(Courtesy of Dr. Nick Sgaglione.)*

corresponding to the footprints should more closely restore the natural function of the ACL.

The ACL arises from a fossa in front of and lateral to the anterior spine in a footprint that averages 11 mm medial to lateral and 17 mm front to back.[16] Its average length is 38 mm, with a width of 10 mm in its midpoint. It inserts on the posterior medial surface of the lateral femoral condyle. Its blood supply is via the middle geniculate artery and it is innervated by branches of the tibial nerve.

Ruptures of the ACL can be complete or partial. Complete ruptures produce patholaxity, with excessive anterior tibial translation and anterior lateral rotation. The latter produces the common pivot shift of the knee on examination. Partial ruptures can be of the anterior medial or posterior lateral bundles. Anterior medial bundle ruptures allow excessive anterior tibial translation but the pivot shift may be minimal or negative when the posterior lateral bundle is intact. Conversely, ruptures of the posterior lateral bundle may allow excessive anterior lateral rotation and a positive pivot shift while anterior translation remains minimal, with an end point that can be felt on Lachman testing. Careful attention to detail during physical examination is necessary to discern the exact injury.

PATIENT EVALUATION

History and Physical Examination

The history of an acute ACL tear usually involves buckling of the knee with hyperextension, a rapid change in direction, or a direct blow. Often, an audible pop can be heard. Rapid onset of acute pain and swelling occurs, but in partial or incomplete tears swelling may be minimal and pain may subside to the point that the athlete tries to resume play.

Patient relaxation and confidence in the examiner are important for performing a good examination. Pain and muscle spasm are most often present in the acute examination and careful explanation of the process to the patient is vital.

Have the patient lie supine, close to the edge of the examination table. Rest the heel of the patient's injured extremity just off the edge of the table, with the calf fully supported on the table (Fig. 20-3A). This position will allow about 10 degrees of knee flexion and usually the thigh muscles will relax. Accessing the presence of even a small effusion is easy by gently pushing side to side on each side of the patella. Performing a Lachman test is also enhanced by this position, along with medial and lateral stability (see Fig. 20-3B).

Next, while seated, gently abduct the hip and flex the knee off the side of the bed to 90 degrees. Keeping the thigh on the table, stabilize the foot between your knees (see Fig. 20-3C). Grasping the proximal tibia with both hands allows a gentle posterior drawer test to be performed.

Bring the knee to 25 degrees of flexion and, with both hands, a quick jerk forward will usually detect the presence or absence of an end point. This maneuver is especially helpful with large patients in whom a routine Lachman test is difficult to perform simply because of the size of the leg or the presence of muscle spasm (see Fig. 20-3D).

With the patient still supine, range of motion can be recorded. A block in full extension or flexion may be a clue to a displaced bucket handle tear of the meniscus. By gently extending the knee from flexion into full extension with internal rotation and a valgus stress, the presence of a pivot shift can be determined. In an acute setting, this test is difficult to administer because of pain and apprehension on the part of the patient. Once the instability of a positive pivot shift has been experienced, patients will instinctively guard against it. In chromic cases, the pivot shift can be more easily evaluated.

All these testing maneuvers are much more sensitive under anesthesia and a final examination with the patient asleep prior to beginning surgery should be mandatory. Subtle instabilities such as a posterior lateral instability can be diagnosed and properly addressed at the time of surgery.

Diagnostic Imaging

Every examination of the knee should include at least four high-quality x-rays—standing anteroposterior (AP) at 0- and 30-degree, lateral, and sunrise patellar views. Subtle bony injuries such as articular and Segond fractures[17] can be identified. A rim fracture of the patella or lateral femoral condoyle can be helpful in differentiating between a patella dislocation and acute ACL tear, both of which may present with hemarthrosis and muscular spasm.

Magnetic resonance imaging (MRI) can be helpful in evaluating ACL tears, especially in diagnosing associated injuries to meniscal and articular surfaces. The posterior cruciate ligament (PCL) is usually distinct on MRI scan because of its saggital orientation, but the ACL can be more indistinct on routine MRI because of its more oblique orientation. An experienced MRI technician may be helpful in obtaining cuts more in line with ACL orientation and increasing the sensitivity of MRI for diagnosing an ACL tear.

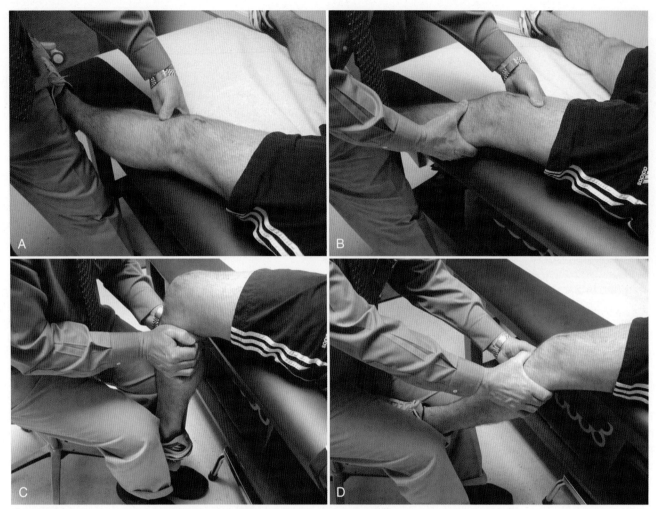

FIGURE 20-3 Physical examination of the ACL. **A,** Rest the heel of the injured extremity just off the edge of the table, with the calf fully supported on the table. **B,** Perform a Lachman test. Bend the knee to about 30 degrees. Then, stabilize the femur with one hand. Place the other hand behind the proximal tibia at the level of the joint line and pull forward. **C,** Gently abduct the hip and flex the knee off the side of the bed to 90 degrees. Keeping the thigh on the examination table, stabilize the foot between your knees. Grasping the proximal tibia with both hands allows a gentle posterior drawer test to be performed. **D,** Bring the knee to 25 degrees of flexion and, with both hands, jerk the knee forward quickly. This will usually detect the presence or absence of an end point. This maneuver is especially helpful with very large patients in whom a routine Lachman test is difficult to perform simply because of the size of the leg or the presence of muscle spasm.

TREATMENT

Conservative Treatment

Nonoperative treatment of ACL tears may be appropriate in older sedentary patients or patients with conditions nonconducive to surgery. The ACL can heal in up to one third of cases,[18,19] with a third having detectable but not debilitating instability and a third having significant functional instability. Results of patients with ACL repair versus nonoperative treatment have shown better objective stability in the surgical groups but no significant difference in patient satisfaction.[20]

When conservative treatment is elected for acute ACL tears, the knee should be immobilized initially to reduce pain. Aspirating the hemarthrosis and liberal use of ice help reduce acute pain and swelling. Prolonged immobilization should be avoided and gentle motion should be started with muscle toning to prevent atrophy in 3 or 4 days. Open-chain quadriceps exercises should be avoided to minimize anterior translation forces on the tibia.

Crutches with partial weight bearing should be instituted as soon as practical. A functional ACL brace may also be helpful for the patient to regain confidence in the knee. After 6 weeks, the patient should be allowed full ambulation without crutches. A periodic examination for clinical instability should be carried out. If persistent functional instability results from this conservative approach, the patient should be counseled about the risk of further injury to the meniscal and articular surfaces.

One study[21] of nonoperative treatment for acute ACL tears with MRI-proven normal menisci, with a goal of early return to sport in an ACL brace, has shown that only 72% returned to their sport at an average of 5.7 weeks postinjury. Patients estimated only an 80% return to their preinjury ability and, at ACL reconstruction, 57% had sustained meniscal tears.

Arthroscopic Technique

Arthroscopic reconstruction of the ACL is a well-proven technique in which the entire ACL is replaced by a tissue graft. Careful attention to surgical detail can achieve clinical success in 90% of patients. A drawback to this technique is that it does not reestablish the complex function of the ACL fibers within its footprints. Recent efforts at double-bundle[22] reconstruction are an effort to reconstruct the functional anatomy of the ACL more closely.

With the evolution of understanding the functional anatomy of the ACL, recent interest in ACL repair and preservation of as much of the normal ligament and bundles as possible has increased.[23-27] With proper patient selection, repair of the ACL can produce good stability, with predictable results.[28] Repair alone or repair of a midsubstance tear is not advisable. The two indications for repair are when the ligament is torn near its proximal attachment or when only one bundle is torn. In the case of proximal tears, the ligament can be repaired with multiple sutures to drill holes in the bone and can be augmented with a soft tissue graft.

After careful examination under anesthesia, routine arthroscopy is carried out through standard portals. The ACL is visualized and probed to assess its potential for repair (Fig. 20-4A). Only ACL tears in the very proximal portion of the ligament should be considered for repair. All other pathology should be corrected prior to proceeding with the ACL repair. Four or five simple sutures are then placed in the ligament with an intra-articular suture device, spacing each suture up and down the unattached ligament as much as possible (see Fig. 20-4B). The two ends of each suture are separated into two groups, one medial and one lateral. Each suture should have one limb in each group.

An accessory incision is made between the lower edge of the iliotibial band and the distal biceps tendon, and a rear entry ACL guide is placed into the knee over the top of the lateral femoral condyle. The tip of the guide is placed 8 mm anterior to the back of the notch in the femoral footprint of the ACL and a guide pin is placed from outside-in. A tunnel is reamed from outside-in to a size corresponding to a previously sized soft tissue graft (usually 6 to 8 mm).

The graft options are the autograft quadriceps tendon, hamstring tendon, and various allografts, including hamstring, anterior tibials, and posterior tibials. The autografts are harvested via small incisions, but the most important step is to size the graft accurately to fit the reamed tunnel, usually 6 to 8 mm. The ends of the graft are secured with strong no. 1 absorbable whipstitches. These sutures will be used to pull the graft into place through the tunnel and to place tension on the graft when it is secured in the tunnel.

The lateral groups of sutures are pulled out through the femoral tunnel while the medial suture ends are pulled out over the top of the femoral condyle. Passage of the medial group of suture is accomplished with the aid of the rear entry guide system, which uses a long C-shaped hook passed via the anterior lateral portal through the notch and over the top of the lateral femoral condyle. This hook helps pass a loop suture back through the knee and out the anterior lateral portal. The suture loop is used to pull the medial group of ACL sutures over the top of the lateral femoral condyle.

Pull the two groups of sutures with sufficient tension to bring the ligament back up to its femoral attachment (Fig. 20-5). With

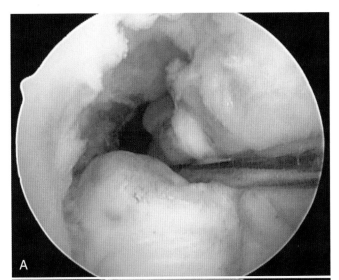

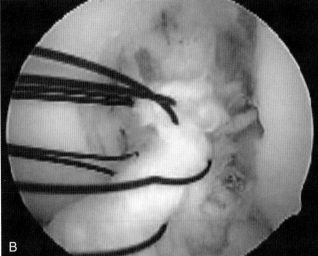

FIGURE 20-4 A, After careful examination under anesthesia, routine arthroscopy is carried out through standard portals. The ACL is visualized and probed to assess its potential for repair. **B,** Four or five simple sutures are placed in the ligament with an intra-articular suture device, spacing each suture up and down the unattached ligament as much as possible.

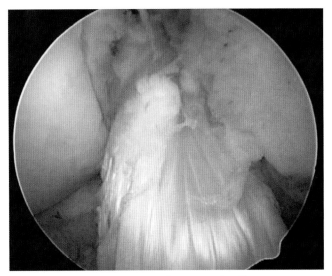

FIGURE 20-5 Pull the two groups of sutures with sufficient tension to bring the ligament back up to its femoral attachment.

the ligament pulled tight, a standard ACL guide is placed in the tibial footprint just at the posterior aspect of the ligament and a 6- to 8-mm tunnel is reamed from outside-in into the posterior aspect of the tibial footprint. Care must be taken at this point not to disrupt the intact ACL fibers with the reamer as it pierces the tibial cortex; slowly advancing the reamer tip or reaming the last 1 to 2 mm with a hand reamer helps prevent damage to the intact ACL fibers. The graft is then passed through the tibial tunnel, out the femoral tunnel using a commercial suture passer, and brought down the femoral tunnel from outside-in and out the tibial tunnel. The tibial side is secured with an interference screw in the tibial tunnel. Tension is applied to the graft with the knee at 30 degrees of flexion and the two suture bundles are tied together over the femoral condyle. Final fixation is accomplished by placing an outside-in interference screw in the femoral tunnel.

The knee is carried through a full range of motion to ensure no impingement of the graft. After routine closure, a sterile dressing is applied.

Repair of an Anterior Medial Bundle Tear

In case of a tear of the anterior medial bundle of the anterior cruciate ligament, an 8-mm soft tissue graft is obtained. After routine arthroscopy and probing of the ACL, which determines that the posterior lateral bundle is intact, a minimal débridement of any loose pieces of anterior medial bundle is done. An 8-mm drill hole is placed with the aid of a tibial guide into the anterior medial aspect of the tibial footprint.

The femoral tunnel is made by using a rear entry outside-in guide to place a guide pin into the posterior superior part of the femoral footprint of the ACL. The tunnel is reamed from outside-in with an 8-mm reamer. As the top of the reamer approaches the cortex of the intercondylar notch when reaming both tunnels, care is taken not to penetrate the notch excessively with the tip of the reamer. This can be done by slowing the reaming process and/or finishing the last few millimeters of the tunnel using a hand reamer. If the tip of the reamer penetrates into the notch, the remaining intact fibers of the ACL can be wound up and destroyed. In case of a tear of the anterior medial bundle of the ACL, an 8-mm soft tissue graft is obtained. Whipstitches are placed in each end of the soft tissue graft for guiding it into place. The tissue graft is passed through the tibial tunnel into the femoral tunnel and both ends are secured in their respective tunnels with interference screws, with the knee in 30 degrees of flexion. The knee is carried through a full range of motion to check for impingement; after routine closure, a sterile dressing is applied.

Repair of the Posterolateral Bundle

After arthroscopic inspection of the joint, probing of the ACL, and determining that a tear of the posterior lateral bundle has occurred and that the anterior medial bundle is intact, the tibial guide is used to place a 6-mm tunnel in the posterior aspect of the tibial footprint. As with anterior medial bundle repair, care must be taken not to damage the remaining intact fibers of the anterior medial bundle. Using an over the top, outside-in guide, a 6-mm tunnel is placed through an accessory lateral incision into the posterior lateral bundle attachment of the femoral footprint of the ACL, which is anterior and inferior on the lateral

femoral condyle. The soft tissue graft is passed from the tibial tunnel into the femoral tunnel and secured with interference screws at 30 degrees of knee flexion. After routine soft tissue closure, a sterile dressing is applied.

PEARLS & PITFALLS

PEARLS

1. Graft harvest and preparation should be complete before drilling so that the tunnels formed are no larger than necessary to accommodate the graft. I prefer is a quadriceps tendon soft tissue graft with whipstitches in each end.
2. Use four or five sutures to repair the proximal ACL tear. Putting the sutures in through a cannula in front of the knee keeps them from becoming crossed on each other and entrapped by anterior soft tissue when passed back into the joint.
3. Ream the femoral tunnel from outside-in to minimize the danger of damaging intact ACL fibers with the end of the reamer.
4. Repair of the AM bundle should be at least 8 mm and of the PL bundle at least 6 mm.
5. Repair sutures should pass from ligament through bone and not from one end of the torn ligament to the opposing end. Sutures placed in one end of a torn ACL into the opposing end are inherently weak and will not keep proper tension on the repaired ligament during healing.

PITFALLS

1. When reaming the tunnels, be careful not to protrude into the notch aggressively with the end of the reamer to minimize damage to the intact ACL fibers.
2. Suture repairs of midsubstance mop-end tears have less chance of success and, with present technology, are better treated with reconstruction.

CONCLUSIONS

Early in the evolution of ACL surgery, primary repair was the preferred procedure. Success was best with proximal tears but because of recurrent instability in many patients, the concept of repairing the ACL was replaced by reconstruction the ACL, usually with bone-tendon-bone (BTB) or hamstring grafts. Reconstruction has resulted in objectively stable knees in 90% of patients and has become the gold standard for treating ACL tears.

Subtle instabilities after ACL reconstruction deemed successful by clinical testing can prevent patients from resuming their preinjury level of ability. These subtle instabilities have heightened interest in ACL anatomy and function of the ACL bundles.

Repairing proximal and one-bundle ACL tears using a soft tissue graft has been successful. Broader footprint attachments of the ACL results from this salvage of ACL tissue. Future developments, such as stimulation of cell migration, addition of growth factors, introducing gene therapy, and using scaffolds, will further refine the concept of ACL repair.

REFERENCES

1. Mayo Robison AW. Ruptured crucial ligaments and their repair by operation. *Ann Surg.* 1903;37:716-718.
2. Andersson C, Odensten M, Good L, Gillquist J. Surgical or non-surgical treatment of acute rupture of the anterior cruciate ligament. A randomized study with long-term follow-up. *J Bone Joint Surg Am.* 1989;71: 965-974.

3. Sanberg R, Balkfors B, Nilsson B, Westlin N. Operative versus non-operative treatment of recent injuries to the ligaments of the knee. A prospective randomized study. *J Bone Joint Surg Am*. 1987;69: 1120-1126.

4. Sherman MF, Lieber L, Bonamo JR, et al. The long-term follow-up of primary anterior cruciate ligament repair: defining a rationale for augmentation. *Am J Sports Med*. 1991;19:243-255.

5. Feagon JA, Curl WW. Isolated tear of the anterior cruciate ligament: 5-year follow-up study. *Am J Sports Med*. 1976;4:95-100.

6. Strand T, Molster A, Hordvik M, Krukhaung Y. Long-term follow-up after primary repair of the anterior cruciate ligament: clinical and radiological evaluation 15-23 years post operatively. *Arch Orthop Trauma Surg*. 2005; 125:217-221.

7. Frank CB, Jackson DW. Current concepts review. The science of reconstruction of the anterior cruciate ligament. *J. Bone Joint Surg Am*. 1997; 79:1556-1576.

8. Murray MM. Effect of the intra-articular environment on healing of the ruptured anterior cruciate ligament. *J Bone Joint Surg Am*. 2001;

9. Marshall JL, Warren RF, Wickiewicz TL. Primary surgical treatment of anterior cruciate ligament lesions. *Am J Sports Med*. 1982;10:103-107.

10. Drogset JO, Grontvedt T, Robak OR, et al. A sixteen-year follow-up of three operative techniques for the treatment of acute ruptures of the anterior cruciate ligament. *J Bone Joint Surg Am*. 2006;88:944-952.

11. Konda E, Yasuda K, Yamanaka M, et al. Effects of administration of exogenous growth factors on biomechanical properties of the elongation-type anterior cruciate ligament injury with partial laceration. *Am J Sports Med*. 2005;33:188-196.

12. Pascher A, Steiner AF, Palmer GD, et al. Enhanced repair of the anterior cruciate ligament by *in situ* gene transfer: evaluation in an in vitro model. *Mol Ther*. 2004;10;2:327-336.

13. Splindler KP, Murray MM, Devin C, et al. The central ACL defect as a model for failure of intra-articular healing. *J Orthop Res*. 2006;24: 401-406.

14. Murray MM, Forsythe B, Chen F, et al. The effect of thrombin on ACL fibroblast interactions with collagen hydrogels. *J Orthop Res*. 2006;24: 508-515.

15. Murray MM, Splinder KP, Devin C, et al. Use of a collagen-platelet rich plasma scaffold to stimulate healing of a central defect in the canine ACL. *J Orthop Res*. 2006;24:820-830.

16. Arnoczky SP. Anatomy of the anterior cruciate ligament. *Clin Orthop Relat Res*. 1983;(172):19-25.

17. Segond P. [Recherches cliniques et experimental les sur les epanchiements sanquin du genou paretorse.] *Prog Med*. 1879;7:297-299.

18. Petrigliano FA, McAllister DR, Wu BM. Tissue engineering for anterior cruciate ligament reconstruction: a review of current strategies. *Arthroscopy*. 2006;24;4:441-451.

19. Meunier A, Odensten M, Good L. Long-term results after primary repair or non-surgical treatment of anterior cruciate ligament rupture: a randomized study with a 15-year follow-up. *Scand J Med Sci Sports*. 2007;17:230-237.

20. Meuffels DE, Favejee M, Vissers M, et al. Ten-year follow-up study comparing conservative versus operative treatment of anterior cruciate ligament ruptures. A matched-pair analysis of high level athletes. *Br J Sports Med*. 2009;43:347-351.

21. Shelton WR, Barrett GR, Dukes A. Early season anterior cruciate ligament tears; a treatment dile mma. *Am J Sports Med*. 25;5:656-658.

22. Fu FH, Irrgang JJ, Bost JE. Re: outcome of single-bundle versus double-bundle reconstruction of the anterior cruciate ligament: a meta-analysis. *Am J Sports Med*. 2009;37:421-422.

23. Steiner ME, Murray MM, Rodeo SA. Strategies to improve anterior cruciate ligament healing and graft placement. *Am J Sports Med*. 2008;36: 176-89.

24. Seitz H, Menth-Chiarai WA, Lang S, Nau T. Histological evaluation of the healing potential of the anterior cruciate ligament by means of augmented and non-augmented repair: an in vitro animal study. *Knee Surg Sports Traumatol Arthosc*. 2008;16:1087-1093.

25. Fleming BC, Carey JL, Spindler KP, Murray MM. Can suture repair of ACL transaction restore normal anteroposterior laxity of the knee? An ex vivo study. *J Orthop Res*. 2008;26:1500-1505.

26. Altman GH, Horan RL, Weitzel P, Richmond JC. The use of long-term bioresorbable scaffolds for anterior cruciate ligament repair. *J Am Acad Orthop Surg*. 2008;16:177-187.

27. Murray MM, Splindler KP, Abreu E, et al. Collagen-platelet rich plasma hydrogel enhances primary repair of the porcine anterior cruciate ligament. *J Orthop Res*. 2007;25:81-91.

28. Buda R, Ferruzzi A, Vannini F, et al. Augmentation technique with semitendinosus and graciliis tendons in chronic partial lesions of the ACL: clinical and arthrometric analysis. *Knee Surg Sports Traumatol Arthrosc*. 2006;14:1101-1107.

CHAPTER 21

Anatomic Single-Bundle Anterior Cruciate Ligament Reconstruction

John C. Richmond

Anterior cruciate ligament (ACL) reconstruction has evolved from the open techniques of the 1970s and early 1980s to current arthroscopic techniques. During the course of that evolution, the endoscopic transtibial reconstructive technique became popular.[1] With this technique, the position of the femoral tunnel is dictated by the direction and position of the tibial tunnel. Unfortunately, not enough attention was paid to this fact and through the 1990s, more transtibial endoscopic ACL reconstructions were done in a very sagittal alignment, resulting in persistent rotatory instability, even if the graft remained intact. Howell and colleagues[2,3] were among the first to recognize this as a clinical problem. They noted that with such an alignment of the graft, one of two problems would ensue, stretching of the graft as it wrapped about the posterior cruciate ligament (PCL) in flexion or failure to regain flexion. They described the coronal angle as the angle in the frontal plane between the axis of the joint line and axis of the tibial tunnel. For coronal angles more than 75 degrees (more vertical), these problems of stretching of the graft or failure to regain motion were encountered. For coronal angles less than 75 degrees, optimal results were obtained.

Raffo and associates[4] have recently described a reproducible anatomic landmark for the starting point of the tibial tunnel on the anteromedial tibia as the point of intersection between the anterior edge of the medial collateral ligament and superior border of the gracilis tendon, as a point that will reproducibly yield a coronal angle of 70 degrees or less. This technique for establishing the tibial tunnel start point is my preference for bone-patellar tendon-bone (B-PT-B) grafts. This allows creation of a femoral socket that will accommodate 30 mm of bone block in the anatomic attachment site of the ACL. Because an interference screw can be placed proximal to the bone block within the socket, the graft can be well positioned near the center of the ACL footprint on the femur. Others have described a similar starting point for the tibial tunnel, but have relied on techniques to identify it[5] that are less reproducible than those I have used.

Fu and coworkers[6] were instrumental in recognizing the issues with the sagittally placed ACL reconstruction, and have exquisitely defined the anatomy of the ACL—in particular, its two-bundle configuration with separate and distinct sites of origin from the femur and insertion onto the tibia. They demonstrated that both anatomically placed double- or single-bundle reconstructions were superior biomechanically and kinematically to nonanatomic techniques.[7,8] Gardiner and coworkers have recently shown in the cadaver laboratory that the anatomic single-bundle technique is kinematically equal to the double-bundle technique.[9] With soft tissue grafts, placing the graft into the center of the footprint of the ACL on the lateral wall of the intercondylar notch and obtaining rigid fixation may best be done through a medial portal technique. This has become my routine for soft tissue grafts. Confirmation of use of the anatomically placed single-bundle reconstructive technique has recently come from a meta-analysis by Meredic and colleagues,[10] which showed no advantage of double-bundle techniques over the anatomic single-bundle procedure.

Graft choice is another variable that may affect ACL outcome. A number of meta-analyses comparing autograft patellar tendon to autograft hamstring tendons have demonstrated that there are distinct differences between the outcomes.[11,12] The patellar tendon graft in these analyses has consistently yielded a higher percentage of stable knees, with a greater percentage of athletes returning to preinjury activities, when compared with the soft tissue alternatives. It is apparent that patellar tendon grafts are not without issues. Anterior knee pain and quadriceps weakness have been identified as problems.[13] These make hamstring grafts an attractive alternative for the patient with less demanding work or athletic pursuits.. Finally, allografts have become more frequently used for ACL reconstruction. In a younger and more active patient, these may lead to significantly greater rates of failure—two or three times greater in a recent meta-analysis—when compared with autograft alterna-

TABLE 21-1 Anterior Cruciate Ligament Graft Selection Algorithm

Patient Characteristics	ACL Graft Choice
Competitive athlete: high school, college, professional	B-PT-B autograft
Recreational athlete <40 yr	Quadrupled hamstring autograft
Recreational athlete >40 yr; mitigating factors (e.g., revision)	Allograft—B-PT-B or tibialis anterior

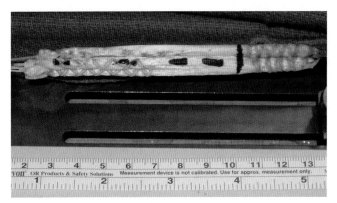

FIGURE 21-1 Soft tissue graft prepared for use with Femoral and Tibial Intrafix devices (DePuy Mitek).

tives.[14,15] All these data considered together have resulted in a graft selection algorithm that I routinely discuss with patients when considering ACL reconstruction (Table 21-1). Autologous B-PT-B is preferred for the high-demand competitive athlete. An autologous four-strand hamstring graft is selected for the moderately demanding recreational athlete, with less time of exposure to high-risk activities. Finally, allograft tissue is reserved forspecial cases, which include age older than 40 years, autologous tendon issues such as failed autograft, or prior tendon injury. Each of these graft choices must be placed in an anatomic location on both the femur and tibia and rigidly fixed to result in a stable knee postsurgery that will allow individuals to pursue their work or recreational activities.

TREATMENT

Arthroscopic Technique: Anatomic Soft Tissue Anterior Cruciate Ligament Reconstruction

Positioning of the leg within the leg holder is crucial to be able to perform anatomic single-bundle ACL reconstruction using a soft tissue graft. The positioning of the leg holder must be such that the knee can be flexed to 120 degrees to drill the femoral socket through the medial portal. The use of a pump to maintain adequate distention with flexion more than 90 degrees is an important key to this technique.

This technique is suited for a soft tissue allograft (e.g., tibialis anterior or posterior tendons) or autologous quadrupled hamstring grafts. When using autologous hamstring tendons, I routinely harvest the semitendinosus and gracilis tendons as the first portion of the procedure. This is done after the diagnosis of complete ACL tear has been confirmed by the presence of a pivot shift test under anesthesia or arthroscopic visualization. This allows preparation of the tendons on the back table while the joint is being prepared for the graft. Because of the elliptic footprint of the ACL on the femur and the relatively short tunnel (25 to 35 mm) with a medial portal technique, I prefer the Femoral Intrafix device (DePuy Mitek; Raynham, Mass) as my standard femoral fixation device. It is made from nonabsorbable plastic, gives high-strength aperture fixation, and maintains two thirds to three quarters of the circumference of the graft in apposition to the femoral bone. Similarly, I prefer the Tibial Intrafix device (DePuy Mitek) for fixation of soft tissue grafts to the tibia. It is also made from nonabsorbable plastic and allows 360 degrees of graft contact to the tibial tunnel while establishing very high-strength fixation.

Preparation of the graft is another important step. For either graft, the overall length is determined by the height of the patient. I routinely double a 21-cm graft (yielding a 10.5-cm construct) for patients 5'8" tall or shorter. For patients between 5'8" and 6'2", I use a 22-cm graft doubled over to yield an 11-cm construct. Finally, for patients taller than 6'2", I use a 23-cm graft doubled over to yield an 11.5-cm overall construct length. These lengths are important, because tensioning the graft on the tibial side with the Intrafix and its tensioner is most easily accomplished with 5 to 10 mm of graft extending from the tibial tunnel when the Intrafix sheath and screw are placed. For the tibialis grafts, I split each end in half for a length of 7 cm to yield four ends for tensioning. I whipstitch with a baseball-type suture configuration using a no. 2 high-strength suture, for a length of 5 cm. The central 5 cm of the graft is whipped together by looping a no. 2 high-strength tie around the graft. This facilitates passage of the sheath for the femoral Intrafix, with its triangular flange between the two bundles. The suture material also improves the fixation properties of the construct, reducing potential slippage of the graft past the device with cyclic loading (Fig. 21-1).

Sizing of the graft for this technique is crucial in that interference fixation is being relied on within the tunnel to maintain tension and prevent slippage. The femoral socket will be drilled to a diameter 1 mm more than the construct size of the looped proximal end of the graft, while the tibial tunnel is drilled to the measured diameter.

Minimal notch preparation is needed for this technique. In a chronic situation, any osteophytes that might potentially impinge on the graft are removed. If the anterior aspect of the notch is narrow, notchplasty to expand this and reduce the likelihood of impingement on the graft is also appropriate. I prefer to preserve the ACL footprint intact on the femur (Video 1), clear it centrally prior to guide pin passage, and mark my preferred guide pin starting point with a curette (Fig. 21-2) (Video 2). Use of an over the back guide of the femoral aimer with an offset to preserve 1.5 to 2 mm of bone posterior to the femoral socket will yield excellent anatomic positioning of the graft.

Prior to placement of the femoral guide pin, it is essential that an adequate amount of the fat pad be resected so that at 120 degrees of flexion, the fat pad does not obstruct vision of the notch (Video 3). Once this is done, the over the back guide is

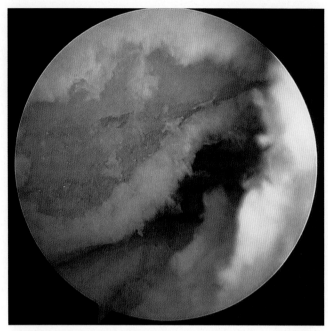

FIGURE 21-2 Starting point for the femoral guide wire in the center of the ACL femoral footprint.

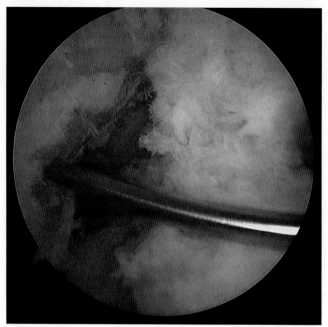

FIGURE 21-4 Flexible 2.4-mm Nitinol wire permits the knee to be moved and the position checked prior to drilling the femoral socket. It can be easily drilled over, and does not shed metal debris like stainless guide wires.

introduced through the medial portal. The medial portal needs to be low (just above the medial meniscus) and medial so that the over the back femoral guide is touching the medial femoral condyle when the guide pin is passed (Fig. 21-3). It is best to identify the anatomic start location for the femoral guide pin with the knee flexed 90 degrees. In this position, the guide pin is directed so that the pin will pass through the ridge separating the foot-

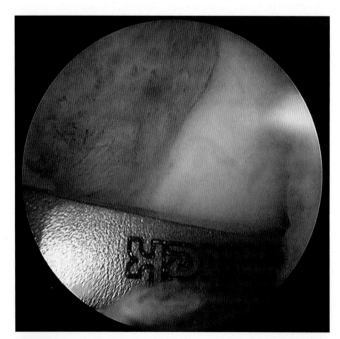

FIGURE 21-3 Over the back guide positioned in contact with the medial femoral condyle as the knee is flexed to 120 degrees.

prints of the anteromedial bundle of the ACL from the posterolateral bundle. While maintaining the guide in that position, the knee is flexed to 120 degrees and the guide pin drilled through the femoral condyle, out through the skin laterally. The guide pin is then immediately removed and switched to a flexible 2.4-mm Nitinol wire. This allows the knee to be extended and the position of the wire inspected to ascertain proper positioning (Fig. 21-4). The acorn drill can be passed into the joint over this flexible wire without damaging the medial femoral condyle by bending the wire away from the condyle as the drill is introduced through the portal. Using a hemostat to spread the portal site along the wire facilitates passage of the cannulated drill. The knee is again flexed to 120 degrees and the socket is established by drilling to the depth of 27 to 30 mm, which is necessary to accommodate the femoral Intrafix (Video). In very small women, this may result in penetration of the lateral cortex of the femoral condyle. This does not present a problem, but one should be careful about to the feel of the drill as it penetrates the cortex. The drill and Nitinol wire are then removed and a large-diameter (5 mm or larger) shaver is used to remove the bone debris from the joint and socket (Fig. 21-5). The socket can then be carefully visualized from the medial portal to ascertain integrity of the posterior cortex and its position in the ACL femoral footprint (Video 6).

The tibial guide pin is then passed. I prefer to maintain a cuff of approximately 5-mm long ACL fibers on the tibia to improve proprioception postsurgery during rehabilitation and return to athletics.[16] The entry site of the guide pin into the tibia needs to be low enough to have adequate tunnel length. I routinely use the superior border of the pes anserine tendons as the starting site, because this will yield a 30 to 40-mm tibial tunnel in all

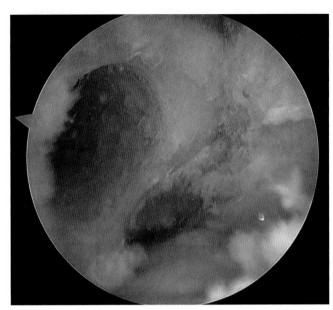

FIGURE 21-5 Femoral socket viewed from the anterolateral portal, showing its location within the ACL footprint.

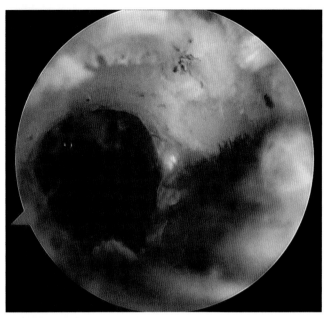

FIGURE 21-6 Sheath placed in the femoral socket only occupies one third or less of the circumference of the hole.

patients. One should aim for an entry site of the guide pin into the joint, which is in the middle of the ACL footprint. For deviations of guide pin placement that are a few millimeters from optimal, the guide pin can initially be overreamed with a small (4.5-mm) cannulated drill and then moved eccentrically within this tunnel when full-size drilling is performed. For greater deviations from optimal for pin placement, use of a parallel guide or complete repositioning of the pin is appropriate.

Once the tibial tunnel has been drilled and the debris removed, the femoral guide pin is reinserted through the medial portal and out through the femoral socket, with the knee flexed to 120 degrees. It is used to retrieve a no. 5 suture through the joint, which is then brought down to exit the tibial tunnel and subsequently used to retrieve the graft transtibially through the joint and into the femoral socket. If the femoral Intrafix device is used for fixation, there is a trial inserter used to separate the two arms of the graft and dilate the tunnel to accept the sheath. If this passes without significant difficulty and can be lightly tapped into place, a standard configuration for sheath and screw can be used. If the bone is hard and it requires significant force to place this trial, the hard bone Femoral Intrafix system is used and the screw that will be placed into the sheath is then downsized by 1 mm.

The sheath is inserted over a Nitinol wire that has been placed anterior in the femoral socket (Video 8). This needs to be fully seated into the femoral socket (Fig. 21-6). The screw is then brought down over this wire and screwed in until it is recessed within the sheath (Video 9). The entire construct should be entirely within the lateral femoral condyle. To maintain the positioning of the graft, I have found that having an assistant maintain tension on both arms of the graft as the socket is dilated and the sheath and screw are inserted is helpful. The two-bundle configuration of the graft as it exits the femur is readily visualized at this point (Fig. 21-7).

The graft is then inspected. I routinely use a probe to position the graft so that it lies in an anterior and posterior plane in the tibial tunnel to mimic the anteromedial and posterolateral bundle configuration of the native ACL. The graft is tensioned using the tibial Intrafix tensioning device. This allows central placement of the sheath and screw on the tibia. I generally tension the grafts with 25 pounds of force on a tensioner and the knee in 0 degree of extension (without hyperextension). Once tibial fixation has been established, the joint can be examined for stability using the Lachman, anterior drawer, and pivot shift tests. If the results are acceptable, final arthroscopic inspection is appropriate prior to closure. By

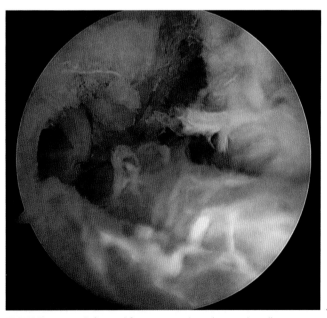

FIGURE 21-7 With femoral fixation complete, the two-bundle configuration of the graft is readily identified.

tensioning the graft at a full 0 degree of extension, with high tension in the graft, full extension and good stability are assured.[17]

For those high-demand patients for whom a B-PT-B autograft has been selected as the graft of choice, variations on this technique are needed. Specifically, the use of a transtibial endoscopic approach for drilling the femur results in a longer femoral socket. This allows recessing of the bone block up into the femoral tunnel to reduce the likelihood of a graft-tunnel mismatch, with the bone block extending out of the tibial tunnel and precluding interference fixation on the tibia.[18] Once ACL insufficiency has been confirmed by examination under anesthesia or by arthroscopy, I harvest the B-PT-B graft prior to preparing the joint. An anterior incision over the patella tendon, which is curved medially at its distal extent, allows placement of the tibial tunnel in the appropriate position just above the intersection of the anteriormost fibers of the medial collateral ligament (MCL) and the superior border of the gracilis tendon. I routinely harvest a minimum width of 10 mm for male patients and 8 mm for female patients, measured at the inferior pole of the patella. In larger patients, I harvest one third or the width of the proximal tendon, up to (but not exceeding) 12 mm. The patellar bone block should be 30 mm in length and 1 cm in depth; this block will ultimately end up in the tibia. The bone block harvested from the tibia will be placed in the femur and should be a total of 33 mm long; this includes an additional 8 mm of bone harvested proximal to the tendon attachment onto the tibia (Fig. 21-8).[17] The graft is prepared on the back table while the joint is being prepared.

The tibial guide pin is passed first using a standard commercially available drill guide. I prefer using a tip guide with the entry site into the tibia on the external cortex of the tibia at the intersection of the leading fibers of the MCL and gracilis tendon.[4] The entry site into the joint should be central in the ACL footprint; guide pin placement can be adjusted, as noted earlier in the discussion of soft tissue ACL reconstruction.

The positioning of this tibial tunnel typically allows placement of the femoral guide wire using a standard, commercially available "over the back" guide. This guide is selected so that it will allow 1 or 2 mm of bone, once overdrilled, as a posterior rim for fixation. The positioning guide wire for the femoral socket in an endoscopic transtibial technique requires that the knee be flexed a minimum of 65 degrees. This is to ensure that adequate bone posterior to the

tunnel is maintained for good interference fixation. I prefer to place the "over the back" guide in this position and then gently flex up to about 75 degrees. When the femoral socket is drilled in this position, one needs to be able to flex the knee to 110 degrees to place the femoral fixation screw. For the femoral socket to be fashioned transtibially, the guide pin should be in the middle of the anteromedial footprint of the ACL on the femur so that when overreamed, the most distal portion of the drill hole will be at the junction of the anteromedial and posterolateral bundles. The guide pin is then overdrilled with an acorn drill to a depth of 40 mm (or until the femoral cortex is encountered) so that there is the opportunity to recess the bone block up into the femoral socket if necessary to maintain distal fixation. The graft is retrieved after the bone debris has been evacuated from the joint.

The bone block is positioned so that the tendinous portion of the graft is central on the femoral footprint and the screw is placed proximal to the bone block over a Nitinol guide wire to push the soft tissue attachment of the tendon to the middle of the ACL femoral footprint (Fig. 21-9). I routinely use titanium screws, because I have encountered a number of screw breakages using composite absorbable screws. This is particularly an issue with the very hard bone of high-performance young male athletes. Biocomposite absorbable screws are a reasonable alternative, but require the additional step of tapping, and may break on insertion if the bone is hard. Using a stainless steel wire in the bone block for tensioning will prevent inadvertent cutting of the tensioning sutures when tapping. When preparing the bone blocks on the back table, I size the block harvested from the tibia that is to be fixed in the femur to ensure a snug fit with less than a 1-mm gap in the sizing block. With this, a 7-mm screw will provide high-strength fixation for the femur, and it is easier to insert past the PCL without injuring the graft when the knee is flexed to 110 degrees. The screw should be 20 mm or longer for adequate strength of fixation.[19]

The graft is tensioned with the knee in full extension, applying maximal manual tension to the graft for fixation. When pre-

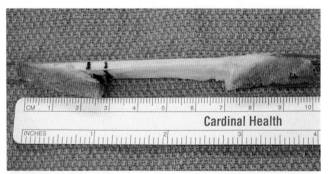

FIGURE 21-8 B-PT-B autograft demonstrating the 8 mm of additional bone harvested proximal to the tibial tubercle (marked in purple on the tendon). This will allow the graft to be recessed into the femoral socket to reduce graft-tunnel mismatch.

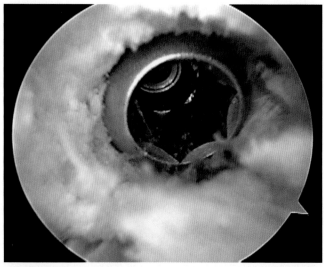

FIGURE 21-9 Titanium screw above the femoral bone block, putting the tendinous attachment in the middle of the ACL femoral footprint.

paring the bone block that was harvested from the patella, to be fixed in the tibia, there should be a 2-mm gap between the bone block and sizing hole. This will ensure that the block will slide in the tibial tunnel without binding as it is tensioned. With this 2-mm gap, a 9-mm interference screw is needed on the tibial side to ensure adequate fixation strength.[19] The screw length is determined by the position of the bone block within the tibial tunnel. At least 20 mm of screw in contact with the bone block is needed, and I try to obtain 25 mm or more, which is adequate length if the block remains in the tunnel. Prior to tensioning and fixing the graft in the tibia, I externally rotate the bone block 90 degrees (toward the fibula). This results in rotation of the flat graft, which mimics the anatomic positioning of the ACL anteromedial and posterolateral bundles on the tibia.[20]

The interference screw is then placed lateral to the bone block, between its cancellous surface and the tunnel wall. Any excess bone block extending out of the tibial tunnel can be cut off with a saw or rongeur.

PEARLS & PITFALLS

PEARLS

1. There should be more than one potential graft source, such as a B-PT-B autograft for high-demand patients, a quadrupled hamstring autograft for moderate-demand patients, and an allograft for lower demand patients or other mitigating circumstances.
2. The knee must be positioned to allow 120 degrees of flexion
3. For B-PT-B autografts, harvest an additional 8 mm of bone proximal to the tendon insertion on the tibia to allow the graft to be recessed into the femoral socket and reduce mismatch of the graft and tunnel lengths.
4. Extensive resection of the fat pad will facilitate visualization for drilling the femoral socket and fixing the graft.
5. Use the medial portal to pass the femoral guide wire and drill the femoral socket for soft tissue graft (transtibial for B-PT-B grafts).
6. For the medial portal technique, switch the Beath pin to a 2.0-mm Nitinol wire prior to drilling the femoral socket.
7. Fix grafts in 0 degree extension with high (25 pounds) of tensioning force to establish appropriate tension and preserve mobility.

PITFALLS

1. If the posterior femoral cortex is violated in drilling the femoral socket, alternative fixation options should be available (e.g., EndoButton; Smith & Nephew Endoscopy; Andover, Mass) or a second incision.
2. Inadequate fat pad resection interferes with visualization, drilling, and fixation for the femur.
3. The medial portal technique, while improving anatomic placement, limits femoral fixation options.
4. Biocomposite screws may break in the hard bone of young male athletes; consider titanium.

Postoperative Rehabilitation

Because the grafts are tensioned in 0 degree of extension, the patient should have no difficulty obtaining this in the immediate postoperative period.[17] My routine rehabilitation protocol keeps the patient in a postoperative adjustable brace locked in extension for 18 hours daily during the first 10 days. During the 6 hours out of the brace, the patient is in a continuous passive motion machine (CPM), stressing full extension to 0 degree and gradually regaining flexion from 40 degrees on the first postoperative day to 90 degrees by day 10, in 5-degree daily increments. Quadriceps setting exercises and straight leg lifts (in full 0-degree extension) out of the brace are used to minimize quadriceps atrophy. Hourly ankle pumps, elastic compression of the calf, and aspirin or a cyclooxygenase-1 (COX-1) nonsteroidal antiinflammatory are used during this period to reduce the risk of thrombophlebitis. At this point (10 days postoperatively), the patient is examined and formal physical therapy is begun, stressing swelling control and maintenance of muscle bulk. I continue use of the postoperative brace with the knee locked in extension for ambulation, but discontinue the brace for all other activities, until 4 weeks after surgery. This allows early revascularization of the graft and healing within the bone tunnels prior to significant stress being applied to the graft. It also allows the patient to regain excellent quadriceps control before being released from the brace to engage in routine daily activities, such as stair climbing and walking on uneven ground.

The remainder of the rehabilitation program is a graduated strength and endurance program designed not to stress the graft through unopposed quadriceps contraction early on, but to promote progressive gain in strength and endurance so that the patient will be adequately rehabilitated to resume high-risk (cutting or pivoting) athletic activities 4½ to 6 months following surgery. Jogging on flat level surfaces may be started at 10 weeks if the patient has adequate quadriceps strength and resolution of the effusion. Young (high school or college) athletes are often ready to return to resume their preinjury sport at this juncture, because they typically have the time to invest in their rehabilitation; however, working adults are often not adequately recovered until after 6 months because of time limits on their rehabilitation program.

REFERENCES

1. Larson RL, Taillon M. Anterior cruciate ligament insufficiency: Principles of treatment. *J Am Acad Orthop Surg.* 1994;2:26-35.
2. Howell SM, Gittins ME, Gottlieb JE, et al. The relationship between the angle of the tibial tunnel in the coronal plane and loss of flexion and anterior laxity after anterior cruciate ligament reconstruction. *Am J Sports Med.* 2001;29:567-574.
3. Simmons R, Howell SM, Hull ML. Effect of the angle of the femoral and tibial tunnels in the coronal plane and incremental excision of the posterior cruciate ligament on tension of an anterior cruciate ligament graft: an in vitro study. *J Bone Joint Surg Am.* 2003;85:1018-1029.
4. Raffo CS, Pizzarello P, Richmond JC, Pathare N. A reproducible landmark for the tibial tunnel origin in anterior cruciate ligament reconstruction: avoiding a vertical graft in the coronal plane. *J Arthrosc Rel Surg.* 2008;24:843-845.
5. Golish SR, Baumfeld JA, Schoderbek RJ, Miller MD. The effect of femoral tunnel starting position on tunnel length in anterior curciate ligament reconstruction: a cadaveric study. *Arthroscopy.* 2007;23:1187-1192.
6. Chhabra A, Starman JS, Ferretti M, et al. Anatomic radiographic, biomechanical and kinematic evaluation of the anterior cruciate ligament and its two functional bundles. *J Bone Joint Surg Am.* 2006;88:2-10.
7. Loh JC, Fukuda Y, Tsuda E, et al. Knee stability and graft function following anterior cruciate ligament reconstruction: comparison between 11 o'clock and 10 o'clock femoral tunnel placement. *J Arthrosc Relat Surg.* 2003;19:297-304.
8. Yagi M, Wong EK, Kanamori A, et al. Biomechanical analysis of an anatomic anterior cruciate ligament reconstruction. *Am J Sports Med.* 2002; 30:660-666.

9. Ho JY, Gardiner A, Shah V, Steiner ME: Equal Kinematics Between Central Anatomic Single-Bundle and Double-Bundle Anterior Cruciate Ligament Reconstructions. *Arthroscopy.* 2009;25:464-472.

10. Meredic RB, Vance KJ, Appleby D, Lubowitz JH. Outcome of single-bundle versus double-bundle reconstruction of the anterior cruciate ligament—a meta analysis. *Am J Sports Med.* 2008;36:1414-1420.

11. Goldblatt JP, Fitzsimmons SE, Balk E, Richmond JC. Reconstruction of the anterior cruciate ligament: meta-analysis of patellar tendon versus hamstring tendon autograft. *Arthroscopy.* 2005;21:791-803.

12. Prodromos CC, Joyce BT, Shi K, Keller BL. A meta-analysis of stability after anterior cruciate ligament reconstruction as a function of hamstring versus patellar-tendon graft and fixation type. *Arthroscopy.* 2005; 21:1202-1208.

13. Poolman RW, Farrokhyar F, Bhandari M. Hamstring tendon autograft better than bone patellar-tendon bone autograft in ACL reconstruction: a cumulative meta-analysis and clinically relevant sensitivity analysis applied to a previously published analysis. *Acta Orthop.* 2007;78:350-354.

14. Prodromos CC, Joyce BT, Shi K, Keller BL. A meta-analysis of stability of autograft compared to allografts after anterior cruciate ligament reconstruction. *Knee Surg Sports Traumatol Arthrosc.* 2007;15:851-856.

15. Singhal MC, Gardiner JR, Johnson DL. Failure of primary anterior cruciate ligament surgery using anterior tibialis allograft. *Arthroscopy.* 2007; 23:469-475.

16. Lee BI, Kwon SW, Kim JB, et al. Comparison of clinical results according to amount of preserved remnant in arthroscopic anterior cruciate ligament reconstruction using quadrupled hamstring graft. *Arthroscopy.* 2008;24:560-568.

17. Nabors ED, Richmond JC, Vannah WM, McConville OR. Anterior cruciate ligament graft tensioning in full extension. *Am J Sports Med.* 1995; 23:488-492.

18. Shaffer B, Gow W, Tibone JE. Graft-Tunnel mismatch in endoscopic anterior cruciate ligament reconstruction: a new technique of intra-articular measurement and modified graft harvesting. *Arthroscopy.* 1993;9: 633-646.

19. Hulstyn M, Fadale PD, Abate J, Walsh WR. Biomechanical evaluation of interference screw fixation in a bovine patellar bone-tendon-bone autograft complex for anterior cruciate ligament reconstruction. *Arthroscopy.*1993;9:417-424.

20. Samuelson TS, Drez Jr. D, Maletis GB: Anterior cruciate ligament graft rotation: reproduction of normal graft rotation. *Am J Sports Med.* 1996; 24:67-71.

SUGGESTED READINGS

Ferretti M, Ekdahl M, Shen W, Fu FH. Osseous landmarks of the femoral attachment of the anterior cruciate ligament: an anatomic study. *J Arthrosc Relat Surg.* 2007;23:1218-1225.

Meredick RB, Vance KJ, Appleby D, Lubowitz JH. Outcome of single-bundle versus double-bundle reconstruction of the anterior cruciate ligament: a meta-analysis. *Am J Sports Med.* 2008;36:1414-1421.

Prodromos CC, Fu FH, Howell SM, et al. Controversies in soft-tissue anterior cruciate ligament reconstruction: grafts, bundles, tunnels, fixation, and harvest. *J Am Acad Orthop Surg.* 2008;16:376-384.

West RV, Harner CD. Graft selection in anterior cruciate ligament reconstruction. *J Am Acad Orthop Surg.* 2005;13:197-207.

Zelle BA, Vidal AF, Brucker PU, Fu FH. Double-bundle reconstruction of the anterior cruciate ligament: anatomic and biomechanical rationale. *J Am Acad Orthop Surg.* 2007;15:87-96.

Double-Bundle Anterior Cruciate Ligament Reconstruction

Joon Ho Wang ● Eric J. Kropf ● Freddie H. Fu

Successful clinical results following single-bundle cruciate ligament (ACL) reconstruction have been reported in 70% to 90% of cases.[1,2] Historically, single-bundle ACL reconstruction techniques have been the standard treatment of choice for the ACL-deficient knee. As more and more patients have been helped through advanced surgical techniques and rehabilitation protocols, the expectations of future patients have risen. Today, almost all patients who suffer an acute ACL injury expect to return to full, unlimited sports activity in a rapid fashion. However, residual rotational instability has been reported in approximately 20% of cases after conventional single-bundle reconstruction.[3] A recent biomechanical study has shown that single-bundle ACL reconstruction can successfully control anterior tibial translation but could not control a combined rotatory load of internal rotation and valgus torque.[4] Similarly, in vivo kinematic studies have shown that ACL reconstruction can restore anteroposterior stability. However, the tibia remains externally rotated relative to the femur during normal kinematics of running.[5] The concept of anatomic ACL reconstruction is predicated on a desire to restore native anatomy more closely and in turn, normal kinematics of the knee.

Multiple anatomic studies have used various methods to demonstrate that the ACL is composed of two distinct functional bundles; the anteromedial (AM) and posterolateral (PL) bundles (Fig. 22-1).[6-8] Biomechanical studies have demonstrated that in situ forces, in response to an anterior tibial and combined rotatory load, are greatest in the PL bundle near full extension and at 60 degrees flexion in the AM bundle, respectively. Studies have also shown that reconstruction of either of the individual bundles alone cannot reproduce the mechanical properties of the native intact ACL.[9,10] Yagi and colleagues[11] have measured the in situ forces in response to an anterior tibial load and a combined rotatory load of internal rotation and valgus torque using a robotic universal force moment sensor testing system. When compared with single-bundle ACL reconstruction, the in situ forces in double-bundle reconstructed knees more closely approximated those of the native ACL.

ANATOMY

The ACL courses from the medial aspect of the lateral femoral condyle (femoral insertion site) to a position on the tibia between the medial and lateral tibial spines (tibial insertion site). For the sake of consistency, this chapter refers to positional relationships with the knee located in the anatomic position or full knee extension. It is important to realize that arthroscopic evaluation of the ACL typically occurs with the knee flexed to 90 degrees. For this reason, the anatomically anterior border of the ACL will appear arthroscopically as the superior border. Similarly, the anatomically posterior extent of the ACL will appear as the arthroscopic inferior border when the knee is flexed to 90 degrees (Fig. 22-2). The femoral insertion site or ACL origin is located at the anatomically posterior aspect of the lateral surface of the femoral intercondylar notch. The length of the femoral footprint of the ACL is 17.7 ± 1.2 mm and the width is 9.9 ± 0.8 mm. The femoral attachment of the AM bundle forms an angle with the PL bundle of 27.6 ± 8.8 degrees.[12] The average length of the femoral AM bundle is 9.8 ± 0.8 mm, and the average length of the femoral PL bundle is 7.3 ± 0.5 mm. The anatomically anterior (arthroscopically superior) border of the femoral insertion of the ACL is defined by an important bony landmark[13] referred to as the lateral intercondylar ridge (see Fig. 22-2). In a surgical observational study, no ACL fibers could be seen attaching anterior to the ridge. The lateral bifurcate ridge, another important osseous landmark, delineates the AM and PL insertion areas. Ferretti and associates[12] arthroscopically visualized the lateral bifurcate ridge in 49 of 60 patients undergoing ACL reconstruction. Of the 49 patients with a discernible lateral bifurcate ridge, 25 had a prominent ridge with a significant change of slope, whereas the other 24 had a relatively smaller but evident ridge.

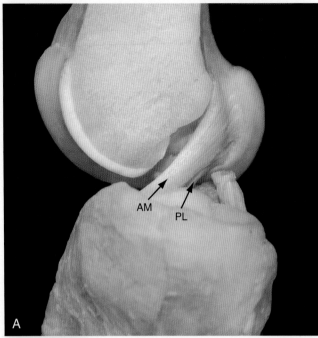

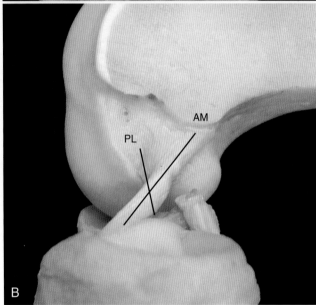

FIGURE 22-1 Cadaveric specimen human knee, sagittal view after the medial femoral condyle has been hemisected and removed. **A,** 0 degree. The AM and PL bundles are seen in parallel. **B,** 90 degrees of flexion. The AM and PL bundles are crossed.

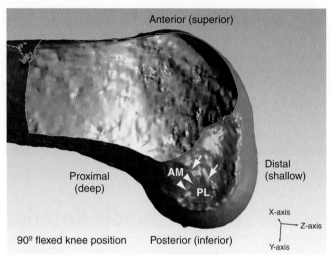

FIGURE 22-2 The surface of the distal femur lateral condyle has been scanned and the femoral insertion sites (AM and PL bundles) have been digitized with a FaroArm Laser scanner (FARO Technologies; Lake Mary, Fla). The lateral intercondylar ridge, or resident's ridge (*arrows*), defines the superior or anterior border of the ACL insertion site. The lateral bifurcate ridge (*arrowheads*) separates the AM and PL bundles. The relative orientation of the insertion sites can be described by two methods: (1) based on the anatomic position, or 0 degree (anterior-posterior-proximal-distal), and (2) arthroscopic view, or 90 degrees (superior-inferior-shallow-deep).

Anatomic ACL reconstruction is based on a comprehensive understanding of normal anatomy. It is important to realize that the course of the AM and PL bundles is distinct, with the bundles lining up in parallel near full extension and then crossing as the knee approaches 90 degrees of flexion (see Fig. 22-1).[6,12,14-16] Specifically, the AM bundle originates at the anatomically posterior and proximal (arthroscopically inferior and deep) aspect of the lateral wall of the intercondylar notch. The PL bundle originates at the anatomically posterior and distal (arthroscopically inferior and shallow) aspect of the lateral wall of the notch (see Fig. 22-2). From the femoral origin, the fibers

of the ACL course down to the tibial insertion site. In its mid-portion, the ACL tapers to a thinner diameter, similar to an hourglass shape. The cross-sectional area of the insertion sites are 3 to 3.5 times larger than the cross-sectional area of the ligament's midsubstance.[8,17] The ACL fibers fan out and insert on the center of the tibial plateau, between the two spines. It is for their relative insertion sites on the tibia that the two bundles of the ACL are named, with the AM tibial insertion site slightly anterior and medial to the PL bundle insertion site (Fig. 22-3.) The mean length of the tibial insertion has been reported in multiple studies[7,18,19] to range from 14 mm (range, 9 to 18 mm) to 29.3 mm (range, 23 to 38 mm). The total area of the tibial insertion has also been reported with great variability, from 114 to 229 mm^2. The area of the AM bundle insertion alone has been reported from 56 to 136 mm^2 and the PL bundle from 52 to 93 mm^2. The tremendous variability in reported size and area of the tibial insertion sites likely stems from the various methods used for taking measurements and the variable size of the cadaveric specimens used.[20]

Biomechanics

Recent biomechanical studies have more clearly defined the specific function of the two individual bundles of the ACL. Selective sectioning studies have shown that transection of the AM bundle increases anterior translation of tibia at 60 and 90 degrees of knee flexion. Conversely, transection of the PL bundle increases anterior translation of the tibia at 30 degrees of flexion. Following PL bundle transection, there was also increased rotation at 0 and 30 degrees in response to a combined rotatory load.[21]

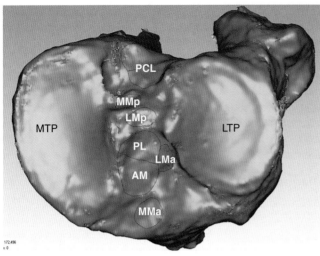

FIGURE 22-3 The surface of the proximal tibia was scanned and the boundaries of the ACL and surrounding structures were digitized with the FaroArm Laser scanner. The boundary of the ACL can be described in relation to the medial and lateral tibial spines, the posterior root of the lateral meniscus (LMp) , the anterior insertion site of the lateral meniscus (LMa), the anterior root of the medial meniscus (MMa). AM, anteromedial bundle of the ACL; LTP, lateral tibial plateau; MMp, posterior insertion of the medial meniscus; MTP, medial tibial plateau; PCL, posterior cruciate ligament; PL, posterolateral bundle of the ACL.

In general, the concept of isometry in ACL reconstruction should be dismissed. The AM and PL bundles do not remain isometric throughout a full functional range of motion. Each bundle of native ACL is exposed to varying degrees of tension at various flexion angles.[22] The AM bundle is slightly more isometric than the PL bundle, remaining taut throughout a greater arc of motion. In contrast, the PL bundle is taut with the knee in extension and is lax when the knee is flexed. Logically, the contribution of the PL bundle to knee stability becomes increasingly important under greater degrees of tension, or near full extension.[9,10,23]

Injury Mechanism and Rupture Pattern

Understanding the mechanism of injury is an important first step in formulating an appropriate treatment strategy. Various injury mechanisms will place differential strains on the AM and PL bundles, thus producing various rupture patterns. Two distinct injury mechanisms of ACL have been classically described by Muller[24]: (1) hyperextension trauma, with resultant stretch of the ACL over the anterior intercondylar notch roof; and (2) moderate extension trauma, during which the AM bundle is taut and a valgus and/or external rotation force is applied. Based on the variable tension patterns exhibited different positions of knee flexion, we have seen a variety of two bundle injury patterns and isolated AM or isolated PL bundle injuries (Fig. 22-4). Isolated PL bundle injury occurs when stress is applied at or near full extension. In greater degrees of flexion (30 to 60 degrees), isolated AM bundle injury can occur.

In a prospective study, 121 consecutive patients were evaluated arthroscopically. with attention directed to determining the pattern of rupture.[25] All patients were evaluated within 120 days of acute injury. There was complete rupture of the AM and PL bundles in 75% of patients. In the remaining 25% of patients, partial tear of the ACL could be seen. In 12% of total patients, no evidence of PL bundle injury could be seen. Therefore, we think that meticulous dissection of the remnant ACL is an important first step prior to proceeding with the reconstructive aspect of ACL surgery. Single-bundle augmentation is performed when appropriate, according to the specific injury pattern.[26] Preservation of intact native tissue has distinct advantages, including preservation of the microvasculature and proprioceptive fibers. Isolated reconstruction of the AM or PL bundle alone requires an awareness of such injury patterns and more precise preoperative and intraoperative diagnostic assessment of the injury pattern.

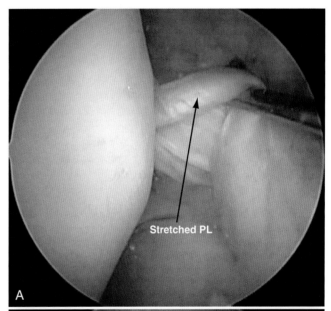

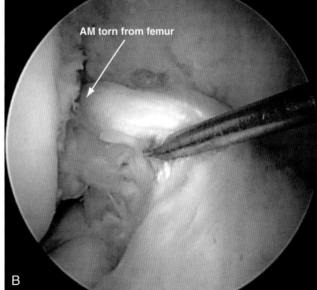

FIGURE 22-4 ACL pattern of injury is variable, depending on the mechanism of injury. **A,** Arthroscopic view of the right knee reveals a stretched but grossly intact PL bundle. **B,** Arthroscopic image from a different patient reveals an AM bundle torn from the femoral side and a partially intact PL bundle.

PATIENT EVALUATION

History and Physical Examination

In cases of acute ACL injury, patients typically present with painful swelling, limp, and an obvious history of trauma. Common mechanisms include landing after jumping, a deceleration change in direction seen in pivoting sports (e.g., soccer, basketball, tennis), and direct blow forces on the lateral side of the knee producing valgus and external rotational force on the tibia. Some patients will report an audible pop or the sensation of tearing at the time of injury. A significant effusion typically occurs within a few hours of injury. A flexed posture of the knee joint can be seen caused by the large hemarthrosis, but should also raise concern for the possibility of mechanical obstruction from the remnant ACL or a bucket handle tear of the meniscus. In patients with a history of trauma followed by hemarthrosis, the most common arthroscopic finding is ACL injury (45% in a study of 320 patients).[27]

In cases of chronic ACL insufficiency, swelling becomes a variable symptom. Recurrent instability or giving way associated with pain and/or limitation of activity and sports typically brings most patients in for clinical evaluation. Recurrent episodes of instability may result in secondary injury, such as meniscal tear or cartilage damage, leading to further pain and complaints.

The clinical evaluation begins when the patient is coming into the room. Gait pattern and overall limb alignment should be assessed and recorded. On first presentation, the entire lower extremity should be evaluated. A detailed examination of the knee then ensues, including inspection, palpation, range of motion, and stability.

A manual assessment of knee laxity includes several tests—the Lachman, anterior drawer, and pivot shift tests. The Lachman test is considered to be the most reliable test for assessment of ACL injury.[28] However, false-negative findings can be seen in acute cases when significant hamstring spasm and guarding are present. To avoid a high false-negative rate, effort should be made to have the patient as relaxed as possible. The Lachman test is performed at 20 to 30 degrees of knee flexion. One hand of the examiner stabilizes the femur and the other hand applies an anteriorly directed force to the proximal tibia. The degree of translation and the quality or firmness of the end point should be noted. Classification of anteroposterior translation is categorized as grade I (3 to 5 mm), grade II (6 to 10 mm), or grade III (more than 10 mm).

The anterior drawer test is performed at 90 degrees of knee flexion with the foot stabilized and an anteriorly directed force applied to the proximal tibia. The examiner should palpate the medial femoral condyle and note the degree of anterior tibial translation relative to the medial femoral condyle. Anterior pseudolaxity can occur in the setting of PCL injury in which the tibia is resting in a posteriorly subluxated position. Reduction of the tibia from the posteriorly subluxated position can be mistakenly perceived as excessive anterior tibial translation.

The pivot shift test is highly specific for the diagnosis of ACL injury, but the sensitivity is low, particularly in the awake patient. Most patients may allow for a single shift to be performed, but will typically guard against allowing the knee to shift thereafter.[28,29] The pivot shift maneuver mimics the giving way or buckling phenomenon that patients experience. A pivot shift test is performed with the patient supine and the hip in slight abduction as a valgus force is applied to the extended knee. In the ACL-deficient knee, the tibia rests in an internally rotated and anteriorly subluxated position. As the knee is flexed to 20 degrees, the tibia reduces, suddenly resulting in the pivot shift. The degree of shift is graded as grade I or pivot glide, grade II or distinct shift, and grade III or transiently locked out. This test can be difficult to perform in the awake patient but is highly sensitive and specific during the examination under anesthesia.[30]

Diagnostic Imaging

Plain radiographs should be included in the initial clinical evaluation of all patients presenting with a history of trauma and acute hemarthrosis. A standard radiographic evaluation of the knee should include the standing anteroposterior (AP), lateral, axial or patellofemoral view (Merchant, Laurin, or sunrise view). These are of far greater usefulness for assessing malalignment, joint space narrowing, and other early signs of degenerative arthritis. At our institution, we typically obtain a single AP view, with the knee in full extension.

In most cases of acute ACL injury, plain radiographs will be negative. Still, radiographs are necessary to rule out combined ligamentous injury, secondary arthritic changes, or physeal injury in the skeletally immature patient. The Segond fracture, or lateral tibial rim avulsion of the meniscotibial ligament, is considered pathognomonic for ACL injury. This lateral capsular avulsion is produced by the stress of knee flexion and internal tibial rotation commonly seen as a mechanism of ACL injury.[31]

Magnetic resonance imaging (MRI) is highly sensitive and specific for the diagnosis of acute ACL tear.[32] However, it is often far more difficult to differentiate partial tears from complete tears or to detect isolated single-bundle tear patterns. There is great variability in clinically available MRI magnets. High-resolution MRI with dedicated ACL sequences greatly increases the sensitivity of MRI. Standard MRI protocols consist of sagittal, coronal, and axial T1- and T2-weighted images (Fig. 22-5). The issue with such sequences is that the ACL does not course through the knee in a perfectly coronal or sagittal plane. Therefore, to improve sensitivity, we use modified oblique coronal and oblique sagittal imaging sequences. When the beam is oriented parallel to the fibers of the ACL, greater detail is appreciated and the AM and PL bundles can be evaluated independently. (Figs. 22-6 and 22-7).

TREATMENT

Arthroscopic Technique

Operating Room Setup and Examination Under Anesthesia

ACL reconstruction can be performed under general or spinal anesthesia based on patient and surgeon preference. The examination under anesthesia can provide additional valuable information and should be performed in all cases. When compared with the office examination, the sensitivity of the pivot shift test is greatly enhanced.[29] Once the patient is under anesthesia, we

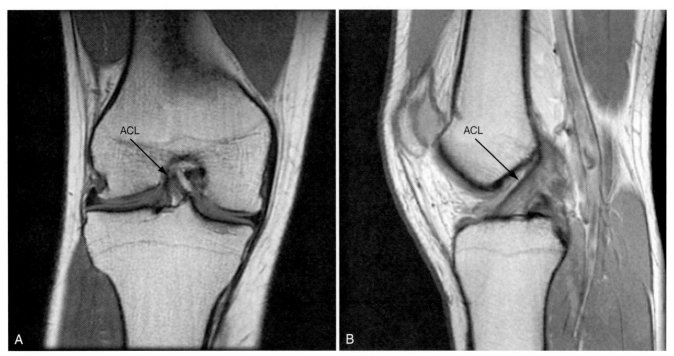

FIGURE 22-5 Conventional T1-weighted MRI scans of the right knee. coronal **(A)** and sagittal **(B)** plane images provide little detail of the anatomy of the native ACL in this case.

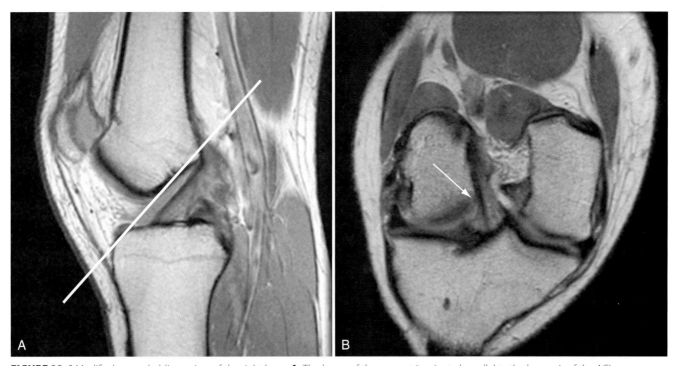

FIGURE 22-6 Modified coronal oblique view of the right knee. **A,** The beam of the magnet is oriented parallel to the long axis of the ACL. **B,** A slightly oblique coronal view is subsequently obtained and greater anatomic detail of the native ACL is seen in this case *(arrow)*.

routinely evaluate the range of motion and perform a comprehensive manual assessment of knee laxity including the pivot shift, Lachman, and anterior and posterior drawer tests to evaluate the degree of anteroposterior laxity.

Once the physical examination is complete, the operative limb is placed in an arthroscopic leg holder with a well-padded

tourniquet placed high on the thigh. The patient must be positioned far down on the bed and the foot of the bed maximally flexed to allow the knee to be ranged from full extension to at least 120 degrees of flexion during various aspects of the procedure (Fig. 22-8). The operative limb should be comfortably positioned so that the knee assumes a position of 90-degree flexion

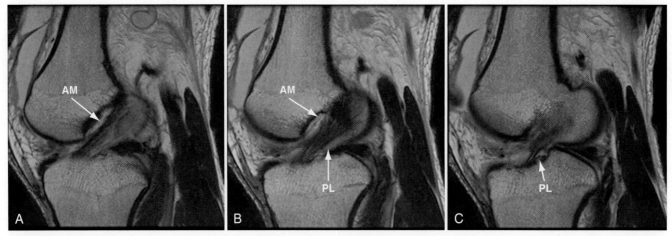

FIGURE 22-7 Modified sagittal oblique view of the right knee. When the beam of the magnet is oriented parallel to the lateral femoral condyle, this plane similarly parallels the axis of the ACL and provides greater anatomic detail of the native ACL. Three successive T2-weighted 1.5-mm cuts are shown here defining the AM bundle alone **(A)**, the AM and PL bundles on one image **(B)**, and the final fibers of the PL bundle alone **(C)**.

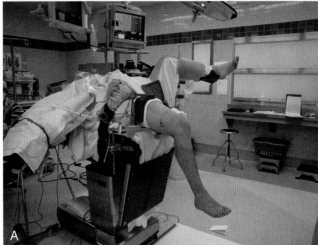

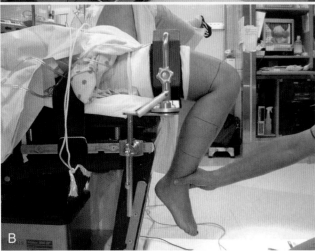

FIGURE 22-8 Operative setup. **A,** The leg is positioned in an arthrocopic leg holder with the contralateral leg well padded and positioned out of the field to allow easy access to the medial side of the knee. **B,** The patient must be positioned to allow for 120 degrees of flexion during later femoral tunnel drilling.

at rest. The nonoperative leg is placed in a well-leg holder with the hip flexed and abducted to allow for unobstructed approach to the operative knee. The operative leg is then prepped in a sterile fashion and draped.

Portal Placement and Diagnostic Arthroscopy

As with all arthroscopic procedures, portal placement is the first and often most important step. Properly placed portals facilitate ease of successful surgery. Conversely, poorly placed portals will only complicate the procedure. In the case of anatomic double-bundle ACL reconstruction, accurately placed portals are necessary to visualize the anatomic landmarks located at the ACL insertion sites properly. With the knee in 90 degrees of flexion, an anterolateral viewing portal is first established just lateral to the patellar tendon (Fig. 22-9). This portal should be placed in a slightly more proximal position, with the distal extent of the portal ending at the level of the inferior pole of the patella. By placing this portal high, less of the patellar fat pad is traversed. Superior visualization of the tibial insertion sites is also achieved. The portal is established with a no. 11 blade and dilated with a straight hemostat to allow easy passage of instruments. The anteromedial portal is established next via 18-gauge needle localization in a similar fashion. This portal will function as both a viewing portal and a working portal. It is positioned at the joint line just above the meniscus and immediately adjacent to the edge of the inferomedial portion of the patellar tendon.

Arthroscopic examination is then performed and associated meniscal or chondral injury is addressed as necessary. The fat pad is débrided to allow clear visualization of the anterior horn of the medial meniscus. Needle localization is again used to establish the accessory medial portal (AMP) at this point. This portal should provide direct access to the most distal and anterior aspects of the lateral intercondylar notch where the PL tunnel will later be drilled (Fig. 22-10). When the needle is introduced, it should be directed toward the PL insertion sited to ensure adequate access for later drilling of the tunnel. The correct position of this portal is significantly more medial than standard medial portals. Therefore, it lies

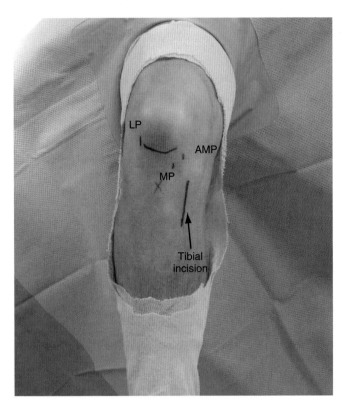

FIGURE 22-9 Three-portal technique. the AL portal is established at the level of the inferior pole of the patella. The medial portal (MP) and accessory medial portal (AMP) are established via needle localization at the level of the joint line. The tibial incision is centered between the crest and the posteromedial border of the tibia at the level of the tubercle.

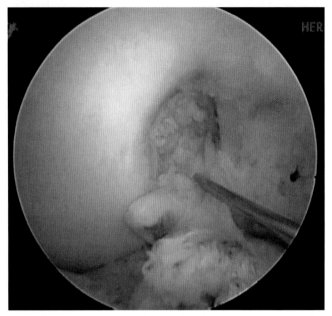

FIGURE 22-10 Accessory medial portal. In this arthroscopic image of a right knee, the accessory medial portal is established via needle localization. Note that the needle enters the notch above the medial meniscus and at a safe distance from the articular cartilage of the medial femoral condyle. The angle of entry allows direct access for later drilling of the PL femoral tunnel.

close to the medial condyle and careful attention must be taken to avoid iatrogenic cartilage injury.

Graft Choice and Preparation

Both autograft and allograft options exist for double-bundle ACL reconstruction.[33-35] However, there are several important factors that should be appreciated when considering double-bundle ACL reconstruction. Most importantly, with autograft tissue, there are inherent limitations on the size and amount of tissue available. Consistent methods for preoperative prediction of hamstring size do not exist. Therefore, it is very likely that the surgeon could be left with insufficient tissue for double-bundle reconstruction with conventional harvest methods. In contrast, allograft tissue affords a greater quantity of tissue without additional donor site morbidity. Still, allograft tissue has several significant drawbacks, including delayed revascularization, tissue reaction, potential risks of disease transmission, high costs and, in some settings, limited availability. Therefore, graft selection should be individualized for each particular situation.

Commonly, two soft tissue allografts (tibialis anterior, tibialis posterior or semitendinosus) provide ample graft for most cases of double-bundle reconstruction. A 24-cm long allograft is doubled over to yield a 12-cm length double-stranded graft of variable diameter. In most cases, the AM bundle is trimmed to a final diameter of 7 to 8 mm and the PL bundle is trimmed to a final diameter of 5 to 7 mm. Both ends of the graft are initially

sutured about 2 to 3 cm with a modified baseball stitch with no. 2 Ticron sutures. It is important to realize that anatomic ACL reconstruction is not dependent on particular types of instrumentation or fixation. Anatomy can be correctly restored with various methods of fixation. We typically use various forms of fixation, including interference screws, suture post fixation, and EndoButtons (Smith & Nephew; Andover, Mass).

For consistency, we will describe our experience using the EndoButton CL (Smith &Nephew), which is probably our most frequently used form of fixation. Per routine, each graft is looped over an EndoButton CL to serve as the femoral fixation point. The length of the EndoButton loop is tailored to ensure that a minimum of 20 mm of graft is engaged within the tunnel. The length of the EndoButton loop is determined by subtracting 20 mm from the total distance from the aperture of the tunnel to the lateral cortex. The tunnel should be dilated to a distance 7 mm longer than the desired length of graft engagement inside the tunnel to allow for ease of flipping the EndoButton. For example, a 15-mm EndoButton can be used after dilating a 27-mm tunnel when the total length from aperture to the lateral femoral cortex is 35 mm. To ensure that the graft is passed and seated properly, two lines are provisionally marked on the femoral end of the graft. The first mark is placed at 20 mm from the end and a second line at 27 mm. The second line marks the point where the graft must be pulled into the tunnel to flip the EndoButton safely, and the first line marks the appropriate final position of

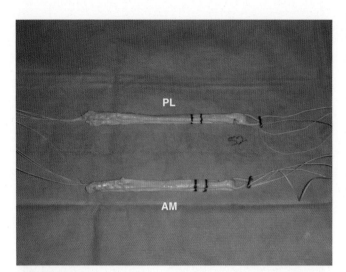

FIGURE 22-11 Final prepared grafts. In this case, two soft tissue allografts are looped over the appropriately sized EndoButton. The graft is marked at two locations. The first line represents the desired position of the fixated graft. The second line represents the distance that the graft must be pulled into the tunnel to flip the EndoButton safely.

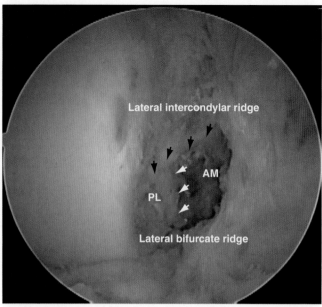

FIGURE 22-12 Arthroscopic image of the right knee viewed through the medial portal. Once the remnant ACL has been carefully débrided, the lateral intercondylar ridge (*black arrows*) and the lateral bifurcate ridge (*white arrows*) are easily visualized defining the borders of the native AM and PL bundles.

the graft when 20 mm is in the tunnel and the graft is secured (Fig. 22-11). In a similar fashion, a hamstring autograft can be used for double-bundle ACL reconstruction. The semitendinosus tendon is typically prepared as the AM bundle and the gracilis tendon is doubled or tripled over to serve as the PL bundle.[33] If this does not provide adequate tissue, the surgeon should be prepared to augment with allograft, as needed.

Identification of the Anterior Cruciate Ligament Insertion Site Footprint

Once the portals have been established and sufficient fat pad has been débrided to visualize the notch clearly, the ACL is closely inspected. The remnant tissue should not be aggressively or quickly débrided, but rather carefully dissected back to the true anatomic insertion sites. In approximately 10% of cases, we have found that one of the bundles is functional and can be preserved. In such cases, the intact bundle is preserved and single-bundle augmentation surgery is performed according to the injury pattern.[36] If it has been decided that no functional tissue remains, a radiofrequency thermal device (ArthroCare; Sunnyvale, Calif) is used to define the anatomic insertion sites clearly. Importantly, notchplasty is not routinely performed. Notchplasty would destroy the normal bony landmark and distort normal anatomic structures.

In cases of chronic ACL injury, the remnant ACL is often not clearly preserved. If it is difficult to delineate the anatomic outer margin of the footprint, osseous landmarks at the femoral origin can be used to define the anatomic insertion sites of two bundles.[12] The lateral intercondylar ridge forms the anterior (or arthroscopically viewed superior) border of the ACL. The lateral bifurcate ridge divides the AM bundle insertion site from the PL bundle insertion site (Fig. 22-12).

The tibial insertion site is then similarly examined. It is typically easier to define the femoral insertion sites and then track the remnant tissue back to the tibial insertion. When significant remnant ACL tissue remains, the PL bundle can be better isolated by viewing from the lateral portal, with the knee in a figure-of-four position. This places the PL bundle under maximal tension, making it clearly visible adjacent to the root of the posterior horn of the lateral meniscus. In cases of chronic ACL deficiency, when the ACL stump has already been resorbed or only fibrous tissue remains, the PCL, intermeniscal ligament, and lateral meniscus attachments provide important intra-articular cues for tibial tunnel positioning. It is important to note that the distance between the PCL and the center of the ACL footprint varies significantly among patients and is not a reliable tool for placement of the tibial tunnel.

Measurement of Footprint Size

After the femoral and tibial footprints have been defined, measurements are taken. A metallic ruler is inserted through the anteromedial portal, with the arthroscope in the lateral portal. We measure the length and width of each insertion site on the tibia and femur (Fig. 22-13). To measure the femoral insertion sites accurately, the arthroscope must be moved to the accessory medial portal while the ruler is kept in the anteromedial portal (Fig. 22-14).

At this point, based on the total length of the footprint, we determine whether to proceed with double-bundle surgery or to perform anatomic single-bundle surgery. If the total length of the femoral insertion site is 14 mm or less, double-bundle surgery is not technically feasible, because the two tunnels would need to be of extremely small diameter or risk collapsing into one another. It is important to realize that the femoral insertion

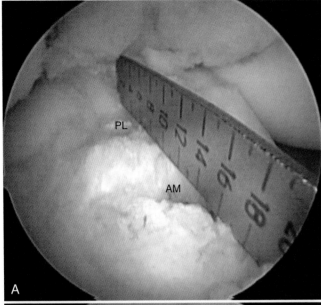

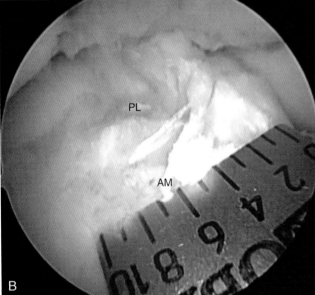

FIGURE 22-13 A, B, With the arthroscope in the anterolateral viewing portal, a ruler is passed through the anteromedial portal. The length and width of the native ACL tibial insertion site are measured and recorded for all cases.

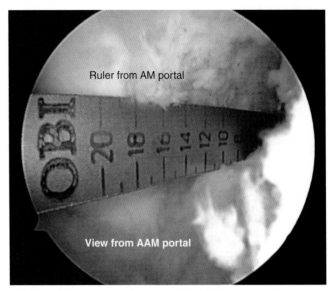

FIGURE 22-14 Arthroscopic image of the right knee. With the arthroscope in the accessory medial portal, the ruler is passed through the medial portal and the width and length of the femoral insertion sites are measured and recorded.

study has revealed that the average length of the femoral AM insertion is 9.8 ± 1 mm and that of the femoral PL insertion is 7.3 ± 0.5 mm.[12] However, realize that the chosen reamer size should be slightly smaller than the actual size of the insertion site due because of the widening effect of the tunnel created by the oblique approach of the reamer to the bony surface of the notch. Generally, we select a reamer 1 to 2 mm smaller than the size of the insertion site to maintain an adequate bone bridge between tunnels (Fig. 22-15).

size is the limiting factor when deciding whether to proceed with double-bundle reconstruction. This occurs for two reasons. First, the total length of the femoral footprint is typically about 2 mm smaller than the tibial footprint. This is because of the manner whereby the ACL fibers fan out at the tibial footprint, with some fibers actually inserting beneath the intermeniscal ligament. Also, as a result of the oblique angle by which the reamer must approach the femur, the size of the drilled tunnel aperture will actually be slightly larger than the true diameter of the reamer.

We individualize the sizes of the AM and PL tunnels based on the size of the native insertion sites in all cases. A recent anatomic

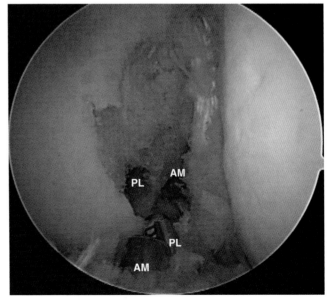

FIGURE 22-15 Arthroscopic image of the right knee viewed from the medial portal. The AM and PL tibial and femoral tunnels have all been created. Note that a small bone bridge exists between the two femoral tunnels.

Tunnel Placement

For creation of the femoral tunnels, the arthroscope is inserted through the anteromedial viewing portal. When the portal has been properly positioned, the trajectory of the arthroscope will look slightly up, allowing for a view of the entire lateral wall of the intercondylar notch. The centers of the femoral insertion sites of the PL and AM bundles are preliminarily marked with a Steadman awl inserted through the accessory anteromedial (AAM) portal). The femoral-sided PL tunnel is made first. A 3.2-mm guide wire is inserted through the AAM portal at 90 degrees of knee flexion and aimed to the previously marked point. The pin is gently tapped with a mallet to engage the pin into the provisional hole at about 3 mm. After engaging the pin, the knee is bent to 110 to 120 degrees. By placing the knee in a deep flexion angle, the trajectory of the pin is aimed more anteriorly. Therefore, the risk of peroneal nerve injury is minimized. When the reamer is passed over the guide pin, the articular cartilage of the medial femoral condyle must be visualized directly. The trajectory of this tunnel is far different than that of conventional ACL reconstruction methods, and the risk of iatrogenic chondral injury is high if care is not taken to protect the medial femoral condyle. A 5-mm cannulated reamer is inserted over the guide wire through the AAM portal and drilled to a 25-mm depth. The 4.5-mm cannulated EndoButton reamer is then drilled out through the lateral cortex. The EndoButton depth gauge is used to measure the distance from the inner aperture to the lateral cortex. The appropriately sized EndoButton is then chosen to ensure that 20 mm of graft is engaged within the tunnel. To avoid excessive widening of the tunnel, we sequentially hand-dilate up from 5 mm in 0.5-mm increments to the final desired tunnel diameter (usually 6 to 7 mm)

Attention is next turned to creation of the tibial tunnels. A 3- to 4-cm vertical skin incision is made over the proximal tibia 1 to 2 cm distal to the joint line and centered over the tibia, 1 to 2 cm medial to the tibial tubercle. Sharp dissection is carried down to the tibia, ensuring that the fibers of the medial collateral ligament (MCL) are not violated. Full-thickness soft tissue flaps are reflected anteriorly and posteriorly to allow a safe distance for the creation of two tibial tunnels. Next, the arthroscope is reinserted through the anterolateral portal and the tibial footprint is visualized directly. An ACL tip guide, set at 45 degrees, is inserted through AAM portal for creation of the PL tibial tunnel. The tip of the guide is centered at the previously marked anatomic insertion site of the PL bundle. The ACL guide is secured externally over the anteromedial cortex of the tibia, just anterior to the leading edge of the superficial MCL. A 3.2-mm guide wire is inserted through the drill sleeve and advanced to the footprint of the PL bundle. The ACL tip guide is then removed from the knee, adjusted to 55 degrees, and reinserted through the AM portal

for creation of the AM tibial tunnel. The tip of the guide is again aimed at the center of the anatomic insertion site of the AM bundle, and the drill sleeve is advanced down to the anteromedial tibial cortex. A minimum of a 1.5-cm bony bridge should be maintained between the two tunnels on the external tibia. Both tibial tunnels are then provisionally drilled with a 5- or 6-mm reamer. The tunnels are hand-dilated up to the final desired tunnel diameter to minimize the risk of excessive tunnel widening.

The femoral AM tunnel is the last tunnel created. The femoral AM tunnel can be drilled through one of three different approaches: (1) transtibial AM; 2) transtibial PL; or (3) accessory medial portal (Fig. 22-16). The deciding factor is always the ability to re-create the true anatomic location. If a transtibial guide wire can safely reach the previously marked true anatomic location, the transtibial technique is preferred because it creates a slightly longer and divergent tunnel relative to the femoral PL tunnel. If this is not possible, the accessory AM portal should be used to place the femoral AM tunnel. A transtibial approach through the tibial PL tunnel works in about 20% of cases. A correctly positioned accessory medial portal approach will provide excellent access to the true femoral AM tunnel position in all cases. Once the appropriate technique is determined, the tunnel is provisionally drilled to a depth of 25 mm with an acorn bit. The far cortex of the AM femoral tunnel is then breached with a 4.5-mm EndoButton drill (Smith & Nephew Endoscopy), and the depth gauge is used to measure the distance to the far cortex. The tunnel is dilated or hand-reamed up to the final desired diameter with the final determined depth for EndoButton fixation, similar to the PL tunnel.

Graft Passage

A Beath pin with a suture loop in its eyelet is first passed through the AAM portal and up through the femoral PL tunnel. The looped suture is retrieved with a suture retriever passed through the PL tibial tunnel. Another Beath pin with a looped suture is similarly passed through the AM femoral tunnel and retrieved through the AM tibial tunnel (Fig. 22-17). The PL graft is passed first, followed by AM graft passage. On the femoral side, an EndoButton CL is used for femoral-sided fixation. In some cases, when the PL femoral tunnel is shorter than 25 mm, an EndoButton Direct is used to maximize the amount of graft in the tunnel. On the tibial side, a bioabsorbable screw that is the same diameter as the drilled tunnel is used for each bundle.

The grafts are pretensioned by flexing and extending the knee through 20 cycles of full motion. Final fixation of the grafts is done at 30 degrees of flexion for the AM bundle and 0 degree for the PL bundle. A final arthroscopic inspection is always performed to confirm correct position and tensioning of the grafts and the absence of graft impingement (Fig. 22-18).

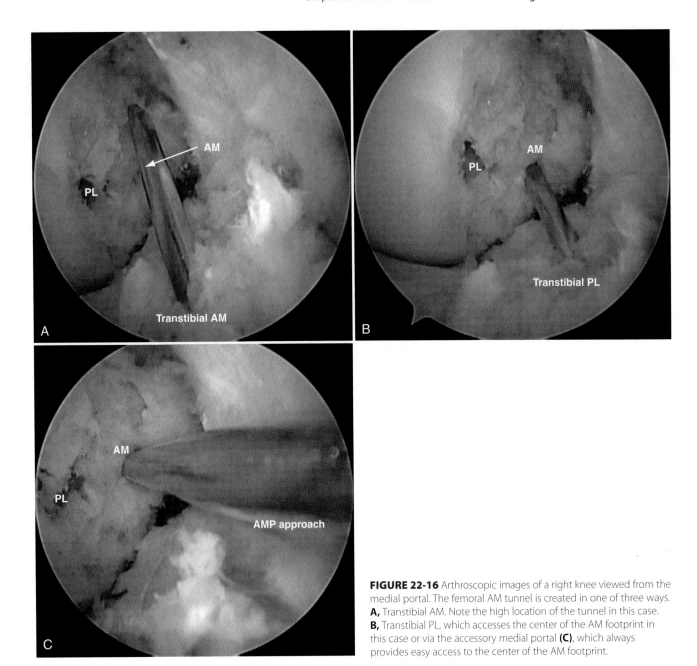

FIGURE 22-16 Arthroscopic images of a right knee viewed from the medial portal. The femoral AM tunnel is created in one of three ways. **A,** Transtibial AM. Note the high location of the tunnel in this case. **B,** Transtibial PL, which accesses the center of the AM footprint in this case or via the accessory medial portal **(C)**, which always provides easy access to the center of the AM footprint.

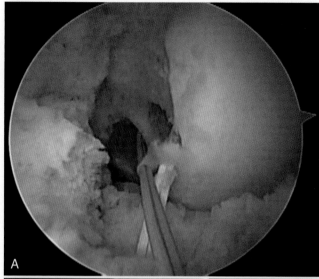

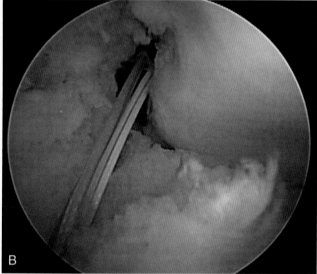

FIGURE 22-17 Two Beath pins are passed with suture loops to shuttle the respective grafts. Note that the suture loops mimic normal graft configuration. **A,** Crossed at 90 degrees of flexion. **B,** Lining up in parallel as the knee is extended.

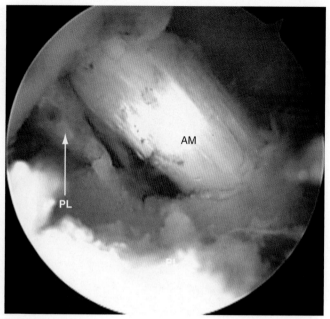

FIGURE 22-18 Final grafts are fixated at 30 degrees for the AM bundle and 0 degree for the PL bundle, respectively. Once the AM graft is passed, the PL will only be visible when viewed from the lateral viewing portal. After the grafts have been passed, the knee is brought into full extension to ensure that impingement does not occur.

PEARLS&PITFALLS

PEARLS

- Prior to prepping the patient, always ensure that the operative knee is positioned to allow for a minimum of 120 degrees of flexion. This is important to ensure safety during later drilling of the femoral tunnels.
- Ensure that the nonoperative leg is placed in the lithotomy position and abducted as far out of the surgical field as safely possible. This allows the surgeon to move to the medial side of the knee freely when drilling via the accessory medial portal (see later).
- The significance of appropriately placed portals cannot be overemphasized. Visualization is the first step to successful surgery.
  - *High position of the AL portal.* This position provides the best view of the anatomic tibial insertion of the ACL. This bird's eye view allows for a slightly wider field of view so that the insertion sites can be visualized relative to other anatomic landmarks, such as the medial and lateral menisci, intermeniscal ligament, and PCL, all at the same time.
  - *Low position of the AM portal.* This position allows the best view of the ACL footprint on the femoral side. The entire surface area of the lateral side of the intercondylar notch, including the osseous ridges of the ACL insertion site, can thus be easily seen.

PITFALL

- *Scarring of remnant ACL.* In chronic ACL injury, the remnant ACL will often be scarred down to a nonanatomic position. This commonly occurs when the ACL is torn from the femoral side and the ligament scars to the PCL or high in the notch. This should not be mistaken as the true insertion site. It is important to discriminate the normal remnant of the ACL from scar tissue. If unsure, recall that the normal ACL has no fibers inserting above the lateral intercondylar ridge.

POSTOPERATIVE REHABILITATION PROTOCOL

Immediately after surgery, the knee is placed into a hinged knee brace locked in full extension for 7 to 10 days. Immediate full weight bearing with crutches is allowed as tolerated based on pain and extent of effusion. The brace is continued for 6 weeks. Continuous passive motion is started immediately after surgery from 0 to 45 degrees of flexion and increased by 5 to 10 degrees daily as tolerated. If a meniscal repair has been performed, flexion beyond 90 degrees is not allowed for 4 weeks postoperatively. Active isometric quadriceps strengthening begins on the first postoperative day. Gradual progression in a structured physical therapy setting continues over the next 3 months. Noncutting, nontwisting activities such as straight line running, cycling, and swimming are generally allowed at 12 weeks after surgery. Functional training begins at 6 months in a supervised setting. Return to unrestricted activity, including contact sports, is allowed at 7 to 9 months. To return to sport, the patient must be pain-free, without effusion, and have a clinically stable knee, full range of motion, and strength grossly equivalent to that of the contralateral side.

CONCLUSIONS

Since the first arthroscopic ACL reconstruction was performed by Dancy in 1980,[37] great technical advances have followed. Generally, most published series detailing clinical outcomes after single-bundle surgery have reported satisfactory results.[38] Still, significant room for improvement exists. As medical science continues to advance, patient expectations only grow higher. Regardless of the severity of injury, most patients expect to return to a full preinjury level of physical function rapidly. As orthopedic surgeons, we need to seek a higher standard of care to meet the increasing demands of our active patients.[39]

The concept of the anatomic double-bundle ACL reconstruction surgery is predicated on a very simple principle—restoration of normal ACL anatomy. Through accurate restoration of native anatomy, we hope to restore normal kinematics and function. A detailed understanding of native ACL anatomy, biomechanics, and injury patterns forms the basis for advanced anatomic double-bundle reconstruction techniques. A recent prospective cohort study of 100 consecutive patients who underwent anatomic double-bundle ACL reconstruction has shown promising early clinical results.[40] Randomized prospective clinical trials are still needed to determine fully the true clinical benefit of anatomic double-bundle surgery compared with conventional single-bundle ACL reconstruction. At present, results of studies using more sensitive advanced imaging modalities and outcomes measures suggest significant early benefits of anatomic ACL reconstruction methods.[6,38]

REFERENCES

1. Freedman KB, D'Amato MJ, Nedeff DD, et al. Arthroscopic anterior cruciate ligament reconstruction: a meta-analysis comparing patellar tendon and hamstring tendon autografts. *Am J Sports Med.* 2003;31:2-11.
2. Yunes M, Richmond JC, Engels EA, Pinczewski LA. Patellar versus hamstring tendons in anterior cruciate ligament reconstruction: A meta-analysis. *Arthroscopy.* 2001;17:248-257.
3. Aglietti P, Giron F, Buzzi R, et al. Anterior cruciate ligament reconstruction: bone-patellar tendon-bone compared with double semitendinosus and gracilis tendon grafts. A prospective, randomized clinical trial. *J Bone Joint Surg Am.* 2004;86:2143-2155.
4. Woo SL, Kanamori A, Zeminski J, et al. The effectiveness of reconstruction of the anterior cruciate ligament with hamstrings and patellar tendon. A cadaveric study comparing anterior tibial and rotational loads. *J Bone Joint Surg Am.* 2002;84:907-914.
5. Tashman S, Collon D, Anderson K, et al. Abnormal rotational knee motion during running after anterior cruciate ligament reconstruction. *Am J Sports Med.* 2004;32:975-983.
6. Ferretti M, Levicoff EA, Macpherson TA, et al. The fetal anterior cruciate ligament: an anatomic and histologic study. *Arthroscopy.* 2007;23:278-283.
7. Girgis FG, Marshall JL, Monajem A. The cruciate ligaments of the knee joint. Anatomical, functional and experimental analysis. *Clin Orthop Relat Res.* 1975;(106)16-231.
8. Harner CD, Baek GH, Vogrin TM, et al. Quantitative analysis of human cruciate ligament insertions. *Arthroscopy.* 1999;15:741-749.
9. Gabriel MT, Wong EK, Woo SL, et al. Distribution of in situ forces in the anterior cruciate ligament in response to rotatory loads. *J Orthop Res.* 2004;22:85-89.
10. Sakane M, Fox RJ, Woo SL, et al. In situ forces in the anterior cruciate ligament and its bundles in response to anterior tibial loads. *J Orthop Res.* 1997;15:285-293.
11. Yagi M, Wong EK, Kanamori A, et al. Biomechanical analysis of an anatomic anterior cruciate ligament reconstruction. *Am J Sports Med.* 2002;30:660-666.
12. Ferretti M, Ekdahl M, Shen W, Fu FH. Osseous landmarks of the femoral attachment of the anterior cruciate ligament: an anatomic study. *Arthroscopy.* 2007;23:1218-1225.
13. Purnell ML, Larson AI, Clancy W. Anterior cruciate ligament insertions on the tibia and femur and their relationships to critical bony landmarks using high-resolution volume-rendering computed tomography. *Am J Sports Med.* 2008;36:2083-2090.
14. Steckel H, Starman JS, Baums MH, et al. Anatomy of the anterior cruciate ligament double bundle structure: a macroscopic evaluation. *Scand J Med Sci Sports.* 2007;17:387-392.
15. Chhabra A, Starman JS, Ferretti M, et al. Anatomic, radiographic, biomechanical, and kinematic evaluation of the anterior cruciate ligament and its two functional bundles. *J Bone Joint Surg Am.* 2006;88(suppl 4):2-10.
16. Fu FH, Jordan SS. The lateral intercondylar ridge: a key to anatomic anterior cruciate ligament reconstruction. *J Bone Joint Surg Am.* 2007;89:2103-2104.
17. Odensten M, Gillquist J. Functional anatomy of the anterior cruciate ligament and a rationale for reconstruction. *J Bone Joint Surg Am.* 1985;67:257-262.
18. Siebold R, Ellert T, Metz S, Metz J. Tibial insertions of the anteromedial and posterolateral bundles of the anterior cruciate ligament: morphometry, arthroscopic landmarks, and orientation model for bone tunnel placement. *Arthroscopy.* 2008;24:154-161.
19. Luites JW, Wymenga AB, Blankevoort L, Kooloos JG. Description of the attachment geometry of the anteromedial and posterolateral bundles of the ACL from arthroscopic perspective for anatomical tunnel placement. *Knee Surg Sports Traumatol Arthrosc.* 2007;15:1422-1431.
20. Kopf S, Musahl V, Tashman S. A systematic review of the femoral origin and tibial insertion morphology of the ACL. *Knee Surg Sports Traumatol Arthrosc.* 2009;17:213-219.
21. Zantop T, Herbort M, Raschke MJ, et al. The role of the anteromedial and posterolateral bundles of the anterior cruciate ligament in anterior tibial translation and internal rotation. *Am J Sports Med.* 2007;35:223-227.
22. Amis A, Dawkins G. Functional anatomy of the anterior cruciate ligament. *J Bone Joint Surg Br.* 1991;73:260-267.
23. Buoncristiani AM, Tjoumakaris FP, Starman JS, et al. Anatomic double-bundle anterior cruciate ligament reconstruction. *Arthroscopy.* 2006;22:1000-1006.
24. Muller W. Form, function, and ligament reconstruction. In: Muller W. *The Knee.* Berlin: Springer; 1982:.
25. Zantop T, Brucker PU, Vidal A, et al. Intraarticular rupture pattern of the ACL. *Clin Orthop Relat Res.* 2007;(454):48-53.
26. Siebold R, Fu FH. Assessment and augmentation of symptomatic anteromedial or posterolateral bundle tears of the anterior cruciate ligament. *Arthroscopy.* 2008;24:1289-1298.
27. Sarimo J, Rantanen J, Heikkila J, et al. Acute traumatic hemarthrosis of the knee. Is routine arthroscopic examination necessary? A study of 320 consecutive patients. *Scand J Surg.* 2002;91:361-364.
28. Benjaminse A, Gokeler A, van der Schans CP. Clinical diagnosis of an anterior cruciate ligament rupture: a meta-analysis. *J Orthop Sports Physical Ther.* 2006;36:267-288.
29. Donaldson WF 3rd, Warren RF, Wickiewicz T. A comparison of acute anterior cruciate ligament examinations. Initial versus examination under anesthesia. *Am J Sports Med.* 1985;13:5-10.
30. Galway HR, MacIntosh DL. The lateral pivot shift: a symptom and sign of anterior cruciate ligament insufficiency. *Clin Orthop Relat Res.* 1980;(414):5-50.
31. Hess T, Rupp S, Hopf T, et al. Lateral tibial avulsion fractures and disruptions to the anterior cruciate ligament. A clinical study of their incidence and correlation. *Clin Orthop Relat Res.* 1994;(303):193-197.
32. Vellet AD, Lee DH, Munk PL, et al. Anterior cruciate ligament tear: prospective evaluation of diagnostic accuracy of middle- and high-field-strength MR imaging at 1.5 and 0.5 T. *Radiology.* 1995;197:826-830.

33. Noh HK, Wang JH, Bada LP, et al. Trantibial anterior cruciate ligament double bundle reconstruction technique: two tibial bundle in one tibial tunnel. *Arch Orthop Trauma Surg.* 2008;128:1245-1250.

34. Yasuda K, Kondo E, Ichiyama H, et al. Anatomic reconstruction of the anteromedial and posterolateral bundles of the anterior cruciate ligament using hamstring tendon grafts. *Arthroscopy.* 2004;20:1015-1025.

35. Kim SJ, Jo SB, Kumar P, Oh KS. Comparison of single- and double-bundle anterior cruciate ligament reconstruction using quadriceps tendon-bone autografts. *Arthroscopy.* 2009;25:70-77.

36. Shen W, Forsythe B, Ingham SM, et al. Application of the anatomic double-bundle reconstruction concept to revision and augmentation anterior cruciate ligament surgeries. *J Bone Joint Surg Am.* 2008; 90(suppl 4):20-34.

37. Strocchi R, de Pasquale V, Gubellini P, et al. The human anterior cruciate ligament: histological and ultrastructural observations. *J Anat.* 1992; 180:515-519.

38. Meredick RB, Vance KJ, Appleby D, Lubowitz JH. Outcome of single-bundle versus double-bundle reconstruction of the anterior cruciate ligament: a meta-analysis. *Am J Sports Med.* 2008;36:1414-1421.

39. Irrgang JJ, Bost JE, Fu FH. Re: Outcome of single-bundle versus double-bundle reconstruction of the anterior cruciate ligament: a meta-analysis. *Am J Sports Med.* 2009;37:421-422.

40. Fu FH, Shen W, Starman JS, et al. Primary anatomic double-bundle anterior cruciate ligament reconstruction: a preliminary 2-year prospective study. *Am J Sports Med.* 2008;36:1263-1274.

Revision Anterior Cruciate Ligament Reconstruction

J. Christopher Shaver ● Darren L. Johnson

Reconstruction of the torn anterior cruciate ligament (ACL) has seen a significant increase in volume over the past 3 decades. It is currently one of the most common procedures performed by orthopaedic surgeons in the United States and across the globe. Current estimates cite approximately 250,000 procedures performed annually in the United States. Although the most of these patients have a fairly uneventful recovery and return to sport and/or work, there are patients who present as clinical failures, with three categories represented by recurrent instability, loss of motion, and pain.[1] With the ever-increasing numbers of primary surgeries performed, it follows that the numbers of failed primary procedures will subsequently increase. Orthopedic surgeons will be required to tackle these challenging situations.

Although the causes of failure may be multifactorial, these failures may be broadly classified into three categories: loss of motion, recurrent instability, and pain.[2] Another potential category may be progressive joint deterioration without the above findings after ACL reconstruction. Any of these factors may play a role in the failure of a reconstruction, but the final goal of revision reconstruction remains constant—provide a stable and functional ACL that most accurately reproduces the normal knee kinematics, allow the individual to return to an active lifestyle, and potentially decrease the development of early osteoarthritis.[3,4]

ANATOMY

Although commonly overlooked throughout the past 1 to 2 decades, recent anatomic studies have further defined our precise understanding of the anatomy of the native ACL, grossly and arthroscopically.[5,6] Recognition of the ACL as a functional two-bundle ligament comprised of distinct anteromedial and posterolateral bundles, as well as their relationship to bony insertion site anatomy, has led to a revolution in discussing ACL reconstruction techniques.[7] It is now understood that re-creation of the native anatomy of the ACL may lead to improved kinematic and

functional results. Prior nonadherence to these principals may be a major root cause of many primary reconstruction failures.[8]

Causes of Reconstruction Failure

Loss of Motion

Loss of motion after reconstruction of the ACL may lead to profound functional disability. Depending on the source, the patient may experience loss of extension, flexion, patellar entrapment, and/or global loss of motion as measured in all three planes. The loss of extension often has a more deleterious functional effect on the patient than loss of flexion, because it leads to difficulty with simple ambulation and restoration of the normal gait cycle by feedback loop inhibition of the extensor mechanism.[9-11] This may also lead to patellofemoral symptoms, referred or secondary joint arthralgias caused by antalgic gait, and loss of athletic performance. Increased forces are experienced in the patellofemoral compartment, leading to early osteoarthritic changes in these young patients. Loss of minor flexion is often asymptomatic and rarely causes significant disability unless total flexion is limited to less than 120 degrees.[10]

The causative factors for motion loss are often complex and may be intimately interrelated. Possible factors include poor technique causing graft impingement, infection, immobilization, inadequate or excessive rehabilitation, capsulitis-arthrofibrosis, and complex regional pain syndrome.[9,10,12] Nonanatomic technique often creates a situation in which the ACL graft is not anatomically positioned in respect to the femoral or tibial insertion sites, or both. This nonanatomic placement may result in a situation in which the graft impinges on the wall of the lateral femoral condyle, roof of the intercondylar notch, or posterior cruciate ligament (PCL), resulting in mechanical loss of motion in flexion or extension and graft attrition, as well as eventual stretching of the graft because of nonanatomic placement of the graft. Loss of flexion may be related to relative anterior placement of the graft on the femoral and tibial sides; conversely, loss of extension may occur with excessive posterior placement of the graft in relation to the tibial and femoral anatomic positions.[1,2,13]

Another cause of mechanical motion loss includes the phenomenon known as the cyclops lesion, which is rather uncommon. This represents fibroproliferative nodules that may occur on the anterior surface of the ACL graft that limit extension by a mechanical block in the final few degrees.[14] These may develop as a result of failure to remove excess debris from the intercondylar notch produced during reaming, or may be a scarring response to repeated impingement of the graft on the roof of the intercondylar notch. Preventive measures against the cyclops lesions include immediate passive and active extension exercises prior to formation of the nodules.

Some patients may experience a condition known as regional capsulitis, or arthrofibrosis, which may also result in loss of motion.[1,15] This may be broken down into primary and secondary conditions, with primary being an idiopathic exaggerated healing response to surgical trauma and secondary representing the results of inappropriate surgical timing and/or rehabilitation. In primary or idiopathic arthrofibrosis, the patient presents with excessive postoperative pain, swelling, warmth, resistance to motion in flexion and extension, and severely limited patellar motion in all planes. Treatment generally focuses on restoration of full motion through gentle rehabilitation modalities while, most importantly, reducing the associated pain and inflammation. Early operative intervention should be avoided, because this often accentuates the process. Eventually, this process may result in permanent or fixed global loss of motion caused by caused by intra-articular adhesions.[16] If initial conservative measures are inadequate for restoration of motion, surgical manipulation and lysis of these adhesions may be considered once the period of acute inflammation has defervesced and pain controlled. Although this may result in improved motion, these patients rarely achieve objective full motion and only occasionally experience clinical recurrent instability.

Technical Errors

Nonanatomic surgical technique in the primary ACL reconstruction represents the most common cause of failure of these procedures.[4] Technical errors include inadequate clearance for the graft in the intercondylar notch, malpositioned nonanatomic tunnels, poor tensioning of the grafts, and inadequate fixation of the graft. Although the concepts of roofplasty and wallplasty are controversial, the surgeon must confirm that the graft is free of bony impingement throughout the full knee range of motion, which may require some degree of bone and soft tissue removal, particularly in the chronic revision ACL-deficient knee.

Placement of tibial and femoral tunnels in nonanatomic positions may result in graft attrition and mechanical entrapment or capture of the knee. Additionally, these errors in tunnel management may result in a graft that allows for persistent or recurrent instability, even in the face of an intact graft. Estimates show that approximately 70% to 80% of failures may be attributed to improper tunnel placement, with nonanatomic femoral locations representing the most commonly encountered error in tunnel placement. Cadaveric and arthroscopic studies have confirmed the topographic bony insertion and origin sites of the ACL and their relationship to the reconstructed ligament. Related studies cast doubt that the common endoscopic transtibial approach to femoral tunnel placement may result in an anatomic location of the femoral insertion of the reconstructed ACL.[17,18] This transtibial endoscopic technique most commonly leads to common mistakes in graft placement, including excessive posterior placement on the tibial side combined with a femoral site too high and/or anterior on the medial wall of the lateral femoral condyle. In the best case scenario, there is a mismatch in graft placement within the native insertion site, more closely recreating the posterolateral (PL) site on the tibia to the anteromedial (AM) site on the femur. This combination results in poor tensioning in relation to overall knee kinematics, possible impingement of the graft on the PCL, and a vertical graft (Figs. 23-1 and 23-2).[19] This situation leaves the graft in

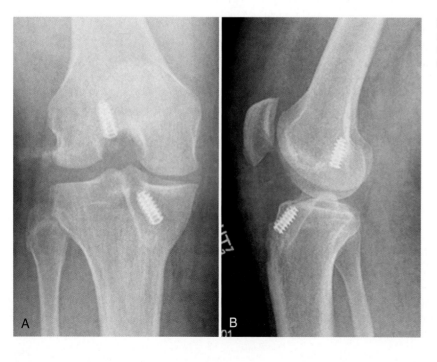

FIGURE 23-1 Failed vertical ACL reconstruction. **A,** AP view. **B,** Lateral view. *(From Shaver J, Johnson D. Revision anatomic double-bundle anterior cruciate ligament surgery. Oper Tech Sports Med. 2008;16:157-164.)*

A   B

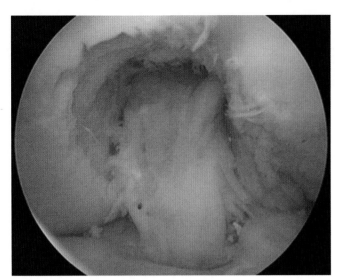

FIGURE 23-2 Failed ACL reconstruction with a vertical intact graft but a grossly positive pivot shift on EUA.

a position that may provide some anteroposterior stability, but sacrifices rotational stability and possibly limits range of motion of the knee. In this case, the knee may actually have been made worse by the reconstruction. Revision surgery is almost inevitably required, depending on the patient's level of activity.

The tibial insertion site may be somewhat more forgiving to mistakes in tunnel placement, but significant deviations from anatomic locations may result in less ideal outcomes. Excessive anterior placement results in superior root impingement in full extension and excessive graft forces in flexion, whereas posterior placement results in flexion laxity and possible impingement on the PCL. Additionally, medial or lateral deviations may result in PCL and/or wall impingement and eventual graft attrition and failure.[20-23]

Failure of Biologic Incorporation

Failure of the graft to incorporate into the host bone may also represent a source of failure of primary ACL reconstruction. This often presents with recurrent instability in the face of an anatomically well-positioned graft. This may be a result of poor fixation on the femoral or, more commonly, the tibial side, excessive forces experienced by the graft during rehabilitation and biologic incorporation, immune responses of the host versus the graft in the case of allografts, or lack of recognition of certain graft-host mismatches. The tibial metaphyseal bone has been identified as the weak link in graft fixation, and therefore additional backup fixation is often recommended, particularly with all soft tissue ACL reconstruction.[24] Excessively aggressive rehabilitation protocols may not allow the proper ligamentization of the graft and may eliminate or delay the reparative process that incorporates the graft with the host bone. Each graft substitute has a biologic timetable of incorporation that must be recognized and rehabilitation tailored to the individual situation.[25,26] Immune responses have been known to occur between host bone and allografts and/or certain fixation devices, which may result in tunnel lysis and failure of incorporation of the graft. Recognized graft-host mismatches include soft tissue allografts and autografts in young

hyperlax females and high-demand athletes, which may stretch out over time and result in recurrent instability.[27-29]

Concurrent Laxity

Another cause of failure of primary ACL reconstructions is lack of recognition of concurrent injuries to the important secondary stabilizers of the ACL. The native ACL is the primary restraint to anterior displacement of the tibia, but must work in concert with multiple other structures to function optimally.[30] This remains true for the reconstructed ACL, and may be even more important because prior to realization of full strength, the graft must undergo incorporation and ligamentization over an extended period of time. If the secondary stabilizers are absent or nonfunctional, nonphysiologic forces are placed on the graft during the ligamentization process, resulting in a nonfunctional lax graft that does not recreate the stability of the native ACL. The secondary stabilizers are numerous, and include the menisci (medial > lateral), medial collateral ligament (MCL), posteromedial corner (including the posterior oblique ligament [POL]), posterior cruciate ligament (PCL), and the posterolateral corner (PLC).[31] These structures may be injured in conjunction with the original ACL injury, or may become lax because of repeated episodes of instability in a chronically ACL-deficient knee.[32] A reconstruction of the ACL in the face of concurrent laxity places nonphysiologic stresses on the graft, and often results in premature failure of these reconstructions.[33,34] Recognition by thorough examination and proper management strategies for these additional sources of laxity must be taken into account in the primary and revision ACL reconstruction situations.

Traumatic Causes

Finally, the well-placed primary graft may simply fail because of traumatic events inherent to the stresses experienced in grafts of many of this active subset of patients. These failures can be caused by excessive strain placed on the immature graft by excessive rehabilitation, premature return to high-level sports or activities, or shear bad luck during high-level sporting activities. These are generally characterized as early failures (less than 1 year), which occur during graft remodeling and incorporation prior to realization of the final graft strength, or late failures (more than 1 year, with no subjective evidence of prior instability).[13] Late failures often present in a similar fashion to their initial traumatic event, often with an acute hemarthrosis and recurrent instability. It is important to evaluate the patient critically who has failed primary surgery and has never returned to high-level sports. These patients often have some component of technical errors that precluded their full return after the index procedure.

PATIENT EVALUATION

The most important aspect of preoperative planning for the revision ACL patient is elucidation of the primary cause of the index surgery's failure, as noted. Another vital component is the patient's expectations and desires following the revision reconstruction. It is imperative that the surgeon and patient have realistic goals in the revision situation, as studies have shown a significantly lower rate of return to high-level sports.[35-37] Some patients may have a degree of injury that makes this goal unrealistic, and the revision may be considered a salvage procedure to limit any further damage.[38] The patient and surgeon must also understand and agree that in the revision situation, a significant investment of time and effort is often required for successful outcomes.

History

As with any patient, a detailed history with thorough knowledge of the primary injury circumstances is paramount to success. This not only includes the actual mechanism of injury, but also prior surgical treatment. The timing of surgery, type of graft used, rehabilitation protocol after the index procedure, subjective and objective results thereafter, and any complications experienced may provide clues about the cause of failure and help design the revision surgeon's plan. The patient may present with a myriad of complaints from symptomatic instability to pain without instability. In most cases, patients with symptoms and examination consistent with recurrent instability have the greatest potential for a successful revision outcome.

Thorough knowledge of the index procedure is essential. This includes review of the initial magnetic resonance imaging (MRI) scans, if available, the primary surgeon's operative record, arthroscopic images from the index procedure, and follow-up imaging after the procedure. This not only educates the surgeon about the overall condition of the knee, but also aids in preoperative preparation for expected pitfalls, such as additional surgeries needed, equipment required, and need for staged procedures.

Physical Examination

The physical examination in the revision ACL situation must include a global assessment of the limb. This includes an evaluation of overall limb alignment and gait, because significant variations such as a varus thrust may compromise the longevity of an ACL reconstruction.[39] Limitations of motion of not only the knee but also the hip and ankle must be taken into account and possibly addressed prior to revision. The condition and any dysfunction of the supporting thigh musculature need to be addressed, because this may be key to rehabilitation after any revision reconstruction. Residual infectious processes must be ruled out in all cases, because this will doom any revision. The locations of previous incisions are taken into account, and future incisions planned to ensure cutaneous tissue viability.

A comprehensive objective evaluation of the knee is imperative, and must include thorough evaluation of not only the function of the ACL, but also the supporting structures. Evaluation of the ACL includes quantifying and qualifying examinations such as the Lachman, pivot shift, and anterior drawer tests and KT1000 arthrometer (MEDmetric; San Diego, Calif) measurements. Secondary evaluation of the menisci, MCL, PLC, and posteromedial corner (PMC) are performed and included in the global assessment of the knee.

Diagnostic Imaging

Good-quality radiographic evaluation of the knee aids significantly in preoperative planning and should always be performed.

These include standing full extension anteroposterior and lateral views of the knee, as well as 45-degree flexion weight-bearing posteroanterior views. Additional examinations that may be of aid include axial views of the patella, full-length mechanical axis views, varus and valgus stress views, and views of the contralateral knee for comparison. These radiographic studies are evaluated for prior tunnel placement, tunnel expansion, location of prior hardware, presence of degenerative changes, and notch geometry.[40] These patients often present with MRI scans, which this may be reviewed for concomitant injury to the secondary stabilizers, condition of the menisci and articular cartilage, and placement and condition of the prior graft.

If tunnel expansion or cystic changes are noted on plain radiographs, additional computed tomography (CT) scans may aid in identification of previous tunnel location and quantification of the bony defects. Three-dimensional CT is particularly useful to look at previous tunnel placement and its implications for revision. This is often the best modality to plan for additional fixation, alternative strategies such as over the top and two incision techniques, and/or a staged procedure in these cases.

Arthroscopic Technique

Staging

When faced with the revision patient, one consideration faced by the surgeon is whether the case can be appropriately managed in one surgical session. Situations such as significant limb malalignment, motion loss, and tunnel osteolysis may represent occasions when a staged procedure must be considered. Addressing limb malalignment with osteotomies concurrently with revision ACL surgery is technically feasible; however, this situation may have a propensity for a difficult rehabilitation and portend poor results in all but the most motivated of patients.[41] The same concept can be applied to addressing significant motion restriction at the time of revision reconstruction. Most would recommend addressing this with surgical manipulation, lysis of adhesions, and/or aggressive physical therapy, with subsequent revision reconstruction when restoration of motion is achieved. Revision surgery proceeds only if true clinical instability is the problem, not instability caused by lack of rehabilitation strength in the extremity.

If the degree of tunnel expansion, osteolysis, or previous hardware placement will not allow both anatomic reconstruction and secure postoperative fixation of the grafts for immediate motion postoperatively, the procedure should be staged. Generally, this includes surgical removal of previous hardware and bone grafting of the tunnels, followed by full motion and quadriceps rehabilitation while protecting the knee from recurrent buckling episodes. Revision surgery may then proceed after incorporation of this bone graft material, typically at 4 to 6 months.[3,42] When possible, autogenous bone graft should be used in preference to allograft substitutes (Fig. 23-3).

Graft Selection

Thus far, no source of graft in the revision situation has been proven to be the gold standard or clinically superior. The choice of graft must be tailored to the patient's age, gender, factors such as hyperlaxity, and the physical demands that the reconstructed

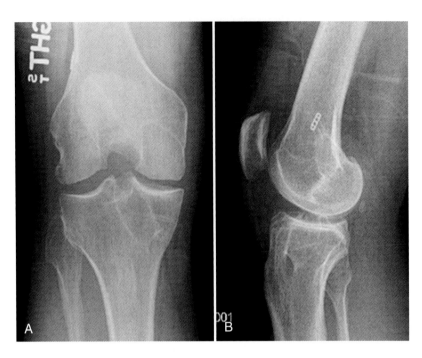

FIGURE 23-3 A, B, Significant tunnel osteolysis and failed vertical ACL reconstruction.

graft will experience, similar to the recommendations for primary ACL surgery. The full spectrum of grafts may be considered with the revision ACL reconstruction, including numerous autograft and allograft choices. Autograft availability may be limited by their prior use, and scarring from prior procedures may make this technically difficult, if not impossible, although contralateral harvest may be a viable choice in these situations. Cases involving bone loss and tunnel expansion may be more suitable for autografts or allografts that have bone attached, because these are thought to provide better tunnel fill and secure graft fixation characteristics.

Advantages to allograft revision reconstruction are numerous. Many revision surgeons believe that this may represent the optimal graft selection. The lack of donor site morbidity, smaller incisions resulting in less soft tissue trauma, less operative theatre time, and ability to customize the graft size dimensions to the revision situation represent some of the major advantages of allografts in revision ACL reconstructions.[43] However, disadvantages such as patient preference, longer incorporation times, and concerns regarding disease transmission remain. Currently, the most common allografts choices include the Achilles tendon-calcaneus and bone-patellar tendon-bone grafts, and all soft tissue grafts such as the anterior and posterior tibialis tendon grafts.

Retained Hardware

Having to plan for and deal with retained hardware or absorbable implants is ubiquitous to revision ACL surgery, and may significantly influence the technical aspects of the procedure. Often, when the primary surgery was performed in a nonanatomic fashion, the hardware may not interfere with anatomic tunnel and graft placement and is therefore retained.[44] If it does interfere, the surgeon should have detailed knowledge of the retained implant and an armamentarium of instruments available that are designed for removal of this hardware. The sur-

geon must also be comfortable with alternative fixation strategies (over the top and two-incision techniques) to deal with the consequences that may occur after removal of offending hardware and technical problems such as short femoral tunnels or posterior wall blowout.

Primary Tunnels

As a result of the primary reconstruction, it is inevitable that the revision surgeon must account for and often incorporate previous tunnels into the surgical plan. These may interfere with the placement of new anatomic tunnels. If they are located in a position significantly away from the planned revision tunnels, surgery may proceed much like a primary reconstruction (Fig. 23-4).

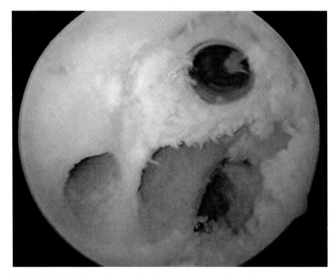

FIGURE 23-4 Vertical tunnel with screw removed and anatomic PL and AM tunnel placement. *(From Shaver J, Johnson D. Revision anatomic double-bundle anterior cruciate ligament surgery.* Oper Tech Sports Med. *2008;16:157-164.)*

If after revision clearance of the notch and visualization of the over the top position the previous tunnels interfere with anatomic placement, there are several management options available. Those situations in which the previous tunnels are appropriate or overlap ideal locations, hardware removal, and customized tunnel expansion can be performed using tunnel dilators. This may allow contouring of the tunnel to the ideal location and subsequent placement of larger grafts, bone-containing grafts, or bone graft material may result in anatomic graft placement.

Another strategy involves use of the concept of divergence to allow the surgeon to miss the previous bony tunnel while incorporating the intra-articular entry and exit points of prior tunnels.[45] On the femoral side, this usually includes the use of additional accessory portals or varying angles of knee flexion while changing the inclination or position of the tunnel on the tibial metaphyseal side. The surgeon may also choose to use outside-in drilling or the two-incision technique.

Previous tunnel placement with expansion may also require the surgeon to alter fixation strategies on the tibial and femoral sides. The surgeon may incorporate over the top or back and two-incision techniques to allow secure femoral sided fixation, as well as tibial metaphyseal fixation using oversized or stacked screws, spiked washers, posts, staples, and dual fixation.

If secure and stable fixation cannot be provided because of previous tunnel location and/or expansion, a staged procedure may be required to avoid another failure.

Required Surgical Instruments

The revision situation requires the surgeon and staff to be prepared for the complexity of the case because of technical challenges that may occur during the procedure. Preparedness includes having a vast armamentarium of equipment not routinely used in primary surgery. Hardware removal devices for the specific previous implants must be available, as well as an assortment of trephines, reamers, picks, and curettes to get to this hardware. Tunnel dilators, single and full fluted drill bits (including half-sizes), and multiple tunnel and backup fixation devices need to be accessible. Availability of bone allografts as well as various bone-containing and soft tissue allografts also aid in surgeon flexibility.

Anatomic Single- Versus Double-Bundle Revision

In regard to the type of revision surgery to perform, there are several considerations. Patient size, instability pattern and degree (grade I vs. grade III pivot shift), intraoperative findings, and surgeon comfort influence this choice tremendously. Patients of small stature may not be ideal candidates for the use of anatomic double-bundle techniques, whereas patients with subtle concurrent secondary laxity (i.e., previous significant medial damage or meniscectomies) may be ideal candidates for this technique. Anatomic double-bundle techniques allow for a greater volume of intra-articular graft volume to counteract the secondary laxity often encountered in revision situations. This has been shown to be superior for the restoration of normal knee kinematics versus traditional single-bundle reconstructions.[8,46,47] However, the anatomic double-bundle technique remains a technically challenging procedure, with a steep learning curve with an increased risk

of intraoperative complications, which further accentuates the difficulty of these already complex revision cases.

Often, previous nonanatomic grafts may lie in a position that adequately controls the anteroposterior motion of the tibia, effectively eliminating the Lachman test and reducing the negative results of the anterior drawer test; however, they experience recurrent rotational instability, clinically expressing the pivot shift test. This may result in significant functional instability in regard to athletic participation. These patients may be candidates for an augmentation procedure to add the second anatomic posterolateral bundle, eliminating the rotational instability.[48] This requires a thorough knowledge of the functional and arthroscopic anatomy of the ACL, with expertise in placing this graft while not damaging the prior graft.

Principles of Revision Procedures

It is our belief that use of the anatomic double-bundle anterior cruciate ligament techniques and principles in revision surgeries is advantageous and the treatment of choice for most of these patients. Adherence to this philosophy will lead to improved restoration of the native kinematics of the knee, thereby improving overall outcomes. The larger volume of tissue counteracts the effects of chronic laxity of the ACL and supporting structures, once again aiding in the restoration of the native environment of the knee. However, certain patient situations may not be conducive to this technique. These include individuals of significantly smaller stature, which will not allow adequate surface area and volume of bone in the lateral femoral condyle that are required to perform a double-bundle reconstruction safely. In these situations, we prefer to revise them to an anatomic single-bundle reconstruction, but still adhere strictly to the principles of tunnel placement previously noted (Fig. 23-5).

Examination Under Anesthesia

A global examination under anesthesia (EUA) should be performed and the condition of not only the degree of ACL laxity but also the supporting structures documented. This should be

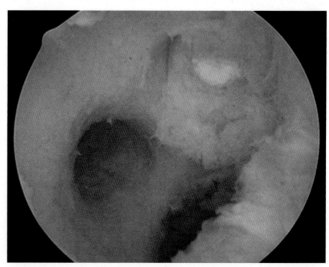

FIGURE 23-5 Anatomic single-bundle placement below previous soft tissue graft (because of patient's small condylar size).

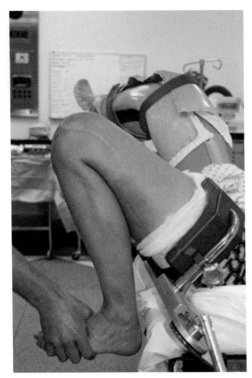

FIGURE 23-6 Surgical positioning allowing hyperflexion. Note hip flexion.

evaluated in comparison to the contralateral knee to determine the true degree of pathologic laxity. It is our experience that the in-office clinical examination is very inconsistent with the EUA, especially in regard to the degree of anterolateral rotatory instability as noted by the pivot shift test. The office examination often underestimates the degree of pathologic laxity.

Patient Positioning

Our preferred setup uses an operating room table that provides full clearance for the lower extremities by a break in the lower half of the bed, with the patient's buttocks positioned at this break. The nonoperative extremity is held in a padded arthroscopic well-leg holder with the hip flexed to approximately 90 degrees and mildly externally rotated, providing clearance for access to the medial side of the operative extremity. A padded tourniquet is placed high on the thigh and the arthroscopic leg holder is placed on the most distal portion of the bed. The leg holder is then flexed to approximately 30 to 45 degrees, providing mild hip flexion and allowing for deep hyperflexion of the knee (Fig. 23-6). This position makes drilling of the femoral tunnels at 110 and 130 degrees possible from the accessory medial portal, which we recommend for anatomic tunnel placement in primary and revision surgery.[49] This also allows full access to the distal half of the thigh, which may be needed to access and remove previous fixation hardware or perform a two-incision technique when required.

Portals and Diagnostic Arthroscopy

Correct portal placement is essential for adequate visualization and allows a significant degree of freedom for alternative visual-

ization during the procedure. The initial anterolateral portal created is high and tight to the patellar tendon, which skirts the inferolateral pole of the patella. After insertion of the arthroscope, a low and tight to patellar tendon anteromedial portal is created under direct visualization of a spinal needle. This should be low enough not to interfere with use of the tip or elbow tibial ACL guide later in the procedure.[49]

An additional accessory far medial portal may be created at this time, or later, to aid in hardware removal and for eventual drilling of the AM and PL femoral tunnels. This portal is created at 90 degrees of knee flexion just superior to the anterior third of the medial meniscus under direct visualization of a spinal needle. The spinal needle should skirt the medial femoral condyle, leaving just enough room not to cause iatrogenic damage during insertion of half-fluted reamers later in the procedure. It should also allow access to the over the back position for creation of the AM bundle. It is also helpful to create this portal horizontally to protect the meniscus and allow medial or lateral translation for insertion of equipment such as reamers.

Diagnostic arthroscopy is then carried out; the condition of the articular cartilage, menisci, and primary graft should be documented with images for later patient education. Additionally, signs of interarticular laxity not related to the ACL, such as stressed medial and lateral drive-through or gap signs, should be noted. Limited areas of notch, fat pad, medial or lateral gutter, or suprapatellar scarring that may cause limitation of motion are dealt with at this time.

Graft Selection and Preparation

In select cases, autograft tissue or a hybrid of autografts and allografts may be used for the anatomic double-bundle revision reconstruction. These may be harvested at this time in standard fashion, and prepared on the back table. Our preferred revision tissue is the calcaneus-Achilles allograft because of its large size and flexibility to meet several revision demands. The larger size often allows it to be split to create the 7- to 8-mm AM bundle and 5- to 6-mm PL bundle, which represents a cost savings to the patient and facility. If needed, the bone plug may be shaped to fill smaller bony deficits on the femoral side or may be removed to create an all–soft tissue graft.

In patients who have initially failed an allograft reconstruction, or have demonstrated a strong desire to return to high-level participation in running and cutting sports, we support revision using autograft tissues. In this situation, we use an 8- to 9-mm central bone-patellar tendon-bone or quadriceps tendon autograft for the AM bundle and a 5- to 6-mm double-looped gracilis or semitendinosus hamstring autograft for the PL bundle. Use of these graft sources may lead to improved early incorporation, decreased risk for later graft relaxation, and earlier return to ACL-dependent activities. This may require contralateral harvest, which is controversial.

Preparation of the Notch

With complete failure of the previous graft or frank nonanatomic prior surgery, the residual graft is removed from the notch to improve visualization. Although the degree of roofplasty and wallplasty performed is controversial, the surgeon must visualize

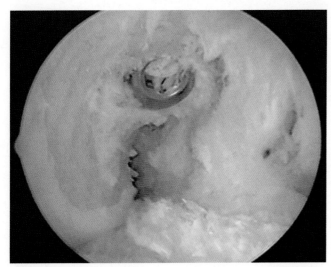

FIGURE 23-7 Retained hardware from primary ACL reconstruction after revision notchplasty. *(From Shaver J, Johnson D. Revision anatomic double-bundle anterior cruciate ligament surgery. Oper Tech Sports Med. 2008;16:157-164.)*

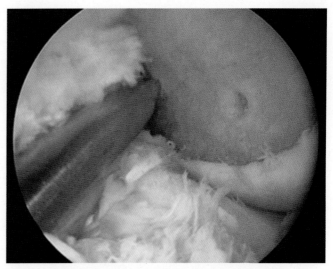

FIGURE 23-8 Marking of PL and AM bundles from accessory medial portal.

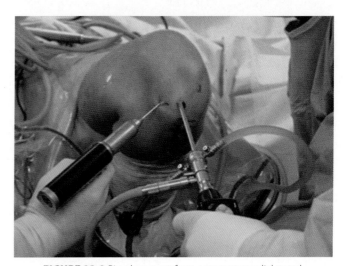

FIGURE 23-9 Pin placement from accessory medial portal.

the entire wall and the over the back position, including the lateral intercondylar and bifurcate ridges, if still recognizable. The notchplasty is only done to allow for visualization and restoration of the native anatomy. It has been shown that the bony notch grows back after ACL reconstruction. Therefore, a notchplasty simply for graft placement is not necessary. Previous tunnels and hardware must be cleared of soft tissue and overgrowth of bone by curettes, osteotomes, and picks to allow for easier removal of previous hardware (if required), with a minimum of bony disruption (Fig. 23-7). We have found that at minimum the most inferior surface of the lateral femoral condyle should be contoured away from the notch to limit any potential impingement on this area after graft placement.

Femoral Tunnels

The arthroscope is then inserted in the low tight AM portal for direct visualization of the lateral wall. If the patient's size and position of previous tunnels allow for two new anatomic femoral tunnels to be created safely, the technique follows as for a standard anatomic double-bundle surgery. Using an arthroscopic awl at 90 degrees of knee flexion, the anatomic positions of the proposed AM and PL tunnels are picked and marked (Fig. 23-8). Guide pins are placed and tunnels reamed at 110 degrees to create first the 5- to 6-mm PL tunnel and next at 130 degrees to create a divergent 7- to 9-mm AM tunnel. Intraoperative fluoroscopy or radiography may be used at this time to assist in placement of tunnels in an anatomic position. These tunnels are both drilled from the accessory medial portal using half-fluted reamers to avoid articular cartilage damage on entry while visualized from the low tight AM portal (Fig. 23-9). Overall length of the PL and AM tunnels are 28 to 34 and 32 to 40 mm, respectively. The integrity of the tunnel walls can then be visualized after removal of bony debris and contouring of the edges using a 5.5-mm shaver to reduce graft impingement (Fig. 23-10).

In patients in whom the previous femoral tunnel interferes with anatomic tunnel placement, usually the AM tunnel, it may be overreamed and contoured to the anatomic position. This is done by placing a guide pin in the desired direction of tunnel expansion and then using subsequently larger and larger reamers to expand the tunnel in this direction. The additional bone from the Achilles-calcaneus allograft may be contoured or used as free graft to fill the deficit left by the previous tunnel. Alternatively, differing angles of knee flexion during drilling may allow creation of a divergent tunnel with the same intra-articular point, but intact bony walls, producing an environment conducive to secure fixation and ingrowth of the graft.

Tibial Tunnels

If the previous scar allows for anatomic placement of the tibial tunnels, this is used to access the primary tibial tunnel and remove hardware as indicated. A guide pin is placed across this prior tunnel, and the primary graft is removed to the interarticular position. This position can be then checked to determine its

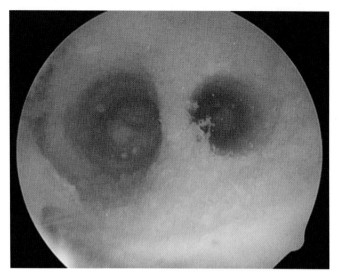

FIGURE 23-10 Anatomic AM and PL tunnel placement with divergent tunnels.

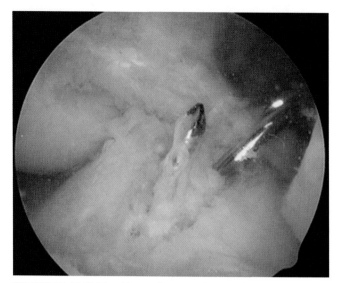

FIGURE 23-12 Tibial guide pins for AM and PL tunnels exiting prior tibial tunnel.

relationship to anatomic tibial tunnels. If in an anatomic or near-anatomic position, this tunnel may be overreamed to remove soft tissue and provide healthy bleeding bone or directionally expanded as described for the femoral tunnels to create the tibial AM tunnel. If previous tunnels are far from anatomic, a new 8- to 9-mm AM tunnel can be created with the guide set at 55 to 60 degrees and perpendicular to the joint line, and the previous tunnel bone grafted with excess bone from the Achilles-calcaneus allograft.

The 5- to 6-mm PL tunnel is created by placing the ACL drill guide through the accessory medial portal or low tight anteromedial portal and referencing off the lateral downslope of the medial tibial spine for its interarticular entry site. The angle of inclination for this guide is approximately 45 degrees, with its entry site at the anterior edge of the MCL on the tibial metaphysis (Fig. 23-11). Once again, intraoperative fluoroscopy or radiography may be of assistance in placement of anatomic tunnels. The AM and PL tunnels may often converge at

the joint line into a singular intra-articular exit point, but with separate bony tunnels for each graft and later incorporation (Fig. 23-12).

In the case of significant tibial tunnel expansion, the previous tunnel may be used for both grafts, although this is not preferred and may lead to incorrect placement of the grafts within the tibial tunnel. In this situation, staged procedures with bone grafting are preferred to allow for anatomic revision surgery.

Graft Passage and Fixation

Passing pins are directed through the femoral tunnels in identical trajectories to drilling from the accessory medial portal, and passing sutures are retrieved through the tibial tunnels using a probe or pituitary ronguer. At this time, anatomic placement of the tunnels can be checked using the exit points of the pins. They should exit the skin 2 to 4 cm apart on the lateral distal femur along the iliotibial band, and should be parallel to each other along the long axis of the femur (Fig. 23-13).

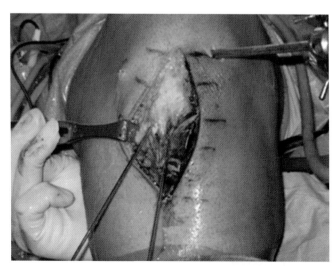

FIGURE 23-11 Tibial guide pin placement for double-bundle revision.

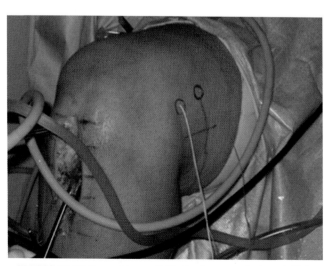

FIGURE 23-13 Pins exit in parallel to the femur on the lateral thigh.

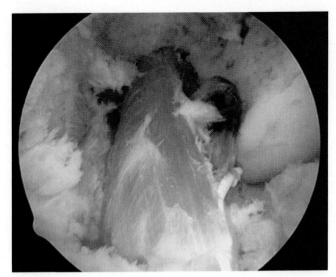

FIGURE 23-14 Passing the AM bundle while tensioning the PL bundle.

The PL bundle is passed first and femoral-sided fixation of this graft is done, usually with a 15-mm EndoButton (Smith & Nephew; Andover, Mass) fixation. Tension is kept on this graft while the AM bundle is passed and femoral-sided fixation is placed. Use of a probe or a 90- degree instrument may aid in passing the AM bundle past the PL graft. The AM bundle fixation is variable, and may be accomplished using an EndoButton or metal–soft tissue interference screw. The grafts are then cycled to evaluate isometry and pretension the grafts. The appropriately placed PL graft should have minimal translation with range of motion, but the AM may have a few millimeters of retraction in full extension (Fig. 23-14).

Our preferred and recommended technique is to tension and provide tibial fixation of the AM bundle first, at 30 to 60 degrees of flexion, using a cannulated bioabsorbable interference screw. The PL bundle is tensioned and fixed in full extension, often in

conjunction with backup anteromedial tibial fixation of the AM bundle using a soft tissue staple or screw and washer.

Final arthroscopic visualization confirms no impingement of the grafts, and postprocedure EUA is compared to the preoperative examination for re-creation of anteroposterior stability and elimination of the pivot shift (Fig. 23-15).

PEARLS&PITFALLS

PEARLS
- Anatomic double-bundle techniques allow for a greater intra-articular graft volume to counteract secondary laxity often encountered in revision situations.
- Hip flexion allows for knee hyperflexion during femoral tunnel drilling, assisting in the creation of anatomic tunnels.
- Anatomic positions of the AM and PL tunnels are determined at 90 degrees of knee flexion.
- Femoral passing pins should exit the skin 2 to 4 cm apart along the iliotibial band in parallel to the long axis of the femur.
- Accelerated physical therapy protocols are slowed to allow anchoring of the grafts in the bone tunnels and sports participation may be delayed until the 9- to 12-month mark.

PITFALLS
- Nonanatomic surgical technique in the primary ACL reconstruction represents the most common cause of failure of these procedures.
- Nonanatomic femoral locations represent the most commonly encountered error in tunnel placement and may be related to the transtibial approach to femoral tunnel drilling.
- A reconstruction of the ACL in the face of concurrent secondary laxity places nonphysiologic stresses on the graft, and often results in premature failure of these reconstructions.
- If the degree of tunnel expansion and osteolysis will not allow anatomic reconstruction or secure postoperative fixation of the grafts, the procedure should be staged.
- The office examination often underestimates the degree of anterolateral rotatory instability (pivot shift).

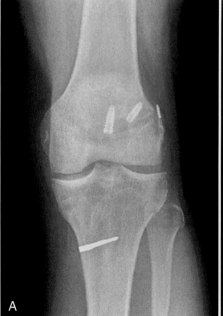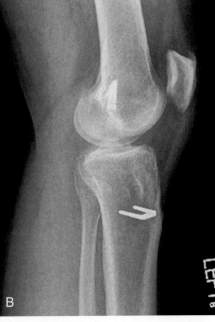

A   B

FIGURE 23-15 X-rays of final anatomic double-bundle revision ACL graft with retained vertical interference screw from primary ACL reconstruction. **A,** AP view. **B,** Lateral view. (From Shaver J, Johnson D. Revision anatomic double-bundle anterior cruciate ligament surgery. Oper Tech Sports Med. 2008;16:157-164.)

POSTOPERATIVE REHABILITATION PROTOCOL

The extremity is placed in a double-hinged knee brace locked in extension for the first 6 weeks while the patient is upright and ambulating. Patients can unlock the brace for seated duties and participation in physical therapy. At approximately 1 week postoperatively, we begin formal rehabilitation. We slightly slow the common accelerated physical therapy protocols because of concerns for anchoring the grafts in the bone tunnels. These protocols may be altered as a result of concomitant reconstruction of secondary stabilizers or additional surgery for meniscal or cartilage pathology. Remaining the same are the goals of maintenance of patellar mobility, almost full range of motion by 6 to 8 weeks, and emphasis on closed-chain lower extremity rehabilitation of all major muscle groups, including the hip. Sports participation follows similar benchmarks as primary surgery, although this may be delayed until the 9- to 12-month mark, allowing for strong graft incorporation and correct remodeling as well as full proprioceptive rehabilitation of the extremity.

CONCLUSIONS

Current published outcomes for revision ACL reconstructions are far from optimal, with only approximately 60% of patients returning to sports participation. Of these who do return, most do so at a level inferior to their previous goals. There are a myriad of causes of a failed primary surgery, but the goal of revision surgery remains the same—to provide a stable and functional ACL that most accurately reproduces the kinematics of the native knee. We believe that adherence to the philosophy, principles, and techniques of anatomic double-bundle anterior cruciate ligament reconstruction in the revision setting will improve overall outcomes, especially in regard to high-level sports participation.

REFERENCES

1. Johnson DL, Fu FH. Anterior cruciate ligament reconstruction: why do failures occur? *Instr Course Lect.* 1995;44:391-406.
2. Johnson DL, Harner CD, Maday MG, Fu FH. Revision anterior cruciate ligament surgery. In: Fu FH, Harner CD, Vince KG, eds. *Knee Surgery.* Baltimore: Williams & Wilkins; 1994;877-895.
3. Getelman MH, Friedman MJ. Revision anterior cruciate ligament reconstruction surgery, *J Am Acad Orthop Surg.* 1999;7:189-198,
4. Wetzler MJ, Getelman MH, Friedman MJ, et al. Revision anterior cruciate ligament surgery: etiology of failures. *Oper Tech Sports Med.* 1998; 6:64-70,
5. Chhabra A, Starman JS, Ferretti M, et al. Anatomic, radiographic, biomechanical, and kinematic evaluation of the anterior cruciate ligament and its two functional bundles. *J Bone Joint Surg Am.* 2006;4(suppl):2-10.
6. Ferretti M, Levicoff EA, Macpherson TA, et al. The fetal anterior cruciate ligament: an anatomic and histologic study. *Arthroscopy* 2007;23: 278-283.
7. Fu FH, Jordan SS. The lateral intercondylar ridge—a key to anatomic anterior cruciate ligament reconstruction. *J Bone Joint Surg Am.* 2007; 89:2103-2104. .
8. Yagi M, Kuroda R, Nagamune K, et al. Double-bundle ACL reconstruction can improve rotational stability. *Clin Orthop Relat Res.* 2007;(454): 100-107.
9. Harner CE, Irrgang JJ, Paul J. Loss of motion after anterior cruciate ligament surgery. *Am J Sports Med.* 1992;20:499-506.
10. Irrgang JJ, Harner CD. Loss of motion following knee ligament surgery. *Sports Med.* 1995;19:150-159.
11. Sachs RA, Daniel DM, Stone ML. Patellofemoral problems after anterior cruciate ligament reconstruction. *Am J Sports Med.* 1989;17:760-765.
12. Bach BR, Wojtys EM, Lindenfeld TN. Reflex sympathetic dystrophy, patella infera contracture syndrome, and loss of motion following anterior cruciate ligament surgery. *Instr Course Lect.* 1997;46:251-260.
13. Maday MG, Harner CD, Fu FH. Revision ACL surgery: evaluation and treatment. In: Feagin JA, ed. *The Crucial Ligaments.* New York: Churchill-Livingstone; 1994;711-723.
14. Jackson DW, Schaefer RK. Cyclops syndrome: loss of extension following intra-articular anterior cruciate ligament reconstruction. *Arthroscopy.* 1990;6:171-178.
15. Shelbourne KD, Wilckens JH, Mollasbashy A. Arthrofibrosis in acute anterior cruciate ligament reconstruction: the effects of timing of reconstruction and rehabilitation. *Am J Sports Med.* 1991;19:332-336.
16. Paulos L, Meislin R. Patellar entrapment following anterior cruciate ligament surgery. In: Jackson DW, Arnoczky SP Woo SLY, eds. *The Anterior Cruciate Ligament: Current and Future Concepts.* New York: Raven Press; 1993;365-372.
17. Arnold MP, Kooloos J, van Kampen A. Single-incision technique misses the anatomical femoral anterior cruciate ligament insertion: a cadaver study. *Knee Surg Sports Traumatol Arthrosc.* 2001;9:194-199.
18. Paessler H, Rossis J, Mastrokalos D, et al. Anteromedial vs. transtibial technique for correct femoral tunnel placement during arthroscopic ACL reconstruction with hamstrings: an in vivo study. *J Bone Joint Surg Br.* 2004;86(suppl):234.
19. Stevenson WW 3rd, Johnson DL. Vertical grafts: a common reason for functional failure after ACL reconstruction. *Orthopedics.* 2007;30: 206-209.
20. Howell SM, Taylor MA. Failure of reconstruction of the anterior cruciate ligament due to impingement on the intercondylar roof. *J Bone Joint Surg Am.* 1993;21:572-581.
21. Howell SM, Barad SJ. Knee extension and its relationship to the slope of the intercondylar roof: implications for positioning the tibial tunnel in anterior cruciate ligament reconstructions. *Am J Sports Med.* 1995;23: 288-294.
22. Jackson DW, Gasser SI. Tibial tunnel placement in ACL reconstruction. *Arthroscopy.* 1994;10:124-131.
23. Muneta T, Yamamoto H, Ishibashi T. The effects of tibial tunnel placement and roofplasty on reconstructed anterior cruciate ligament knees. *Arthroscopy.* 1995;11:57-62.
24. Kurosaka M, Yoshiya S, Andrish JT. A biomechanical comparison of different surgical techniques of graft fixation in anterior cruciate ligament reconstruction. *Am J Sports Med.* 1987;15:225-229.
25. Schepsis A, Getelman MH, Zimmer J. Revision ACL reconstruction: overall results and a comparison between autograft and allograft. Paper presented at: Book of Abstracts and Instructional Courses of the 14th Annual Meeting of the Arthroscopy Association of North America; May 4-7, 1995; San Francisco.
26. Rodeo SA, Arnoczky SP, Torzilli PA, et al. Tendon-healing in a bone tunnel: a biomechanical and histological study in the dog, *J Bone Joint Surg Am.* 1993;75:1795-1803.
27. Gobbi A, Domzalski M, Pascual J. Comparison of anterior cruciate ligament reconstruction in male and female athletes using the patellar tendon and hamstring autografts. *Knee Surg Sports Traumatol Arthrosc.* 2004;12:534-539.
28. Barrett GR, Noojin FK, Hartzog CW, et al. Clinical comparison of intra-articular anterior cruciate ligament reconstruction using autogenous semitendinosus and gracilis tendons in men versus women. *Am J Sports Med.* 2000;28:783-789.
29. Kim SJ, Kim TE, Lee DH, et al. Anterior cruciate ligament reconstruction in patients who have excessive joint laxity. *J Bone Joint Surg Am.* 2008;90:735-741.
30. Muller W. Kinematics. In: Muller W. *The Knee: Form, Function, and Ligament Reconstruction.* New York: Springer-Verlag; 1983:8-20.
31. Noyes FR, Stowers SF, Grood ES. Posterior subluxations of the medial and lateral tibiofemoral compartments: an in vitro ligament sectioning study in cadaveric knees. *Am J Sports Med.* 1993;21:407-414.
32. Gersoff WK, Clancy WG. Diagnosis of acute and chronic anterior cruciate ligament tears. *Clin Sports Med.* 1988;7:835-848.
33. Papageorgiau CD, Woo SLY, Fu FH. The biomechanical interdependence between the anterior cruciate ligament replacement graft and the medial meniscus. *Am J Sports Med.* 2001;29:1-6.
34. Paulos LE, Rosenberg TD, Parker RD. The medial knee ligaments: pathomechanics and surgical repair with emphasis on the external-rotation pivot-shift test. *Tech Orthop.* 1987;2:37-46.

35. Johnson DL, Swenson TM, Irrgang JJ, et al. Revision anterior cruciate ligament surgery: experience from Pittsburgh. *Clin Orthop Relat Res.* 1996;(325):100-109.

36. Uribe JW, Hechtman KS, Zvijac JE, Tjin-A-Tsoi EW. Revision anterior cruciate ligament surgery: experience from Miami. *Clin Orthop Relat Res.* 1996;325:91-99.

37. Grossman MG, El Attrache NS, Shields CL, Glousman RE. Revision anterior cruciate ligament reconstruction: three- to nine-year follow-up. *Arthroscopy.* 2005;21:418-423.

38. Johnson DL, Coen MJ. Revision ACL surgery: etiology, indications, techniques, and results. *Am J Knee Surg.* 1995;8:155-167.

39. Noyes FR, Schipplein OD, Andriacchi TP. The anterior cruciate ligament deficient knee with varus alignment: an analysis of gait adaptations and dynamic joint loadings. *Am J Sports Med.* 1992;20:707-716.

40. Gomoll AH, Bach Jr BR. Managing tunnel malposition and widening in revision anterior cruciate ligament surgery. *Oper Tech Sports Med.* 2006; 14:36-44.

41. Gilbart MK, Chhabra A, Harner CD. ACL surgery-the Pittsburgh experience. *Sports Med Arthrosc.* 2005;13:79-85.

42. Thomas NP, Kankate R, Wandless F, et al. Revision anterior cruciate ligament reconstruction using a two-stage technique with bone grafting of the tibial tunnel. *Am J Sports Med.* 2005;33:1701-1709.

43. Olsen EJ. Use of soft tissue allografts in sports medicine. *Adv Oper Orthop.* 1993;1:111-128.

44. Miller M. Revision cruciate ligament surgery with retention of femoral interference screws. *Arthroscopy.* 1998;14:111-114.

45. Dworsky B, Jewell BF, Bach BR Jr. Interference screw divergence in endoscopic anterior cruciate ligament reconstruction, *Arthroscopy.* 1996; 12:45-49.

46. Seon JK, Song EK, Bae BH, Park SJ. Kinematic study following double-bundle anterior cruciate ligament reconstruction. *Int Orthop.* 2007;31: 623-628.

47. Yasuda K, Kondo E, Ichiyama H, et al. Clinical evaluation of anatomic double bundle anterior cruciate ligament reconstruction using hamstring tendon grafts: comparisons among three different procedures. *Arthroscopy.* 2006;22:240-251.

48. Brophy RH, Selby RM, Altchek DW. Anterior cruciate ligament revision: double bundle augmentation of a primary vertical graft. *Arthroscopy.* 2006;22:683.

49. Cohen SB, Fu FH. Three-portal technique for anterior cruciate ligament reconstruction: use of a central medial portal. *Arthroscopy.* 2007; 23:325.

SUGGESTED READING

Shen W, Forsythe B, Ingham SM, et al. Application of the anatomic double-bundle reconstruction concept to revision and augmentation anterior cruciate ligament surgeries. *J. Bone Joint Surg Am.* 2008;90(suppl 4): 20-34.

Transtibial Single-Bundle Posterior Cruciate Ligament Reconstruction

Samuel P. Robinson ● Kevin F. Bonner

Injuries to the posterior cruciate ligament (PCL) are increasingly being recognized in athletes and trauma patients. The past decade has seen an increase in the diagnosis, treatment, and study of these injuries. Depending on the patient population being evaluated, there is a wide range reported for the incidence of PCL injuries. The incidence of PCL injury varies between 3% in an athletic population to 37% in the emergency room trauma setting.[1-3] Many of these patients have multiple ligament involvement including anterior cruciate ligament (ACL), posterolateral corner (PLC), and medial-sided injuries. Clinical and cadaveric studies have established that grade 3 PCL injuries usually involve concurrent injury to the posterolateral corner.[4]

In this chapter, we will describe the anatomy of the posterior cruciate ligament, pertinent aspects of the history and physical examination in evaluating patients with a potential PCL injury, diagnostic imaging, treatment options, and our single-bundle transtibial reconstruction technique. There is much debate surrounding PCL reconstruction, including timing and the optimal technique. This chapter describes our preferred transtibial technique in detail, but we are aware that several successful reconstructive techniques may yield equivalent outcomes.[5-12]

ANATOMY

Structure

The posterior cruciate ligament is an extra-articular ligament. Although it is clearly visualized arthroscopically, there is a thin layer of synovium that reflects from the posterior capsule and surrounds the PCL. The PCL is between 32 and 38 mm in length and its cross-sectional area at its midsubstance is 32.2 mm² (approximately 1.5 times larger than the ACL).[13] The insertion sites of the PCL are approximately three times larger than the midsubstance cross-sectional area, giving the PCL an hourglass ap-

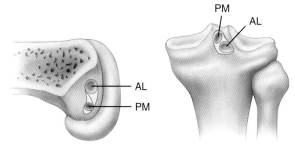

FIGURE 24-1 Anatomy of the PCL femoral (*left*) and PCL insertion (*right*) sites.

pearance. The fibers of the PCL attach on the tibia approximately 1.0 to 1.5 cm below the joint line in a lateral to medial direction (Fig. 24-1). On the femoral side, the PCL fibers attach to the medial femoral condyle in an anterior to posterior direction, adjacent to the anterior margin of the articular cartilage.

There are three main components of the PCL—the anterolateral bundle (AL), the posteromedial bundle (PM), and the meniscofemoral ligaments.[14-17] These components each have unique bony insertions as well as anatomic and biomechanical properties. The anterolateral bundle has a maximum load of 1120 N and a stiffness of 120 N/mm, the posteromedial bundle has a maximum load of 419 N and a stiffness of 57 N/mm, and the meniscofemoral ligaments have a maximum load of 297 N and a stiffness of 49 N/mm.[16] The anterior meniscofemoral ligament (ligament of Humphrey) and the posterior meniscofemoral ligament (ligament of Wrisberg) arise from the posterior horn of the lateral meniscus and sandwich the PCL bundles. Because the meniscofemoral ligaments are attached to the mobile lateral meniscus, it is possible for the PCL to be ruptured while the meniscofemoral ligaments remain intact. Their anatomic location and relative strength allow them to provide a scaffold for an injured PCL ligament while it attempts to heal. The AL bundle has twice the cross-sectional area of the PM bundle and 150% of the stiffness and strength, so it is considered the most important component of the PCL and the focus of single-bundle reconstructions.[18]

The vascular supply to the posterior cruciate ligament is from the popliteal artery via the middle geniculate artery. The synovial sleeve covering the PCL is well vascularized and is a major contributor to the blood supply of the ligament.[19,20] The synovial sleeve that provides a rich vascular supply to the PCL, as well as the meniscofemoral ligaments, gives some PCL injuries the potential to heal. Both the PCL and its synovial sleeve are innervated by nerve fibers from the popliteal plexus. The plexus receives contribution from the posterior articular nerve, a prominent branch of the posterior tibial nerve, and from the terminal portions of the obturator nerve.[21] Golgi organ–like structures have been observed near ligament origins beneath the synovial sheath and are thought to have a proprioceptive function in the knee.[22] Ruffini's corpuscles (pressure receptors), Vater-Pacini corpuscles (velocity receptors), and free nerve endings (pain receptors) have also been found in the PCL on histologic study.[23] Therefore, disruption of the PCL not only alters knee kinematics, but also alters the sensation and, probably, proprioception.[24]

Injuries to the posterolateral corner are commonly associated with PCL injuries. It is highly unlikely that a patient has a grade 3 PCL injury without a significant injury to the posterolateral corner.[4] The structures of the PLC have been studied at length and there remains some debate as to which structures are included. Traditionally, the structures of the posterolateral corner are the popliteus tendon, popliteofibular ligament, and lateral collateral ligament.[25-27] However, other structures that have been described as part of the posterolateral corner include the joint capsule, arcuate ligament, and fabellofibular ligaments.

Function

The kinematics of the posterior cruciate ligament reflects the two-bundle anatomy. The larger anterolateral bundle is tight in flexion and slackens with knee extension.[14,17] The posteromedial bundle is tight in extension and slackens with knee flexion. With deep knee flexion, the PM bundle moves anterior and away from the tibial plateau so that it becomes taut again in deep knee flexion.[28] Midranges of flexion recruit fibers from both bundles so that neither bundle is completely slack. When studied independently, however, neither bundle is completely isometric.

Biomechanical studies have shown that the PCL is the primary restraint to posterior drawer forces and is a secondary restraint to external rotation.[25-27] Isolated section of the PCL, without damage to the posterior capsule, results in a small degree of increased posterior laxity in full extension, with more pronounced increases in posterior laxity with flexion to 90 degrees.[29,30] In these studies, there were only minimal changes in rotation or varus-valgus laxity from isolated PCL sectioning.

The structures of the posterolateral corner each have an independent kinematic profile that comes together in a complex pattern to provide resistance to tibial external rotation and posterior tibial translation.[4,25-27] Individually, the lateral collateral ligament

(LCL) is the primary restraint to varus stress and does not significantly contribute to anterior/posterior translational control. The popliteofibular ligament complex, which comprises the popliteus and popliteofibular ligament, is relatively isometric and controls external tibial rotation at all angles of knee flexion.[31] It tightens in full extension to provide restraint to posterior tibial translation at full extension. Combined sectioning of the PCL and posterolateral corner results in significantly increased posterior laxity when compared with isolated sectioning of the PCL or the posterolateral corner alone.[32] Therefore, injuries to either structure when both are damaged will result in increase stress on the remaining structure or reconstruction.[33]

PATIENT EVALUATION

History

Evaluation of any patient begins with a careful history to delineate the specific mechanism of injury. This helps the physician determine the injury pattern, severity, acuity, and possible associated injuries. The mechanism of injury to the PCL is usually the result of an external force placed on the knee. The classic description of a dashboard injury results from a posteriorly directed force being placed on the tibia, with the knee in a flexed position. Noncontact injuries to the PCL, although rare, can result from hyperflexion or hyperextension mechanisms. Many patients with isolated lower grade PCL injuries do not report the sensation of a "pop" when injuring their knee. They often report swelling, stiffness, and mild posterior knee pain. Some patients may continue to participate in sports after the injury occurs. Higher grade multiligamentous knee injuries may result from severe trauma or from a seemingly benign mechanism with minimal evidence of trauma on physical examination. It is important to maintain a high index of suspicion.

Physical Examination

Physical examination should begin with evaluation for deformity, skin abrasions or contusions, limb alignment, gait pattern (if ambulatory), swelling, and range of motion. It is not uncommon for patients with isolated PCL injuries to have a moderate amount of swelling, an antalgic gait, and loss of up to 20 degrees of knee flexion. Patients typically have severe pain with multiligamentous injuries but, with lower grade injuries, may have just mild to moderate discomfort over the posterior aspect of their knee with knee flexion or posterior drawer examination. The presence of alignment or dynamic gait abnormalities are important to note in the chronic setting because the treatment plan may be altered in their presence.

Careful evaluation of the ligamentous structures of the knee is crucial. Because isolated PCL injuries are rare, and isolated grade 3 tears perhaps nonexistent, a multiligamentous injury should be suspected whenever a PCL injury is identified. The usual clinical testing of the ACL, medial collateral ligament (MCL), and LCL should be carried out. In an unstable knee, it is critical to perform these tests with the knee starting in a reduced position. If the test is performed from a subluxed position, the examiner may mistake the cause of laxity—for example, reporting a positive anterior drawer in the setting of a PCL tear because the anterior drawer test was initiated from a posteriorly subluxed position.

A posterior drawer test is the most accurate clinical test for PCL injuries.[34,35] The patient is placed supine with the knee flexed to 90 degrees and the tibia neutrally rotated. A posteriorly directed force is placed on the proximal tibia. This can also be performed with the tibia in external rotation (posterolateral drawer) and internal rotation (posteromedial drawer) to assist in evaluation of the posterolateral and posteromedial corners, respectively. The extent of posterior translation of the tibia with respect to the femur is measured by evaluating the relationship and change in position of the proximal tibia and medial femoral condyle. Normally, the medial proximal tibia is positioned approximately 1 cm anterior to the medial femoral condyle, but comparison with the contralateral side, if uninjured, can provide an accurate reference point. In addition to degree of translation, the quality of the end point is important in the evaluation of the PCL injury.

Grade I injuries are partial thickness tears that have a palpable but diminished step-off of the tibia with respect to the femur. This corresponds to 0 to 5 mm of posterior tibial translation. Grade II injuries are partial-thickness tears in which patients have lost the normal tibial step-off, but the proximal tibia does not translate posteriorly to the medial femoral condyle. This corresponds to 5 to 10 mm of posterior tibial translation. More than 10 mm of posterior tibial translation corresponds to a grade III injury, which is consistent with a complete PCL rupture.[33] The proximal tibia will translate posterior to the medial femoral condyle without a good end point in this setting. Grade III injuries are associated with PLC injury in most, if not all cases.[4]

The posterior sag test (Godfrey test) is performed with the hip and knee flexed to 90 degrees. The examiner supports the lower extremity by holding the foot and observes the proximal tibia with respect to the femur. In the setting of a complete PCL tear, gravity will pull the proximal tibia posteriorly. By comparing the anterior profile of the injured knee and proximal tibia with the normal side, very subtle posterior translations can be seen. The quadriceps active test is performed with the patient supine and the knee flexed to 60 degrees. While the examiner stabilizes the foot, the patient contracts the quadriceps muscle. With PCL insufficiency, the tibia will initially lie posteriorly subluxed when the knee is relaxed, but with isometric quadriceps contraction, the tibia will translate anteriorly and attempt to reduce relative to the femur. The reverse pivot shift test is performed by passively extending the knee from a flexed position with the foot externally rotated and a valgus force applied to the tibia. The tibia will initially be subluxed posterolaterally if the PCL-PLC is not functional, but will abruptly reduce with respect to the femur at 20 to 30 degrees of knee flexion as the knee comes into extension.[36] Additional tests for injury to the PCL and posterolateral corner have been described. See the chapter on the posterolateral corner for an in-depth review of this topic (Chapter ••).

A careful neurovascular examination is critical for evaluating patients with PCL injuries. The structures of the popliteal fossa include the popliteal artery, popliteal vein, tibial nerve, and peroneal nerve. The popliteal artery is tethered proximally at the adductor hiatus and distally at the soleus arch, and therefore vulnerable to injury from dislocation of the knee. The peroneal nerve is at risk for injury because of the course it takes around the fibular head, especially in the setting of associated varus injury. The incidence of neurovascular injury ranges from 14% to 49%.[26,29,30] Because many knee dislocations "autoreduce" before they are examined or imaged, the physician must be careful to monitor for injury and to get appropriate studies if injury is suspected.

Diagnostic Imaging

Radiography

A standard knee series, including bilateral standing anteroposterior (AP), AP flexion 45-degree weight-bearing, lateral, and Merchant patellar radiographs, should be evaluated for evidence of posterior tibial subluxation, avulsion fractures, and associated knee injury. Subtle posterior tibial subluxation may be the only finding on these films. The unopposed pull of the hamstrings causes posterior tibial subluxation, which can become fixed within a short time. Stress lateral radiography performed in neutral rotation and the knee flexed to 90 degrees with and without a posterior drawer force may show increased tibial translation with respect to the femur when compared with the contralateral knee (Fig. 24-2).

Magnetic Resonance Imaging

Magnetic resonance imaging (MRI) has become the diagnostic study of choice for evaluation of the knee with clinical suspicion of a PCL injury (Fig. 24-3). MRI and stress radiography have been shown to corroborate the severity of the PCL injury as identified on physical examination.[37] Normally, the PCL appears curvilinear and dark on both T1- and T2-weighted sequences, representing the relatively lax anterolateral component. The sensitivity of an MRI scan for determining acute PCL tears has been reported to be between 96% and 100%.[38-40] The sensitivity of MRI, however, is not nearly as good for the evaluation of a chronic PCL injury. It is not uncommon for the PCL to look attenuated but intact, even in the setting of chronic grade III instability. MRI is also helpful for evaluating and determining the appropriate treatment course for associated injuries to the knee.

TREATMENT

Indications and Contraindications

Each patient is treated individually based on age, activity level, and associated injuries, but the following are our general guidelines.

Indications

Patient with low-grade PCL injuries that can be treated successfully with conservative treatment are not indicated for PCL reconstruction.[41,42] Most isolated grades I and II PCL injuries do well with conservative management, including a rehabilitation program that focuses on quadriceps strengthening while eliminating any hamstring strengthening through a flexed knee.[26,43,44] Insertion site avulsions from the femur or tibia may be treated successfully if acute anatomic repair is possible and typically

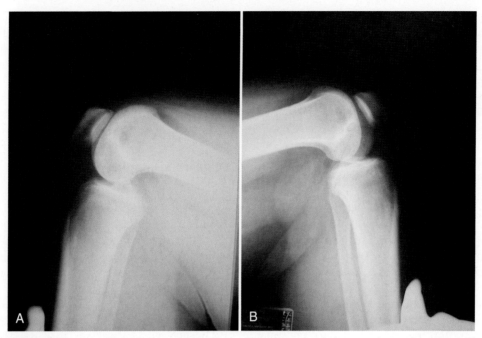

FIGURE 24-2 Stress radiographs of a grade III PCL tear (**A**) compared with the normal contralateral knee (**B**).

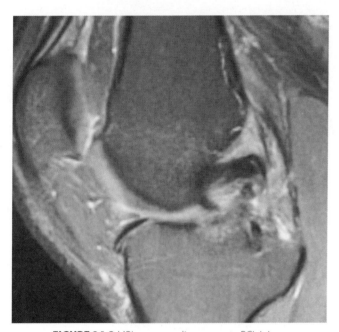

FIGURE 24-3 MRI scan revealing an acute PCL injury.

yield results superior to reconstruction. Acute grade III PCL tears combined with a PLC injury and/or other multiligamentous injuries is generally considered an indication for surgery. Associated ligament injuries, especially to the posterolateral corner, also need to be evaluated and treated appropriately. Posterolateral corner injuries and insertion site avulsions are best treated with acute direct repair (within 3 weeks of injury). Patients with chronic grade III PCL injuries that fail conservative treatment and cause symptomatic functional instability are candidates for PCL reconstruction.

Contraindications

In the chronic setting, patients with significant malalignment or visual gait disturbances should not be treated with isolated PCL reconstruction. Long-term successful treatment of these problems may require more than an isolated soft tissue reconstruction. In situations in which both bony malalignment and ligamentous laxity exist, the bony component must be addressed first or at the time of ligamentous reconstruction to maximize the healing potential of the soft tissue work. Revision cases must have adequate bone stock to support tunnels and bone-tendon healing. Additional procedures, such as additional ligament reconstructions, may be performed concurrently with PCL reconstruction or may require staged reconstruction.

Conservative Management

Nonoperative treatment for grades I and II PCL injuries has been shown to have a high rate of success.[33,43,44] We use a four-phase rehabilitation protocol for nonoperative treatment of grades I and II PCL injuries. Phase I involves a brace locked in extension for 6 to 8 weeks after the initial injury. The patient is weight bearing as tolerated while in the brace and uses crutches as needed for assistance. The patient may remove the brace for physical therapy and a home exercise program. The key to this phase is to avoid posterior tibial translation and active knee flexion while the PCL heals. Phase II begins with discontinuation of the brace and crutches when gait has normalized. Physical therapy focuses on restoring range of motion and quadriceps strength through a progressive step up program. Open-chain hamstring exercises are discouraged. Phase III begins active knee flexion without resistance, a progressive step-down program, and proprioception activities. The goals of phase III include full range of motion and functional progression with adequate strength. Phase IV is sport-specific training with aggressive functional strengthening, gradual return to running, agility exercises, and plyometric training.

Arthroscopic Technique

The patient is placed on the table in the supine position with the knee placed beyond the break in the table to allow space behind the knee once the foot of the table is dropped down. Both knees are examined under anesthesia to confirm the surgical plan. A tourniquet is applied to the proximal thigh. Position the leg to allow access for intraoperative fluoroscopy or radiography.

Our graft of choice is a fresh-frozen Achilles allograft, which is prepared for 12-mm femoral and tibial tunnels. We may go down to 11-mm tunnels in the setting of a small patient. We use the calcaneal bone portion of the graft to create a 12- by 25-mm bone plug, which will be placed in the femoral tunnel. The graft is prepared at the beginning of the procedure by the surgeon or assistant. Alternatively, if an autograft is preferred, the graft may be obtained by harvesting the quadriceps, patellar, or hamstring tendon. Tunnels would have to be downsized accordingly based on autograft selection and size.

Standard anterior knee arthroscopy portals are used for the procedure. When establishing the anterior medial portal, make sure that there is adequate access to the posterior aspect of the joint when the knee is in flexion, without obstruction of the medial femoral condyle. A spinal needle can be used to optimize portal placement. The arthroscope is placed in the anterior lateral portal and instruments are placed through the anterior medial portal. A posterior medial portal is typically required, except in cases of concurrent ACL reconstruction, when it is not always necessary. This portal is located approximately 1 cm above the joint line and allows access to the tibial footprint of the PCL. A cannula is kept in this portal and a 70-degree arthroscope can be valuable for visualization.

A posteromedial safety incision, as described by Fanelli,[45] can be valuable not only for avoiding injury, but also for expediting proper tibial tunnel placement (Fig. 24-4). A 2.0- to 2.5-cm incision is made approximately 3 cm distal to the joint line. The crural fascia is incised in a longitudinal fashion anterior to the medial head of the gastrocnemius muscle. This is the same interval commonly used for the tibial inlay approach. A gloved finger can be used to dissect the interval bluntly under the medial head of the gastrocnemius, over the popliteus muscle belly, and proximally along the tibia up to the PCL insertion site. In this location, the gloved finger will be extracapsular, with the neurovascular structures lying just posterior. This enables the surgeon to check the proper placement of the PCL tibial guide and guide pin while protecting the neurovascular structures behind the finger during the reaming. A malleable ribbon retractor can also be used in this interval to help protect the neurovascular bundle.

FIGURE 24-4 Fanelli safety incision. **A,** Proper placement below the joint line. **B, C,** The proper anatomic intervals for the safety incision (lateral and axial views). (**A** *adapted from Biomet Sports Medicine, Warsaw, Ind.*)

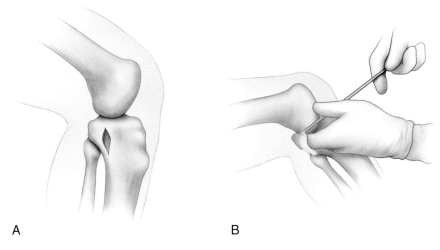

A   B

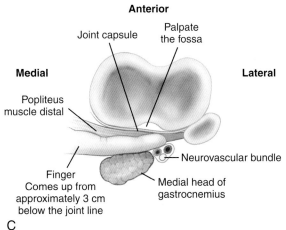

C

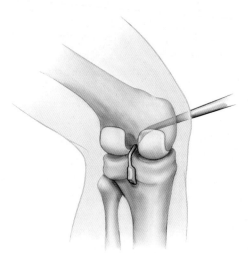

FIGURE 24-5 Posterior capsular elevation with curved PCL instruments through the medial portal. *(Adapted from Biomet Sports Medicine, Warsaw, Ind.)*

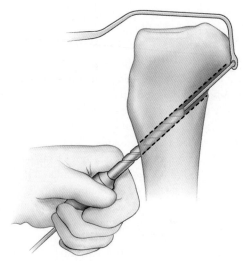

FIGURE 24-7 The tibial guide pin is capped during reaming of the tibial tunnel. *(Adapted from Biomet Sports Medicine, Warsaw, Ind.)*

It is critical to perform a diagnostic arthroscopy to evaluate and treat coexisting pathology, which needs to be addressed in the setting of a grade III PCL injury. The remnant of the torn PCL is débrided using standard synovial shavers but maintaining a small footprint on the femoral side. This will serve as a guide for appropriate femoral tunnel placement. With the arthroscope in the anterior lateral portal, the anterior and posterior medial portals can be used to débride the remnant of the PCL tibial stump. This needs to be done carefully, with the blade of the shaver always facing away from the thin posterior capsule. Curved PCL instruments are used through the anteromedial portal to elevate the posterior capsule off of the tibia (Fig. 24-5). The posteromedial safety incision can be used to ensure that the curettes are properly positioned on the bone.

The curved PCL guide is placed through the anterior medial portal and over the back of the tibia into the PCL fossa (Fig. 24-6) with the assistance of the surgeon's finger through the posteromedial safety incision. The guide pin is placed in the tibial insertion site of the PCL with a vertical orientation when compared with a standard ACL reconstruction tunnel. A 3-cm incision is made on the anteromedial aspect of the tibia for placement of the tibial tunnel. The guide is initially placed to determine the proper location of the anteromedial incision. The tibial guide pin is placed using extreme caution under fluoroscopy to ensure proper pin placement and avoid injury to the neurovascular structures. Placing the arthroscope in the posteromedial portal may offer improved visualization of the guide pin.

The tip of the guide pin is covered with a curved curette to prevent its advancement and the tibial tunnel is reamed with a standard constant diameter cigar reamer (Fig. 24-7). Fluoroscopy and a finger in the posterior medial safety incision can be used to make sure that the guide pin is not advancing. Fanelli has recommended that surgeons stop reaming once at the inner portion of the posterior cortex, leave the cigar reamer in place, remove the guide wire, and replace it with the blunt end going up into the reamer to the posterior cortex.[45] This technique will help avoid injury to the neurovascular structures if the guide pin is inadvertently advanced (Fig. 24-8). When reaming through the posterior cortex, the reamer may be used without power to provide additional safety. The reamer will initially penetrate the distal posterior cortex, which is typically out of the arthroscopic visualization field. Once again, the neurovascular bundle can be protected with a malleable retractor or with a finger through the safety incision. When reaming is completed, a rasp is used to smooth the sharp edges along the edge of the tunnel (Fig. 24-9).

Although the femoral tunnel can be established via an inside-out or outside-in method, we currently prefer the inside-out technique. An accessory low anterolateral portal is made with the aid of a spinal needle. Inside-out femoral guides are commercially available (Biomet Sports Medicine; Warsaw, Ind) and placed through the low anterolateral portal. The aiming guide allows direct visualization of the ultimate position of the femoral tunnel. For the single-bundle PCL reconstruction, the guide (and subsequent tunnel) is centered over the femoral anterolateral bundle footprint (Fig. 24-10). If the footprint is difficult to visualize, the single-bundle tunnel will be at approximately the 10:30 position on a left knee and 1:30 on a right knee, with the

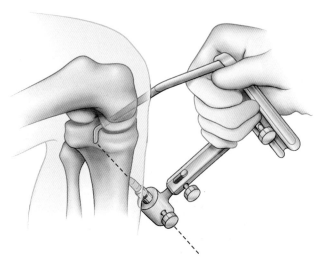

FIGURE 24-6 PCL guide positioned for proper placement of the transtibial guide pin. *(Adapted from Biomet Sports Medicine, Warsaw, Ind.)*

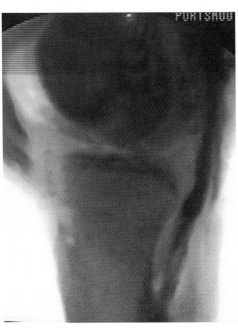

FIGURE 24-8 Lateral x-ray with contrast in the artery and vein showing the proximity of the vascular structures to the posterior tibia.

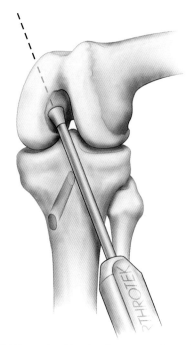

FIGURE 24-10 Femoral guide wire placement using an inside-out guide. *(Adapted from Biomet Sports Medicine, Warsaw, Ind.)*

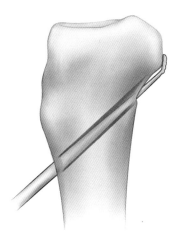

FIGURE 24-9 The tunnel edges are chamfered after reaming. *(Adapted from Biomet Sports Medicine, Warsaw, Ind.)*

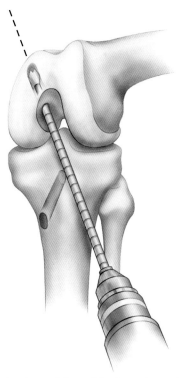

FIGURE 24-11 Inside-out drilling of the femoral tunnel through an accessory low anterolateral portal. *(Adapted from Biomet Sports Medicine, Warsaw, Ind.)*

knee in 90 degrees of flexion. Make sure that the tunnel does not violate the articular cartilage of the medial femoral condyle; however, the edge of the tunnel will typically be within 3 to 5 mm of the articular surface. As an example, for a 12-mm tunnel, the guide pin will be placed approximately 10 mm from the articular surface (6-mm tunnel radius plus 4 mm). Drill the femoral guide pin through the aiming guide, through the femur, and out of the lateral skin. An acorn reamer is then used to drill from inside-out through the accessory anterolateral portal (Fig. 24-11) while being careful not to injure the cartilage on the lateral femoral condyle during this step. A rasp is again used to smooth the edges of the tunnel.

Alternatively, an outside-in PCL femoral guide may be used. The guide is placed through the inferomedial portal so that the guide pin exits through the center of the anterolateral footprint (Fig. 24-12). The guide should be angled so the guide pin

will enter through the medial aspect of the metaphysis, proximal to the epicondyle and medial to the trochlea (Fig. 24-13). Confirm that the femoral tunnel will not violate the articular surface of the trochlear groove and drill from outside-in with the appropriately sized cannulated cigar reamer (Fig. 24-14). Cap the guide pin with a curette and use care not to injure the ACL or

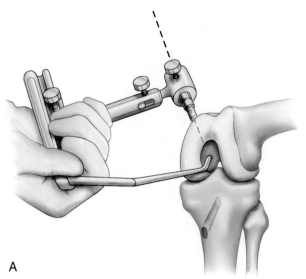

A

FIGURE 24-12 The PCL guide is positioned from outside-in through the anteromedial portal. *(Adapted from Biomet Sports Medicine, Warsaw, Ind.)*

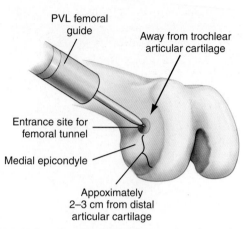

PVL femoral guide

Away from trochlear articular cartilage

Entrance site for femoral tunnel

Medial epicondyle

Appoximately 2–3 cm from distal articular cartilage

FIGURE 24-13 Proper entry point for the outside-in femoral guide pin and tunnel.

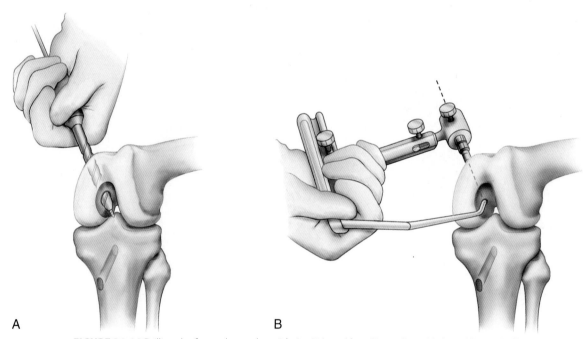

A   **B**

FIGURE 24-14 Drilling the femoral tunnel outside-in. *(Adapted from Biomet Sports Medicine, Warsaw, Ind.)*

other intra-articular structures when entering the joint with the reamer. Remove bony debris and smooth the edges of the tunnel with a rasp.

The optimal graft delivery technique depends on the surgeon's preferred femoral fixation method. When using graft fixation to the outer cortex of the femoral metaphysis for primary or backup fixation, the graft can be delivered outside-in through the femur, across the joint, and into the tibial tunnel. A looped 18-gauge wire is advanced through the tibial tunnel and pulled into the joint with a grasper placed through an anterior arthroscopy portal. Passage of the wire into the joint can be made easier by placing a finger through the posteromedial safety incision and reducing the tibia with an anterior drawer force. The grasper is then placed into the joint through the femoral tunnel and used to pull the wire loop up through the femoral tunnel. The wire loop can now be used to pass the graft proximally to distally (Fig. 24-15). Alternatively, a commercially available suture-passing device (Magellan suture passer; Biomet) can be used in a similar manner.

We alternatively use a graft delivery technique that uses the accessory inferolateral portal (see Fig. 24-15B). The looped 18-gauge wire is delivered through the tibia similarly to the previously described technique, except that the wire is delivered out the accessory inferolateral portal. A Beath pin is placed through the same portal, through the femoral tunnel, and exits through the skin. Because we typically use a large Achilles allograft with a bone plug, the bone plug sutures are placed through the Beath pin eyelet (femoral side) and

the sutures holding the soft tissue end of the graft are passed through the 18-gauge wire loop (tibial side). The Beath pin and 18-gauge wire are both advanced to deliver the bone plug into the femoral tunnel and the soft tissue side of the graft into the tibial tunnel, respectively. It is important to make sure that the sutures are delivered through the tibial tunnel before attempting to pass the large soft tissue graft itself. Occasionally, soft tissue from the fat pad can get caught between the Beath pin and wire loop. This soft tissue must be débrided prior to graft passage to prevent the graft from getting caught. One way to avoid this problem is to place an arthroscopy cannula into the accessory inferolateral portal before the wire loop and Beath pin are passed through the portal. Once the suture shuttles are delivered, the cannula is removed before the sutures and graft are passed. This alternative graft passage technique uses a femoral interference screw at the intra-articular aperture for fixation and obviates the need to drill the femoral tunnel all the way through the femoral metaphysis and the need to make an additional incision. However, this technique does not provide for backup femoral fixation.

Once the graft is passed, the femoral side is fixed first with a metal or bioabsorbable interference screw. This can be accomplished inside-out, to obtain aperture fixation (our preferred method), or outside-in. If fixation is thought to be suboptimal, backup fixation is used on the outer cortex. Once the femoral side is fixed, a commercially available graft-tensioning device (Biomet) is used to assist the surgeon in maintaining proper graft tension and joint reduction during

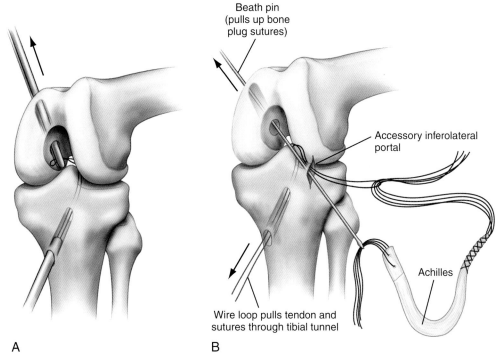

A   B

FIGURE 24-15 A, A wire loop is used to pass the graft proximally to distally. **B,** Schematic showing passage of the graft through the accessory anterolateral portal.

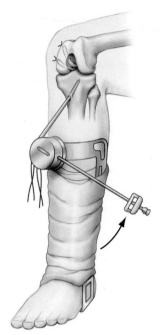

FIGURE 24-16 Knee ligament graft-tensioning boot assists the surgeon during graft tensioning and fixation. *(Adapted from Biomet Sports Medicine, Warsaw, Ind.)*

tibial fixation (Fig. 24-16). The ends of the sutures from the tibial side of the graft are attached to the tensioning device and traction is applied through a ratcheting mechanism. The tibial step-off is reduced to normal and the knee is cycled 20 to 25 times throughout a full range of motion. The tibial side of the graft is secured primarily with a bioabsorbable interference screw placed over a guide wire up to the posterior cortex of the tibia, with the knee between 70 and 90 degrees of flexion. Backup fixation is provided by a screw with a washer on the tibial cortex (Fig. 24-17).

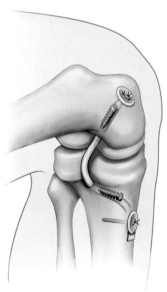

FIGURE 24-17 Final fixation of the graft. Alternatively, backup fixation may be also be used on the outer cortex of the femur.

PEARLS&PITFALLS

PEARLS
1. Grade 3 PCL tears are typically associated with a posterolateral corner injury; both need to be addressed at the time of surgery.
2. Ask a vascular surgeon to be available in the event of an inadvertent vascular injury.
3. Have patience when débriding the remnant of the tibial stump and stripping the posterior capsule. This will take some time and it is important that this be done carefully.
4. Use fluoroscopy to confirm proper tibial tunnel placement. The proper location is typically more distal than surgeons often expect.
5. Be careful when reaming the tibial tunnel. Consider placing the blunt end of the guide wire posteriorly.
6. Use the safety incision to retract and protect the neurovascular structures.
7. Reducing the tibia manually with an anterior drawer force will assist in the passage of a wire loop and the graft itself.
8. Recovery and rehabilitation are slower and more conservative than with an ACL.

PITFALLS
1. Make sure the tibial tunnel is appropriately distal.
2. Always rule out concomitant injuries, especially posterolateral corner injury.
3. Proceed conservatively with postoperative rehabilitation.

Postoperative Rehabilitation

Postoperatively, patients are placed in a brace locked in extension. Initially, care is taken during the rehabilitation protocol to avoid posterior tibial translation and active knee flexion. Patients are partial weight bearing for the first 2 weeks and gradually progress to full weight-bearing by week 5. This, however, may be modified based on concomitant reconstructive procedures. Braces and crutches are used until the quadriceps are adequately strengthened and gait has normalized, approximately week 6. Goals for the first 5 weeks include range of motion from 0 to 90 degrees using active assisted range of motion extension from 70 to 0 degrees and passive range of motion for flexion. Range of motion is gradually increased from weeks 6 to 12 and a progressive step-up/step-down program is implemented. Open-chain hamstring exercises are not initiated until week 12 and resistive knee flexion exercises are not initiated until week 20. As long as progression with rehabilitation falls within the expected guidelines, patients may start running in a straight line 6 months postoperatively with expected return to sport at from 8 to 12 months.

REFERENCES

1. Miyasaka D, Daniel D, Stone M. The incidence of knee ligament injuries in the general population. *Am J Knee Surg.* 1991;4:85-96.
2. Fanelli GC. Posterior cruciate ligament injuries in trauma patients. *Arthroscopy.* 1993;9:291-294.
3. Fanelli GC, Edson CJ. Posterior cruciate ligament injuries in trauma patients: part II. *Arthroscopy.* 1995;11:526-529.
4. Sekiya JK, Whiddon DR, Zehms CT, Miller MD. A clinically relevant assessment of posterior cruciate ligament and posterolateral corner injuries. Evaluation of isolated and combined deficiency. *J Bone Joint Surg Am.* 2008;90:1621-1627.

5. Sekiya JK, West RV, Ong BC, et al. Clinical outcomes after isolated arthroscopic single-bundle posterior cruciate ligament reconstruction. *Arthroscopy.* 2005;21:1042-1050.
6. MacGillivray JD, Stein BE, Park M, et al. Comparison of tibial inlay vs. transtibial techniques for isolated posterior cruciate ligament reconstruction: minimum 2-year follow-up. *Arthroscopy.* 2006;22:320-328.
7. Seon JK, Song EK. Reconstruction of isolated posterior cruciate ligament injuries: a clinical comparison of the transtibial and tibial inlay techniques. *Arthroscopy.* 2006;22:27-32.
8. Chen CH, Chen WJ, Shih CH, Chou SW. Arthroscopic posterior cruciate ligament reconstruction with quadriceps tendon autograft: minimal 3 years follow-up. *Am J Sports Med.* 2004;32:361-368.
9. Wang CJ, Weng LH, Hsu CC, Chan YS. Arthroscopic single vs. double bundle posterior cruciate ligament reconstructions using hamstring autograft. *Injury.* 2004;35:1293-1299.
10. Ahn JH, Yoo JC, Wang JH. Posterior cruciate ligament reconstruction: double-loop hamstring tendon autograft vs Achilles tendon allograft. Clinical results of a minimum 2-year follow-up. *Arthroscopy.* 2005;21: 965-969.
11. Wu CH, Chen AC, Yuan LJ, et al. Arthroscopic reconstruction of the posterior cruciate ligament by using a quadriceps tendon autograft: a minimum 5-year follow-up. *Arthroscopy.* 2007;23:420-427.
12. Hatayama K, Higuchi H, Kimura M, et al. A comparison of arthroscopic single and double bundle posterior cruciate ligament reconstruction: review of 20 cases. *Am J Orthop.* 2006;35:568-571.
13. Girgis FG, Marshall JL, Monajem A. The cruciate ligaments of the knee joint. Anatomical, functional, and experimental analysis. *Clin Orthop Relat Res.* 1975;(106):216-231.
14. Harner CD, Xerogeanes JW, Livesay GA, et al. The human posterior cruciate ligament complex: an interdisciplinary study. Ligament morphology and biomechanical evaluation. *Am J Sports Med.* 1995;23: 736-45.
15. Harner CD, Livesay GA, Kashiwaguchi S. et al. Comparative study of the size and shape of the human anterior and posterior cruciate ligaments. *J Orthop Res.* 1995;13:429-434.
16. Race A, Amis AA. Loading of the two bundles of the posterior cruciate ligament: an analysis of bundle function in AP drawer. *J Biomech.* 1996; 29:873-879.
17. Amis AA, Gupte CM, Bull AM, Edwards A. Anatomy of the posterior cruciate ligament and the meniscofemoral ligaments. *Knee Surg Sports Traumatol Arthrosc.* 2006;14:257-263.
18. Inderster A, Benedetto KP, Klestil T, et al. Fiber orientation of posterior cruciate ligament: an experimental morphological and functional study. Part 2. *Clin Anat.* 1995;8:315-322.
19. Arnoczky SP, Rubin RM, Marshall JL. Microvasculature of the cruciate ligaments and its response to injury. An experimental study in dogs. *J Bone Joint Surg Am.* 1979;61:1221-1229.
20. Scapinelli R. Studies on the vasculature of the human knee joint. *Acta Anat (Basel).* 1968;70:305-331.
21. Kennedy JC, Alexander IJ, Hayes KC. Nerve supply of the human knee and its functional importance. *Am J Sports Med.* 1982;10:329-335.
22. Schultz RA, Miller DC, Kerr CS, Micheli L. Mechanoreceptors in human cruciate ligaments. A histological study. *J Bone Joint Surg Am.* 1984; 66:1072-1076.
23. Katonis PG, Assimakopoulos AP, Agapitos MV, Exarchou EI. Mechanoreceptors in the posterior cruciate ligament. Histologic study on cadaver knees. *Acta Orthop Scand.* 1991;62:276-278.
24. Safran MR, Allen AA, Lephart SM, et al. Proprioception in the posterior cruciate ligament deficient knee. *Knee Surg Sports Traumatol Arthrosc.* 1999;7:310-317.
25. Grood ES, Stowers SF, Noyes FR. Limits of movement in the human knee. Effect of sectioning the posterior cruciate ligament and the posterolateral structures. *J Bone Joint Surg Am.* 1988;70:88-97.
26. Veltri DM, Deng XH, Torzilli PA, et al. The role of the popliteofibular ligament in stability of the human knee. A biomechanical study. *Am J Sports Med.* 1996;24:19-27.
27. Gollehon DL, Torzilli PA, Warren RF. The role of the posterolateral and cruciate ligaments in the stability of the human knee. A biomechanical study. *J Bone Joint Surg Am.* 1987;69:233-242.
28. Van Dommelen BA, Fowler PJ. Anatomy of the posterior cruciate ligament. A review. *Am J Sports Med.* 1989;17:24-29.
29. Fox RJ, Harner CD, Sakane M, et al. Determination of the in situ forces in the human posterior cruciate ligament using robotic technology. A cadaveric study. *Am J Sports Med.* 1998;26:395-401.
30. Markolf KL, Feeley BT, Tejwani SG, et al. Changes in knee laxity and ligament force after sectioning the posteromedial bundle of the posterior cruciate ligament. *Arthroscopy.* 2006;22:1100-1106.
31. Sugita T, Amis AA. Anatomic and biomechanical study of the lateral collateral and popliteofibular ligaments. *Am J Sports Med.* 2001;29: 466-472.
32. Harner CD, Baek GH, Vogrin TM. et al. Quantative analysis of human cruciate ligament insertions. *Arthroscopy.* 1999;15:741-749.
33. Harner CD, Hoher J. Evaluation and treatment of posterior cruciate ligament injuries. *Am J Sports Med.* 1998;26:471-482.
34. Clancy WG Jr, Shelbourne KD, Zoeliner GB, et al. Treatment of knee joint instability secondary to rupture of the posterior cruciate ligament: Report of a new procedure. *J Bone Joint Surg Am.* 1983;65:310-322.
35. Covey DC, Sapega AA. Injuries to the posterior cruciate ligament. *J Bone Joint Surg Am.* 1993;75:1376-1386.
36. Jakob R, Hassler H, Staeubli H. Observations on rotatory instability of the lateral compartment of the knee: Experimental studies on the functional anatomy and the pathomechanism of the true and reversed pivot shift sign. *Acta Orthop Scand Suppl.* 1982;91:1-32.
37. Schulz MS, Steenlage ES, Russe K, Strobel MJ. Distribution of posterior tibial displacement in knees with posterior cruciate ligament tears. *J Bone Joint Surg Am.* 2007;89:332-338.
38. Esmaili J, et al. Accuracy of MRI in comparison with clinical and arthroscopic findings in ligamentous and meniscal injuries of the knee. *Acta Orthop Belg.* 2005;71:189-96.
39. Grover JS, Bassett LW, Gross ML, et al. Posterior cruciate ligament: MR imaging. *Radiology.* 1990;174:527-530.
40. Polly DW Jr, Callaghan JJ, Sikes RA, et al. The accuracy of selective magnetic resonance imaging compared with the findings of arthroscopy of the knee. *J Bone Joint Surg Am.* 1988;70:192-198.
41. Torg JS, Barton TM, Pavlov H, Stine R. Natural history of the posterior cruciate ligament-deficient knee. *Clin Orthop Relat Res.* 1989; (246):208-216.
42. Boynton MD, Tietjens BR. Long-term follow-up of the untreated isolated posterior cruciate ligament-deficient knee. *Am J Sports Med.* 1996; 24:306-310.
43. Shelbourne KD, Davis TJ, Patel DV. The natural history of acute, isolated, nonoperatively treated posterior cruciate ligament injuries: A prospective study. *Am J Sports Med.* 1999;27:276-283.
44. Shelbourne KD, Muthukaruppan Y. Subjective results of nonoperatively treated, acute, isolated posterior cruciate ligament injuries. *Arthroscopy.* 2005;21:457-461.
45. Fanelli GC, ed. *Posterior Cruciate Ligament Injuries: A Practical Guide To Management.* New York: Springer-Verlag; 2004.

SUGGESTED READINGS

Fanelli GC, Orcutt DR, Edson CJ. Current concepts: the multiple ligament-injured knee. *Arthroscopy.* 2005;21:471-486.
Fanelli GC, Edson CJ, Reinheimer KN. Arthroscopically assisted posterior cruciate ligament reconstruction. In: Jackson DW, ed. *Master Techniques in Orthopaedic Surgery: Reconstructive Knee Surgery.* 3rd ed. Philadelphia: Lippincott, Williams & Wilkins; 2008:223-239.

Double-Bundle Posterior Cruciate Ligament Reconstruction

David McGuire ● Stephen Hendricks

Injuries to the posterior cruciate ligament (PCL), although infrequent, often present as complex problems that can result in severe disability because of the relationship between posterior instability and rotatory instability, combined with other ligamentous injury and cartilage degeneration. It is rare that PCL injuries occur in isolation; they frequently present in conjunction with anterior cruciate ligament (ACL) or posterolateral corner injuries.[1] Both the rare isolated and concomitant PCL lesions are often misdiagnosed or overlooked altogether because PCL-specific symptoms can be difficult to distinguish or can be confounding when presenting with additional injuries.[2]

Joint function impairment in PCL-deficient knees correlates positively with chronicity.[3-6] A PCL failure over time imposes additional medial compartment forces, resulting in increased pain and joint effusion. Functional limitations become increasingly frequent, especially with coexisting ligament injuries.[7,8] Better understanding of PCL biomechanics has led to improvements in clinical evaluation and resulted in earlier recognition of PCL insufficiency. With earlier diagnoses and improvements in PCL reconstruction techniques, surgical indications for this type of injury have expanded markedly.[9-13]

ANATOMY

Anatomic descriptions of the PCL vary by degree of detail. The ligament is commonly described as consisting of two fiber bundles, the anterolateral (AL) and posteromedial (PM), with each defined by their relative femorotibial insertion sites, respectively. The anterior section comprises the bulk of the fibers, with the cross-sectional mass almost four times larger than the posterior section. The AL bundle is taut in flexion and becomes lax when approaching extension, whereas the significantly smaller PM bundle is tight in extension (Figs. 25-1 and 25-2) and relaxes toward flexion.[14]

In close conjunction with the PCL, two meniscofemoral ligaments can be present in some knees. Although their presence can vary, their attachments are uniform. Both ligaments attach distally to the posteromedial aspect of the lateral meniscus. The anterior meniscofemoral ligament (ligament of Humphry) passes diagonally anterior to the PCL and inserts on the lateral aspect of the medial femoral condyle in the roof of the intercondylar notch. The posterior meniscofemoral ligament (ligament of Wrisberg) passes at almost the same angle posterior to the PCL

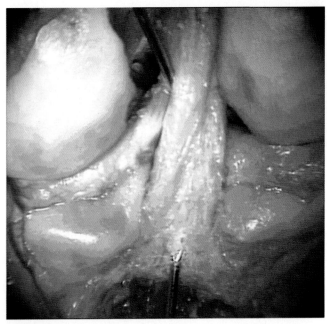

FIGURE 25-1 In this posterior image, the PCL is visualized and the PM bundle is seen crossing posteriorly to the AL bundle as it travels diagonally and superior from the tibial attachment on the posterior aspect of the femoral insertion with the knee in extension.

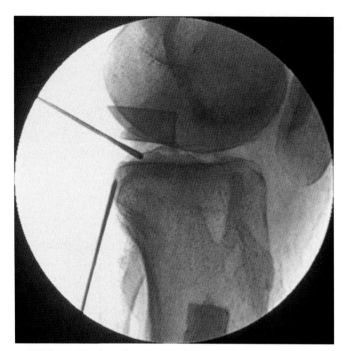

FIGURE 25-2 This lateral x-ray view of the previous image shows the relative position of the guide wires used to identify the positional anatomy in the photograph. In this knee angle, the PL bundle is almost vertical.

to the femur, blending with the attachment of the posterior longitudinal group of PCL fibers. Literature reviews[15-17] have shown that Humphry ligaments are present alone in 25% to 38%, Wrisberg ligaments present alone 39% to 50%, both present in 17% to 20%, and neither in 3% to 8% of knees. Both meniscofemoral ligaments have roles as secondary restraints to posterior tibial translation, which has been noted subsequent to complete transection of the PCL.[18,19] With their cross-sectional area at about 10 mm^2 and each ligament comprising an estimated 22% of the PCL cross section, the extent of any ligament function potential will vary by the comparative size of the PCL and the presence or absence of either meniscofemoral ligament.

Functional Biomechanics

When the knee is flexed and approaches 45 degrees, the AL bundle fibers tighten and are aligned to resist posterior tibial force. In contrast, the PM bundles exhibit reciprocal behavior, are tight in extension and, when the knee is flexed, begin to slacken. The angle of the PM bundle is not suitable to resist posterior tibial force while tight during knee extension and only provides secondary restraint to resist hyperextension. Once flexion meets or exceeds 120 degrees, the PM bundle femoral attachment moves anteriorly in relation to the tibia so that it is tight and aligned to resist posterior tibial forces, which illustrates its function in deep knee flexion. As complete knee flexion is approached, the AL fibers wrap against the intercondylar notch roof, becoming almost vertical to the tibial plateau, and are thus poorly aligned to control posterior tibial translation. In the presence of collateral ligament and posterolateral corner pathology, PCL injuries have additional rotatory laxity, valgus instability, and posterior tibial translation.[20,21]

PATIENT EVALUATION

Clinical Assessment

The posterior drawer test is a reliable clinical assessment tool and should be performed at both 30 and 90 degrees for PCL assessment. Begin by defining the distance (usually 1 cm) of the medial tibial plateau from the medial femoral condyle at 90 degrees of flexion. Grade I injuries are not associated with significantly abnormal joint motion and have a palpable but diminished step-off (0 to 5 mm). Grade II injuries are indicated with slight to moderate joint motion and have lost their step-off, but the medial tibial plateau cannot be pushed beyond the medial femoral condyle (5 to 10 mm). Grade III injuries are usually associated with markedly abnormal joint motion and an absent medial step-off, and the tibia can be moved posterior to the medial femoral condyle (>10 mm). Obvious positive posterior sag is present in these cases. To perform the posterior sag test, the hip and knee are flexed to 90 degrees; with complete tears, the tibia sags and becomes obviously posteriorly subluxed relative to the femur and by comparison to the other knee.

Note that some normal laxity is seen in patients with physiologic genu recurvatum. If posterior translation is normal at 90 degrees but slightly increased at 30 degrees, a PLC injury is likely. Not all patients with PCL tears have a positive posterior drawer test on physical examination.[22] Although the PCL is commonly evaluated by performing the posterior drawer test at 90 degrees,[23-26] it can also be assessed by other methods, including the dynamic posterior shift test,[27] the quadriceps active test, the posterior sag sign, the prone posterior drawer test, and the reverse pivot-shift test.[28] Using the quadriceps active test in the presence of a PCL tear, the active contraction of the quadriceps muscle with the knee from 60 to 90 degrees of flexion produces anterior tibial movement and a posterior tibial sag is eliminated.

Diagnostic Imaging

Plain radiography with five views—anteroposterior (AP), lateral, sunrise notch, weighted AP, and Merchant views—is preferred for knee assessments. The identification of any insertion site avulsion fractures, fragments, or small tibial plateau fractures are additional signs of combined ligament injuries. A lateral view may demonstrate posterior subluxation of the tibia and, when obvious, is pathognomonic for a PCL lesion.

To characterize PCL injury by magnetic resonance imaging (MRI), three planes should be used—axial, coronal, and sagittal. The use of a dedicated knee coil improves signal-to-noise ratio and a small field of view (10 to 14 cm) helps improve spatial resolution.[29] The most sensitive views for evaluating the PCL are obtained with the sagittal oblique plane. With MRI, evaluations of PCL tears can be delineated into intrasubstance, partial, complete, or avulsion. Hemorrhage and edema are evident interstitially in intrasubstance tears. Partial tears are evident by interruption of a portion of one of the margins of the ligament and may present a circumferential ring of hemorrhage or edema (halo sign) around the margins. Complete tears have portions of the ligament that are completely absent and may include hemorrhage and edema blurring the margins or in focal areas in lieu of the ligament at tibial or femoral attachments. Avulsions are usually at the tibial insertion and the PCL will retract away with its bone fragment.

When precise physical examination is complicated by pain, MRI is helpful for diagnosing acute lesions and also contributes to the diagnosis of concomitant injuries. Diagnostic arthroscopy is usually not required to evaluate PCL tears with the advent of MRI, which has excellent specificity and sensitivity for soft tissue diagnoses. However, in some cases, the presence of metallic foreign bodies, intracranial surgical clips, pacemaker wires, patient size, or motion limitations may preclude the use of MRI.

Isolated Posterior Cruciate Ligament Injuries

When isolated PLC injury occurs, the following conditions are typically found:

1. Abnormal posterior laxity less than 10 mm
2. Abnormal posterior laxity decreases with tibial internal rotation
3. No abnormal varus
4. Abnormal external rotation of the tibia on the femur less than 5 degrees compared with the uninvolved side tested with the knee at 30 and 90 degrees of flexion.

Posterior Cruciate Ligament–Posterolateral Corner Injury Combination

A combined injury to the PCL and PLC structures will typically be manifested as follows:

1. Abnormal posterior laxity more than 20 to 25 mm; tibial step-off absent and negative
2. Abnormal varus displacement at 30 degrees
3. Abnormal external rotation thigh-foot angle of more than 10 to 15 degrees in comparison to the normal lower extremity tested at 30 and 90 degrees

TREATMENT

Conservative Management

In the past, it was assumed that patients with an isolated PCL rupture did well with nonoperative treatment.[30,31] Shelbourne and colleagues[32] have studied chronic PCL injury nonoperated patients; 170 patients were untreated for their grade II or lower acute isolated PCL injuries. They stated that "...their conditions didn't deteriorate over time as a group." However, 20% reported giving way with activities of daily living, 26% reported giving way with strenuous activity, and 54% reported that they did not experience any instability. It is important to note that isolated PCL grade II or lower injuries are atypical. Nonoperative management for isolated PCL injuries (rarely occurring) is not a standard that should be applied universally to multiple ligament injuries.

Arthroscopic Technique

Most single-strand techniques attempt to reconstruct the larger anterolateral bundle.[33,34] The posteromedial bundle, and the stability it provides in extension, is ignored. Double-bundle techniques have arisen in an attempt to address both the anterolateral and posteromedial bundles.[35-37] In vitro research[36,38] has sug-

gested that these double-bundle reconstructions can eliminate joint laxity in flexion and extension.

A tibial tunnel drill guide used in the present technique for the PCL known as the Tundra system (Smith & Nephew Endoscopy; Andover, Mass) uses coring reamers (trephines) that are externally guided instead of using internal cannulation with a guide wire. A guide wire is not required for the placement of the tibial tunnel with this system. The point of contact on the guide arm by the trephine is a small plate (backsplash). In the lateral view, it looks like a triangular wedge. It is round, 11 mm in diameter; it prevents the trephine from passing beyond it and protects the posterior structures from injury. When used in conjunction with an Achilles graft in the present double-bundle technique, difficulty with graft passage around the "killer turn" is obviated.

This arthroscopic technique for double-bundle PCL reconstruction uses an Achilles tendon allograft. This graft source anatomically mimics the PCL insertion and, when prepared into two bundles, can be used to reconstruct the AL and PM ligament components of the PCL. This arthroscopic reconstruction is secured with anatomic fixation by three bioabsorbable interference screws using a single-incision, five-portal technique.

Patient Preparation

The patient is placed in a supine position and a tourniquet is applied, with a leg holder placed sufficiently proximal to permit posteromedial cannula placement. Access through this cannula with a rotary shaver is crucial and requires the noninvolved extremity to be positioned sufficiently lateral.

Graft Preparation

Prepare a double-bundle Achilles tendon allograft at a side table. Divide the tendinous portion of the graft into two 7- × 250-mm bundles. Place a 5-cm long series of whipstitches at the end of each bundle to provide for advancement of the graft. The bony portion of the graft is typically trimmed to a length of 25 mm and sized to fit a 12-mm tunnel. Once trimmed, attach a wire suture to the bone plug to allow for positioning and tensioning (Fig. 25-3).

Portal Establishment and Posterior Cruciate Ligament Resection

Establish standard anteromedial, proximal anterolateral, and midanterolateral arthroscopic portals initially. The distolateral and posteromedial arthroscopic portals are added later (Fig. 25-4). The midanterolateral portal must be placed sufficiently proximal and near the patella to allow for arthroscope access to the posterior medial compartment. Improper placement of this portal will also

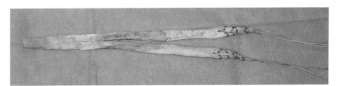

FIGURE 25-3 An Achilles allograft is shown with the bone plug sized to 12 mm and the individual bundles sized to 7 mm. A hole is placed into the bone plug and surgical wire is threaded to retain the plug in the tibial tunnel and to apply tension during fixation. Use of a suture instead of the wire may risk laceration by the screw during insertion.

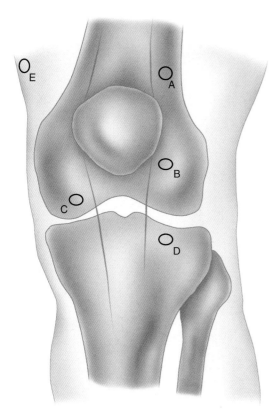

FIGURE 25-4 The proximal lateral portal (A) is located 1 cm proximal to the patella and parallel to the dorsal surface of the femur laterally. The midanterolateral portal (B) is positioned at the apex of the triangle formed by the lateral femoral condyle, the lateral border of the patella, and the lateral border of the patellar ligament. The anteromedial portals (C) are placed 1 cm proximal to the joint line medially and approximately 1 cm medial to the medial border of the patellar ligament. The PCL-specific inferior distal anterolateral portal (D) is located at the joint line and a spinal needle is used to approximate the portal location. The portal location must allow clearance of the lateral femoral condyle and the anterior horn of the lateral meniscus, and still allow creation of the femoral tunnels. It is in the same vertical axis distal to the anterolateral portal (B). The midanterolateral portal must be placed sufficiently proximal and near the patella to allow for arthroscope access to the posterior medial compartment. Improper placement of this portal will also interfere with arthroscope placement while drilling the femoral tunnels through the distolateral portal. Supplemental visualization of the posterior aspect of the tibia is obtained through the posteromedial portal (E) located at the conjunction of the sartorius and vastus medialis muscles.

interfere with arthroscope placement while drilling the femoral tunnels through the distolateral portal.

Resect the torn PCL using an arthroscopic shaver. Then position the posteromedial portal approximately 13 to 15 cm proximally to the joint line and anterior to the hamstring tendons at the posterior margin of the vastus medialis muscle. From this position, direct the portal toward the tibial PCL attachment (Fig. 25-5). Begin by inserting a spinal needle, observing its position with the arthroscope. Once positioned properly, follow the needle with a scalpel to make space for switching stick insertion. Place a 10-mm cannula over the switching stick through the posteromedial portal. This portal provides access to the PCL tibial fovea for the arthroscope or rotary shaver, as required. Place the shaver through the posteromedial portal and débride the stump of the PCL.

Drill the Tibial Tunnel

Make a 2.5-cm vertical incision 1 cm medially and 3 to 4 cm distally to the crest of the tibial tubercle and extend it distally (Fig. 25-6). Use the Tundra PCL drill guide (Smith & Nephew) to place the tibial tunnel. With the Tundra guide body and PCL arm assembly adjusted to the closed (smallest angle) setting, insert the drill guide through the anteromedial portal and direct it to the anatomic insertion of the PCL on the posterior tibia. Once in this position, readjust the arm to a larger angle setting to achieve the maximum possible between the 54- and 57-degree marks on the arm. Position the distal end of the drill guide over the medial tibial incision and lock it firmly in place by adjusting the force on the outriggers. Using fluoroscopic visualization, verify the correct guide position (Fig. 25-7). Advance the trephine until it exits through the tibia posteriorly and contacts the backsplash (Fig. 25-8).

Drill the Femoral Tunnels

Flex the knee to 90 degrees. Débride the femoral stump and use its margins as a reference for Beath pin placement. Approach through the distolateral portal and place two chisel-point, slot-eyed Beath pins near the distal and proximal margins of the femoral footprint of the PCL (posterior and anterior margins when the knee is extended; Fig. 25-9). The slot in the eye of the pins permit graft suture placement without threading sutures through the eyelet. Direct the pins proximally and medially so that they exit the thigh medially, approximately 7 to 10 cm proximal to the joint line. Advance a cannulated 7-mm trephine over the previously placed slot-eyed pins. Beginning with the posterior tunnel (for the PM tendon bundle), drill it through the medial femoral cortex. Use the grasper to hold the slot-eyed pin in place while backing out the trephine. Repeat the procedure for the anterior femoral tunnel (for the AL tendon bundle), leaving both pins in place.

Graft Insertion and Fixation

Advance each pin until its slotted eye is drawn into the joint space and protrudes slightly from its respective femoral tunnel (Fig. 25-10). Reposition the graspers flush with the skin to prevent the slot-eyed pins from shifting or falling out while the sutures are threaded. Débride the soft tissue from the orifice of each tunnel. Orient the graft so that the tendinous side of the bone block is posterior, with one bundle exiting medially and one bundle laterally. Pass the PM tendon bundle sutures into the tibial tunnel with a grasper and transfer them to a ringed grasper just proximal to the posterior tunnel aperture (Fig. 25-11). Draw the sutures anterior with the ring grasper and remove the ring grasper out of the anteromedial portal. Using a grasper, insert it into the anteromedial portal, grasp the sutures, and lay them into the slot eye of the Beath pin (Fig. 25-12). Advance the pin to bring the sutures medially to exit the skin and release the sutures being held with the tibial tunnel grasper to allow tension to be applied to the graft (Fig. 25-13). Transfer the Kocher clamp from the pin to the tensioned sutures. Repeat the process with anterolateral bundle sutures to the slot-eyed pin in the anterior femoral tunnel until they exit the skin medially; transfer the Kocher clamp from that pin to those sutures.

Advance the tendinous portion of the Achilles allograft through the tibial tunnel simultaneously (Fig. 25-14). Apply

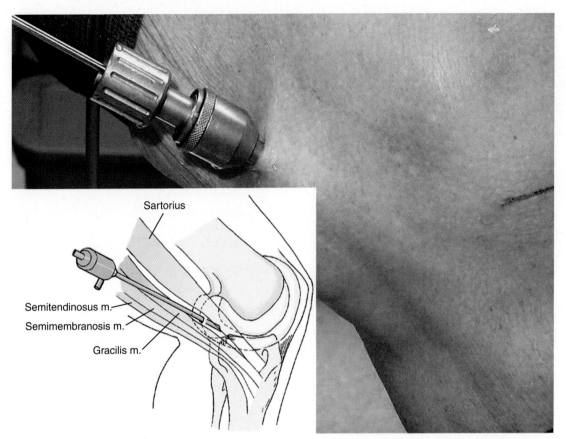

Sartorius

Semitendinosus m.

Semimembranosis m.

Gracilis m.

FIGURE 25-5 A cannula placed through this portal provides rotary shaver or direct arthroscope access to prepare or inspect the tibial fovea. Note that the angle of the cannula insertion requires significant access medially. Prior to making any incisions, the noninvolved leg must be positioned sufficiently lateral to provide both insertion and work room for these instruments.

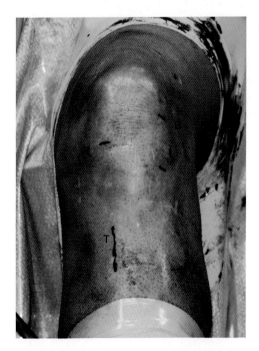

FIGURE 25-6 A vertical incision provides access for the distal tibial tunnel (T). The proximal point is positioned 1 cm medially and 3 to 4 cm distally to the crest of the tibial tubercle and extended distally. This incision, and the tunnel placed through it, are sufficiently distal to permit another incision placed more proximally to accommodate an ACL reconstruction. Note that the midanterolateral portal (B) must be placed sufficiently proximal and near the patella to allow for proper access. Improper placement of this portal will cause problems with arthroscope access to the posteromedial compartment and will also interfere with femoral tunnel drilling through distolateral portal.

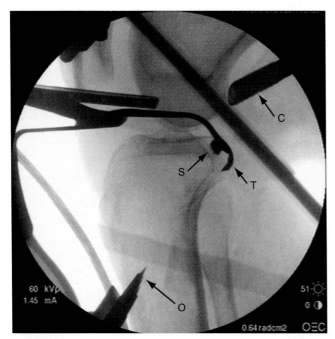

FIGURE 25-7 The tibial guide arm is positioned approximately parallel to the tibial plateau with the tang (T) shown placed at the distal edge of the posterior compartment, the backsplash (S) positioned over the tibial footprint fovea, and the outriggers (O) ratcheted firmly against the anterior tibia within the medial tibial incision. The posterior cannula (C) is shown in position.

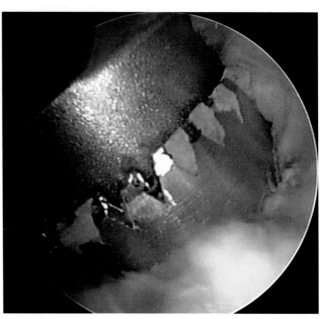

FIGURE 25-8 The backsplash is visualized arthroscopically positioned in the posterior compartment over the tibial footprint fovea. The backsplash is shown with the trephine in contact around its outer surface. This configuration allows the bone core to be completely cut through the cortical bone, without the production of attached bone fragments common with fully fluted trephines. This feature obviates débriding these fragments.

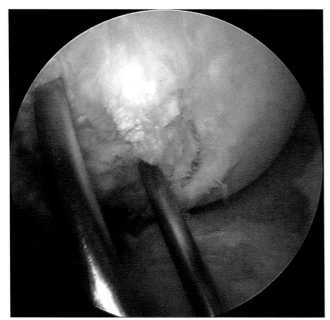

FIGURE 25-9 The lateral aspect of the medial femoral condyle with both slot-eyed Beath pins inserted into their anterior and posterior positions within the femoral footprint is shown. The pins are placed at least 4 mm from the medial femoral condyle articular margins so that the 7-mm tunnels drilled over them are close to the articular margins without encroaching into the articular cartilage.

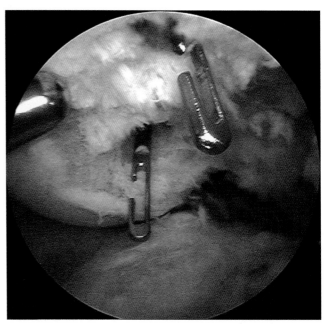

FIGURE 25-10 The 7-mm tunnels have been drilled and the pins are shown advanced with the slot eyes protruding slightly from each tunnel into the compartment, ready to receive the bundle suture ends for graft passage.

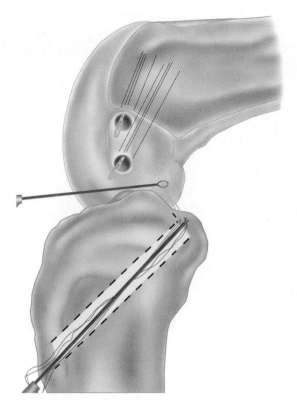

FIGURE 25-11 The posteromedial tendon bundle sutures being passed into the tibial tunnel with a grasper and transferred to a ringed grasper just proximal to the posterior tunnel aperture are shown. Note the slot-eyed Beath pins partially exposed in the femoral tunnels.

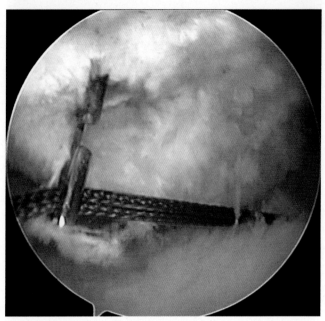

FIGURE 25-12 The posteromedial tendon bundle sutures are both laid into the slot of the slot-eyed Beath pin.

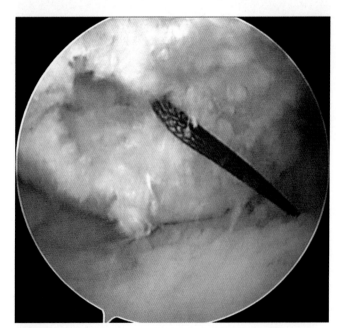

FIGURE 25-13 The posteromedial tendon bundle sutures are shown drawn through and out the posterior femoral tunnel and are held by a clamp on the medial side of the knee.

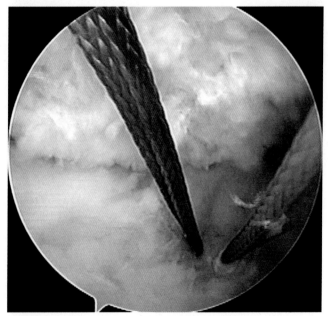

FIGURE 25-14 Shown is a posterior view of the two graft bundles and their passing sutures. Proper sizing permits light tension to draw the graft bundles to exit the tibial tunnel posteriorly and be drawn over the "killer turn" and across the knee compartment into place. The sutures on the posteromedial bundle have been colored dark blue for identification.

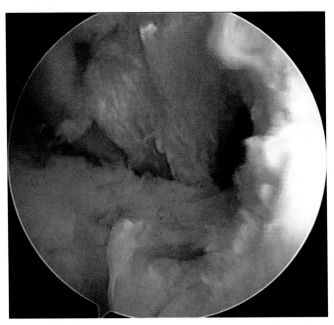

FIGURE 25-15 Both graft bundles have been drawn into place and ready to begin tensioning prior to securing the graft with headless cannulated bioabsorbable interference screws (HCIS).

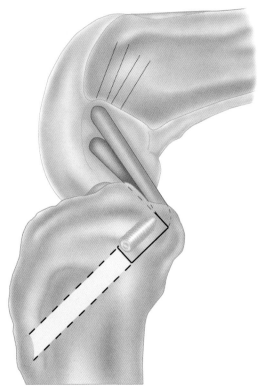

FIGURE 25-16 The 7- × 25-mm HCIS is in position with the bone plug and screw at the posterior aperture of the tibial tunnel.

tension on the tendon bundle sutures. Avoid advancing either bundle significantly further than the other (Fig. 25-15). Adjust the distal-proximal position of the graft so that the proximal end of the bone block is flush with the posterior aperture of the tibial tunnel. Advance a guide wire anteriorly within the tibial tunnel, positioning it between the cancellous side of the bone block and tibial tunnel wall. Advance a 7- × 25-mm cannulated bioabsorbable screw along the guide wire until the screw makes solid purchase with the bone block and tibial tunnel wall (Fig. 25-16). This maneuver can be fluoroscopically monitored.

Manipulate the knee vigorously and apply anterior force to the tibia, with traction maintained on both bundles. The PM bundle is tensioned and secured with interference screw fixation near extension, typically in 20 degrees of flexion (Fig. 25-17). Direct a guide wire through the distal anterolateral portal and position it anterior to the bundle in the distal femoral tunnel. With traction applied to the PM bundle located in the posterior femoral tunnel, advance a 7- × 25-mm cannulated bioabsorbable screw over the guide wire through the distal anterolateral portal alongside the graft until it is seated completely within the tunnel, thereby providing direct tendon to bone fixation. The AL bundle, located in the anterior femoral tunnel, is tensioned and secured in 90 degrees of flexion. Fixation is accomplished with a 7- × 25-mm cannulated bioabsorbable screw also directed through the distal anterolateral portal over its respective guide wire.

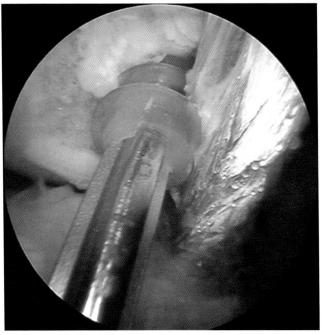

FIGURE 25-17 The posteromedial bundle, under tension at 20 degrees of flexion, is being secured by a 7- × 25-mm HCIS, with the anterolateral bundle shown adjacent to it.

PEARLS&PITFALLS

1. *Pitfall:* The leg holder is placed too distally. This will make the creation of and access to the posteromedial portal impossible.
   Pearl: Place the leg holder proximal to the midpoint of the femur and potentially higher on smaller patients.
2. *Pitfall:* The noninvolved leg is positioned too close to the index knee prior to commencing the procedure. This causes access problems for the arthroscope and rotary shaver through the posteromedial portal.
   Pearl: Position the noninvolved leg sufficiently lateral to provide insertion and work room for these instruments.
3. *Pitfall:* The midanterolateral portal is malpositioned. This causes arthroscope access problems to the posterior medial compartment and interferes with femoral tunnel drilling through the distolateral portal.
   Pearl: This portal must be placed sufficiently proximal and near the patella.
4. *Pitfall:* Not resecting the PCL prior to the initiation of the posteromedial portal can result in difficulty viewing the spinal needle, scalpel, switching stick, and cannula during posteromedial portal creation and access setup.
   Pearl: Resect the bulk of the PCL from the femoral attachment to as far posterior as possible with a rotary shaver through the anterior portal.
5. *Pitfall:* The tibial guide access incision is initiated too proximally. This precludes the proper access angle for the Tundra guide without lengthening the incision, which would thus be longer than required.
   Pearl: Make sure that the proximal end of the incision begins at least 3 cm distal to the crest of the tibial tubercle.
6. *Pitfall:* There is guide insertion difficulty in the medial tibial incision. This could damage the cartilage during insertion through the skin into the medial compartment.
   Pearl: Make sure that the guide is closed (lowest angle setting) and positioned horizontally (parallel with the floor) until it is in the compartment; then rotate and extend it posteriorly.
7. *Pitfall:* Drilling the femoral tunnels so that one extends into the articular margin could result in chondral collapse.
   Pearl: The tunnels must be placed near the distal and proximal margins without extending into the articular margin.
8. *Pitfall:* The bone plug is not completely prepared or was swollen post-sizing, which could lead to increased difficulty when inserting the graft into the desired location.
   Pearl: Round the ends with a rongeur and confirm graft size with tunnel diameter matched sizing tube. Do not continue to hydrate once sized; the plug can swell.
9. *Pitfall:* Anteromedial or posterolateral cross-bundle insertion could lead to reverse bundle orientation and result in graft failure.
   Pearl: Mark the sutures of the one bundle with a dark surgical marker. Our preference is posteromedial; in any sequence it is always first.
10. *Pitfall:* The interference screw insertion torque is too low, which leads to increased risk of fixation failure.
    Pearl: Use the next larger screw size or use a second screw of the same size.

Postoperative Management

Post-tourniquet control, incisions are closed in a subcuticular fashion and Steri-Strips are applied to all incisions. Knees are dressed and wrapped with a 6-inch Ace wrap and placed in a hinged brace for variable control of flexion and extension.

All patients use crutches and are non–weight bearing for the first week. Partial weight bearing is permitted in extension weeks 2 and 3, and full weight bearing thereafter. Knees are maintained in extension in the brace except during range-of-motion (ROM) exercises for 8 weeks. Brace ROM is set at 0 to 30 degrees (extension-flexion) during the first week. The brace ROM settings are changed to 0 to 60 degrees during week 2, 0 to 90 degrees during week 3, and 0 to 120 degrees from week 4 on. ROM exercises are initially limited with a continuous passive motion (CPM) device for the first 7 days and progress to passive-assisted heel slides thereafter. CPM ROM is increased from 0 to 30 degrees initially to 0 to 45 degrees on day 2 to 0 to 60 degrees on day 4. Cryotherapy is prescribed for all patients for the first 2 weeks, with a cuff used in conjunction with a continuous flow motorized thermos. Cryotherapy is applied continuously for the first 4 days and then as needed through week 2. Postoperative pain and inflammation are controlled with oral medication.

REFERENCES

1. Fanelli GC, Edson CJ. Posterior cruciate ligament injuries in trauma patients: Part II. *Arthroscopy.* 1995;11:526-529.
2. Pearsall AW, Hollis JM. The effect of posterior cruciate ligament injury and reconstruction on meniscal strain. *Am J Sports Med.* 2004;32: 1675-1680.
3. Parolie JM, Bergefd JA. Long-term of nonoperative treatment of isolated posterior cruciate ligament injuries in the athlete. *Am J Sports Med.* 1986; 14:35-38.
4. Logan M, Williams A, Lavelle J, et al. The effect of posterior cruciate ligament deficiency on knee kinematics. *Am J Sports Med.* 2004;32: 1915-1922.
5. Clancy WG. Repair and reconstruction of the posterior cruciate ligament. In: Chapman M, ed. *Operative Orthopedics.* Philadelphia: JB Lippincott; 1998:1651-65.
6. Hughston JC, Bowden JA, Andrews JR, Norwood LA. Acute tears of the posterior cruciate ligament: results of operative treatment. *J Bone Joint Surg Am.* 1980;62:438-450.
7. Clancy W, Shelbourne D, Zoellinger G. Treatment of knee joint instability secondary to rupture of posterior cruciate ligament. *J Bone Joint Surg Am.* 1983;65:310-322.
8. Keller PM, Shelbourne KD, McCarroll JR, Retting AC. Non-operatively treated isolated posterior cruciate ligament injuries. *Am J Sports Med.* 2004;12:420-428.
9. Dandy D;Pusey R. The long-term results of unrepaired tears of the posterior cruciate ligament. *J Bone Joint Surg Am.* 1982;64:92-94.
10. Covey DC, Sapega AA, Marshall RC. The effects of varied joint motion and loading conditions on posterior cruciate ligament fiber length behavior. *Am J Sports Med.* 2004;32:1866-1872.
11. Park SE, Stamos BD, DeFrate LE, et al. The effect of posterior knee capsolotomy on posterior tibial translation during posterior cruciate ligament tibial inlay reconstruction. *Am J Sports Med.* 2004;32:1514-1519.
12. Chen CH, Chou SW, Chen WJ, Shih CH. Fixation strength of three different grafts used in posterior cruciate ligament reconstruction. *Knee Surg Sports Traumatol Arthrosc.* 2004;12:371-375.
13. Zaffagnini S, Martelli S, Garcia L, Visani A. Computer analysis of PCL during range of motion. *Knee Surg Sports Traumatol Arthrosc.* 2004;12: 420-428.
14. Amis AA. Anatomy and biomechanics of the posterior cruciate ligament. *Sports Med Arthrosc Rev.* 1999;7:225-234.
15. Makris CA, Georgoulis AD, Papageordiou, et al. Posterior cruciate ligament architecture: Evaluation under microsurgical dissection. *Arthroscopy.* 2000;16:627-632.

16. Heller L, Langman J. The menisco-femoral ligaments of the human knee. *J Bone Joint Surg Br.* 1964;46:307-313.

17. Yamamoto M, Hinohara K. Anatomical study on the meniscofemoral ligaments of the knee. *Kobe J Med Sci.* 1991;37:209-226.

18. Gergis FG, Marshall JL, Monajem ARS. The cruciate ligaments of the knee joint. Anatomical functional and experimental analysis. *Clin Orthop Relat Res.* 1975;(106):216-231.

19. Harner JD, Höher J. Evaluation and treatment of posterior cruciate ligament injuries *Am J Sports Med.* 1998;26:471-482.

20. Nielsen S, Helmig. The static stabilizing function of the popliteal tendon in the knee. An experimental study. *Arch Orthop Trauma Surg.* 1986;104:357-362.

21. Nielsen S, Ovesen J, Rasmussen O. The posterior cruciate ligament and rotatory knee instability. An experimental study. *Arch Orthop Trauma Surg.* 1985;104:53-56.

22. Hughston JC. The absent posterior drawer test in some acute posterior cruciate ligament tears of the knee. *Am J Sports Med.* 1988;16:39-43.

23. Noyes FR, Stowers SF, Grood ES, et al. Posterior subluxations of the medial and lateral tibiofemoral compartments. An in vitro sectioning study in cadaveric knees. *Am J Sports Med.* 1993;21:407-414.

24. Gollehon DL, Torzilli PA, Warren RF. The role of the posterolateral and cruciate ligaments in the stability of the human knee. A biomechanical study. *J Bone Joint Surg Am.* 1987;69:233-242.

25. Grood E, Stowers S, Noyes F. Limits of movement in the human knee: effect of sectioning the posterior cruciate ligament and posterolateral structures. *J Bone Joint Surg Am.* 1988;70:88-97.

26. Henry MH, Berend ME, Feagin JA Jr. Clinical diagnosis of acute knee ligament injuries. *Ann Chir Gynaecol* 1991;80:120-126.

27. Covey DC, Sapega AA, Sherman GM. Testing for isometry during reconstruction of the posterior cruciate ligament. Anatomic and biomechanical considerations. *Am J Sports Med.* 1996;24:740-746.

28. Jakob RP, Hassler H, Stäubli HU. Observations on rotatory instability of the lateral compartment of the knee: experimental studies on the functional anatomy and pathomechanism of the true and reverse pivot shift sign. *Acta Orthop Scand Suppl.* 1981;191:1-32.

29. Grover JS, Bassett LW, Gross ML, et al. Posterior cruciate ligament: MRI imaging. *Radiology.* 1990;174:527-530.

30. Parolie JM, Bergfeld JA. Long-term results of nonoperative treatment of isolated posterior cruciate ligament injuries in the athlete. *Am J Sports Med.* 1986;14:35-38.

31. Torg JS, Barton TM, Pavlov H, Stine R. Natural history of the posterior cruciate ligament-deficient knee. *Clin Orthop Relat Res.* 1989;(133):208-216.

32. Shelbourne KD, O'Shea JJ, Patel DV. The natural history of nonoperatively treated posterior cruciate ligament injuries. *Am J Sports Med.* 1999;27:276-283.

33. Furie E. Risk factors of arthroscopic popliteal artery laceration. *Arthroscopy.* 1995;11:324-327.

34. Veltri DM, Warren RF, Silver G. Complications in posterior cruciate ligament surgery. *Oper Tech Sports Med.* 1993;1:154-158.

35. Berg EE. Posterior cruciate ligament tibial inlay reconstruction. *Arthroscopy.* 1995;11:69-76.

36. Border PS, Nyland JA, Caborn DNM. Posterior cruciate ligament reconstruction (double bundle) using anterior tibialis tendon allograft. *Arthroscopy.* 2001;17:e14.

37. Campbell RB, Jordan SS, Sekiya JK. Arthroscopic tibial inlay for posterior cruciate ligament reconstruction. *Arthroscopy.* 2007;23:1356.

38. Chen CH, Chen WJ, Shih CH. Arthroscopic double-bundled posterior cruciate ligament reconstruction with quadriceps tendon-patellar bone autograft. *Arthroscopy.* 2000;16:780-782.

Inlay Posterior Cruciate Ligament Reconstruction

Chealon D. Miller ● Luke Choi ● Mark D. Miller

Treatment of posterior cruciate ligament (PCL) injuries has faced debate and continues to evolve. Debate is caused by the sparse number of PCL injuries available for surgical standardization of technique and the relative heterogeneity of these injuries. Posterior cruciate ligament tears are often not diagnosed because they are often asymptomatic. However, studies have shown that PCL injuries are more common than previously thought and can comprise up to 3% of knee injuries in the general population and 37% of trauma patients with an acute hemarthrosis.[1,2] As the detection of such injuries improves, there will be a corresponding rise in the number of basic science and clinical studies investigating these injuries. The result will be improved understanding of the proper techniques for treatment and standardization of operative procedures. However, one issue that may continue to be subjective and thus more controversial is the indication for surgical intervention.

ANATOMY

Knee stability requires the intact integrity of four ligaments—the anterior cruciate ligament (ACL), PCL, medial collateral ligament (MCL), and lateral collateral ligament (LCL). The PCL is the primary structure that confers static stabilization against posterior translation of the tibia with respect to the femur. The PCL averages 38 mm in length and 13 mm in width and is believed to be the stronger of the two cruciate liagments.[3] Selective division of the PCL has shown that it is most important in flexion, although it acts as a check during hyperextension when the anterior cruciate ligament has been compromised.[4] The PCL originates from the posterolateral aspect of the medial femoral condyle in the intercondylar notch and inserts on the posterior aspect of the tibial plateau (Fig. 26-1).[5,6] The PCL is more vertically than obliquely oriented and the midpoint of its femoral attachment is 1 cm posterior to the articular cartilage.[7] The insertion of the

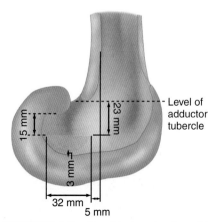
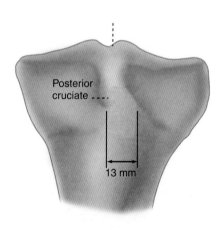

FIGURE 26-1 Drawing of the lateral surface of the right medial femoral condyle (*left*) and posterior tibia (*right*) showing the average measurements and relationships of the PCL attachments. (*Adapted from Girgis M: The cruciate ligaments of the knee joint: anatomical, functional and experimental analysis.* Clin Orthop. *1975;106: 216-231.)*

ligament is within a central depression about 1.0 to 1.5 cm distal to the articular surface of the posterior tibia in an area known as the PCL facet, or fovea.[8] This posterior insertion is a major factor in anatomic reconstructive techniques because of its proximity to the popliteal vessels that may be injured during posterior approaches to the knee.

The posterior cruciate ligament has two major bands, also known as bundles. These bundles are named for their specific insertion on the femur (anterior or posterior) and tibia (lateral or medial).[9] The anterolateral band is tight in flexion and loose in extension, and the posteromedial band is loose in flexion and tight in extension. The posteromedial band is half the size of the anterolateral band in cross section. The anterolateral band is reconstructed during single-bundle reconstruction. The PCL is also composed of meniscofemoral ligaments, the ligament of Humphry, which is located anteriorly, and the ligament of Wrisberg, located on the posterior aspect. These ligaments travel from the posterior horn of the lateral meniscus to the posteromedial femoral condyle.[10]

PATIENT EVALUATION

History and Physical Examination

Most patients with posterior cruciate ligament injuries do not report a pop or any feeling of subjective instability, which is distinctly different from anterior cruciate ligament injuries. Instead, most patients will complain of knee pain, swelling, or a " funny feeling " in the knee. The physician should inquire about to the chronicity of symptoms to classify the injury as acute or chronic. One of the most common mechanisms of PCL injury is the dashboard injury. This term is used to describe the phenomenon of the anterior tibia sustaining a posteriorly directed force from the dashboard with the knee in 90 degrees of flexion. In the case of an athlete, the history usually includes a direct blow to the anterior tibia or a fall on a flexed knee with the foot in plantar flexion. This is in contrast to a fall on a dorsiflexed foot, which causes patellofemoral injury. Isolated partial tears in athletes are often secondary to hyperflexion injuries, which can occur, for example, during a football tackle.[10,11]

On physical examination, several considerations must be made. Such considerations include the possibility of multiple ligament injuries, most notably the effect of a concurrent posterolateral corner (PLC) or ACL injury. When examining a knee with a PCL injury, it is often missed that the tibia is starting in a subluxed position and further posterior stress does not lead to additional translation. An anterior drawer does result in anterior translation and the diagnosis of an ACL tear can be erroneously made. Despite this, the most accurate clinical test of PCL integrity is the posterior drawer test. This is performed by placing the patient supine and placing a posteriorly directed force to the anterior tibia (Fig. 26-2) with the knee flexed at 90 degrees. The examiner palpates the medial joint line before applying force to determine the location of the tibia in relation to the medial femoral condyle.

Documentation of the examination should include the amount of translation and the presence of an end point. Traditional teaching described tibial translation in numeric terms. PCL injury was described as grade I for 0 to 5 mm of tibial translation, grade II

for 5 to 10 mm of translation, and grade III for more than 10 mm of translation. However, many have suggested classifying PCL injuries based on the medial tibial plateau–medial femoral condyle position.[12] The tibial plateau is usually 1 cm anterior to the femoral condyle. In the positional classification system, grade I injuries have some preservation of the anterior position of the tibia in relation to the femur, grade II injuries occur when the tibia is flush with the medial femoral condyle, and grade III injuries are manifested by displacement of the anterior tibia posterior to the medial femoral condyle. The ligament of Wrisberg and the ligament of Humphry are a part of the posterior cruciate ligament. These ligaments can confer stability with internal rotation and lead to a decrease in posterior laxity in this position.[13]

Other tests for PCL integrity include the posterior sag test (Godfrey test), quadriceps active test, and reverse pivot shift test.[14] The posterior sag test involves flexing the hip to 45 degrees and the knee to 90 degrees and noting the posterior pull of gravity creating a sag or dimple at the joint line, indicating the posterior location of the tibia on the femur. The quadriceps active test involves watching for a reduction of this displacement by asking the patient to contract the quadriceps muscle. If the patient does not understand this request, one can ask the patient to try to extend the knee or kick the leg out while the examiner holds the foot down. The reverse pivot shift test is similar to the pivot shift evaluation performed with ACL injury.[15] The position of the hands on the knee is the same as for the pivot shift examination (valgus force on an externally rotated foot) with an axial load. However, instead of starting in extension, the examiner starts in 90 degrees of flexion and brings the leg into complete extension; a palpable reduction of the tibial plateau is observed between 20 and 30 degrees of flexion. The external rotation recurvatum and posterolateral drawer tests can also serves as adjuncts to these tests, but are rarely used in isolation because of their high false-positive rate.[16,17]

Diagnostic Imaging

The initial evaluation of a patient with knee complaints should include plain radiography. Subtle posterior subluxation of the tibia on the femur and avulsion fractures of the tibia can be seen on plain radiographs. In trauma patients, plain radiographs are important to evaluate for osseous injury, dislocation, and other associated injuries. Stress posterior drawer radiographs and comparisons to the contralateral side are important for increasing the sensitivity when attempting to detect PCL injuries and are also helpful for measuring PCL reconstruction results. Stress radiographs are taken with the knee in 90 degrees of flexion. A side to side difference measured from the medial femoral condyle to the posterior plateau of the tibia of more than 8 mm is considered indicative of a PCL tear (Fig. 26-3).[17-19] Anteroposterior (AP) films, standing AP films with the patient in 45 degrees of flexion, and a sunrise view can be helpful to detect arthritis in patients with chronic PCL injuries. Moreover, plain radiographs may be necessary in patients with claustrophobia or metallic implants that prevent the use of magnetic resonance imaging (MRI).[8,10]

MRI is the advanced imaging modality of choice for suspected PCL and soft tissue injuries of the knee. MRI has a sensitivity from 96% to 100% in diagnosing PCL tears. It has the added

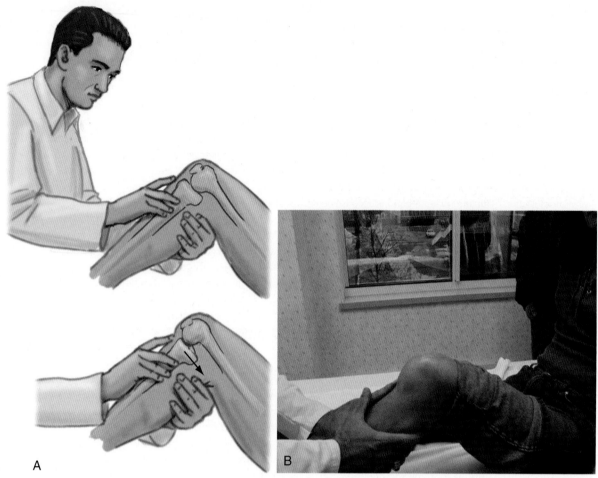

FIGURE 26-2 A, Posterior drawer test. The examiner places a finger on the anteromedial joint line while a posterior load is applied. **B,** PCL injury as seen on examination. (**A** *adapted from Miller MD, Harner CD, Koshiwaguchi S. Acute posterior cruciate ligament injuries. In: Fu FH, Vince KG, Harner CD, eds.* Knee Surgery. *Baltimore: Williams & Wilkins; 1991:749-767.)*

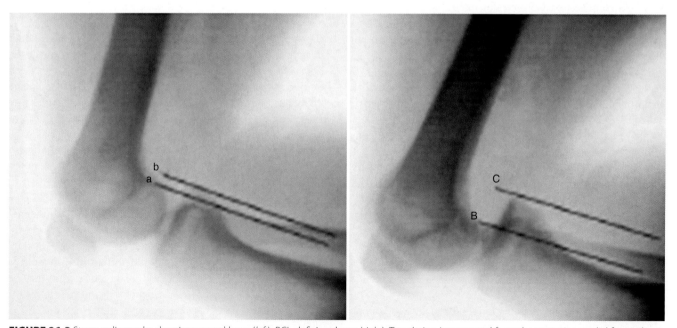

FIGURE 26-3 Stress radiographs showing normal knee (*left*), PCL-deficient knee (*right*). Translation is measured from the posterior medial femoral condyle to the posterior tibial plateau. a, ; b, ; B, ; C,. (*From Margheritini F, Mancini L, Mauro CS, Mariani PP. Stress radiography for quantifying posterior cruciate ligament deficiency.* Arthroscopy. *2003;19:706-711.)*

effect of being able to detect associated injuries, such as postero-lateral corner injuries.[9,20] There has been evidence to suggest that PCL injuries can heal and look relatively normal on MRI scans.[21] MRI has also been helpful in establishing the fact that PCL injures have a decreased likelihood of meniscal tears and bone bruise patterns as compared with ACL injuries.[2]

Other advanced techniques such as radionuclide bone scans can be helpful in patients with chronic PCL tears. Because these patients are at increased risk of patellofemoral and medial compartment arthritis, bone scans can be helpful for the detection of early arthritis. If the history and physical examination do not directly indicate PCL reconstruction, but the bone scan demonstrates increased uptake in susceptible knee compartments, the patient may be a more suitable candidate for surgery.[20,22]

TREATMENT

Multiple factors must be considered when formulating a plan for treatment. The activity level of the patient and the patient's subjective instability are major factors in the decision for treatment of isolated PCL injuries. Patient's expectations should also be discussed. Finally, associated injuries must be investigated and properly identified because they will have an effect on the decision to proceed with surgical intervention.

Conservative Management

Conservative treatment is mostly reserved for patients with advanced degenerative changes of the knee and those with isolated grade I and symptomatic grade II PCL injures.[11] Numerous studies have shown that up to 80% of isolated PCL injuries have good to excellent results when treated conservatively.[23,24] Quadriceps strengthening and motion are the cornerstones of conservative treatment. Quadriceps strengthening helps in keeping the tibia reduced under the femur and decreases the tension on the injured PCL. Strengthening exercises include quadriceps sets, straight leg raises, and partial weight bearing in extension. These patients usually recover strength fairly quickly and are able to return to activity in 4 weeks.[9] Bracing is generally ineffective in controlling PCL laxity. Because grade III injuries are often associated with other injuries, especially posterolateral corner injuries, they are largely treated surgically. If conservative treatment is elected for grade III injuries, the knee is splinted in full extension for 2 to 4 weeks.[9] Children with PCL injuries often undergo similar treatment with cast immobilization in extension; however, these injuries are infrequent in this patient population.[8] Failed conservative treatment usually manifests as continued knee pain rather than instability, because persistent tibial subluxation causes increased stress on the patellofemoral and medial compartments of the knee.[25]

Arthroscopic Technique

Operative treatment of PCL injuries are usually found in situations that include displaced avulsion injuries of the PCL, combined ligamentous injuries, and symptomatic grade II or III injuries that fail rehabilitation and in active patients unwilling to alter their lifestyle in compliance with conservative management.[6] Preoperative planning includes the presence or absence

of repairable meniscus tears or chondral lesions and affected limb alignment.[26] In the presence of the former, operative intervention should include treatment of the associated injuries to prevent future arthrosis. In the latter case, an osteotomy may be needed to prevent failure of the reconstruction.[27] Once operative treatment has been decided on, the manner in which surgery is performed is determined by the site of injury. Primary repair is indicated for fractures from the origin or insertion site; however, repair of midsubstance tears has been shown to result in poorer outcomes and is generally not recommended.[12] Reconstructive methods are divided into two categories, transtibial reconstruction and tibial inlay reconstruction. Tibial inlay reconstruction has the advantage of avoiding the "killer turn," postoperative laxity, and late graft failure seen in transtibial techniques.[12]

The patient is placed in the lateral decubitus position with the operative leg up and the contralateral leg, or well leg, padded in its entirety using a bed roll technique. The operative leg is placed in an ankle-foot orthosis-type leg holder (Fig. 26-4). A well-padded tourniquet is placed as far proximal as possible on the operative thigh and all extremities are padded, with particular attention paid to the axilla (axillary roll), the peroneal nerve of the contralateral leg, and the ulnar nerves. The leg is examined under anesthesia to assess for associated ligamentous laxity before prepping and draping the operative extremity. The leg is positioned for graft harvest and arthroscopy by rotating the hip and placing the foot eccentrically in the foot holder (Fig. 26-5). Standard arthroscopic portals are used for this procedure. The inferior lateral portal is the primary viewing portal and the inferior medial portal is the primary instrumentation portal. A diagnostic arthroscopy confirms the absence of the PCL from the

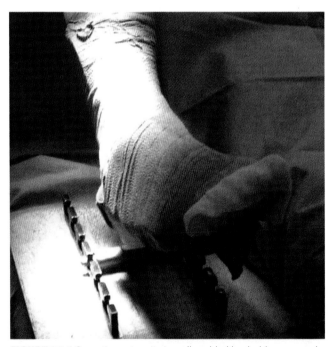

FIGURE 26-4 Operative extremity in well-padded leg holder wrapped in Coban. *(From Miller MD, Harner CD, Koshiwaguchi S. Acute posterior cruciate ligament injuries. In: Fu FH, Vince KG, Harner CD, eds.* Knee Surgery. *Baltimore: Williams & Wilkins; 1991:749-767.)*

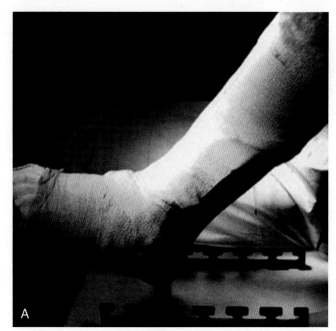

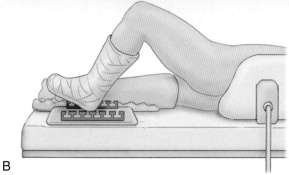

FIGURE 26-5 External rotation of leg (**A**) and placement in leg holder (**B**) in preparation for arthroscopy and graft harvest. *(From Miller MD, Harner CD, Koshiwaguchi S. Acute posterior cruciate ligament injuries. In: Fu FH, Vince KG, Harner CD, eds.* Knee Surgery. *Baltimore: Williams & Wilkins; 1991:749-767.)*

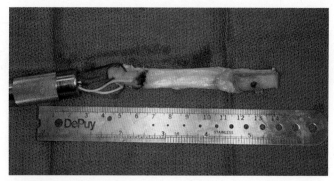

FIGURE 26-7 Bone-patellar tendon-bone autograft—tibial side (*right*) in rectangular shape with drill hole; patellar side (*left*) with tapered bone plug and perpendicular sutures.

Graft harvest begins by making a central anterior knee incision just medial to the midline from the middle of the patella down to approximately 2 cm distal to the tibial tubercle. This incision is carried down through the subcutaneous tissue until the peritenon layer is identified around the patellar tendon. The peritenon layer is incised along the entire length of the patellar tendon and saved for later closure. Once the medial and lateral borders of the patella tendon have been established from the midpatella proximally to the tibial tubercle distally, a sharp blade is used to take the central third of the patella tendon. A sagittal saw is used to take the bone plugs, measuring approximately 25 mm in length from both the tibia and patella. The sagittal saw is angled to protect the articular cartilage and prevent fracture. During graft preparation, a flat surface is made on the tibial side of the harvested graft so that it can be laid onto the tibia. This bone block must also be prepared to accept a 4.5-mm bicortical screw by drilling and tapping. The patellar portion of the graft is contoured in a cylindric fashion and the tip sculpted in a bullet shape to facilitate graft passage. The graft should be at least 18 mm long and perpendicular sutures passed into the ends to avoid suture cut-out during graft fixation (Fig. 26-7).

Preparation for acceptance of the graft can occur simultaneously as the graft itself is being prepared. The arthroscopic shaver is used to débride the lateral aspect of the medial femoral condyle (medial wall), the injured PCL, and the soft tissue in the notch. There must be a clear arthroscopic view from the anterior notch to the posterior

lateral aspect of the medial femoral condyle and can determine the presence of associated injuries. Arthroscopic indicators of PCL injury include hemorrhage, decreased tension, and pseudo-laxity of the ACL (Fig. 26-6). Once the PCL tear is confirmed, the surgeon proceeds with graft harvest.

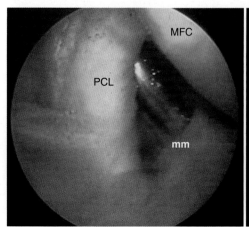

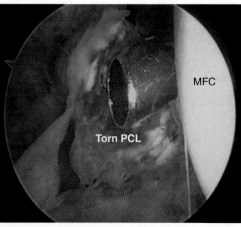

FIGURE 26-6 Intact PCL (*left*); torn PCL with hemorrhage (*right*). MFC, medial femoral condyle.

capsule for successful graft passage. Once the soft tissue has been cleared, a commercially available PCL guide is placed approximately 6 to 8 mm from the articular surface on the anteromedial portion of the intercondylar notch at the 11 or 1 o'clock position. The guide is used to determine the incision that is made on the medial portion of the knee at the medial femoral condyle along Langer's lines. This incision is approximately 2 cm in length and is carried down through the subcutaneous tissue until of the inferior border of the vastus medialis oblique is identified. A subvastus approach is used with electrocautery to encounter the bone of the medial condyle, with protection of the musculature at all times. Once contact is made with bone, the guide wire is placed using a drill and the correct position inside the intercondylar notch is confirmed (Fig. 26-8). The guide pin is then overdrilled with a drill bit sized appropriately for the graft. The posterior aspect of the tunnel is rasped to reduce graft abrasion. An 18-gauge guide wire or commercially available graft passer is then introduced into the femoral tunnel and the posterior aspect of the knee joint to facilitate future graft passage from the posterior incision that will be made.

After preparing the femoral tunnel, arthroscopic instruments are removed and the leg is rotated with the hip and knee extended, allowing the patient to be fully in the lateral decubitus position (Fig. 26-9). An incision is marked for a modified posterior approach to the knee. A horizontal incision is made in the crease of the popliteal fossa. The interval between the medial head of the gastrocnemius and the semimembranosus is developed. Lateral retraction of the gastrocnemius using Steinmann pins bent laterally provides access to the posterior capsule of the knee and simultaneously protects the neurovascular structures of the popliteal fossa (Fig. 26-10). This allows for excellent visualization and exposure of the sulcus between the medial and lateral tibial plateaus posteriorly. Electrocautery can then be used to clear the soft tissue from the sulcus and to expose as laterally as possible through the window. With the use of an osteotome, burr, and tamp, a unicortical window is made at the site of the tibial insertion of the PCL to match the size of the tibial side of the graft prepared earlier. A

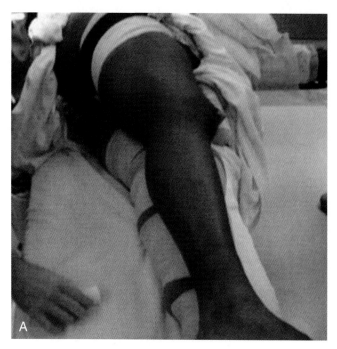

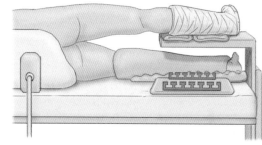

FIGURE 26-9 A, B, Lateral decubitus position in preparation for posterior approach to the knee. *(From Miller MD, Harner CD, Koshiwaguchi S. Acute posterior cruciate ligament injuries. In: Fu FH, Vince KG, Harner CD, eds. Knee Surgery. Baltimore: Williams & Wilkins; 1991:749-767.)*

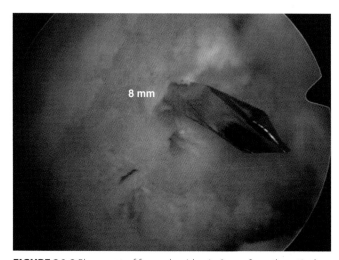

FIGURE 26-8 Placement of femoral guide pin 8 mm from the articular surface of the medial femoral condyle.

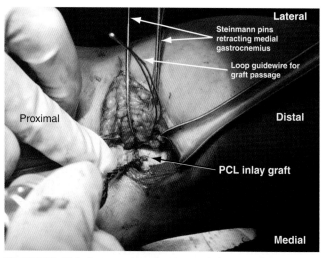

FIGURE 26-10 Steinmann pins retracting medial gastrocnemius. A looped guide wire is used for graft passage. *(From Miller MD, Cole BJ. PCL tibial inlay and posterolateral corner reconstruction. In: Gill SS, Cohen SB, Miller MD, eds. Philadelphia: WB Saunders; 2004:.)*

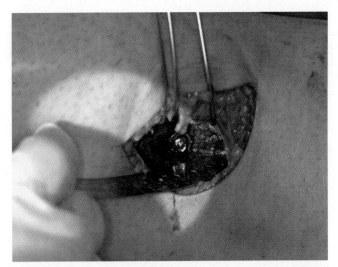

FIGURE 26-11 Posterior to anterior screw with washer in tibial trough.

posterior arthrotomy can then be performed sharply and carried proximally enough to ensure passage of the bone block. The arthrotomy will allow for visualization of the guide wire placed posteriorly in previous steps and a clamp is used to grasp the looped wire for passage through the posterior arthrotomy. On the preparation table, one or two guide pins are placed through the bone block of the tibia to allow for provisional fixation and assess screw length for definitive fixation. The graft, with the provisional pins, are brought to the surgical field and placed in the trough that is created. The two pins are inserted through the anterior tibial cortex and adjusted for proper length. Once the correct length has been determined, the screw sizes are measured and a cannulated drill bit is used to overdrill the guide pins; 4.5-mm cortical screws and a flat washer of appropriate length are then placed to lag the tibial bone block to the tibia (Fig. 26-11).

The patellar end of the tendon graft is then pulled through the posterior arthrotomy into the joint and up into the femoral tunnel using the prepositioned looped guide wire (Fig. 26-12). This

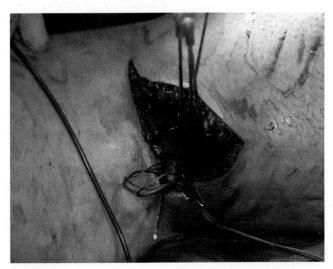

FIGURE 26-12 Looped 18-gauge wire used for passage of patellar end through arthrotomy.

maneuver can be done in two steps, if needed. First, the graft is passed into the notch by passing the sutures from the bony end of the graft through the anteromedial portal. Second, another loop is passed from the femoral tunnel out of the same portal and is used to the pull the bone plug into the femoral tunnel. Once the bone block on the patellar side is in the femoral tunnel, the location of the bone plug tendon junction is evaluated. The junction should be at the articular margin of the femoral tunnel. Once the position of the bone plug in the femoral tunnel is complete, a maximum amount of tension is applied (knee angle) to the sutures on the femoral side and an anterior drawer force is applied while a 9- × 20-mm metal interference screw is fully seated into the femoral tunnel. Once the interference screw is placed, a posterior drawer test confirms that PCL stability has been restored.

The bone graft, which is saved during graft preparation and femoral tunnel drilling, is packed into the patella and the tibial tubercle if enough remains. Wounds are closed in layered fashion, with care taken to irrigate all wounds copiously, especially the posterior arthrotomy. Radiographs should be taken before the patient exits the operating room to ensure that the graft and hardware placement are appropriate (Fig. 26-13). The knee is braced in extension after the dressing is placed. Bracing should support the posterior tibia to prevent posterior translation.

PEARLS & PITFALLS

PEARLS

- Be prepared. Have a plan A, B, and C. Make sure that you have all equipment readily available
- Recognize combined injuries ahead of time.
- Do not be fooled by a lax ACL. Perform an anterior drawer test and this laxity will resolve.
- Mobilize the vastus medialis oblique and place the femoral tunnel through a subvastus approach.
- Mobilize the medial head of the gastrocnemius with blunt dissection and retract it as far laterally as possible.
- Use $\frac{3}{32}$-inch pins that are drilled from posterior to anterior and bent over as retractors.
- Extend your inlay proximal, make a generous posterior arthrotomy in line with it, and make sure that the two are contiguous.
- Pass the graft part way into the joint before fixing into the trough. Be careful not to capture soft tissue with the drill.
- Using cannulated screws allows the surgeon to measure the lengths first and then advance the wire and clamp it anteriorly so that it will not get caught in the cannulated drill bit.
- After final passage of the graft, cycle the knee to ensure that there are no kinks.
- Place an anterior drawer force to reproduce the normal tibial step-off prior to fixation.
- Back up the fixation on the femoral side.
- Do not change your mind about the need to perform a PLC reconstruction after your PCL surgery is complete.
- Rehabilitation should emphasize prone range of motion early and quadriceps rehabilitation later.

PITFALLS

- Be careful in the workup regarding indications and patient selection.

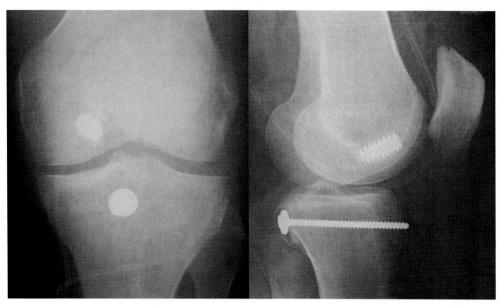

FIGURE 26-13 Postoperative AP (*left*) and lateral (*right*) views of tibial inlay fixation. *(From Miller MD, Harner CD, Koshiwaguchi S. Acute posterior cruciate ligament injuries. In: Fu FH, Vince KG, Harner CD, eds.* Knee Surgery. *Baltimore: Williams & Wilkins; 1991:749-767.)*

- Make sure that the lateral femoral starting point is at least 15 to 20 mm from the articular cartilage of the femur to avoid "blow-out."
- Check regularly for tight compartments in the thigh and calf to avoid iatrogenic compartment syndrome.
- Make sure that the medial head of the gastrocnemius is protecting the neurovascular structures to avoid injury
- Use fluoroscopy if there is any question regarding wires, hardware, or grafts.

Postoperative Rehabilitation

The PCL reconstruction fixation is not as robust as a typical ACL fixation and requires prevention of posterior translation throughout the first 8 weeks of rehabilitation. The goals of rehabilitation are full knee range of motion (ROM), pain and edema reduction, enhancement of quadriceps muscle recruitment, and prevention of posterior translation. Pertinent aspects of the initial rehabilitation protocol include 50% weight bearing with crutches in a brace and prone or side-lying ROM for the first month.

Rehabilitation begins when the patient is taken off the operating room table. A knee brace with adjustable limits to flexion is placed on the operative extremity. The brace is locked at 0 degree for the first 2 weeks at all times except for passive ROM exercises by the physical therapist or athletic trainer. After the first 2 weeks, the brace is advanced to allow for 0 to 90 degrees of motion. ROM exercises are performed in the prone or side-lying position and anterior pressure is applied proximally to the tibia while flexing the knee by gripping the heads of the gastrocnemius-soleus muscle group. Patella mobilizations and scar management are performed as therapists advance ROM as tolerated. To improve quadriceps strength, 10 sets of 10 repetition quadriceps contractions or straight-leg raises are performed three times daily. To prevent posterior sag, this exercise is done with assistance until complete quadriceps contraction can be done by the patient independently.

The first month also includes seated calf exercises, Russian stimulation (alternating currents), and a home quadriceps exercise program. The patient may begin stationary bike exercises at 2 weeks after the operation and leg press exercises with both legs and leg extensions at 3 weeks. Physical therapy is done at least twice weekly and no hamstring isometrics are allowed during the first 7 weeks.

During the fifth week of rehabilitation, the patient may begin aquatic therapy, emphasizing normal gait. The brace is discontinued and full weight bearing is encouraged, allowing for discontinuation of crutches. Prone flexion is increased to 120 degrees and treadmill walking is initiated. The patient is taught single-leg stands for balance and proprioception on an Airex balance pad or trampoline. Unilateral step-ups are started with 2-inch heights and progress to normal step height, as tolerated. Chair and wall squats are performed with the tibia kept perpendicular to the floor. At 8 weeks of rehabilitation, the patient begins lateral stepping, standing leg curls with cuff weights, or seated leg curls. No crossover stepping or shuffling should be performed and, if ROM is not progressing, the surgeon should be notified. Stairmaster exercises, slide boards, VersaClimber, elliptical trainers, and Nordic track use can begin at 10 weeks postoperatively.

The patient may begin jogging on a treadmill at 3 months postoperatively, with lateral movements, stepping, shuffling, and hopping supervised by a physical therapist or athletic training. At 14 to 16 weeks, sport-specific activities and plyometrics are initiated under supervision. Plyometrics focused on low-intensity vertical and lateral hopping begins with both feet, with transition to one foot as soon as possible. The volume for plyometric exercises is adjusted based on the intensity of the exercise and is focused on strengthening, not conditioning. Beginning at 4 months, progression of therapy proceeds with running and sport-specific drills. Strength and power development are emphasized and isokinetic tests for quadriceps strength differences and unilateral hamstring-to-quadriceps strength ratio are performed. The goal for quadriceps strength differences and unilateral hamstring-to-quadriceps strength ratio is less than 15 % and 65 % or better, respectively. The patient is tested monthly until isokinetic tests are passed and then functional testing begins if the person is to return to advanced recreational activities or sports.

Complications

The most common complication following PCL reconstruction is the return of objective posterior laxity on physical examination.[12,28] Also, acute PCL reconstruction in the setting of multiligamentous knee reconstruction or repair can result in arthrofibrosis and extensive scarring. Other complications include anterior knee pain, infection, heterotopic ossification, and painful hardware.[29] Recent studies have shown that the use of bioabsorbable screws can decrease the effects of painful hardware and eliminate future hardware removal.[30] There have also been reports of avascular necrosis of the medial femoral condyle. Therefore, tunnel placement should be proximal to the articular margin.

CONCLUSIONS

There continues to be an evolution of knowledge regarding posterior cruciate ligament injuries and their treatment. A thorough understanding of the anatomy of the PCL is critical to understanding its function when planning for proper treatment. It is well known that the PCL consists of an anterolateral bundle and a posteromedial bundle and interest has increased regarding double-bundle PCL reconstruction and all-arthroscopic inlay techniques.[31] However, double-bundle PCL reconstruction has been shown to be comparable to single-bundle PCL reconstruction in providing posterior stability for knees with an intact posterolateral corner.[32] The history and physical examination allow the surgeon to assess the most appropriate diagnostic tests and provide information on chronicity and severity of injury. When diagnostic tests confirm PCL disruption, the degree of laxity and associated injuries will aid in the decision to undergo surgery. Once the decision to proceed with intervention is made, preoperative planning is important to ensure a successful operation and postoperative rehabilitation. The tibial inlay technique described attempts to re-create the anatomy of the PCL and restore its biomechanical function while decreasing the intraoperative complications observed in alternative techniques. Whether conservative or surgical treatment is chosen, the key to a functional recovery after PCL injury is strong quadriceps musculature and a competent extensor mechanism. Information regarding PCL injuries continues to evolve and, as studies focusing on the multitude of factors that affect outcome improve, more standardized treatment algorithms will arise.

REFERENCES

1. Fanelli GC, Edson CJ. Posterior cruciate ligament injuries in trauma patients: part II. *Arthroscopy*. 1995;11:526-529.
2. Shelbourne KD, Davis TJ, Patel DV. The natural history of acute, isolated, nonoperatively treated posterior cruciate ligament injuries. A prospective study. *Am J Sports Med*. 1999;27:276-283.
3. Covey CD, Sapega AA. Injuries of the posterior cruciate ligament. *J Bone Joint Surg Am*. 1993;75:1376-1386.
4. Noyes FR, Stowers SF, Grood ES, et al. Posterior subluxations of the medial and lateral tibiofemoral compartments. An in vitro ligament sectioning study in cadaveric knees. *Am J Sports Med*. 1993;21:407-414.
5. •••. The posterior cruciate ligament. In: DeLee JC, Drez D, Miller MD, eds. *DeLee & Drez's Orthopaedic Sports Medicine: Principles and Practice*. 2nd ed. Philadelphia: WB Saunders; 1994:1374-1400.
6. Miller MD, Harner CD, Koshiwaguchi S. Acute posterior cruciate ligament injuries. In: Fu FH, Vince KG, Harner CD, eds. *Knee Surgery*. Baltimore: Williams & Wilkins; 1991:749-767.
7. Miller RH, Azar FM. Knee injuries. In: Canale ST, Beaty JH, eds. *Campbell's Operative Orthopaedics*. Philadelphia: Elsevier; 2008.
8. Cosgarea AJ, Jay PR. Posterior cruciate ligament injuries: evaluation and management. *J Am Acad Orthop Surg*. 2001;9:297-307.
9. Harner CD, Hoher J. Evaluation and treatment of posterior cruciate ligament injuries. *Am J Sports Med*. 1998;26:471-482.
10. Skinner HB. Current diagnosis and treatment in orthopedics. In: *Knee Injuries*. New York: Lange Medical Books/McGraw-Hill; 2003.
11. Miller MD, Cole BJ. PCL tibial inlay and posterolateral corner reconstruction. In: Gill SS, Cohen SB, Miller MD, eds. Philadelphia: WB Saunders; 2004.
12. Miller MD, Bergfeld JA, Fowler PJ, et al. The posterior cruciate ligament injured knee: principles of evaluation and treatment. *Instr Course Lect*. 1999;48:199-207.
13. Clancy WG Jr, Shelbourne KD, Zoellner GB, et al. Treatment of knee joint instability secondary to rupture of the posterior cruciate ligament. Report of a new procedure. *J Bone Joint Surg Am*. 1983;65:310-322.
14. Daniel DM, Stone ML, Barnett P, Sachs R. Use of the quadriceps active test to diagnose posterior cruciate-ligament disruption and measure posterior laxity of the knee. *J Bone Joint Surg Am*. 1988;70:386-391.
15. Jakob R, Warne, J. Lateral and posterolateral rotatory instability of the knee. In: Jakob RP, Staubli H, eds. *The Knee and the Cruciate Ligaments: Anatomy, Biomechanics, Clinical Aspects, Reconstruction, Complications, and Rehabilitation*. New York: Springer; 1992:463-494.
16. Cooper DE. Tests for posterolateral instability of the knee in normal subjects. Results of examination under anesthesia. *J Bone Joint Surg Am*. 1991;73:30-36.
17. Hughston JC, Norwood LA Jr. The posterolateral drawer test and external rotational recurvatum test for posterolateral rotatory instability of the knee. *Clin Orthop Relat Res*. 1980;(147):82-87.
18. Hewett TE, Noyes FR, Lee MD. Diagnosis of complete and partial posterior cruciate ligament ruptures. Stress radiography compared with KT-1000 arthrometer and posterior drawer testing. *Am J Sports Med*. 1997;25:648-655.
19. Margheritini F, Mancini L, Mauro CS, Mariani PP. Stress radiography for quantifying posterior cruciate ligament deficiency. *Arthroscopy*. 2003; 19:706-711.
20. Fanelli GC, Giannotti BF, Edson CJ. Arthroscopically assisted combined posterior cruciate ligament/posterior lateral complex reconstruction. *Arthroscopy*. 1996;12:521-530.
21. Shelbourne KD, Jennings RW, Vahey TN. Magnetic resonance imaging of posterior cruciate ligament injuries: assessment of healing. *Am J Knee Surg*, 1999;12:209-213.
22. Petrie RS, Harner CD. Evaluation and management of the posterior cruciate injured knee. *Oper Tech Sports Med*. 1999;7:93-103.
23. Tietjens BR. Posterior cruciate ligament injuries. *J Bone Joint Surg Br*. 1985;67:674.
24. Parolie JM, Bergfeld JA. Long-term results of nonoperative treatment of isolated posterior cruciate ligament injuries in the athlete. *Am J Sports Med*. 1986;14:35-38.
25. Torg JS, Barton TM, Pavlov H, Stine R. Natural history of the posterior cruciate ligament-deficient knee. *Clin Orthop Relat Res*. 1989;(246): 208-216.
26. Shino K, Horibe S, Nakata K, et al. Conservative treatment of isolated injuries to the posterior cruciate ligament in athletes. *J Bone Joint Surg Br*. 1995;77:895-900.
27. Noyes FR, Roberts CS. High tibial osteotomy in knees with associated chronic ligament deficiencies. In: Jackson DW, ed. *Reconstructive Knee Surgery*. New York: Raven Press; 1995:185-210.
28. Miller MD, Olszewski AD. Posterior cruciate ligament injuries. New treatment options. *Am J Knee Surg*. 1995;8:145-154.

29. Jung YB, Lee YS, Jung HJ. Heterotopic bone formation after posterior cruciate ligament reconstruction using inlay method and posterolateral corner sling with tibia tunnel: report of one case. *Knee Surg Sports Traumatol Arthrosc.* 2007;15:729-732.

30. Gupta A, Lattermann C, Busam M, et al. Biomechanical evaluation of bioabsorbable versus metallic screws for posterior cruciate ligament inlay graft fixation: a comparative study. *Am J Sports Med,* 2009;37: 748-753.

31. Campbell RB, Jordan SS, Sekiya JK. Arthroscopic tibial inlay for posterior cruciate ligament reconstruction. *Arthroscopy.* 2007;23:1356.

32. Whiddon DR, Zehms CT, Miller MD, et al. Double compared with single-bundle open inlay posterior cruciate ligament reconstruction in a cadaver model. *J Bone Joint Surg Am.* 2008;90:1820-1829.

Anatomic Reconstruction of the Posterolateral Corner

James Bicos ● Daniel Purcell ● Robert Arciero

Injuries to the posterolateral corner (PLC) of the knee have received increased attention in recent years, with its elusive diagnosis, and potential surgical approaches to guide repair and/or reconstruction are still highly debated. Most injuries to the PLC occur in combination with disruption of the posterior cruciate ligament (PCL) or, to a lesser extent, the anterior cruciate ligament (ACL).[1-8] Failure to identify and treat these combined injuries has been reported to cause premature failure of cruciate ligament reconstruction, yet despite numerous surgical advancements enhancing cruciate ligament repair, results regarding PLC reconstruction remain far less predictable.[9-17] Perhaps secondary to its complex, often variable anatomy, lack of consensus guiding repair and/or reconstruction, or absence of current methods to assess treatment success, much controversy remains regarding optimal recognition and treatment of these injuries.[18,19]

Common causes of PLC injury include sports-related trauma, motor vehicle accidents, and falls.[1,4,20] Both contact and noncontact injuries have been recounted.[21] Injury of the PLC in combination with other ligamentous injuries occurs by a number of different mechanisms, typically involving a combination of knee hyperextension, external rotation, and varus rotation.[2,3,7,8,22-25] Posterolateral instability can also follow knee dislocation, and careful physical examination is required to rule out associated neurovascular complication. The incidence of neurovascular damage, most commonly involving the peroneal nerve, have been estimated to be from 12% to 29% following injuries to the PLC.[26-27]

Clinical manifestations of posterolateral corner insufficiency most notably include functional instability with the knee in extension. This is apparent with stair activity, slopes, or activities that require pivoting or change of direction.[28] Gait analysis may reveal a varus or hyperextension thrust, partially compensated for by walking with a slightly flexed knee.[3] Stress testing may reveal abnormal tibial external rotation, varus instability, as well as pathologic anterior or posterior translation with concomitant ACL or PCL injuries.[1-4,6,20-22,25,29-32]

Isolated injury to the PLC is uncommon, and a high degree of suspicion must exist to recognize these often subtle clinical findings skillfully. DeLee and colleagues,[4] in a comprehensive review of 735 knees with ligamentous injuries, found that only 1.6% of these subjects had acute isolated posterolateral deficiency. The greatest opportunity to achieve optimal results has been attributed to early repair, usually within 3 weeks from the date of injury, with the goal of obtaining anatomic repair of all injured structures.[6,29,33] Stannard and associates[18,19] have recommended augmentation, even at the time of primary repair, because of poor success rates. With respect to chronic injuries (more than 3 weeks postinjury), direct repair of individual structures is impractical, and invariably requires reconstructive techniques that should ideally mimic intrinsic anatomic function. Extensive scar tissue formation, secondary physiologic changes to involved structures, and potential alterations in weight-bearing and force-loading kinematics make this a formidable challenge, a monumental task for even the best of surgical technicians.

Numerous techniques to repair or augment the structures of the posterolateral corner have been described, but poor outcomes have been reported in 9% to 37% in clinical series.[5,18,19,34] Previous accounts have included advancement and recession of the lateral collateral ligament and arcuate complex, biceps tenodesis, augmentation of the biceps femoris or iliotibial band, autogenous or allograft reconstruction through a transfibular tunnel, and use of a transtibial tunnel technique.[9,13,17,35-38] All are performed in an attempt to recreate native fibular (lateral) collateral ligament function, considered the primary restraint to varus loads at full knee extension.

Advancement procedures have also been advocated, premised on tightening PLC structures by proximal relocation on the femur or by distal advancement on the tibia. However, these procedures have traditionally been nonanatomic and/or nonisometric, overconstraining knee motion or creating residual pathologic laxity; both can lead to suboptimal function and potential graft failure with repeated cycling.[6,9,13,15,18,19] Furthermore, this technique is dependent on good residual tissue for advancement. Thus, in the absence of bony avulsion or with midsubstance ruptures that create tissue ends not amenable to anatomic repair, most authors recommend anatomic reconstruction. Unfortunately, despite many techniques having been advocated, a glaring lack of objective data exists to support these immeasurable claims.[17,35-37]

Newer techniques used for reconstruction are based on the creation of dual femoral tunnels that attempt to approximate the anatomic footprints of the popliteus and lateral collateral ligament (LCL) on the lateral femoral condyle.[26] Similarly, current transfibular techniques describe a tunnel made in a strictly anterior to posterior direction in the fibula, along with a single isometric femoral tunnel providing two limbs to address varus laxity and abnormal increases in tibial external rotation. Moreover, patients with marked varus alignment and/or a lateral thrust in the stance phase of gait may require a valgus-producing tibial osteotomy prior to ligament reconstruction to re-create more conventional mechanical alignment, enhance repair kinematics, and decrease overall risk of graft failure.[9,39]

Our goal here is to describe a more anatomic approach to aid in the restoration of comparatively native biomechanics and weight-bearing properties following isolated PLC or coupled cruciate ligament reconstruction. It involves the creation of dual femoral sockets and two separate limbs of soft tissue graft to reproduce LCL and popliteal-fibular function. The unique element of this technique is the orientation of the transfibular bone tunnel, which is though to place the reconstructed LCL in a more anatomic location on the femur. It is directed in an anterolateral to posteromedial course, allowing the graft to assume a more conventional orientation in the coronal plane with the LCL. Furthermore, the posterior limb of the soft tissue graft travels in concert with the popliteus tendon–popliteofibular component, directly traversing the hiatus into a separate femoral socket just anterior and distal to the insertion of the popliteus tendon. This helps restore relatively inherent kinematic properties of the popliteofibular functional complex necessary to restrict pathologic external tibial rotation. Finally, imbrication of the posterolateral capsule is performed to augment stability further, ensuring heightened graft competence and longevity following reconstruction.

This chapter will provide a concise description of the PLC, including its anatomic structure and function, clinical and imaging diagnostic tools, and treatment and rehabilitative guidelines concerning chronic reconstruction. In addition, we will describe our preferred surgical technique, and the results of an unpublished series describing intermediate results involving this technique will also be presented.

ANATOMY

The anatomic features of the PLC are extremely complex, considerably variable, and likely represent the least understood functional compartment of the knee. Inconsistent terminology, confusing nomenclature, and demonstrable changes in anatomic relationships, specifically evolutionary alterations regarding structures associated with the fibular head, have caused much

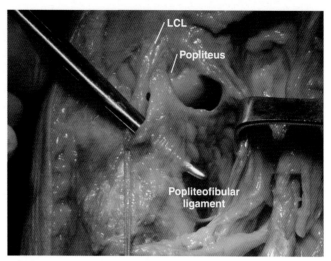

FIGURE 27-1 Gross anatomic depiction of the posterolateral corner demonstrating the relationship between the LCL, popliteus tendon, and popliteofibular ligament (under scissors).

deliberation concerning its organization.[40-42] Terry and LaPrade have provided much clarity to this exposure through cadaveric dissection and study.[43]

The key elements include the fibular (lateral) collateral, popliteus, and popliteofibular ligaments (Fig. 27-1) Functioning as a unit, these structures, along with associated capsular components, prevent abnormal posterior translation, varus rotation, and coupled external rotation of the tibia.[24,31,44,45] In addition, by preventing abnormal translation and rotation, the PLC has a secondary function of protecting the cruciate ligaments from abnormally high tensile loads, which can potentially disrupt the normal healing process following cruciate repair, leading to premature graft failure.[3,14,46]

The PLC is commonly depicted in terms of its soft tissue arrangement, remarkably defined within the context of the layer concept by Seebacher and coworkers[47] and the three-fascia incision technique popularized by Terry and LaPrade[43] (Figs. 27-2 and 27-3). The most superficial layer, or layer I, contains the lateral fascia, iliotibial band, and biceps femoris tendon. The middle layer includes the quadriceps retinaculum, patellofemoral ligaments, and patellomeniscal ligament, whereas the deepest layer, or layer III, contains the lateral joint capsule, popliteal muscle-tendon unit, and fibular collateral ligament. The fabellofibular and arcuate ligaments, which are variable in terms of their size and contributions to stability, also reside in the deepest layer.

The PLC can also be divided into primary and secondary stabilizers. Primary stabilizers include the LCL and popliteus complex, whereas less prominent contributors include the arcuate complex, posterolateral capsule, and various connections to the lateral meniscus.[2,23,46] Similarly, these primary stabilizers can be broken down into static and dynamic stabilizers, with the popliteus tendon complex considered a prime example. The dynamic component includes the popliteus muscle and tendon unit proper, controlling the screw-home mechanism; the static component includes several branching ligamentous structures that insert into the tibia, fibula, and lateral meniscus, respectively.

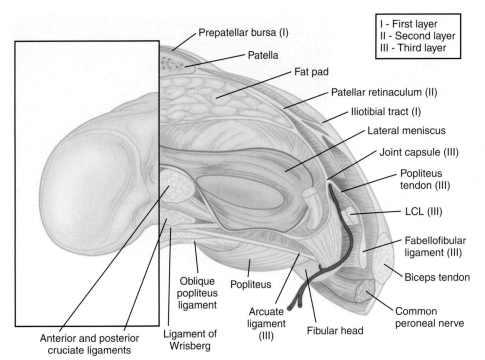

| I - First layer |
| II - Second layer |
| III - Third layer |

Prepatellar bursa (I)

Patella

Fat pad

Patellar retinaculum (II)

Iliotibial tract (I)

Lateral meniscus

Joint capsule (III)

Popliteus tendon (III)

LCL (III)

Fabellofibular ligament (III)

Biceps tendon

Common peroneal nerve

Oblique popliteus ligament

Popliteus

Arcuate ligament (III)

Fibular head

Anterior and posterior cruciate ligaments

Ligament of Wrisberg

FIGURE 27-2 Cross-sectional view demonstrating the three layers of the knee and associated anatomic structures of the posterolateral aspect of the knee.

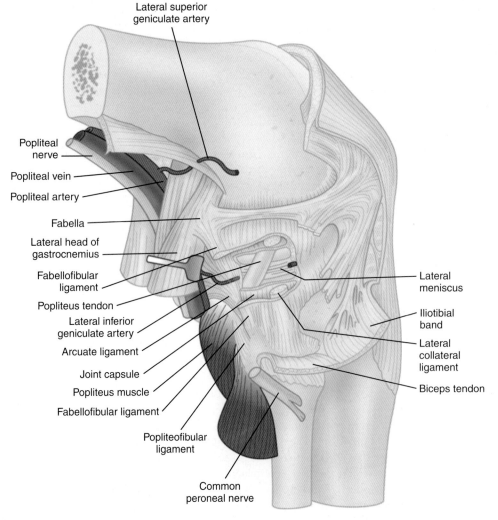

Lateral superior geniculate artery

Popliteal nerve

Popliteal vein

Popliteal artery

Fabella

Lateral head of gastrocnemius

Fabellofibular ligament

Popliteus tendon

Lateral inferior geniculate artery

Arcuate ligament

Joint capsule

Popliteus muscle

Fabellofibular ligament

Popliteofibular ligament

Common peroneal nerve

Lateral meniscus

Iliotibial band

Lateral collateral ligament

Biceps tendon

FIGURE 27-3 Lateral view of the posterolateral corner demonstrating relationships of the anatomic structures within the three layers of the knee.

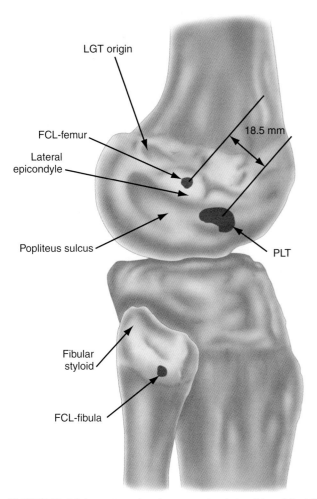

FIGURE 27-4 Relevant insertion site anatomic relationships of the LCL, popliteus tendon, and popliteofibular ligament.

The strength of the posterolateral compartment can be viewed as a composite effort by its constituents, but the main contributors include the fibular collateral ligament, tendinoaponeurotic portion of the popliteus muscle, and posterolateral capsule. The fibular collateral ligament (FCL) originates just proximal and posterior to lateral femoral epicondyle, slightly anterior to the femoral attachment of the lateral head of the gastrocnemius tendon. It follows an oblique course to insert on the lateral aspect of the fibular head, anterior and distal to the tip of the fibular styloid process (Fig. 27-4). It provides stability against varus loads, most notably at terminal knee extension, and as a secondary restraint to combined external rotation and posterior displacement of the knee. It is a distinct entity from the joint capsule and, unlike the medial collateral ligament, has no attachments to its corresponding meniscus.[3,44,45,48]

The popliteus muscle arises from the posteromedial proximal tibia, just above the soleal line, extending superiorly and laterally to form a tendinous structure as it courses through the popliteal hiatus. It then inserts on the lateral femoral condyle, anterior and distal to the LCL origin, resisting pathologic external rotation of the tibia from 20 to 130 degrees and excessive varus rotation from 0 to 90 degrees. It also sends fibers to the posterior horn of the lateral meniscus, helping to restrict its excessive forward displacement as the knee assumes a more extended position.[49]

The popliteofibular ligament originates near the popliteus musculotendinous junction and courses distally and laterally, attaching to the medial aspect of the fibular styloid process.[48-50] Anatomic studies have shown it to be present 93% to 100% of the time.[23,24] It can be easily be differentiated from the arcuate ligament by the orientation of its fibers, with the proximal third coursing obliquely and fusing with the popliteal tendon, and the remaining distal fibers running vertically, similar to the pattern of the LCL (Fig. 27-5). It helps prevent excessive posterior translation, varus angulation, and primary and coupled tibial external rotation.[43] Remarkably, it is as wide as or even wider than the popliteus tendon proper.

The arcuate ligament forms a Y-shaped pattern that begins distally on the styloid process of the fibula, with the medial and lateral limbs both extending proximally. The lateral limb coalesces with the lateral joint capsule and the medial limb attaches to the posterior capsule of the knee.[21,23,26,47,48] Studies have shown it to be present in only 24% of cadaveric specimens, whereas the equally as variable fabellofibular ligament has been found to be present in approximately 68%.[49] Both act in complementary fashion to stabilize the PLC further when present.

Biomechanics

To understand the PLC fully, one must review the complex interplay between the static and dynamic stabilizers of the knee. Numerous biomechanical studies implementing selective ligament cutting protocols have demonstrated that injury to the PLC results in increased primary external rotation, primary varus rotation, primary posterior translation, and coupled external rotation.[3,8,51] In terms of varus rotational stability, the PLC acts as a restraint at lesser degrees of knee flexion, with maximal restraint at 30 degrees.[46] Regarding external rotational instability, sectioning of the LCL and PLC capsule has been shown to result in greater posterolateral rotary instability than isolated sectioning of either structure alone.[31,44,45] Concerning posterior translational instability, the PLC resists posterior translation at lesser degrees of knee flexion with maximal restraint at 30 degrees, whereas the PCL resists posterior tibial translation at higher degrees of knee flexion, with maximal restraint at 90 degrees.[52]

Forces on the intact ligaments of the knee after PLC injury can be substantial. The PCL experiences significant increases in forces between 45 to 90 degrees of knee flexion after complete sectioning of the PLC and tibial varus or external rotation.[53] Harner and colleagues[12] have found a significant increase in the force on a PCL reconstruction graft in PLC-deficient knees, with the PCL graft rendered almost ineffective and, as expected, predisposing it to failure. Combined PCL and PLC injuries have also been shown to produce increased contact pressures in the patellofemoral joint when compared to isolated PCL injuries alone.[54] Similarly, tension on the ACL is also increased with PLC injury, particularly with tibial internal rotation in the range of 0 to 20 degrees of knee flexion.

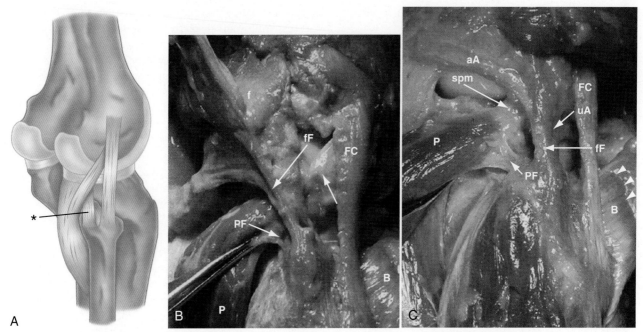

FIGURE 27-5 A, The popliteofibular ligament (*) can be seen arising from the posterior aspect of the fibula and inserting onto the popliteus tendon. **B,** This dissection of the PLC of the knee shows the popliteofibular ligament (PF) extending from the fibula to the popliteus muscle (P). The *black arrow* points to the popliteus tendon. Just anterior and slightly lateral to the PFL is the fabellofibular ligament (fF), and further anterolaterally on the fibula is the fibular collateral ligament (FC). **C,** This view of the PLC of the knee shows the popliteus muscle (P) retracted medially revealing the popliteofibular ligament (PF). One can also see the superior popliteomeniscal fascicle (spm), the fabellofibular ligament (fF), and the fibular collateral ligament (FC).

PATIENT EVALUATION

PLC injuries can be subtle and are easily missed if a high degree of suspicion for injury does not exist. Symptoms invariably depend on timing and severity of injury, degree of associated instability, and other sustained defects. Injuries are often classified as grade I, II, or III sprains, corresponding to minimal, partial, or complete tearing, respectively. Quantification of the degree of joint opening in response to varus stress is also commonly used, with a score of 3+ describing an opening of more than 10 mm, with a soft or no appreciable end point.[3,10] Patients with evidence of injury, but without significant pathologic laxity or functional limitations, corresponding to grade I and II injuries, are often treated with rehabilitation and observation.[55,56] However, patients with grade III injuries, which typically reflect abnormal joint motion, are advised to undergo primary repair, augmentation, or reconstruction.[4,18,19,32]

Diagnostic evidence of PLC injury can come in a wide variety, and includes physical signs, imaging, or both. Gait abnormalities may be present, particularly in chronic injuries, and may include standing varus alignment of the knee and/or a hyperextension-varus thrust during the stance phase of gait. Patients may attempt to walk with the knee slightly flexed or modify footwear to help decrease symptoms of pain and instability.[2,3,22]

Along with physical examination parameters, which includes meticulous evaluation of the cruciate ligaments, specific tests to detect PLC injury include the varus load, posterolateral drawer, and Dial tests. They all attempt to assess increased external rotation of the tibia relative to the femur. When there is an isolated injury to the posterolateral structures with an intact PCL, there is maximally increased varus, external rotation, and posterior translation at 30 degrees of flexion because of a minimal amount of PCL fibers tensed at low knee flexion angles (Fig. 27-6). In contrast, at 90 degrees of flexion, all intact PCL fibers are tightened and help provide a secondary restraint against external rotation and varus forces, including providing the primary restraint to posterior tibial translation. With specific reference to the Dial test, increased external rotation at 30 but not at 90 degrees indicates an isolated PLC injury, whereas increased external rotation at both suggests injury to both structures. An increase of 10 degrees from the normal knee is also considered a significant finding (Fig. 27-7).[1-3,20,22,28,32,48,57]

Diagnostic Imaging

Imaging studies can provide an objective identification of PLC injuries, and popular modalities include standard radiography, stress radiography (Telos stress device; Telos Medical USA; Keene, NH), and magnetic resonance imaging (MRI). Increased joint space widening and abnormalities associated with the fibular head on plain x-ray may suggest PLC pathology, whereas a Segond fracture (lateral capsular avulsion), usually pathognomonic for acute ACL rupture, can indicate disruption of one or both structures. Regarding chronic PLC injury, degenerative changes may be present across all compartments; however, the lateral compartment is usually the most affected.

Stress radiography has recently been popularized in the literature, and may be a useful adjunct to diagnosis of more imprecise PLC injuries. It involves the application of a standardized force in an effort to produce abnormal joint displacement. It has been

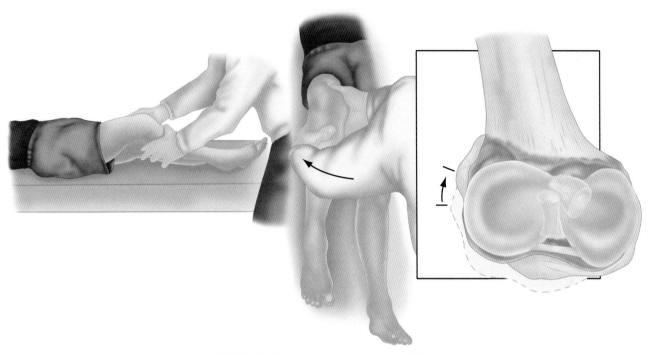

FIGURE 27-6 Posterolateral Lachman test at 30 degrees.

shown to be a reliable measure of posterior joint laxity in patients with PCL injuries, and was recently found to be a good predictor of concomitant disruption to the PLC.[58,59] Sekiya and associates[7] have found that a grade 3 posterior drawer test and more than 10 mm of tibial translation on stress radiography correlate with a complete disruption of the PCL, in addition to PLC injury. This reported association should help raise examiner suspicion to the possibility of damage to the PLC so often overlooked in combined ligamentous injuries.

Regarding MRI, perhaps the most sensitive marker of all, recent studies have shown that either T1- or T2-weighted coronal oblique images through the knee, which include the entire fibular head and styloid process, provide the best visualization of the individual structures of the PLC (Fig. 27-8).[60] Moreover, it can also detect associated injuries, most importantly, concomitant ACL and PCL tears that will directly influence surgical planning and associated patient rehabilitation. Furthermore, in the acute setting, when physical examination may not be possible secondary to patient discomfort, the use of MRI to qualify disruption of the PLC structures can be of utmost importance to aid in acute diagnosis and facilitate early intervention.

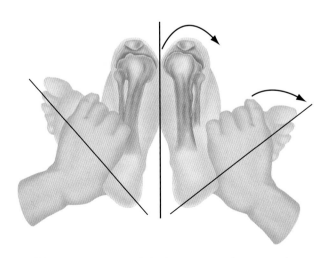

FIGURE 27-7 Supine external tibial rotation or Dial test at 30 degrees of knee flexion.

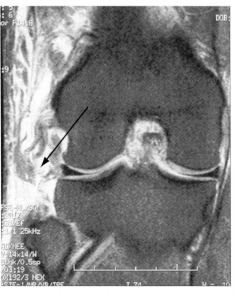

FIGURE 27-8 Coronal MRI scan showing an acute avulsion of biceps tendon and lateral collateral ligament *(arrow)*.

TREATMENT

Timing is of critical importance in the surgical management of isolated PLC or combined injuries.[1,4,22,28,56] Acute events, defined as within 3 weeks of injury, have generally demonstrated greater enduring success than operative management of chronic PLC injuries. However, many still favor primary reconstruction over attempted repair, even in the acute setting, arguing that repair and/or augmentation of the fibular collateral ligament is indicated only for patients with bony avulsions potentially amenable to internal fixation.[18,19,23,36] In either case, it is imperative to detect and treat PLC injuries early to avoid physiologic and biomechanical changes that accompany chronic injuries, and are professed to generate inferior functional long-term results. When combined injuries are involved, preoperative planning must select for appropriate patient positioning, graft availability and/or harvest technique, and sequential surgical instrumentation to guide the repair and/or reconstruction.

In cases in which there is marked varus malalignment and/or a lateral thrust in the stance phase of gait, initially performing a valgus tibial osteotomy may prevent increased targeted loads on the newly reconstructed lateral capsular structures, potentially enhancing repair mechanics and decreasing the risk of graft failure. Diagnostic and therapeutic arthroscopy is also an invaluable adjunct, and should be performed prior to initiation of PLC and/or cruciate ligament reconstruction. Its value cannot be overestimated regarding direct evaluation of soft tissue disruption, detection of associated injuries, and primary role in meniscal or chondral débridement or repair.

Arthroscopic Technique

Here we will describe reconstruction of the PLC through implementation of a free soft tissue graft, introduced through a transfibular tunnel. An autograft or allograft can be used. Principal features include the construction of dual femoral sockets, with two separate limbs created to reproduce LCL and popliteal-fibular function individually. The transfibular tunnel will be created in an anterolateral to posteromedial direction, allowing for graft tensioning to resume more appropriate anatomic positioning. Furthermore, the posterior limb of the graft will course through the hiatus in a more representative fashion of the native popliteus tendon–popliteofibular component. Overall, we believe that this technique represents a more anatomic reconstruction of the PLC, more closely resembling native PLC structure and function.

Following patient preparation and placement in the supine position, with all bony prominences protected, the three-fascia incision technique popularized by Terry and LaPrade[43] is initiated. A curvilinear or hockey stick–type incision is gently created over the lateral aspect of the knee. It should be centered over the lateral epicondyle and extend distally to the anterior fibular head, midway between the fibular head and Gerdy's tubercle. The first fascial incision is distal to expose the peroneal nerve and mobilize it away from the proximal fibula. The peroneal nerve should then be identified and dissected free, from just inferior to the biceps tendon to the posterior aspect of the

fibular head. It must be protected throughout the entire procedure to ensure optimal post-operative function. Using a blunt elevator, the muscle and soft tissue on the posterior aspect of the fibula are gently reflected to expose the posterior bony surface of the fibula. The LCL insertion on the fibula is then identified. This ligament inserts on the lateral aspect of the fibula in a small sulcus. It can be found by making a small linear incision in the biceps fascia, spreading and exposing the ligament, as described by LaPrade. The fibular head is then exposed just anterior and distal to the insertion site and a ³/₃₂-inch guide wire is drilled from this spot posteromedially. A 6- or 7-mm bone fibular tunnel is created with a cannulated reamer and a looping suture is placed for future graft passage. The angle of this tunnel is unique to this reconstruction; it is thought to reconstruct the LCL more anatomically compared with the traditional method of drilling this tunnel from a more anterior to posterior direction (Fig. 27-9).

The second fascial incision is then made, exposing the lateral capsular region, extending from the superoanterior border of the short head biceps tendon to the inferior border of the iliotibial

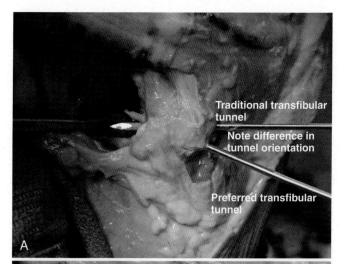

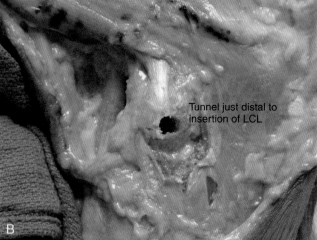

FIGURE 27-9 A, Preferred transfibular tunnel placement. Note the orientation from anterolateral to posteromedial. **B,** Tunnel position shown just inferior to the lateral collateral ligament insertion.

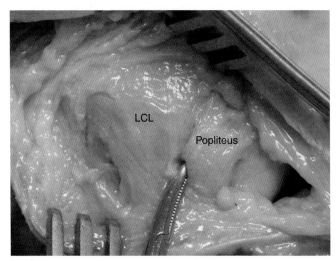

FIGURE 27-10 Femoral attachment site for the LCL and popliteus tendon.

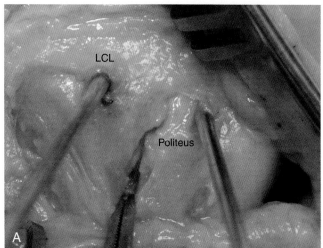

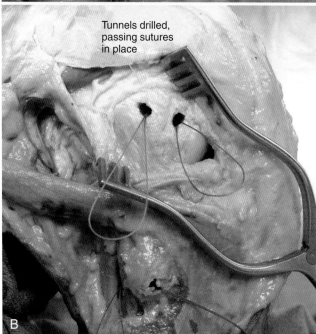

FIGURE 27-11 A, ³⁄₃₂-inch guide wire placed in the appropriate location for the femoral tunnels of the LCL and popliteus tendons. **B,** Both tunnels after drilling.

(IT) band. A posterior arthrotomy is made and no. 2 nonabsorbable sutures are placed for reefing of the posterolateral capsule at the end of the procedure. Finally, the IT band should be incised centrally over the lateral femoral epicondyle and continued anteriorly and slightly distally. Often, a thickened bursal layer will obscure the LCL origin, and should be separated to gain proper exposure of the femoral attachment site of the LCL.. An anterior arthrotomy then allows for identification of the origin of popliteus tendon on the femur (Fig. 27-10). This incision is made vertically to expose the distal lateral condylar articular surface and peripheral edge of the anterolateral meniscus. Gentle retraction will allow for visualization of the popliteus tendon coming in an oblique fashion and inserting distally on the lateral femur, close to the articular surface.

A second guide wire is then directed approximately 3 to 4 mm anterior to the central origin of the LCL, creating a 7- to 8-mm femoral socket about 30 to 35 mm in length. It should be directed toward the medial cortex, even penetrating the medial cortex to aid in graft passage. A passing suture can be placed and clamped. In the case of combined PCL reconstruction, the tunnel should be angled slightly more proximally so as to not encroach on the femoral insertion for the PCL.

The popliteofibular tunnel is now created, with a pin inserted approximately 3 to 4 mm distal and slightly anterior to the femoral attachment for the popliteus tendon. It is aimed medially, but only requires a depth of 25 to 30 mm. A 7- to 8-mm cannulated reamer is used to prepare the femoral socket for the popliteus limb. The dual femoral tunnels should be separated by approximately 18 mm, according to the anatomic insertions of the LCL and popliteus tendon (Fig. 27-11. Also see Fig. 27-10).[43]

A graft of suitable length (we prefer a posterior tibialis allograft or semitendinosus autograft), typically 24 to 26 cm, is then chosen, and its free ends tagged with a baseball stitch over a distance of approximately 25 to 30 mm with a no. 2 nonabsorbable suture. The graft is then passed through the transfibular tunnel and firmly tensioned with an equal length of graft limbs, both anterior and posterior. The posterior limb is then tunneled along the posterior aspect of the fibula, through the popliteal hiatus, and into its respective femoral tunnel. An 8- or 9- × 23-mm biotenodesis screw (Arthrex; Naples, Fla) is then used for fixation. This unicortical tunnel and graft fixed in this fashion obviates the need for drilling across the femur, which could potentially interfere with other tunnels created for cruciate ligament reconstruction. The other limb is now tunneled deep to the biceps femoris tendon insertion, adjacent to the native or remnant LCL. Using the passing suture already in place for the LCL tunnel, the anterior limb is then transferred into its femoral socket. With the knee in approximately 30 degrees of flexion, slight internal rotation, and slight valgus, firm tension is then applied medially to tighten this limb of the re-

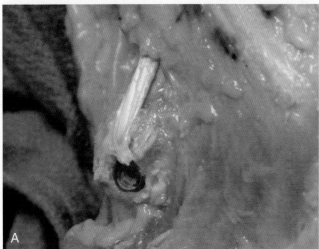

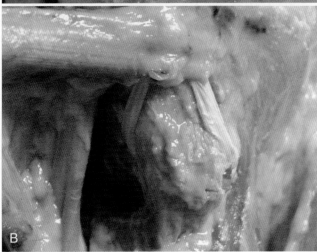

FIGURE 27-12 A, Free tendon graft passed through the fibular tunnel and secured with a bioabsorbable screw (anterior view). Note the orientation in line with the native LCL. **B,** Posterolateral view of the reconstruction with the LCL limb to the right and the popliteus-PFL limb to the left. LCL = lateral collateral ligament; PFL = popliteofibular ligament.

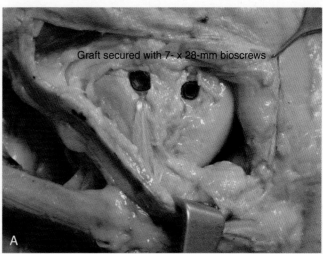

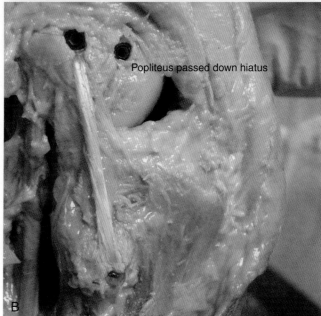

FIGURE 27-13 A, LCL graft limb and popliteus graft limb secured with bioabsorbable tenodesis screws. **B,** Finished repair.

construction. A 7- to 8-mm × 28-mm bioabsorbable interference screw is then placed into each tunnel, definitively securing the graft (Figs. 27-12 and 27-13). The wounds are copiously irrigated, closed in layers, and the knee placed in a hinged brace and locked in full extension.

COMPLICATIONS

Complications of surgical management of PLC injuries can include injury to the peroneal nerve, wound problems, postoperative knee stiffness (most commonly, loss of flexion), hamstring weakness (particularly in biceps tenodesis repair or advancement procedures), soft tissue graft failure, and hard-

ware issues.[2,3] Meticulous preoperative planning, expert surgical technique, and a strict rehabilitation protocol can help diminish their potential occurrence. The risk of peroneal nerve injury can be skillfully decreased by careful identification, fastidious dissection, and watchful protection throughout the surgical process. Knee stiffness, a common sequela, especially in the early postoperative setting, can develop into advanced arthrofibrosis, requiring manipulation under anesthesia and/or arthroscopic release of adhesions to enhance long-term flexibility. Proper tensioning techniques should help bolster graft strength and predicted durability; however, following stringent rehabilitation parameters is the overall key to minimize the chance of catastrophic failure.

PEARLS & PITFALLS

- Position the patient distal enough on the table to obtain unobstructed access to the lateral knee. Also, if this procedure is being performed with other ligament reconstruction (e.g., ACL, PCL), the well leg should be positioned in a soft knee support with the foot supported to prevent nerve traction or compression injuries from a prolonged surgical procedure.
- Take your time with dissection to develop the three lateral windows. The first window will allow visualization of the common peroneal nerve. This must be protected. Dissect it distally enough so that it is released around the fibular head.
- The dissection through the second lateral window is between the biceps femoris and iliotibial band. This should give you access to the posterior fibula. Make sure that you can palpate the posterior tibiofibular joint. There is a sulcus on the posteromedial side of the fibular head that is the landmark for the fibular tunnel exiting posteriorly.
- A small 5-mm incision through the longitudinal fibers of the biceps tendon, directly over the lateral aspect of the fibular head, and spreading these fibers will permit identification of the LCL on the fibula for proper guide wire placement and direction of the fibular tunnel. This will maximize anatomic positioning of the LCL portion of the reconstruction.
- The orientation of the fibular tunnel is not anterior to posterior. It is anterolateral to posteromedial. The starting point is just distal and anterior to the anterior portion of the LCL attachment on the fibula previously exposed.
- In addition, when drilling the fibular tunnel, two technical errors can occur: (1) too much of a medial to lateral orientation can cause inadvertent violation of the proximal tibiofemoral joint; and (2) because the starting point is slightly anterior to the midlateral aspect of the fibular head (and anterior to the fibular attachment site of the LCL), if the angle of orientation is too much in an anterior to posterior direction, a violation of the lateral cortex of the fibula can occur.
- The distance between the popliteal and lateral collateral femoral tunnels is consistently defined, approximately 18 to 19 mm. It will help restore anatomic placement of the tunnels.
- The center of the femoral attachment site for the LCL is not the lateral epicondyle. It is 3 to 5 mm proximal and slightly posterior to the epicondyle.
- The use of a biotenodesis screw for the fixation of the popliteus limb of the reconstruction on the femur obviates the need for a complete transfemoral guide wire or socket. This is important for minimizing the number of tunnels in the distal femur, especially because this reconstruction is frequently performed in concert with ACL and/or PCL reconstructions.
- Failure to appreciate a varus thrust or varus malalignment with preoperative standing and hip to ankle mechanical alignment radiographs, and failure to address varus malalignment, will compromise the surgical result of the PLC reconstruction.

Postoperative Rehabilitation

Following surgical intervention, immediate mobilization is initiated with protected weight bearing (PWB) to safeguard the repair. The patient is placed in a hinged knee brace, locked in full extension. Gentle range of motion (ROM) is not typically done prior to 3 weeks. Static quadriceps exercises and straight leg raises are permitted. Patellar mobilization and gaining full extension are important. Weight bearing is restricted for the first 6 weeks, usually 20 to 40 pounds of PWB. Specific goals during the early recovery period include minimizing postoperative inflammation and associated fibrosis while concomitantly working to prevent quadriceps atrophy. At 6 weeks, patients enter the next phase of rehabilitation, premised on demonstrating active ROM of at least 0 to 115 degrees and quadriceps strength at least 60% of the contralateral leg referenced as a control. Once this is achieved, the hinged brace is discontinued and patients can begin proprioceptive skills training. Weight bearing is then progressed to full weight-bearing status by the week 8. At approximately 3 months, further strengthening exercises, specifically, closed-chain exercises, can be safely initiated. Return to competitive sports and/or heavy labor is permitted at approximately the 6-month mark if patients have achieved quadriceps strength of 80% of the unaffected leg and appropriate proprioceptive ability has been established.

CONCLUSIONS

The combined structures of the PLC have greater tensile strength than any of the other major knee ligaments and act in combination with the PCL to resist posterior translation and external and varus rotation of the tibia on the femur. Functional outcomes following nonoperative management of the multiple ligament–injured knee are considered to be poor at best. Disruption of the PLC with an intact PCL results in increased varus and external rotation of the knee, most pronounced at 30 degrees of knee flexion, whereas disruption of the PCL with an intact PLC results in increased posterior translation of the tibia, most pronounced at 90 degrees of knee flexion.[2,3] Moreover, cruciate ligament disruption can lead to increased compartment pressures, accelerating the risks of associated degenerative joint disease.[54,61]

Prompt recognition and treatment of PLC injuries are important to potentiate the success of PLC repair or reconstruction, in addition to the results of combined cruciate ligament reconstruction. Repair or reconstruction of the PLC specifically attempts to recreate the LCL for varus stability and the popliteus and popliteofibular ligament for stability in external rotation. Management should be dictated by the severity of injury, timing of diagnosis, and associated functional requirements of each individual. Surgical intervention should be determined based on a thorough understanding of the biomechanics of the injury, along with the application of anatomic repair principles.

Numerous reconstruction techniques have been described in the medical literature using a variety of grafts to reinforce or replace the fibular collateral ligament, posterolateral capsule, popliteus tendon, or popliteofibular ligament with anatomic or nonanatomic anchor repair and/or reconstruction sites. Nonanatomic reconstructions, in particular, have produced variable results, whereas anatomic reconstructions offer the most promise by restoring normal knee stability and kinematics. Our goal was to describe a more anatomic approach to PLC reconstruction regarding chronic injuries considered to be more than 3 weeks postinjury.

The principal features of this reconstruction include dual femoral sockets with two separate limbs of soft tissue graft to reproduce the native function of the lateral collateral ligament and popliteal fibular ligament. Second, the orientation of the transfibular tunnel is directed in an anterolateral to posteromedial direction, assuming a more anatomic orientation in the coronal plane with the lateral collateral ligament. Furthermore, the posterior limb travels in a similar direction as the popliteus tendon–popliteofibular ligament component, coming directly into the hiatus and into a separate femoral socket just anterior and distal to the popliteus tendon insertion.

Early results of an unpublished case series using this technique as a component of multiligamentous reconstruction have demonstrated good intermediate term success at a minimum of 2 years postoperatively. Using patient-oriented validated outcome scores and accompanying clinical and stress radiography examination parameters, 22 patients with a mean age of 19.5 years at a median of 4 months following injury underwent primary reconstruction of chronic PLC injuries. This was performed by a single surgeon, using a single surgical technique that involved reconstructing the lateral collateral ligament, popliteus tendon and popliteofibular ligament. Subjects were reevaluated at an average of 41 months. At the most recent follow-up, there were no reported graft failures or other major complications. Patient-oriented validated outcome measures demonstrated that 16 of 22 had good and/or excellent Lysholm scores, the mean Tegner activity level was 6, and the mean SF-12 score was 42. No abnormal varus stress or prone external rotation tests were discovered, with all patients exhibiting tibial external rotation within 10 degrees of the contralateral knee at 30 and 90 degrees of flexion, respectively. The mean KT arthrometry measurement was 1.5 mm (a side to side difference less than 3 mm is considered within normal limits). Nineteen patients had varus stress radiography of the reconstructed and normal knee performed with the knee in 20 degrees of flexion. Side to side differences in the lateral joint line opening, evaluated by Telos stress radiography, demonstrated less than 3 mm difference in 18 of 19 knees and a 4.1-mm difference in the remaining knee. To our knowledge, this study will be the first to report on chronic PLC injuries treated by a single surgeon using a single primary reconstruction technique and evaluating subjects using multiple validated knee ligament scales, KT arthrometry, and varus and posterior stress radiography.

Pasque,[33] in a cadaveric study under defined loading conditions, has demonstrated the importance of repairing all associated PLC structures. No individual component demonstrated an ability to act as a primary restraint to external rotation, varus rotation, and posterior tibial translation from 0 to 120 degrees. With an applied external rotation tibial force applied, LCL reconstruction alone was not sufficient enough to reduce PCL graft forces to normal. Addition of a popliteus or popliteofibular reconstruction was necessary to reduce PCL graft forces to near-normal values.

There is ample evidence to support anatomic reconstruction of the PLC versus other attempted salvage and/or advancement procedures, and every attempt should be made to restore almost native function in consideration of preinjury structural biomechanics. Concomitantly, the PLC must be addressed in situations in which the potential for combined ligamentous injuries exist; suspicion for disruption should always be evaluated in association with cruciate ligament evaluation. Untreated posterolateral corner instability is possibly the most common identifiable cause of ACL reconstruction failure—biomechanical studies of PCL grafts have shown these grafts to be rendered ineffective and overloaded in the setting of deficient PLC structures because of increases in situ forces that occur during tensioning.

In patients with both chronic PLC and cruciate ligament deficiency, cruciate ligament reconstruction should be performed collectively with PLC reconstruction because of the potential for better long-term functional outcome. Failure to address instability of the PLC can increase tensile forces at cruciate ligament graft sites, contributing to graft failure through the generation of higher forces associated with varus loading at varying degrees of flexion, not observed in those with intact PLC structures. Anatomic reconstruction allows for the greatest potential of resuming functional independence and should be the procedure of choice for chronic isolated or combined posterolateral and cruciate ligament injuries.

REFERENCES

1. Baker CL Jr, Norwood LA, Hughston JC. Acute posterolateral instability of the knee. *J Bone Joint Surg Am.* 1983;65:614-628.
2. Chen FS, Rokito AS, Pitman MI. Acute and chronic posterolateral instability of the knee. *J Am Acad Orthop Surg.* 2000;8:97-110.
3. Covey DC. Injuries of the posterolateral corner of the knee: anatomy, biomechanics, and the management of injuries. *J Bone Joint Surg Am.* 2001;83:106-118.
4. DeLee JC, Riley MB, Rockwood CA Jr. Acute posterolateral instability of the knee. *Am J Sports Med.* 1983;11:199-207.
5. Noyes FR, Barber-Westin SD. Surgical reconstruction of severe chronic posterolateral complex injuries of the knee using allograft tissues. *Am J Sports Med.* 1995;23:2-12.
6. Ranawat A, Baker CL 3rd, Henry S, Harner CD. Posterolateral corner injury of the knee: evaluation and management. *J Am Acad Orthop Surg.* 2008;16:506-518.
7. Sekiya JK, Whiddon DR, Zehms CT, Miller MD. A clinically relevant assessment of posterior cruciate ligament and posterolateral corner injuries. Evaluation of isolated and combined deficiency. *J Bone Joint Surg Am.* 2008;90:1621-1627.
8. Veltri DM, Deng XH, Torzilli PA, et al. The role of the cruciate and posterolateral ligaments in stability of the knee. A biomechanical study. *Am J Sports Med.* 1995;23:436-443.
9. Arciero R. Anatomic posterolateral corner reconstruction. *Arthroscopy.* 2005;21:1147.
10. Fanelli GC. Surgical reconstruction for acute posterolateral injury of the knee. *J Knee Surg.* 2005;28:157-162.
11. Freeman RT, Duri ZA, Dowd GS. Combined chronic posterior cruciate and posterolateral corner ligamentous injuries: a comparison of posterior cruciate ligament reconstruction with and without reconstruction of the posterolateral corner. *Knee.* 2002;9:309-312.
12. Harner CD, Vogrin TM, Hoher J, et al. Biomechanical analysis of a posterior cruciate ligament reconstruction: deficiency of the posterolateral structures as a cause of graft failure. *Am J Sports Med.* 2000;28:32-39.
13. Khanduja V, Somayaji HS, Harnett P. et al. Combined reconstruction of chronic posterior cruciate ligament and posterolateral corner deficiency. A two- to nine-year follow-up study. *J Bone Joint Surg Br.* 2006; 88:1169-1172.
14. LaPrade RF, Johansen S, Wentorf FA. et al. . An analysis of an anatomical posterolateral knee reconstruction: an in vitro biomechanical study and development of a surgical technique. *Am J Sports Med.* 2004;32: 1405-1414.
15. LaPrade RF, Muench C, Wentorf F, Lewis JL. The effect of injury to the posterolateral structures of the knee on force in a posterior cruciate ligament graft: a biomechanical study. *Am J Sports Med.* 2002;30: 233-238.

16. McGuire DA, Wolchok JC. Posterolateral corner reconstruction. *Arthroscopy*. 2003;19:790-793.

17. Yoon KH, Bae DK, Ha JH, Park SW. Anatomic reconstructive surgery for posterolateral instability of the knee. *Arthroscopy*. 2006;22:159-165.

18. Stannard JP, Brown SL, Farris RC. et al. The posterolateral corner of the knee: repair versus reconstruction. *Am J Sports Med*. 2005;33:881-888.

19. Stannard JP, Brown SL, Robinson JT, et al. Reconstruction of the posterolateral corner of the knee. *Arthroscopy*. 2005;21:1051-1059.

20. Fleming RE Jr, Blatz DJ, McCarroll JR. Posterior problems in the knee. Posterior cruciate insufficiency and posterolateral rotary insufficiency. *Am J Sports Med*. 1981;9:107-113.

21. Davies H, Unwin A, Aichroth P. The posterolateral corner of the knee. Anatomy, biomechanics, and the management of injuries. *Injury*. 2004;35:68-75.

22. Larson RV, Tingstad E. Lateral and posterolateral instability of the knee in adults. In: DeLee JC, Drez DJ, eds. *DeLee and Drez's Orthopaedic Sports Medicine. Principles and Practice*. 2nd ed. Philadelphia: WB Saunders; 2003:1969-1994.

23. Shahane SA, Ibbotson C, Strachan R, Bickerstaff DR. The popliteofibular ligament. An anatomical study of the posterolateral corner of the knee. *J Bone Joint Surg Br*. 1999;81:636-642.

24. Veltri DM, Deng XH, Torzilli PA, et al. The role of the popliteofibular ligament in stability of the human knee. A biomechanical study. *Am J Sports Med*. 1996;24:19-27.

25. Veltri DM , Warren RF. Anatomy, biomechanics, and physical findings in posterolateral knee instability. *Clin Sports Med*. 1994;13:599-614.

26. LaPrade RF, Ly TV, Wentorf FA, Engebretsen L. The posterolateral attachments of the knee: a qualitative and quantitative morphologic analysis of the fibular collateral ligament, popliteus tendon, popliteofibular ligament, and lateral gastrocnemius tendon. *Am J Sports Med*. 2003;31:854-860.

27. Noyes FR, Grood ES, Torzilli PA. Current concepts review. The definitions of terms for motion and position of the knee and injuries of the ligaments. *J Bone Joint Surg Am*. 1989;71:465-472.

28. Hughston JC, Jacobson KE. Chronic posterolateral instability of the knee. *J Bone Joint Surg Am*. 1985;67:351-359.

29. Cooper DE WR, Warner JP. The posterior cruciate ligament and posterolateral structures of the knee: anatomy, function, and patterns of injury. *Instr Course Lect*. 1991;40:249-270.

30. Daniel DM, Akeson WH, O'Connor JJ. *Knee Ligaments: Structure, Function, Injury, and Repair*. New York: Raven Press; 1990.

31. Nielsen S, Ovesen J, Rasmussen O. The posterior cruciate ligament and rotatory knee instability. An experimental study. *Arch Orthop Trauma Surg*. 1985;104:53-56.

32. Ross G, DeConciliis GP, Choi K, Scheller AD. Evaluation and treatment of acute posterolateral corner/anterior cruciate ligament injuries of the knee. *J Bone Joint Surg Am*. 2004;86(suppl 2):2-7.

33. Pasque C. The role of the popliteofibular ligament and tendon of the popliteus in providing stability in the human knee. *J Bone Joint Surg Br*. 2003;85:292-298.

34. Kim SJ, Shin SJ, Jeong JH. Posterolateral rotary instability treated by a modified biceps rerouting technique: technical considerations and results in cases with and without PCL insufficiency. *Arthroscopy*. 2003;19:493-499.

35. Buzzi R, Aglietti P. Vena LM, Giron F. Lateral collateral ligament reconstruction using a semitendinosus graft. *Knee Surg Sports Traumatol Arthrosc*. 2004;12:36-42.

36. Latimer HA, Tibone JE, ElAttrache NS, McMahon PJ. Reconstruction of the lateral collateral ligament of the knee with patellar tendon allograft: report of a new technique in combined ligament injuries. *Am J Sports Med*. 1998;26:656-662.

37. Noyes FR, Barber-Westin SD. Posterolateral knee reconstruction with an anatomical bone-patellar tendon-bone reconstruction of the fibular collateral ligament. *Am J Sports Med*. 2007;35:259-273.

38. Sekiya JK, Kurtz CA. Posterolateral corner reconstruction of the knee: surgical technique utilizing bifid Achilles tendon allograft and a double femoral tunnel. *Arthroscopy*. 2005;21:1400.

39. Arthur A, LaPrade RF, Agel J. Proximal tibial opening wedge osteotomy as the initial treatment for chronic posterolateral corner deficiency in the varus knee: a prospective clinical study. *Am J Sports Med*. 2007;11:1844-1850.

40. Dye SF. An evolutionary perspective of the knee. *J Bone Joint Surg Am*. 1987;69:976-983.

41. Herzmark MH. The evolution of the knee joint. *J Bone Joint Surg Am*. 1938;20:77-84.

42. Maynard MJ, Deng X, Wickiewicz TL, Warren RF. The popliteofibular ligament. Rediscovery of a key element in posterolateral stability. *Am J Sports Med*. 1996;24:311-316.

43. Terry GC, LaPrade RF. The posterolateral aspect of the knee. Anatomy and surgical approach. *Am J Sports Med*. 1996;24:732-739.

44. Nielson S, Helming P. The static stabilizing function of the popliteal tendon in the knee. An experimental study. *Arch Orthop Trauma Surg*. 1986;104:357-362.

45. Nielson S, Helming P. Posterior instability of the knee joint. *Arch Orthop Trauma Surg*. 1986;105:121-125.

46. Gollehon DL. The role of the posterolateral and arcuate ligaments in stability of the human knee. A biomechanical study. *J Bone Joint Surg Am*. 1987;69:233-242.

47. Seebacher JR. The structure of the posterolateral aspect of the knee. *J Bone Joint Surg Am*. 1982;64:536-541.

48. Watanabe Y, Moriya H, Takahashi K. et al. Functional anatomy of the posterolateral structures. *Arthroscopy*. 1993;9:57-62.

49. Sudasna S, Harnsiriwattanagit K. The ligamentous structures of the posterolateral aspect of the knee. *Bull Hosp Jt Dis Orthop Inst*. 1990;50:35-40.

50. Wadia FD, Pimple M, Gajjar SM, Narvekar AD. An anatomic study of the popliteofibular ligament. *Int Orthop*. 2003;27:172-174.

51. Grood ES, Stowers SF, Noyes FR. Limits of movement in the human knee. Effect of sectioning the posterior cruciate ligament and posterolateral structures. *J Bone Joint Surg Am*. 1988;70:88-97.

52. Noyes FR, Stowers SF, Grood ES, et al. Posterior subluxations of the medial and lateral tibiofemoral compartments. An in vitro sectioning study in cadaveric Knees. *Am J Sports Med*. 21;1993:407-414.

53. Markolf KL, Wascher DC, Finerman GA. Direct in vitro measurement of forces in the cruciate ligaments. Part II: the effect of sectioning of the posterolateral structures. *J Bone Joint Surg Am*. 1993;75:387-394.

54. Skyhar MJ, Warren RF, Ortiz GJ, et al. The effects of sectioning of the posterior cruciate ligament and the posterolateral complex on the articular contact pressures within the knee. *J Bone Joint Surg Am*. 1993;75:694-699.

55. Kannus P. Nonoperative treatment of grade II and III sprains of the lateral ligament compartment of the knee. *Am J Sports Med*. 1989;17:83-88.

56. Krukhaug Y, Mølster A, Rodt A, Strand T. Lateral ligament injuries of the knee. *Knee Surg Sports Traumatol Arthrosc*. 1998;6:21-25.

57. Hughston JC, Norwood LA Jr. The posterolateral drawer test and external rotational recurvatum test for posterolateral rotatory instability of the knee. *Clin Orthop Relat Res*. 1980:(147);82-87.

58. LaPrade RF, Heikes C, Bakker AJ, Jakobsen RB. The reproducibility and repeatability of varus stress radiographs in the assessment of isolated fibular collateral ligament and grade-III posterolateral knee Injuries. *J Bone Joint Surg Am*. 2008;90:2069-2076.

59. Vinson EN, Major NM, Helms CA. The posterolateral corner of the knee. *AJR Am J Roentgenol*. 2008;190:449-458.

60. Schulz MS, Russe K, Lampakis G, Strobel MJ. Reliability of stress radiography for evaluation of posterior knee laxity. *Am J Sports Med*. 2005;33:502-506.

61. Anderson DD. Effects of sectioning of the PCL complex on the articular contact pressures within the knee. *J Bone Joint Surg Am*. 1995;77:649.

SUGGESTED READING

Fanelli GC, Orcutt DR, Edson CJ. The multiple-ligament injured knee: evaluation, treatment, and results. *Arthroscopy*. 2005;21:471-486.

Multiple-Ligament Knee Injuries and Management of Knee Dislocations

Gregory C. Fanelli ● John D. Beck ● Raffaele Garofalo

The combined anterior cruciate ligament–posterior cruciate ligament (ACL-PCL) injured (dislocated) knee is a severe injury that can result from high- or low-energy trauma. Both cruciates are torn, plus one or both collateral ligament complexes. The frequency of popliteal artery injuries occurs with the same frequency in bicruciate knee ligament injuries and frank tibiofemoral dislocations. Nerve injuries, associated fractures, other structural injuries, functional instability, and post-traumatic arthrosis may all occur with this injury complex.[1,2]

ANATOMY

Knee dislocations can be classified by the direction of tibial displacement, anatomic classification, open or closed injury status, and the energy level associated with the knee dislocation.[3] Hyperextension of the tibiofemoral joint leads to anterior tibiofemoral dislocation. This mechanism may result in popliteal artery stretch, leading to intimal arterial damage, delayed thrombus formation, and ultimate arterial occlusion. The dashboard knee mechanism of injury leads to abrupt posterior tibial dislocation with the knee at 90 degrees of flexion, and may result in arterial transection. Varus force inducing tibiofemoral dislocation may result in peroneal nerve injury.[1-3]

PATIENT EVALUATION

History and Physical Examination

Initial evaluation of the acute bicruciate ligament injured knee includes evaluation of the deformity, location of abrasions or contusions, neurovascular status of the extremity, and presence or absence of a dimple sign. The presence of normal pulses, normal Doppler, and normal capillary refill in the presence of a reduced bicruciate (dislocated) knee does not guarantee the absence of vascular injury. Serial physical examinations, ankle

brachial indices, and arteriography all must be used as necessary to document intact arterial circulation to the injured lower extremity.[4-19]

Physical examination of the ACL-PCL–injured knee will demonstrate abnormal anterior posterior tibiofemoral laxity at 30 and 90 degrees of knee flexion. The pivot shifting phenomenon will be present. The tibial step-off will be negative, the posterior drawer will be positive, and there will be abnormal varus and/or valgus laxity at full extension and 30 degrees of knee flexion.

Diagnostic Imaging

Imaging studies used in the evaluation of the acute and chronic PCL-based multiple-ligament injured knee include plain radiography, magnetic resonance imaging, arteriography, and venographys. Emergent surgical indications include irreducible dislocation, vascular injury, compartment syndrome, inability to maintain reduction, and open dislocations.

TREATMENT

Indications and Contraindications

The current consensus indicates that surgical treatment yields better results than nonsurgical treatment of the multiple-ligament injured knee.[20-25] Technical advancements in the procurement, processing, and use of allograft tissue, arthroscopic surgical instruments, graft fixation methods, and improved surgical techniques, and an improved understanding of the ligament structures and the biomechanics of the knee, have led to more predictable and successful results in the treatment of these complex knee injuries. Various studies have published excellent results with return to preinjury level of function documented with physical examination, arthrometer measurements, knee ligament rating scales, and stress radiography.[2,26-33]

Arthroscopic Technique

Surgical Timing

Surgical timing in the acute bicruciate multiple-ligament injured knee is dependent on the vascular status of the involved extremity, collateral ligament injury severity, degree of instability, and postreduction stability. Delayed or staged reconstruction of 2 to 3 weeks postinjury has demonstrated a lower incidence of arthrofibrosis.[30,31]

Surgical timing in acute ACL-PCL lateral side injuries is dependent on the lateral side classification.[34] We have described three types of posterolateral instability, A, B, and C.[34] Posterolateral instability (PLI) type A has increased external rotation only, corresponding to injury to the popliteofibular ligament and popliteus tendon. PLI type B presents with increased external rotation and mild varus of approximately 5 to 10 mm, with increased lateral joint line opening to varus stress at 30 degrees of knee flexion. This occurs with damage to the popliteofibular ligament and popliteus tendon, and attenuation of the fibular collateral ligament. PLI type C presents with increased tibial external rotation and varus instability of 10 mm more than the normal knee tested at 30 degrees of knee flexion with varus stress. This occurs with injury to the popliteofibular ligament, popliteus tendon, fibular collateral ligament, and lateral capsular avulsion in addition to cruciate ligament disruption. The intact medial collateral ligament, tested with valgus stress at 30 degrees of knee flexion, is the stable hinge in the ACL-PCL- posterolateral corner (PLC)–injured knee.

Arthroscopic combined ACL-PCL reconstruction with lateral side repair and reconstruction can be performed within 2 to 3 weeks postinjury in knees with types A and B lateral posterolateral instability. Type C lateral posterolateral instability combined with ACL-PCL tears is often treated with staged reconstruction. The lateral posterolateral repair or reconstruction is performed within the first week after injury, followed by arthroscopic combined ACL-PCL reconstruction 3 to 6 weeks later.

Surgical timing in acute ACL-PCL medial side injuries is also dependent on the medial side classification. Some medial side injuries will heal with 4 to 6 weeks of brace treatment, provided that the tibiofemoral joint is reduced in all planes. Other medial side injuries require surgical intervention. Types A and B medial side injuries are repaired or reconstructed as a single-stage procedure with combined arthroscopic ACL-PCL reconstruction. Type C medial side injuries combined, with ACL-PCL tears are often treated with staged reconstruction. The medial posteromedial repair or reconstruction is performed within the first week after injury, followed by arthroscopic combined ACL-PCL reconstruction 3 to 6 weeks later.[1,2,30,31,35,36]

Surgical timing may be affected by factors beyond the surgeon's control, and may cause the surgical treatment to be performed earlier or later than desired. These include injured extremity vascular status, open or closed injury, reduction stability, skin conditions, multiple system injuries, other orthopedic injuries, and meniscal and articular surface injuries.[1,2]

Chronic bicruciate multiple ligament knee injuries often present to the orthopedic surgeon with progressive functional instability, and possibly some degree of post-traumatic arthrosis. Considerations for treatment require the definition of all structural injuries. These may include ligaments injured, meniscal injuries, bony malalignment, articular surface injuries, and gait abnormalities. Surgical procedures under consideration may include proximal tibial or distal femoral osteotomy, ligament reconstruction, meniscus transplantation, and osteochondral grafting.

Graft Selection

Our preferred graft for the posterior cruciate ligament is the Achilles tendon allograft for single-bundle PCL reconstructions and an Achilles tendon and tibialis anterior allografts for double-bundle PCL reconstructions. We prefer an Achilles tendon allograft or other allograft for the ACL reconstruction. The preferred graft material for the PLC is allograft tissue combined with a primary repair, or a posterolateral capsular shift procedure. Our preferred method for MCL and posteromedial reconstructions is a primary repair and/or posteromedial capsular shift, with allograft supplementation as needed.

Patient Positioning

The patient is placed on the operating room table in the supine position and, after satisfactory induction of anesthesia, the operative and nonoperative lower extremities are carefully examined. A tourniquet is applied to the upper thigh of the operative extremity, a lateral post is used for extremity control, and that extremity is prepped and draped in a sterile fashion. Allograft tissue is prepared prior to bringing the patient into the operating room. Autograft tissue is harvested prior to beginning the arthroscopic portion of the procedure. The Achilles tendon allograft is trimmed and tabularized with purple size 0 Vicryl suture to facilitate intraoperative positioning. Two no. five permanent braided sutures are woven through each end of the Achilles tendon allograft to serve as traction and back up fixation sutures. There is no bone plug on the Achilles tendon allograft. Platelet-rich fibrin matrix (Musculoskeletal Transplant Foundation; Edison, NJ) is woven into the grafts during preparation to enhance biologic healing. The graft is placed on the Biomet graft-tensioning boot (Biomet; Warsaw, Ind) on the back table under 10 pounds of force for pretensioning.

The arthroscopic instruments are inserted with the inflow through the superolateral patellar portal. Instrumentation and visualization are achieved through inferomedial and inferolateral patellar portals, and can be interchanged as necessary. Additional portals are established as necessary. Exploration of the joint consists of evaluation of the patellofemoral joint, medial and lateral compartments, medial and lateral menisci, and intercondylar notch.

When there is a posterior cruciate ligament tear, the tear of the PCL is identified and the intact anterior cruciate ligament is confirmed. The residual stump of the posterior cruciate ligament is débrided with the synovial shaver and hand tools, as necessary. In the case of a combined ACL-PCL injury, the residual stumps of both the anterior and posterior cruciate ligaments are débrided. In patients with combined ACL-PCL injuries, the notchplasty for the ACL portion of the procedure is performed at this time.

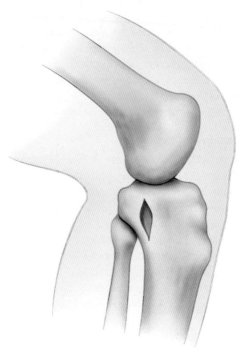

FIGURE 28-1 Posteromedial safety incision used to protect the neurovascular structures and confirm accuracy of the tibial tunnel. *(Adapted from Fanelli GC. Rationale and Surgical Technique for PCL and Multiple Knee Ligament Reconstruction. 2nd ed. Warsaw, Ind: Biomet Sports Medicine; 2008.)*

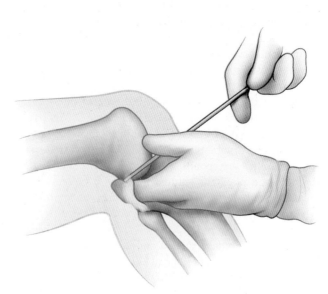

FIGURE 28-2 Surgeon's finger in posteromedial safety incision used to protect the neurovascular structures and confirm accuracy of the tibial tunnel. *(Adapted from Fanelli GC. Rationale and Surgical Technique for PCL and Multiple Knee Ligament Reconstruction. 2nd ed. Warsaw, Ind: Biomet Sports Medicine; 2008.)*

Initial Incision

An extracapsular extra-articular posteromedial safety incision is made by creating an incision approximately 1.5 to 2 cm long, starting at the posteromedial border of the tibia approximately 1 inch below the level of the joint line and extending distally (Fig. 28-1). Dissection is carried down to the crural fascia, which is incised longitudinally. Care is taken to protect the neurovascular structures. An interval is developed between the medial head of the gastrocnemius muscle posterior and the capsule of the knee joint anterior. The surgeon's gloved finger is able to position the neurovascular structures posterior to the finger and the capsule anterior to the finger (Fig. 28-2). In this way, the surgeon can monitor tools such as the over the top PCL instruments and the PCL-ACL drill guide as it is positioned in the posterior aspect of the knee. This also allows for accurate placement of the guide wire in medial lateral and proximal distal directions. The PCL and ACL reconstructions are performed with the knee in approximately 70 to 90 degrees of knee flexion.

Elevating the Capsule.   The curved over the top PCL instruments are used to lyse adhesions in the posterior aspect of the knee sequentially and elevate the capsule from the tibial ridge posteriorly. This will allow accurate placement of the drill guide and correct placement of the tibial tunnel (Fig. 28-3).

Positioning of the Guide

The arm of the PCL-ACL guide is inserted through the inferior medial patellar portal. The tip of the guide is positioned at the inferior lateral aspect of the PCL anatomic insertion site. This is below the tibial ridge posterior and in the lateral aspect of the PCL

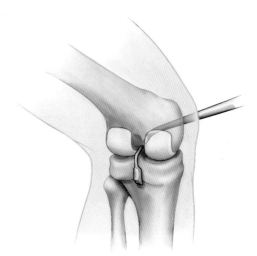

FIGURE 28-3 Elevation of posterior knee joint capsule to prepare for transtibial PCL tunnel creation. *(Adapted from Fanelli GC. Rationale and Surgical Technique for PCL and Multiple Knee Ligament Reconstruction. 2nd ed. Warsaw, Ind: Biomet Sports Medicine; 2008.)*

anatomic insertion site. The bullet portion of the guide contacts the anteromedial surface of the proximal tibia at a point midway between the posteromedial border of the tibia and the tibial crest anterior, approximately 1cm below the tibial tubercle (Fig. 28-4). This will provide an angle of graft orientation so that the graft will turn two very smooth 45-degree angles on the posterior aspect of the tibia and will not have an acute 90-degree angle turn, which may cause pressure necrosis of the graft. The tip of the guide, in the posterior aspect of the tibia, is confirmed with the surgeon's finger through the extracapsular extra-articular posteromedial

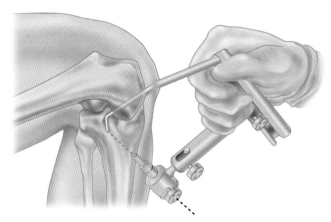

FIGURE 28-4 PCL-ACL drill guide positioned to create PCL tibial tunnel *(Adapted from Fanelli GC. Rationale and Surgical Technique for PCL and Multiple Knee Ligament Reconstruction. 2nd ed. Warsaw, Ind: Biomet Sports Medicine; 2008.)*

safety incision. Intraoperative anteroposterior (AP) and lateral x-rays may also be used. When the PCL-ACL guide is positioned in the desired area, a blunt spade-tipped guide wire is drilled from anterior to posterior. The arthroscope, in the posterior medial portal, visualizes the tip of the guide wire. The surgeon's finger confirms the position of the guide wire through the posterior medial safety incision. This is a double safety check.

Tunnel Drilling

Drilling the Tibial Tunnel. The appropriately sized standard cannulated reamer is used to create the tibial tunnel. The curved PCL closed curette is positioned to cup the tip of the guide wire. The arthroscope, which may be positioned in the posterior medial portal, visualizes the guide wire being cupped, which protects the neurovascular structures. The surgeon's finger through the extracapsular extra-articular posteromedial incision is monitoring the position of the guide wire. When the drill is engaged in bone, the guide wire is reversed, with the blunt end pointing

posterior, for additional patient safety. The drill is advanced until it comes to the posterior cortex of the tibia. The chuck is disengaged from the drill and the tibial tunnel is completed by hand. This gives an additional margin of safety for completion of the tibial tunnel. The tunnel edges are then chamfered and rasped with the PCL-ACL system rasp.

Drilling the Femoral Tunnel Outside-In: Single- and Double-Bundle Posterior Cruciate Ligament Reconstruction. The PCL-ACL drill guide is positioned to create the femoral tunnel. The arm of the guide is introduced through the inferomedial patellar portal and is positioned so that the guide wire will exit through the center of the stump of the anterior lateral bundle of the posterior cruciate ligament (Fig. 28-5A). The blunt spade-tipped guide wire is drilled through the guide and, just as it begins to emerge through the center of the stump of the PCL anterior lateral bundle, the drill guide is disengaged. The accuracy of the placement of the wire is confirmed arthroscopically with probing and visualization. Care must be taken to ensure that the patellofemoral joint has not been violated by arthroscopically examining the patellofemoral joint prior to drilling. The appropriately sized standard cannulated reamer is used to create the femoral tunnel. A curette is used to cap the tip of the guide wire so that there is no inadvertent advancement of the guide wire, which could damage the anterior cruciate ligament or articular surface. As the reamer is about to penetrate interiorly, the reamer is disengaged from the drill and the final reaming is completed by hand. This adds an additional margin of safety. The reaming debris is evacuated with a synovial shaver to minimize any fat pad inflammatory response, with a subsequent risk of arthrofibrosis. The tunnel edges are chamfered and rasped.

When the double-bundle PCL reconstruction is performed, the PCL-ACL drill guide is positioned to create the second femoral tunnel. The arm of the guide is introduced through the inferior medial patellar portal and is positioned so that the guide wire will exit through the center of the stump of the posterior medial bundle of the PCL (see Fig. 28-5B). The blunt spade-tipped guide wire is drilled through the guide and, just as it begins to emerge through

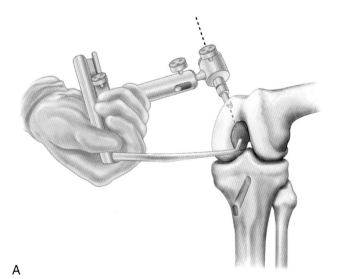

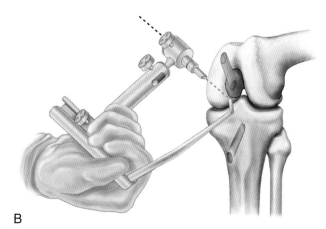

A   B

FIGURE 28-5 Outside-in anterolateral bundle (**A**) and posteromedial bundle (**B**) femoral tunnel creation using PCL-ACL drill guide. *(Adapted from Fanelli GC. Rationale and Surgical Technique for PCL and Multiple Knee Ligament Reconstruction. 2nd ed. Warsaw, Ind: Biomet Sports Medicine; 2008.)*

the center of the stump of the PCL posterior medial bundle, the drill guide is disengaged. The accuracy of the placement of the wire is confirmed arthroscopically with probing and visualization. Care must be taken to ensure that there will be an adequate bone bridge (approximately 5 mm) between the two femoral tunnels prior to drilling. This is accomplished using the calibrated probe and direct arthroscopic visualization. The appropriately sized standard cannulated reamer is used to create the posterior medial bundle femoral tunnel. A curette is used to cap the tip of the guide wire so that there is no inadvertent advancement of the guide wire, which could damage the anterior cruciate ligament, or articular surface. As the reamer is about to penetrate interiorly, the reamer is disengaged from the drill and the final reaming is completed by hand. This adds an additional margin of safety. The reaming debris is evacuated with a synovial shaver to minimize fat pad inflammatory response with subsequent risk of arthrofibrosis. The tunnel edges are chamfered and rasped.

Drilling the Femoral Tunnel Inside-Out: Single- and Double-Bundle Posterior Cruciate Ligament Reconstruction. The PCL single- or double-bundle femoral tunnels can be made from inside-out using the double-bundle aimers. Inserting the appropriately sized double-bundle aimer through a low anterior lateral patellar arthroscopic portal creates the PCL anterior lateral bundle femoral tunnel. The double-bundle aimer is positioned directly on the footprint of the femoral anterior lateral bundle PCL insertion site (Fig. 28-6A). The appropriately sized guide wire is drilled through the aimer, through the bone, and out a small skin incision. Care is taken to ensure that there is no compromise of the articular surface. The double-bundle aimer is removed and an acorn reamer is used to drill endoscopically from inside-out the anterior lateral PCL femoral tunnel. The tunnel edges are chamfered and rasped. The reaming debris is evacuated with a synovial shaver to minimize fat pad inflammatory response with subsequent risk of arthrofibrosis. When the surgeon chooses to perform a double-bundle double femoral tunnel PCL reconstruction, the same

process is repeated for the posterior medial bundle of the PCL (see Fig. 28-6B). Care must be taken to ensure that there will be an adequate bone bridge (approximately 5 mm) between the two femoral tunnels prior to drilling. This is accomplished using the calibrated probe and direct arthroscopic visualization (Fig. 28-7).

Tunnel Preparation, Graft Passage, and Posterior Cruciate Ligament Femoral Fixation. A Magellan suture retriever is introduced through the tibial tunnel into the joint and retrieved through the femoral tunnel. The traction sutures of the graft material are attached to the loop of the Magellan suture retriever and the graft is pulled into position. The graft material is secured on the femoral side using the Biomet BioCore screw for primary aperture opening fixation, and a Biomet polyethylene ligament fixation button is used for cortical suspensory fixation.

Posterior Cruciate Ligament Graft Tensioning and Tibial Fixation

Tension is placed on the PCL graft distally using the Biomet graft-tensioning boot with the knee in full extension, and the tension is set for 20 pounds (Fig. 28-8). This restores the anatomic tibial step-off. The knee is cycled through a full range of motion 25 times to allow pretensioning and settling of the graft. In double-bundle PCL reconstructions, both the anterolateral and posteromedial bundles have final fixation in 70 to 90 degrees of knee flexion. The process is repeated until there is no further change in the torque setting on the graft tensioner, indicating that all laxity is removed from the system. The knee is placed in 70 to 90 degrees of flexion; fixation is achieved on the tibial side of the PCL graft with a Biomet BioCore interference screw and cortical suspensory fixation with a bicortical screw and spiked ligament washer (Fig. 28-9).

Anterior Cruciate Ligament Reconstruction Procedures

With the knee in approximately 90 degrees of flexion, the ACL tunnels are created using the PCL-ACL drill guide single-incision endoscopic surgical technique. The arm of the drill guide enters

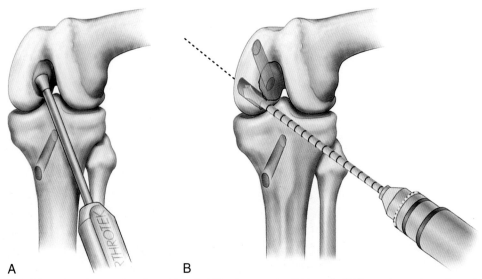

A   B

FIGURE 28-6 Inside-out anterolateral bundle (**A**) and posteromedial bundle (**B**) femoral tunnel creation using double-bundle aimers. *(Adapted from Fanelli GC. Rationale and Surgical Technique for PCL and Multiple Knee Ligament Reconstruction. 2nd ed. Warsaw, Ind: Biomet Sports Medicine; 2008.)*

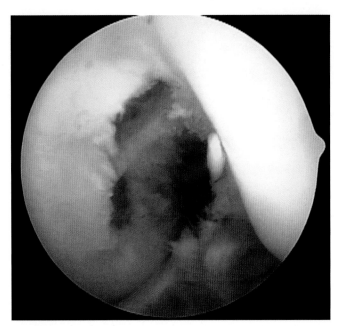

FIGURE 28-7 Intraoperative arthroscopic photograph of anterolateral and posteromedial femoral tunnels for PCL reconstruction. *(Courtesy of Dr. Gregory C. Fanelli.)*

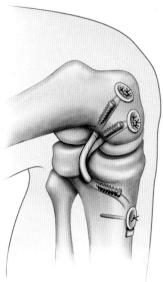

FIGURE 28-9 PCL final fixation using Biomet BioCore resorbable interference screw aperture opening fixation and cortical suspensory fixation with polyethylene ligament fixation buttons, screws, and spiked ligament washers. *(Adapted from Fanelli GC. Rationale and Surgical Technique for PCL and Multiple Knee Ligament Reconstruction. 2nd ed. Warsaw, Ind: Biomet Sports Medicine; 2008.)*

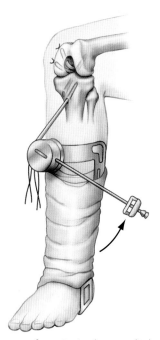

FIGURE 28-8 Biomet graft-tensioning boot applied to PCL reconstruction grafts *(Adapted from Fanelli GC. Rationale and Surgical Technique for PCL and Multiple Knee Ligament Reconstruction. 2nd ed. Warsaw, Ind: Biomet Sports Medicine; 2008.)*

With the knee in approximately 90 degrees of flexion, an over the top femoral aimer is introduced through the tibial tunnel and used to position a guide wire on the medial wall of the lateral femoral condyle. The femoral tunnel is created to approximate the ACL anatomic insertion site, and the offset of the femoral aimer will leave a 1- to 2-mm posterior cortical wall so interference fixation can be used. The ACL graft is positioned; fixation is achieved on the femoral side using a Biomet BioCore interference screw and cortical suspensory fixation with a polyethylene ligament fixation button.

The ACL graft is tensioned on the tibial side using the Biomet graft-tensioning boot, with the knee in full extension. Traction is placed on the ACL graft sutures and tension is set for 20 pounds. The knee is then cycled through 25 full flexion and extension cycles to allow settling of the graft. The process is repeated until there is no further change in the torque setting on the graft tensioner, indicating that all laxity is removed from the system. The knee is placed in 30 degrees of flexion; fixation is achieved on the tibial side of the ACL graft with a Biomet BioCore interference screw and cortical suspensory fixation with a Biomet polyethylene ligament fixation button. The arthroscopic examination shows the completed reconstruction in the intercondylar notch (Fig. 28-10).

Lateral Posterolateral Reconstruction

One surgical technique for posterolateral reconstruction is the free graft figure-of-eight technique using a semitendinosus autograft or allograft, Achilles tendon allograft, or other soft tissue allograft material (Fig. 28-11). This procedure requires an intact proximal tibiofibular joint and the absence of a hyperextension external rotation recurvatum deformity. This technique combined with capsular repair and/or posterolateral capsular shift procedures (Fig. 28-12), mimics the function of the popliteofibular ligament

the knee joint through the inferior medial patellar portal. The bullet of the drill guide contacts the anterior medial proximal tibia externally at a point 1 cm proximal to the tibial tubercle, midway between the posterior medial border of the tibia and the tibial crest anteriorly. The guide wire is drilled through the guide to emerge through the center of the stump of the ACL tibial footprint. A standard cannulated reamer is used to create the tibial tunnel.

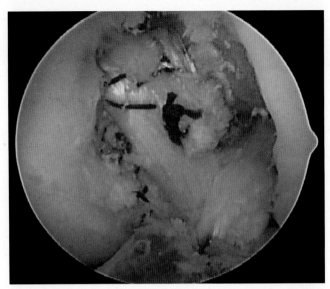

FIGURE 28-10 Intraoperative arthroscopic photograph of combined PCL-ACL reconstruction in the multiple-ligament injured knee. *(Courtesy of Dr. Gregory C. Fanelli.)*

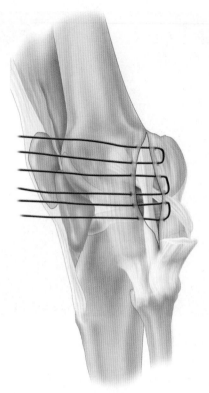

FIGURE 28-12 The posterolateral capsular shift procedure to correct posterolateral capsular redundancy or detatchment is used in conjunction with strut grafting. *(Adapted from Fanelli GC.* Rationale and Surgical Technique for PCL and Multiple Knee Ligament Reconstruction. *2nd ed. Warsaw, Ind: Biomet Sports Medicine; 2008.)*

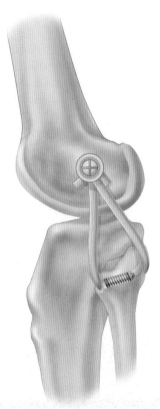

FIGURE 28-11 Fibula-based figure-of-eight reconstruction for posterolateral instability. The posterolateral capsular shift procedure is used to correct posterolateral capsular redundancy or detatchment and is done in conjunction with strut grafting. *(Adapted from Fanelli GC.* Rationale and Surgical Technique for PCL and Multiple Knee Ligament Reconstruction. *2nd ed. Warsaw, Ind: Biomet Sports Medicine; 2008.)*

and lateral collateral ligament, tightens the posterolateral capsule, and provides a post of strong autogenous tissue to reinforce the posterolateral corner. When there is a disrupted proximal tibio-fibular joint or hyperextension external rotation recurvatum deformity, a two-tailed (fibular head, proximal tibia) posterior lateral reconstruction is required (Fig. 28-13). For a comprehensive review of posterolateral reconstruction techniques, see Chapter 27.

Medial Posteromedial Reconstruction

Posteromedial and medial reconstructions are performed through a medial hockey stick incision. Care is taken to maintain adequate skin bridges between incisions. The superficial medial collateral ligament is exposed and a longitudinal incision is made just posterior to the posterior border of the superficial MCL (Fig. 28-14). Care is taken not to damage the medial meniscus during the capsular incision. The interval between the posteromedial capsule and medial meniscus is developed. The posteromedial capsule is shifted anterosuperiorly. The medial meniscus is repaired to the new capsular position and the shifted capsule is sewn into the medial collateral ligament. When superficial MCL reconstruction is indicated, this is performed using allograft or autograft tissue (Fig. 28-15). This graft material is attached at the anatomic insertion sites of the superficial medial collateral ligament on the femur and tibia using a screw and spiked ligament washer or suture anchors. The posteromedial capsular advancement is performed and sewn into the newly reconstructed MCL (Fig. 28-16). The final graft-tensioning position is approximately 30 to 40 degrees of knee flexion.

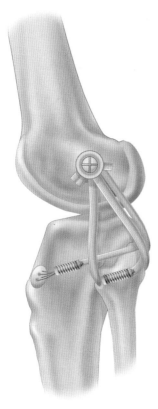

FIGURE 28-13 Fibula-based figure-of-eight reconstruction combined with tibia-based popliteus reconstruction for posterolateral reconstruction. The posterolateral capsular shift procedure to correct posterolateral capsular redundancy or detatchment is used in conjunction with strut grafting. *(Adapted from Fanelli GC. Rationale and Surgical Technique for PCL and Multiple Knee Ligament Reconstruction. 2nd ed. Warsaw, Ind: Biomet Sports Medicine; 2008.)*

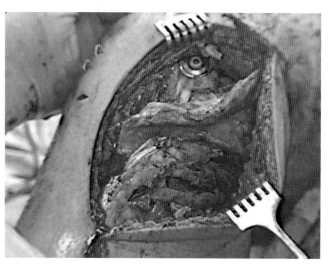

FIGURE 28-14 Intraoperative photograph of posterolateral reconstruction. Note peroneal nerve neurolysis. *(Courtesy of Dr. Gregory C. Fanelli.)*

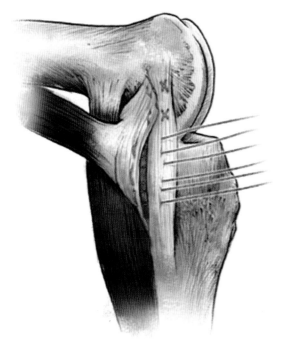

FIGURE 28-15 Posteromedial capsular shift procedure to address medial posteromedial instability. *(Adapted from Fanelli GC. Rationale and Surgical Technique for PCL and Multiple Knee Ligament Reconstruction. 2nd ed. Warsaw, Ind: Biomet Sports Medicine; 2008.)*

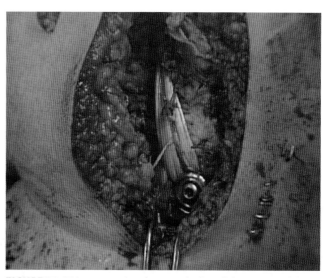

FIGURE 28-16 Intraoperative photograph of medial posteromedial reconstruction. *(Courtesy of Dr. Gregory C. Fanelli.)*

PEARLS & PITFALLS

- The PCL is reconstructed first, followed by the ACL and then the posterolateral complex and medial ligament complex.
- Tension is placed on the PCL graft distally using the Biomet knee ligament-tensioning device, and the tension is set for 20 pounds with the knee in full extension. This restores the anatomic tibial step-off. The knee is cycled through a full range of motion 25 times to allow pretensioning and settling of the graft. The knee is placed in 70 degrees of flexion; fixation is achieved on the tibial side of the PCL graft with a Biomet Bio Core bioabsorbable interference screw and screw and spiked ligament washer.
- The Biomet knee ligament-tensioning device is applied to the ACL graft and set to 20 pounds with the knee in full extension, and the knee is cycled through a full range of motion 25 times to allow pretensioning and settling of the graft. The knee is placed in 30 degrees of flexion, and final fixation of the ACL graft is achieved with a Biomet Bio Core bioabsorbable interference screw and Biomet polyethylene knee ligament fixation button for cortical suspensory fixation.
- Tensioning the central pivot grafts at full extension enables the convex-concave relationship of the tibiofemoral joint to maintain the neutral position of the knee.
- The knee is placed in 30 degrees of flexion, the tibia slightly internally rotated, slight valgus force applied to the knee, and final tensioning and fixation of the posterolateral corner are achieved.
- The MCL reconstruction is tensioned with the knee in 30 degrees of flexion, with the leg in a figure-of-four position. Full range of motion is confirmed on the operating table to ensure that the knee is not captured by the reconstruction.
- The posteromedial safety incision protects the neurovascular structures, confirms accurate tibial tunnel placement, and allows the surgical procedure to be done at an accelerated pace.
- The single-incision ACL reconstruction technique prevents lateral cortex crowding and eliminates multiple through and through drill holes in the distal femur, reducing a stress riser effect.
- It is important to be aware of the two tibial tunnel directions, and to have a 1-cm bone bridge between the PCL and ACL tibial tunnels. This will reduce the possibility of fracture. We have found it useful to use primary aperture fixation and cortical suspensory back-up fixation.
- Primary fixation is with Biomet BioCore interference screws, and cortical suspensory back-up fixation is performed with a screw and spiked ligament washer and Biomet ligament fixation buttons. Secure fixation is critical to the success of this surgical procedure.
- Full range of motion is confirmed on the operating table to ensure that the knee is not captured by the reconstruction.

Postoperative Rehabilitation

Outcomes after PCL reconstructive surgery have historically been inferior to outcomes after reconstruction of the ACL. As such, some surgeons may be reluctant to recommend reconstruction of the PCL. However, recent technologic advances have substantially improved PCL reconstructive surgical outcomes. These advances include the following: better understanding of PCL diagnosis and surgical indications; recognition of the need for repair or reconstruction of associated injuries, especially injuries to the posterolateral and posteromedial corners of the knee; PCL-specific surgical instruments, including mechanical tensioning devices to restore anatomic tibial step-off; improved graft fixation techniques, including primary and back-up methods of fixation; use of strong graft materials, including advances in the procurement, processing, and usage of allograft tissue; improved surgical techniques; and advances in the understanding of knee ligament structure and biomechanics, resulting in more accurate surgical tunnel placement to achieve anatomic graft insertion sites while minimizing graft bending. Today, PCL reconstructive surgery often results in excellent function with return to preinjury level of activity.

Surgeons tend to focus on advances in surgical techniques. However, with regard to PCL outcomes, improved understanding of rehabilitation may be an equally critical factor in our current ability to restore knee stability and function. In contrast to ACL rehabilitation, accelerated PCL postoperative rehabilitation is entirely undesirable. Rather, using a slow and deliberate postoperative rehabilitation program is vital to a successful PCL surgical reconstructive outcome. General principles include appropriate immobilization, avoidance of overstressing of healing tissues, and staged progression of individualized rehabilitation based on basic science and clinical research. In summary, we must protect posterior cruciate and collateral ligament reconstructions until early healing has occurred.

Our specific rehabilitation program is as follows. The knee is kept locked in a long leg brace in full extension for 5 weeks, with non–weight bearing using crutches. The brace is unlocked at the end of postoperative week 5. Progressive range of motion is initiated during postoperative week number 6. Progressive weight bearing at 20% body weight per week begins during postoperative week 6, and progresses through postoperative week 10. Crutches are discontinued at the end of postoperative week 10 when the patient is fully weight bearing and has enough quadriceps control for unassisted ambulation. Progressive strengthening and proprioceptive skill training are initiated while protecting the healing grafts. Return to sports and heavy labor occurs 6 to 9 months postoperatively, when sufficient strength, range of motion, and proprioceptive skills have returned.[37,38]

Posterior cruciate ligament reconstruction performed according to the surgical techniques and rehabilitation program described has led to successful results. Documentation of these results has been performed by physical examination, arthrometer (KT-1000) measurements, knee ligament rating scales, and stress (Telos) radiography. PCL reconstruction in 41 chronic PCL-PLC reconstructions has resulted in 70% normal posterior drawer test and tibial step-off for the overall study group, and 92% normal posterior drawer and tibial step-off in a subgroup using a mechanical graft-tensioning boot.[3] PCL reconstruction in 15 consecutive combined PCL–ACL-collateral ligament (multiple-ligament injured knee) reconstructions has resulted in 87% normal posterior drawer test and tibial step-off in these combined central pivot reconstructions using a mechanical graft-tensioning device.[5]

CONCLUSIONS

The results of surgical treatment of the bicruciate multiple-ligament injured (dislocated) knee have demonstrated excellent functional results, often achieving return to preinjury level of function. This has been demonstrated with physical examination, arthrometer measurements, knee ligament rating scales, and stress radiographs.[2,26-33] Comparisons of single- and double-bundle PCL reconstructions in the multiple-ligament injured knee have demonstrated no superior surgical procedure.[39-46] Both the single-bundle and double-bundle arthroscopically assisted transtibial posterior cruciate ligament reconstruction techniques are successful surgical procedures. Statistically significant improvements from preoperative to postoperative status evaluated by physical examination, knee ligament rating scales, arthrometer measurements, and stress radiography have been demonstrated. Factors contributing to the success of these surgical procedures include identification and treatment of all pathology (especially posterolateral and posteromedial instability), accurate tunnel placement, placement of strong graft material at anatomic graft insertion sites, minimizing graft bending, performing final PCL graft fixation at 70 to 90 degrees of knee flexion using the graft-tensioning boot, using primary and backup fixation, and the appropriate postoperative rehabilitation program.

The multiple-ligament injured knee is a severe injury that may also involve neurovascular injuries and fractures. Surgical treatment offers good functional results documented in the literature by physical examination, arthrometer testing, stress radiography, and knee ligament rating scales. Mechanical tensioning devices are helpful with cruciate ligament tensioning. Some low-grade medial collateral ligament complex injuries may be amenable to brace treatment, whereas high-grade medial side injuries require repair or reconstruction. Lateral posterolateral injuries are most successfully treated with surgical repair or reconstruction. Surgical timing in acute multiple-ligament injured knee cases depends on the ligaments injured, vascular status of the injured extremity, skin condition of the extremity, degree of instability, and the patient's overall health. Allograft tissue is preferred for these complex surgical procedures. Delayed reconstruction of 2 to 3 weeks may decrease the incidence of arthrofibrosis, and it is important to address all components of the instability. Currently, there is no conclusive evidence that double-bundle PCL reconstruction provides superior results to single-bundle PCL reconstruction in the multiple-ligament injured knee.

REFERENCES

1. Fanelli GC, Orcutt DR, Edson CJ. The multiple-ligament injured knee: evaluation, treatment, and results. *Arthroscopy.* 2005;21:471-486.
2. Fanelli GC, Edson CJ, Orcutt DR, et al. Treatment of combined anterior cruciate-posterior cruciate ligament-medial-lateral side knee injuries. *J Knee Surg.* 2005;18:240-248.
3. Burke R, Walker D, Schenck RC, et al. The dislocated knee: a new classification system. *South Med J.* 1992;85(suppl):3S-S61.
4. Abou-Sayed H, Berger DL. Blunt lower-extremity trauma and popliteal artery injuries: revisiting the case for selective arteriography. *Arch Surg.* 2002;137:585-589.
5. Dennis JW, Jagger C, Butcher JL, et al. Reassessing the role of arteriograms in the management of posterior knee dislocations. *J Trauma.* 1993;35:692-695.
6. Hollis JD, Daley BJ. 10-year review of knee dislocations: is arteriography always necessary? *J Trauma.* 2005;59:672-675.
7. Kaufman SL, Martin LG. Arterial injuries associated with complete dislocation of the knee. *Radiology.* 1992;184:153-155.
8. Kendall RW, Taylor DC, Salvian AJ, O'Brien PJ. The role of arteriography in assessing vascular injuries associated with dislocations of the knee. *J Trauma.* 1993;35:875-878.
9. Klineberg EO, Crites BM, Flinn WR. et al. The role of arteriography in assessing popliteal artery injury in knee dislocations. *J Trauma.* 2004; 56:786-790.
10. Martinez D, Sweatman K, Thompson EC. Popliteal artery injury associated with knee dislocations. *Am Surg.* 2001;67:165-167.
11. Stannard JP, Sheils TM, Lopez-Ben RR, et al. Vascular injuries in knee dislocations: the role of physical examination in determining the need for arteriography. *J Bone Joint Surg Am.* 2004;86:910-915.
12. Treiman GS, Yellin AE, Weaver FA, et al. Examination of the patient with a knee dislocation. The case for selective arteriography. *Arch Surg.* 1992;127:1056-1062.
13. Miranda FE, Dennis JW, Veldenz HC, et al. Confirmation of the safety and accuracy of physical examination in the evaluation of knee dislocation for injury of the popliteal artery: a prospective study. *J Trauma.* 2002;52:247-251.
14. Wascher DC. High-velocity knee dislocation with vascular injury. Treatment principles. *Clin Sports Med.* 2000;19:457-477.
15. Sawchuk AP, Eldrup-Jorgensen J, Tober C, et al. The natural history of intimal flaps in a canine model. *Arch Surg.* 1990;125:1614-1616.
16. Stain SC, Yellin AE, Weaver FA, Pentecost MJ. Selective management of nonocclusive arterial injuries. *Arch Surg.* 1989;124:1136-1401.
17. Welling RE, Kakkasseril J, Cranley JJ. Complete dislocations of the knee with popliteal vascular injury. *J Trauma.* 1981;21:450-453.
18. Witz M, Witz S, Tobi E, et al. Isolated complete popliteal artery rupture associated with knee dislocation. Case reports. *Knee Surg Sports Traumatol Arthrosc.* 2004;12:3-6.
19. Mills WJ, Barei DP, McNair P. The value of the ankle-brachial index for diagnosing arterial injury after knee dislocation: a prospective study. *J Trauma.* 2004;56:1261-1265.
20. Dedmond BT, Almekinders LC. Operative versus nonoperative treatment of knee dislocations: a meta-analysis. *Am J Knee Surg.* 2001;14: 33-38.
21. Liow RY, McNicholas MJ, Keating JF, Nutton RW. Ligament repair and reconstruction in traumatic dislocation of the knee. *J Bone Joint Surg Br.* 2003;85:845-851.
22. Harner CD, Waltrip RL, Bennett CH, et al. Surgical management of knee dislocations. *J Bone Joint Surg Am.* 2004;86:262-273.
23. Wascher DC, Becker JR, Dexter JG, Blevins FT. Reconstruction of the anterior and posterior cruciate ligaments after knee dislocation. Results using fresh-frozen nonirradiated allografts. *Am J Sports Med.* 1999;27: 189-196.
24. Talbot M, Berry G, Fernandes J, Ranger P. Knee dislocations: experience at the Hopital du Sacre-Coeur de Montreal. *Can J Surg.* 2004;47:20-24.
25. Yeh WL, Tu YK, Su JY, Hsu RW. Knee dislocation: treatment of high-velocity knee dislocation. *J Trauma.* 1999;46:693-701.
26. Shapiro MS, Freedman EL. Allograft reconstruction of the anterior and posterior cruciate ligaments after traumatic knee dislocation. *Am J Sports Med.* 1995;23:580-587.
27. Noyes FR, Barber-Westin SD. The treatment of acute combined ruptures of the anterior cruciate and medial ligaments of the knee. *Am J Sports Med.* 1995;23:380-389.
28. Noyes FR, Barber-Westin SD. Reconstruction of the anterior and posterior cruciate ligaments after knee dislocation. *Am J Sports Med.* 1997; 25:769-778.
29. Wascher DC. Becker JR. Dexter JG, Blevins FT. Reconstruction of the anterior and posterior cruciate ligaments after knee dislocation. Results using fresh-frozen nonirradiated allografts. *Am J Sports Med.* 1999;27: 189-196.
30. Fanelli GC, Gianotti BF, Edson CJ. Arthroscopically assisted combined anterior and posterior cruciate ligament reconstruction. *Arthroscopy.* 1996;12:5-14.
31. Fanelli GC, Edson CJ. Arthroscopically assisted combined ACL/PCL reconstruction. 2-10 year follow-up. *Arthroscopy.* 2002;18:703-714.
32. Fanelli GC, Edson CJ. Arthroscopically assisted combined PCL-posterolateral reconstruction. 2-10 year follow-up. *Arthroscopy.* 2004; 20(4):339-345.
33. Harner CD. Waltrip RL. Bennett CH, et al. Surgical management of knee dislocations. *J Bone Joint Surg Am.* 2004;86:262-273.

34. Fanelli GC, Feldmann DD. Management of combined anterior cruciate ligament/posterior cruciate ligament/posterolateral complex injuries of the knee. *Oper Tech Sports Med.* 1999;7:143-149.

35. Fanelli GC, Harris JD. Surgical treatment of acute medial collateral ligament and posteromedial corner injuries of the knee. *Sports Med Arthrosc Rev.* 2006;14:78-83.

36. Fanelli GC, Harris JD. Late MCL (medial collateral ligament) reconstruction. *Tech Knee Surg.* 2007;6:99-105.

37. Edson CJ, Rehabilitation of the multiligament-reconstructed knee. *Sports Med Arthrosc Rev.* 2001;9:247-254.

38. Fanelli GC. Posterior cruciate ligament rehabilitation: how slow should we go? *Arthroscopy.* 2008;24:234-235.

39. Levy B, Fanelli GC, Whalen D, et al. Modern perspectives for the treatment of knee dislocations and multiligament reconstruction. *J Am Acad Orthop Surg.* 2009;17:197-206.

40. Levy B, Dajani KA, Whalen DB, et al. Decision making in the multiple ligament injured knee: an evidence-based systematic review. *Arthroscopy.* 2009;25:430-438.

41. Fanelli GC, Edson CJ, Reinheimer KN, Beck J. Arthroscopic single bundle vs. double bundle posterior cruciate ligament reconstruction. *Arthroscopy.* 2008;24(suppl):e26.

42. Fanelli GC, Edson CJ, Reinheimer KN. Evaluation and treatment of the multiple ligament injured knee. *Instr Course Lect.* 2009;58:389-395.

43. Fanelli GC, Edson CJ, Reinheimer KN, Garofalo R. Posterior cruciate ligament and posterolateral corner reconstruction. *Sports Med Arthrosc Rev.* 2007;15:168-175.

44. Fanelli GC, ed. *Posterior Cruciate Ligament Injuries: A Practical Guide To Management.* New York: Springer-Verlag; 2001.

45. Fanelli GC, ed. *The Multiple Ligament Injured Knee. A Practical Guide to Management.* New York: Springer-Verlag; 2004.

46. Garafallo R, Jolles BM, Moretti B, Siegrist O. Double-bundle transtibial posterior cruciate ligament reconstruction with a tendon-patellar bone-semitendinosus tendon autograft: clinical results with a minimum 2 years' follow-up. *Arthroscopy.* 2006;22:1331-1338.

Index

Note: Page numbers followed by f refer to figures; page numbers followed by t refer to tables; page numbers followed by b refer to boxes.

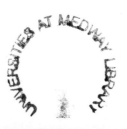